Foundations of Biomedical Ultrasound

Foundations of
Biomedical
Ultrasound

Richard S. C. Cobbold
University of Toronto

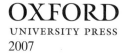

OXFORD
UNIVERSITY PRESS
2007

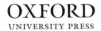

OXFORD
UNIVERSITY PRESS

Oxford University Press, Inc., publishes works that further
Oxford University's objective of excellence
in research, scholarship, and education.

Oxford   New York
Auckland   Cape Town   Dar es Salaam   Hong Kong   Karachi
Kuala Lumpur   Madrid   Melbourne   Mexico City   Nairobi
New Delhi   Shanghai   Taipei   Toronto

With offices in
Argentina   Austria   Brazil   Chile   Czech Republic   France   Greece
Guatemala   Hungary   Italy   Japan   Poland   Portugal   Singapore
South Korea   Switzerland   Thailand   Turkey   Ukraine   Vietnam

Published by Oxford University Press, Inc.
198 Madison Avenue, New York, New York 10016

www.oup.com

Oxford is a registered trademark of Oxford University Press.

Library of Congress Cataloging-in-Publication Data

Cobbold, Richard S. C., 1931–
    Foundations of biomedical ultrasound / Richard S. C. Cobbold.
       p. ; cm. — (Biomedical engineering series)
    Includes bibliographical references and index.
    ISBN-13 978-0-19-516831-0
    ISBN 0-19-516831-3
    1. Ultrasonic imaging.   I. Title.
    II. Series: Biomedical engineering series (Oxford University Press)
    [DNLM: 1. Ultrasonography.   2. Ultrasonics.   WN 208 C654f 2006]
    QM25.C63 2006
    616.07′543—dc22   2005024193

9 8 7 6 5 4 3 2 1

Printed in the United States of America
on acid-free paper

Preface

In an effort to develop a means for detecting the presence of enemy submarines during the First World War, the famous French physicist Paul Langevin designed a 150 kHz source for generating intense ultrasound beams. As noted in 1917, he observed that small fish were killed when entering the beam and that intense pain was caused when a hand was placed in its path. Although the generation and detection of ultrasound had been pursued in the previous century, this aspect of Langevin's work is often regarded to be the inception of modern ultrasound and its biological applications.

Ultrasound is a sub-discipline of acoustics, whose mathematical and physical foundations were developed in the 18th and 19th centuries. An important part of this sub-discipline is the more recent interdisciplinary area of biomedical ultrasonics, which involves mechanics, electrical engineering, physics, biology, and medicine. Specifically, it is concerned with the application of ultrasound techniques for biological and medical purposes, particularly for diagnostic and therapeutic use. Some students beginning to study and research this field find it difficult to determine the most appropriate path for obtaining a good grasp of the fundamentals along with applications and recent developments. A primary purpose of this book is to provide a study path by building on the mathematical foundation that graduate students in physics and engineering should have gained in their undergraduate years. Moreover, it should serve as a useful resource-base for those in industry or academia that are actively engaged in ultrasound research and system development. Much of this base is recorded in a variety of publications, but little has been assembled in a form suited for its use in formal or informal education programs.

This book developed from a graduate course in ultrasound that the author has given for more than 20 years. It evolved initially from extensive course notes and reprints from the literature but in more recent years from compact disk versions provided to students. It should be well suited for a university course, as well as for concentrated training programs in industry and hospitals.

The book consists of 10 chapters that bridge the spectrum from the fundamental properties of wave propagation through to the clinical systems. The first four chapters describe linear and nonlinear propagation and methods for calculating the field produced by transducers of various designs. A number of problems designed to test the reader's understanding, and which are well suited for formal class assignments, accompany these chapters. The topics of ultrasound scattering and transducer design are addressed in Chapters 5 and 6. The final four chapters address methods of imaging and flow measurement. Some 350 drawings, graphs, sketches, and color images have been used. These, together with many tables, have been used to illustrate the various topics covered, a substantial portion of which appears for the first time in published form.

I am particularly indebted to many graduate students and research associates whom I have had the privilege of supervising. From them I have learnt more than they will ever realize. The master's and doctoral students include Marty Hager, Bruno Maruzzo, Larry Korba, Mike Kassam, Oliver Fastag, Jim Arenson, Jerry Arenson, Peter Arato, Rick Appugliese, Benny Lau, Peter Zuech, Donald MacHattie, John Grant, Carl Walker, Kent Poots, Claude Royer, Jim Mehi, Larry Mo, Joe Facca, Weimin Chen, Clement Fung, William Gibson, Peter Bascom, Peter Vaitkus, Ramez Shehada, Theofanis Maniatis, Nirav Shah, Yi Dai, Andrew Hill, David Surat, Yen Lu, Dominic Calla, Brian Lim, Pinar Crombie, Kwok Lam, Roger Zemp, Adam Weathermon, Aaron Steinman, Howard Ginsberg, Elaine Lui, Alfred Yu, Renee Warriner, and Roozbeh Arshadi. Postdoctoral fellows and research associates were a vital part of our research team, and these include Helen Routh, Tadashi Tamura, Yu Fi Law, Jahan Tavakkoli, Jerry Myers, Alex Karpelson, and Nikolai Sushilov. In addition, I wish to thank Peter Veltink, Jan Koers, Bernt Roelfs, and Renee Aarnink, all of whom made significant contributions. They were students from the Netherlands who joined our group to do their final-year thesis research. I should also like to mention the special help that Larry Mo provided through his continuing collaboration with our research group. His insights into the practical and physical aspects of ultrasound pulsed wave flow estimation systems has been particularly helpful in improving the final chapter.

My introduction to ultrasound and its clinical use was in 1973 through the initiatives of an academic and clinical-based colleague, Wayne Johnston. Our collaborative research has now extended to over 30 years, and I am particularly grateful for his encouragement in this major project. Moreover, the research grants that we have jointly held from the Medical Research Council of Canada (currently the Canadian Institutes Heath Research) and the Canadian Heart and Stroke Foundation have played a vital role. Other research grants that have supported our ultrasound research are from the Natural Sciences and Engineering Research Council of Canada and the Hospital for Sick Children Foundation. There are several other academic colleagues that I should like to thank, and these include Matadial Ojha, Ross Ethier, Peter Burns, and Stuart Foster. In addition, I am grateful to the previous and current Director of our Institute for providing essential services and research space. Finally, to my wife, who has again tolerated long periods of temporary absence through my disappearance to the basement office, I am indebted to her for encouragement.

Contents

Detailed Contents

Foundations of Biomedical Ultrasound

1

Introduction

The past 50 years have seen important advances in the understanding, development, and application of ultrasound methods for medical and industrial uses. For medical diagnostic applications, a major advantage accrues from the ability of ultrasound to penetrate biological tissue and to return signals that contain information from which the acoustic structure can be determined. Provided the intensity is not too great, it can do this without causing micro- or macroscopic damage. For medical therapeutic applications, the use of ultrasound can be traced to the mid-1930s, when it was used in physiotherapy for deep tissue heating.

Many of the advances can be attributed to a combination of experimental observations, theoretical developments, and ingenious design. With the availability of high-speed computers and display systems, simulation methods have enabled the design and performance of ultrasound systems to be investigated without the need for costly experimental research. The basis of good simulation methods is a theoretical understanding of the different components of a system, especially the manner in which acoustic waves propagate in liquid and solid media. Much of the theoretical basis of linear and nonlinear acoustic wave propagation was established in the 18th century by Euler (Leonhard, 1707–1783), D'Almbert (Jean-le-Rond, 1717–1783), and Lagrange (Joseph Louis, 1736–1813). In the 19th century, major contributions were made by Poisson (Simeon Denis, 1781–1840), Navier (Claude Louis Marie Henri, 1785–1836), Helmholtz (Hermann Ludwig Ferdinand, 1821–1894), Earnshaw (Rev. Samuel, 1805–1888), Kirchhoff (Gustav Robert, 1824–1887), Stokes

(George Gabriel, 1819–1903), Riemann (Bernhard, 1826–1866), Lebedev (Petr Nikoloevich, 1866–1912), and Lord Rayleigh (John William Strutt, 1842–1919). Perhaps the most important milestone in understanding the fundamental physics of acoustic wave propagation was the classic two-volume treatise by Rayleigh [1] entitled *The Theory of Sound*, which was published in 1877 and 1878. It remains a frequently cited text.

The period beginning around 1916 is considered by some to mark the start of modern ultrasonics development. Langevin (Paul, 1872–1946) was a major contributor to this, but a good deal of his work was unpublished [2], though some was subsequently reported by those who had attended his lectures. Along with Boyle (Robert William, 1883–1955) and a coworker, Constantin Chilowski, Langevin was responsible for many important practical contributions. Wood (Robert Williams, 1868–1955) appears to be the first to report investigations on the effects of high-power ultrasound on biological media, and his work [3] on this topic, published in conjunction with Loomis (Alfred Lee, 1887–1975), can be considered to be the forerunner of modern medical therapeutic applications. All of the above, together with other developments, have been reported by Graff [4] in a comprehensive account of the history of ultrasonics to the immediate post-WWII period.

This chapter aims to provide a mathematical and physical introduction to wave propagation in biological media and should form a foundation for subsequent chapters dealing with theory and applications. It begins with a description of the various forms of wave motion, leading to the development of equations that describe propagation in liquid and solid media. The effects of abrupt changes in the medium characteristics on the propagation, along with the effects of diffraction, are then considered. The final sections are devoted to the effects of absorption and scattering on propagation.

1.1 Physical Nature of Acoustic Wave Motion

1.1.1 Wave Propagation in a Semi-Infinite Medium

Acoustic waves can arise from the application of a time-varying stress to a medium. For an isotropic[1] homogeneous[2] material, the simplest forms of wave motion are those arising from a stress normal to the material surface, giving rise to a longitudinal (compressional) wave. If the medium is solid, application of a unidirectional time-varying shear stress will gives rise to a simple transverse wave that is polarized in the direction of the stress. To provide a physical picture of the effects of such stresses, it is helpful to introduce the concept of an acoustic *particle*.

When a medium is subject to a time-varying stress, the coupling forces between the atoms and molecules of the medium are perturbed and very small

---

1. In an *isotropic* medium, the physical properties are independent of direction.
2. For a *homogeneous* medium, the acoustic properties are constant throughout the propagation region.

displacements result. However, this is a much oversimplified picture of what really happens at an atomic or molecular level. Let us consider the simple crystalline solid illustrated in Fig. 1.1. Such a system of springs and masses will possess many degrees of freedom and as a result will have many normal modes of oscillation. Under equilibrium conditions the thermal energy will cause oscillations: the resulting temperature-dependent spectrum of frequencies is characteristic of the medium. Quantum mechanics requires that acoustic energy be quantized into elementary units of energy called phonons. In the absence of free electrons, virtually all the thermal energy is carried by phonons, whose frequency spectrum generally ranges from frequencies corresponding to the maximum sample linear dimension, up to around 10^{13} Hz. If the medium is disturbed by the application of a time-varying stress, the phonon frequency distribution will be affected: in fact, the passage of a wave through the medium can be considered to correspond to the passage of a group of coherent phonons. The discrete nature of the medium needs to be considered in characterizing the propagation of ultrasonic waves only when the wavelength approaches the inter-atomic or molecular spacing. This occurs when the ultrasonic (hypersonic) frequency is in the order of 100 GHz, with wavelengths around 10^{-8} m. As will be seen, to account for the loss of energy loss during propagation, molecular processes and structural order in the medium can play an important role. If a medium is to be treated as a continuum, then it is convenient to define an acoustic *particle* to be a small volume element whose dimensions are large compared to the inter-atomic spacing and are much

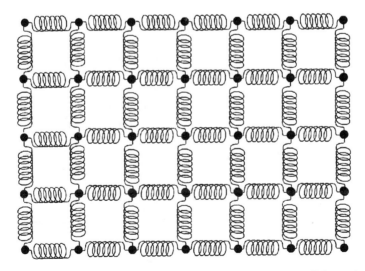

Figure 1.1 2-D representation of a simple crystal lattice. Many possible modes of vibration are possible. Under equilibrium conditions the thermal energy will be distributed over a wide range of frequencies, with wavelengths ranging from the dimensions of the medium to the interatomic spacing.

smaller than the wavelength. In discussing the movement and properties of a given fluid particle, we are really speaking of the movement and properties of all the matter contained within the volume element. Thus, within the volume of given acoustic particle, we assume that all of the physical quantities remain constant.

1.1.2 Longitudinal and Transverse Waves

The simplest form of acoustic wave propagation is that of a plane longitudinal (also called compressional) wave propagating in a homogeneous isotropic medium of semi-infinite extent. As illustrated in Fig. 1.2a, the passage of such a wave is associated with regions of compression and rarefaction that propagate with a speed determined primarily by the properties of the medium. Associated with the wave propagation will be changes in the particle displacement, velocity, density, pressure, and temperature. The speed[3] with which the wave propagates (which must be distinguished from the particle velocity) depends on the properties of the medium. For a fairly stiff medium the wave will propagate faster than for one that is highly elastic (a perfectly incompressible medium would have an infinite propagation speed). Associated with compression and rarefaction of wave propagation will be temperature changes, making it necessary to consider whether isothermal or adiabatic (constant entropy) conditions can be assumed. It might be thought that at lower frequencies, because there would be more time for heat to flow, a longitudinal wave should behave less adiabatically. However, the reverse is true. When the angular frequency ω is decreased, the distance between the crests and valleys increases, and as a result the irreversible heat transfer by conduction can be shown to be proportional to ω^2. This does not compensate for the $1/\omega$ factor that arises from the increased time between cycles at lower frequencies; hence, a compressional wave behaves more adiabatically at lower frequencies [6, p. 275; 7, p. 45]. Indeed, it is a good approximation[4] to assume that the propagation process is adiabatic for frequencies below 10^9 Hz.

A second simple form of wave propagation in a solid medium occurs when the particle movement is at right angles to the direction of propagation. In Fig. 1.2b the particle motion is in the y-direction, with the wave propagating in the z-direction. Such a wave is a y-polarized transverse (also called shear) wave. In contrast to the changes in acoustic particle volume that occur for longitudinal waves, no density change occurs for shear waves, even though there is a transformation of the acoustic particle volume shape. It is also evident from this figure that a shear wave could also propagate in the same direction but with particle displacements in the x-direction. If both components were

---

3. The term *speed* is used to describe the scalar quantity, while *velocity* is used for a velocity vector.

4. For media with a very high thermal conductivity this may not be true: the propagation would then be closer to isothermal.

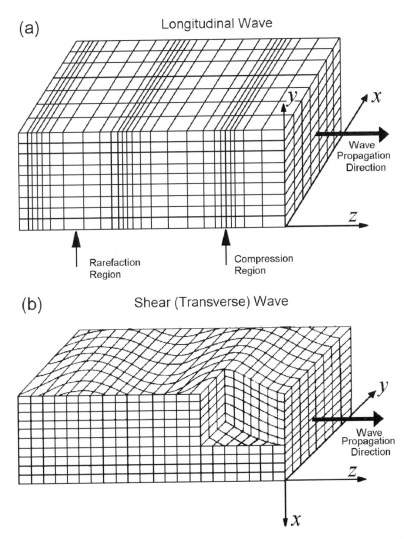

(a)   Longitudinal Wave

Rarefaction
Region

Compression
Region

Wave
Propagation
Direction

(b)   Shear (Transverse) Wave

Wave
Propagation
Direction

Figure 1.2 Snapshot view of "particle" displacements for waves propagating in the z-direction of an isotropic solid medium: (a) a plane longitudinal wave, (b) a y-polarized wave shear wave. The "particles" are assumed to be small volume elements. For the waves illustrated the "particles" move in the z-direction for the longitudinal wave and in the y-direction for the shear wave. (Reproduced from Ristic [5], *Principles of Acoustic Devices*, © 1983 Wiley. This material is used by permission of John Wiley & Sons Limited.)

present, the result would be an elliptically polarized shear wave with a major to minor axis ratio that depends on the relative component amplitudes. Both longitudinal and shear waves may be present in solid media, but in liquids, because shear waves are not supported, only longitudinal waves can propagate.

1.1.3 Rayleigh and Lamb Waves

If the plane boundary of a semi-infinite solid separates the solid from a rarefied medium such as a gas, then wave propagation can occur close to the boundary through a coupling of longitudinal and transverse waves at the interface. Such waves, first described by Rayleigh in 1885, are often referred to as *Rayleigh waves*. As indicated in Fig. 1.3a, the amplitude of the particle displacement for these waves decays very rapidly with distance from the interface: at a depth of two Rayleigh wavelengths (λ_R), the amplitude is virtually zero. Each particle moves in an elliptical orbit whose direction of polarization changes at a depth of about $0.2\lambda_R$ from the interface.

   Other forms of wave motion can occur in plates and rods, and depending on the dimensions a variety of propagation modes are possible. The simplest case occurs when the thickness and width are much less than a wavelength so that only the lowest-order mode is possible. For example, if one end of a thin rod were excited with low-frequency axial vibrations, an *extensional* wave would be propagated, with particle motion both along and perpendicular to the rod axis. As illustrated in Fig. 1.3b, on the free surface of the rod the normal component of the stress is zero; consequently, the stress component in the rod perpendicular to its axis will also be zero. The wave propagates without any changes occurring in the volume associated with a particle, though of course its shape changes. On the other hand, if the material is an infinitely wide flat plate, shear motion can occur in both the width and thickness directions. The waves that result from all possible modes, including the extensional wave mode, are called Lamb waves.

1.2 Properties of Isotropic Media

In our subsequent discussions of wave propagation in an isotropic medium, certain mechanical properties of the medium will be needed for describing the propagation. These will now be defined and equations that relate them to the wave propagation speed will be introduced.

1.2.1 Compressibility and Bulk Modulus: Liquids and Gases

If an equilibrium volume V_o of an isotropic medium is subject to an increase in pressure dp, the volume will decrease by dV and work will done. If the compression is performed under isothermal conditions, the change in volume will normally differ from that occurring under adiabatic conditions; consequently it is necessary to distinguish between the two processes. The *adiabatic compressibility* is defined by

(1.1) $$\text{Adiabatic compressibility} = \kappa = -\frac{1}{V_o}\left.\frac{\partial V}{\partial p}\right|_s,$$

or, since density ρ is the mass per unit volume, i.e., $\rho \propto 1/V$, this can be expressed as

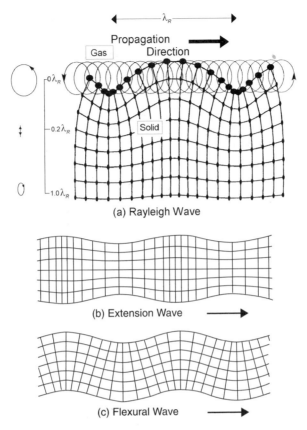

Figure 1.3 Snapshot of particle displacements for (a) Rayleigh wave, (b) extensional (Lamb) wave in a thin rod, and (c) flexural (antisymmetric) Lamb wave in a thin plate. (a, reproduced, with permission, from Hassan and Nagy [8], *J. Acoust. Soc. Am.*, 104, 3107–3110, © 1998, Acoustical Society of America. b and c, reprinted by permission of Elsevier from Kuttruff [9], *Ultrasonics: Fundamentals and Applications*, © 1991 Elsevier.)

(1.2)
$$\kappa = \frac{1}{\rho_o} \frac{\partial \rho}{\partial p}\bigg|_s ,$$

where ρ_o is the equilibrium density and s indicates a constant entropy corresponding to a reversible adiabatic process. A similar definition is used for the *isothermal compressibility* κ_T, except that now the partial derivative is evaluated for a constant temperature. The inverse of the adiabatic compressibility is the *adiabatic bulk (elastic) modulus* $(K = 1/\kappa)$. The variations of the two compressibilities for water as a function of temperature are illustrated in Fig. 1.4. Some of the data shown in Table 1.1 shows that very large differences can exist between the adiabatic compressibilities of different types of media. For example, air is approximately 15,000 times more compressible than water.

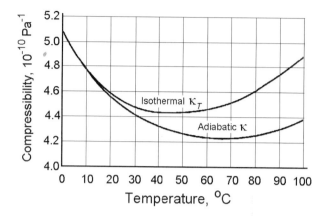

Figure 1.4 Isothermal (κ_T) and adiabatic (κ) compressibility of water as a function of temperature. Based on the values given by Zemansky and Dittman [10].

As previously noted, for most media the effects of thermal conduction between regions of compression and rarefaction during the passage of a longitudinal wave can be expected to be very small, and consequently it is reasonable to assume that *isentropic* (s = const) conditions are maintained throughout the propagation process. For plane wave propagation in a liquid or a gas, all acoustic particles that lie on a given plane normal to the direction of propagation will be subject to the same incremental pressure change. The fractional change in their volume will be proportional to the adiabatic compressibility of the medium. It is therefore reasonable to expect that the speed of propagation[5] (the phase speed) of a small-amplitude longitudinal wave in a liquid or gas should be directly related to the adiabatic compressibility and, as will be subsequently shown, it is given by

$$(1.3) \qquad\qquad c_o = 1/\sqrt{\kappa \rho_o} \, ,$$

where the subscript o has been used to indicate that it is the small-signal speed for quasi-equilibrium conditions. Since the propagation process in most liquids is sufficiently close to adiabatic, measurement of the propagation speed is often used for determining the adiabatic compressibility.[6]

Accurate (± 0.015 m/s) measurements on the propagation speed in pure water over a temperature range from 0.001 to 95°C at 5 MHz and interpolated

5. More generally, for an isentropic process the propagation speed in a gas or fluid is defined by $c^2 = (\partial P/\partial \rho)_s$. Under large signal conditions the non-linearity of the relation between P and ρ must be accounted for, which makes the speed dependent on the instantaneous value of the pressure and hence on the instantaneous particle velocity (see Chapter 4).

6. For certain fluids that are of an additive nature, the compressibility is linearly related to the density. In blood, for example, the net density is the result of the plasma and red blood cell densities, and similarly for the compressibility. Both relations involve the hematocrit, which, when eliminated between the two, yields a linear relation between the compressibility and density that has been verified experimentally [11].

Table 1.1. Approximate Properties of Selected Liquid, Solid, and Gas Media

Medium	T, °C	Density ρ, kg/m³	Adiabatic Compressibility κ, GPa⁻¹	Longitudinal Speed c_L m/s	Transverse Speed c_T m/s	Poisson's Ratio σ, or Ratio of Specific Heats, γ	Young's Modulus E GPa	Absolute Viscosity μ, cPoise ≡ 10⁻³ × kg/(m.s)
Pure water[a]	20	998.2	0.4559	1482.34*	—	$\gamma = 1.0152$	—	1.002
Pure water[a]	30	995.7	0.4410	1509.13*	—	$\gamma = 1.0152$	—	0.798
Blood, whole Human[c], Hct = 40%	36	1055	0.380	1580*	—			~3.5
Bone, fresh Bovine phalanx[d]	NR	1960		4030*	1660*	$\sigma = 0.40$	22	—
Aluminum[b]		2700	0.00912	6374	3111	$\sigma = 0.345$	70	—
Steel (mild)[b]		7800	0.00361	5960	3235	$\sigma = 0.29$	212	—
Dry air (1 atm)[b]	20	1.204	7047	343.3	—	$\gamma = 1.4018$	—	0.01813

* Measured at 5 MHz.
NR, Not reported.
[a] [10].
[b] Kay, G.W.C, and Laby, T.H., *Tables of Physical and Chemical Constants and Some Mathematical Functions*, 15th Edn., Longman, London, 1995.
[c] Gross et al., *JASA*, 64, 423, 1978.
[d] Measured along the long axis: Lang, *IEEE Trans. BME*, 17, 101, 1970.

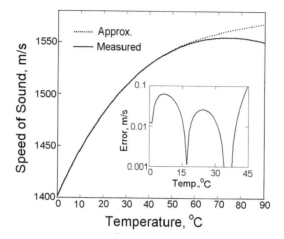

Figure 1.5 Speed of sound in pure water as a function of temperature. The measured values at 5.0 MHz [12] have been interpolated and are accurate to ±0.015 m/s. The insert shows the magnitude of the difference between the values from the approximation given by (1.4) and those measured over the range from 0 to 45°C.

by means of a fifth-order polynomial have been reported by Del Grosso and Mader [12]. These are widely regarded as a standard.[7] The interpolated curve is shown in Fig. 1.5 along with that obtained from the following approximation as given by Temkin [14, p. 47]:

(1.4) $$c_o = 1402.40 + 5.01T - 0.055T^2 + 0.00022T^3.$$

It can be seen that this equation is accurate to <0.1 m/s over the temperature range from 0 to 40°C. Other approximations have been reviewed by Lubbers and Graaff [15].

For an ideal gas, the speed can also be expressed in terms of the pressure by noting that under adiabatic conditions the gas law can be expressed as pV^γ = const., where $\gamma = C_P/C_V$ is the ratio of the specific heat at a constant pressure to that at a constant volume. By differentiating this expression and denoting the equilibrium pressure by p_o, we obtain $dV/V = -dp/(p_o\gamma)$, which by comparison with (1.1) enables the adiabatic compressibility to be expressed as $\kappa = 1/(p_o\gamma)$. By substituting this into (1.3) the wave speed can be written in terms of the ambient pressure and density:

(1.5) $$c_o = \sqrt{p_o\gamma/\rho_o}.$$

The measured values for the propagation speed versus those calculated provide information on the question previously addressed as to whether the passage of an ultrasonic wave can be regarded as an adiabatic or isothermal process. For dry air at atmospheric pressure and 20°C, $\gamma = 1.40$, so that the

7. Based on the adoption of a new (1990) international temperature scale, some corrections have been made; these are reported in [13].

assumption of isothermal propagation (γ = 1.0) leads to an error that approaches 20%. On the other hand, for water at 30°C, γ is very close to unity (γ = 1.0152) and as a result the speed of sound calculated from the isothermal compressibility is in error with respect to that measured or calculated by less than 1%.

1.2.2 Solids: Young's Modulus, Poisson's Ratio, and Shear Modulus

As illustrated in Fig. 1.2a, the propagation of a plane longitudinal wave in an infinite isotropic solid involves no particle motion normal to the propagation axis. For a solid of finite dimensions, this can occur only if appropriate lateral stresses are present on the surface to prevent a dimensional change in the lateral direction. A simple way of visualizing this situation is to consider a thin cylindrical rod of length z to which a compressive stress is applied in the axial direction. Not only will the length of the rod decrease, but there will also be an increase in the radius. The axial strain can be found from knowing *Young's modulus E* for the medium. This is defined as the ratio of the stress to the axial strain (fractional change in length) for a thin rod. In addition, the strain in the radial direction can be found from a second property of the material, namely *Poisson's ratio* σ, which is defined as the ratio of the lateral strain to the longitudinal strain. These two definitions can be written as

$$(1.6) \qquad \text{Young's modulus} = E = \frac{\text{Longitudinal Stress}}{\text{Longitudinal Strain}} = \frac{T_z}{\delta z/z},$$

$$(1.7) \qquad \text{Poisson's Ratio} = \sigma = \frac{-\text{Lateral Strain}}{\text{Longitudinal Strain}} = \frac{-\delta r/r}{\delta z/z},$$

where T_z is the applied axial stress on a rod and $\delta r/r$ and $\delta z/z$ are the strains in the radial and axial directions, respectively.

For an ideal *fluid*, if the strain in the z-direction for a certain small volume element is $\delta z/z$, then, since there can be no net volume change and the lateral strains in the y- and x-directions are equal, it can be readily seen that $\delta z/z = -2\delta x/x$, so that $\sigma = 0.5$. At the other extreme, for a medium in which no lateral strain results from a longitudinal strain, $\sigma = 0$. Consequently, the possible range in values for Poisson's ratio is $0 < \sigma < 0.5$.

If a sinusoidal axial stress is applied to a thin rod, at a sufficiently low frequency so that the wavelength is much greater than the rod diameter, then an extensional wave will be propagated, as illustrated in Fig. 1.3b. In this case the appropriate elastic property governing the speed of propagation is Young's modulus and, as will be shown, the speed given by

$$(1.8) \qquad c_E = \sqrt{E/\rho_o}.$$

On the other hand, if the rod diameter is prevented from changing by the application of an appropriate compressive stress to the surface of the rod, it is evident that for the same axial stress, the axial strain will be reduced, i.e., the rod now behaves in a more rigid manner, and as a result longitudinal waves have a higher speed than extensional waves. Thus, an additional material property can be defined: specifically, the *axial modulus* is given by

$$(1.9) \qquad \text{Axial modulus} = \chi = \frac{\text{Longitudinal Stress}}{\text{Longitudinal Strain}} = \frac{T_z}{\delta z / z}\bigg|_{r=const.}$$

under the condition that there be no lateral strain ($\delta r / r = 0$). Consequently, the speed of a longitudinal wave is given by

$$(1.10) \qquad c_L = \sqrt{\chi / \rho_o}.$$

Alternatively, since $\chi = \dfrac{E(1-\sigma)}{(1-2\sigma)(1+\sigma)}$, this can be written as

$$(1.11) \qquad c_L = \sqrt{\frac{E(1-\sigma)}{\rho_o(1-2\sigma)(1+\sigma)}},$$

which, by comparison with (1.8) and noting that $0 < \sigma < 0.5$, shows that $c_L \geq c_E$.

Since the propagation of transverse waves involves a shearing motion, it is to be expected that the *shear modulus* μ_ℓ, defined by

$$(1.12) \qquad \mu_\ell = \frac{\text{Shear Stress}}{\text{Shear Strain (angular deformation)}},$$

governs the propagation speed. As will be shown, the speed is given by

$$(1.13) \qquad c_T = \sqrt{\mu_\ell / \rho_o},$$

but, because $\mu_\ell = E/\{2(1+\sigma)\}$, the speed can also be expressed in terms of the same two elastic constants used previously, yielding

$$(1.14) \qquad c_T = \sqrt{\frac{E}{2\rho_o(1+\sigma)}}.$$

1.2.3 Temperature Effects

Temperature changes will accompany the pressure changes due to a plane wave propagating under adiabatic conditions. As shown in the following derivation, the amplitude of the temperature changes can be readily calculated from the pressure amplitude. Let T be the absolute temperature, $\gamma = C_P/C_V$, and κ and κ_T be the adiabatic and isothermal compressibilities, respectively. By making use of thermodynamic equations [10], we find that for a reversible adiabatic process (constant entropy s), the second $T\,ds$ equation [10, p. 265] can be written as

$$T\,ds = 0 = C_p\,dT - T\frac{\partial V}{\partial T}\bigg|_p dp,$$

in which V is the volume, and hence

(1.15) $$C_p dT = TV \beta \, dp,$$

where β is the volume expansivity given by $\beta = \dfrac{1}{V}\dfrac{\partial V}{\partial T}\bigg|_p$. Now since $C_P - C_V = TV\,\beta^2/\kappa_T$ [10, p. 270] and $\gamma = C_P/C_V = \kappa_T/\kappa$ [10, p. 271], (1.15) simplifies to

(1.16) $$\frac{\partial P}{\partial T}\bigg|_s = \frac{\beta}{(\gamma - 1)\kappa}.$$

Now for a gas or a liquid $pV = nRT(1 + Bp + Cp^2 + \ldots)$, where B and C are the virial coefficients, n is the number of moles and R is the gas constant [10, p. 106]. Taking the partial derivative of this expansion at a constant pressure and comparing the result with the definition of the volume expansivity, yields $\beta = 1/T$, enabling (1.16) to be written as

$$\frac{\partial P}{\partial T}\bigg|_s = \frac{1}{T(\gamma - 1)\kappa}.$$

Hence, for a small change in pressure Δp, under adiabatic conditions the temperature change is given by

(1.17) $$\Delta T = \Delta p\,(\gamma - 1)T\,\kappa.$$

As an example, consider a plane wave whose amplitude is $2\,\text{kPa}$ traveling in water at $30°\text{C}$. From Table 1.1, $\Delta T = 2 \times 10^3(1.0152 - 1)(273 + 30)4.41 \times 10^{-10} = 4.1\,\mu°\text{C}$, which is very small indeed. Very much higher values can be obtained for propagation in a gas due to the much larger values of the compressibility and $(\gamma - 1)$. For example, the same plane wave propagating in dry air at $20°\text{C}$ results in $\Delta T = 1.6°\text{C}$.

1.3 Equations Governing Wave Propagation in Fluids

The state of a fluid in motion can be mathematically described by a knowledge of the particle velocity function $\mathbf{v} = \mathbf{v}(\mathbf{r}:t)$ together with two[8] thermodynamic functions, such as the density $\rho = \rho(\mathbf{r}:t)$ and pressure $p = p(\mathbf{r}:t)$, at all spatial locations $\mathbf{r}$ and at any instant of time t. By establishing and solving the equations that describe the behavior of these three functions subject to the initial and boundary conditions, the flow field can be fully determined. For the purpose of describing wave motion under adiabatic conditions we shall obtain three equations: an equation of motion, the continuity equation, and an equation of state. As will be seen, these enable equations to be obtained for the particle velocity and thermodynamic functions. We shall start by deriving an equation of motion, though, for rather special conditions.

---

8. Two thermodynamic quantities together with an equation of state are sufficient to determine all other such quantities.

1.3.1 Euler's Equation of Motion

An ideal fluid is one for which the effects of viscosity and thermal conductivity can be neglected. The equation that was first derived by Euler in 1755, and that bears his name, characterizes the motion of an ideal fluid and forms one of the cornerstones of fluid dynamics. This will be first derived since it forms a stepping stone to the derivation of the more complex Navier-Stokes equation that describes the motion of a nonideal fluid.

The stress principle discovered by Cauchy forms the starting point of our derivation. It has been expressed by Truesdell [17] in the following way: "upon any imagined closed surface S there exists a distribution of stress vectors τ whose resultant and moment are equivalent to those of the actual forces of material continuity exerted by the material outside S upon the inside." It therefore follows that we can determine the resultant stress and moment acting on an acoustic particle by examining the stresses acting on a small volume of fluid enclosed by the surface S. For simplicity, we will assume that the effects of body forces such as gravity and electromagnetic forces acting on this volume can be neglected. Under non-equilibrium conditions the surrounding fluid will exert stresses on the surface of the volume causing it to be displaced and changed in shape. In general, for a viscous fluid both tangential (shear) and normal component stresses will be present over the surface, but, because the fluid has been assumed to be inviscid, all tangential components will be zero and the moment will be zero. The remaining normal components are simply a distribution of pressures on the surface. Because the resulting force on the volume due to these pressures will generally be non-zero, the volume will be displaced and may change its shape.

Rather than determining equations governing a given fluid property at a fixed spatial location, it is simpler to focus on the properties of a moving particle as they change (Fig. 1.6) under the action of the various forces. Equations that characterize the properties in this manner are said to be expressed in a Lagrangian form. It will be shown how the Eulerian form, which expresses the property at a fixed spatial location, can be obtained from the Lagrangian form by means of a simple transform relation.[9]

If $p(\mathbf{r}:t)$ represents the pressure distribution on the surface of a fluid volume V, then the resulting vector force $\mathbf{F}$ is given by

$$(1.18) \qquad \mathbf{F} = -\iint_S p\,\tilde{\mathbf{n}}\,dS,$$

where the integral is over the entire surface area S of the fluid volume and $\tilde{\mathbf{n}}$ is an outward-directed normal unit vector on the elementary surface area dS. By making use of a well-known vector relation,[10] this surface integral can be transformed into an integral over the volume V yielding

---

9. The Lagrangian and Eulerian coordinate systems are sometimes referred to as material and spatial coordinate systems, respectively.

10. See Appendix D: from Gauss' Divergence theorem, $\iiint_V \operatorname{div}\mathbf{A}\,dv = \iint_S \mathbf{A}\cdot\tilde{\mathbf{n}}\,dS$, it can be readily shown that $\iiint_V \operatorname{grad}B\,dv = \iint_S B\tilde{\mathbf{n}}\,dS$.

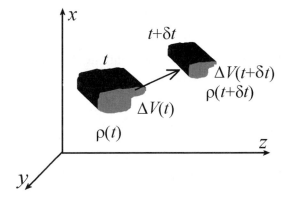

Figure 1.6 Lagrangian description showing a small volume element (an acoustic particle) at a time t and at a subsequent time of $t + \delta t$. The displacement is due to the particle velocity in the direction of the arrow. The density is shown as having increased and the volume as having decreased.

$$\mathbf{F} = - \iiint_V \mathbf{grad}\, p\, dV,$$

in which $\mathbf{grad} \equiv \nabla$ is the gradient operator.[11] It therefore follows that the force per unit volume of the fluid is simply $-\mathbf{grad}p \equiv -\nabla p$. Now, by Newton's second law the force per volume is equal to the product of density and acceleration, yielding

(1.19)
$$\rho \frac{D\mathbf{v}}{Dt} = -\nabla p,$$
(Lagrange)

where $\mathbf{v}$ is the vector velocity of a fluid particle and the use of the capital D on the left side of this equation specifies that the derivative is the rate of change of the velocity of the moving particle, which in general differs from the derivative evaluated at a fixed point in space. On the other hand, the right-hand side is expressed in terms of the stationary coordinate system. This equation is the Lagrangian form of *Euler's equation* of motion.

To obtain an equation in terms of what happens to a fixed point in space, it is necessary to consider how any given property of the particle, such as its velocity and density, changes as the particle moves. Let us suppose that the property (which can be a scalar, a vector, or a tensor) is denoted by f. There are two contributions to the change in f as the particle moves by an incremental vector distance $D\mathbf{r}$ in a time increment of Dt. The first arises from the change that occurs at a fixed spatial location and is equal to $(\partial f / \partial t)Dt$. The second is due to the change in f that occurs over the spatial distance $D\mathbf{r}$, and this can be written in Cartesian coordinates as

---

11. In Cartesian coordinates, $\nabla = \tilde{\mathbf{x}} \dfrac{\partial}{\partial x} + \tilde{\mathbf{y}} \dfrac{\partial}{\partial y} + \tilde{\mathbf{z}} \dfrac{\partial}{\partial z}$, where $\tilde{\mathbf{x}}$, $\tilde{\mathbf{y}}$, and $\tilde{\mathbf{z}}$ are unit vectors along the x-, y- and z-directions.

$$\frac{\partial f}{\partial x}dx+\frac{\partial f}{\partial y}dy+\frac{\partial f}{\partial z}dz=(D\mathbf{r}\cdot\nabla)f.$$

Consequently, by adding these two contributions, dividing by Dt, and noting that the particle velocity is defined by $\mathbf{v}=D\mathbf{r}/Dt$, we obtain

(1.20) $$\underset{\text{Material Derivative}}{\frac{Df}{Dt}}\quad=\quad\underset{\text{Local Derivative}}{\frac{\partial f}{\partial t}}\quad+\quad\underset{\text{Convective Part}}{(\mathbf{v}\cdot\nabla)f}\quad.$$

This equation allows us to relate the rate of change of a given property as seen by an observer moving with the particle to that occurring at a fixed spatial location.

A transformation of (1.19) to a fixed coordinate system can be achieved by first replacing f in (1.20) by $\mathbf{v}$ and then substituting the result into (1.19), yielding the Eulerian form:

(1.21) $$\boxed{\rho\left[\frac{\partial\mathbf{v}}{\partial t}+(\mathbf{v}\cdot\nabla)\mathbf{v}\right]=-\nabla p.}\qquad\text{(Euler)}$$

This is *Euler's equation* of motion for an ideal fluid in the absence of any gravitational forces. It characterizes the time and spatial behavior of the velocity vector in terms of the density and pressure, both of which are generally time- and space-dependent. If the fluid is incompressible the density will be space- and time-invariant, but Euler's equation remains unchanged. The two additional equations that are needed for the state of an inviscid fluid to be fully determined for a given set of boundary and initial conditions, will now be discussed.

1.3.2 Continuity Equation

The continuity equation simply expresses the conservation of mass. It can be derived by assuming that the arbitrary fluid volume V_o shown in Fig. 1.7 remains constant and is at fixed spatial location. Over the surface area S_o enclosing this volume the mass of fluid flowing in must equal that flowing out. If dS is an element of surface area at the location $\mathbf{r}$, $\mathbf{v}(\mathbf{r}:t)$ is the fluid velocity, $\rho(\mathbf{r}:t)$ is the density, and $\tilde{\mathbf{n}}$ is a unit vector pointing outwards from dS, then the net mass that flows out of the volume V_o in a small time increment Δt is equal to $\Delta t\iint_{S_o}\rho\mathbf{v}\cdot\tilde{\mathbf{n}}\,dS$. Now since the rate of increase of the fluid mass inside V_o is given by

$$\frac{\partial}{\partial t}\iiint_{V_o}\rho(\mathbf{r}:t)dV,$$

the conservation of mass requires that

$$\frac{\partial}{\partial t}\left[\iiint_{V_o}\rho dV\right]\Delta t=-\left[\iint_{S_o}\rho\mathbf{v}\cdot\tilde{\mathbf{n}}\,dS\right]\Delta t.$$

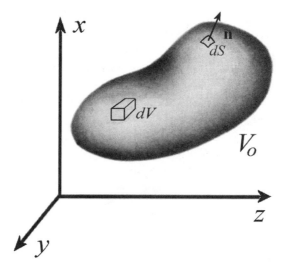

Figure 1.7 Showing a volume V_o of fluid fixed in space, a unit vector ñ normal to an element dS of the surface that encloses the volume, and an elemental volume dV within V_o.

Transforming the RHS to a volume integral and rearranging yields

$$\iiint_{V_o} \frac{\partial \rho}{\partial t} dV = -\iiint_{V_o} \text{div}(\rho \mathbf{v}) dV,$$

in which div $(\mathbf{u}) \equiv \nabla \cdot \mathbf{u}$. But, since this equation must hold true for an arbitrarily small volume, we obtain the Euler form of the continuity equation:

(1.22) $$\frac{\partial \rho}{\partial t} + \text{div}(\rho \mathbf{v}) = 0.$$ (Euler)

The Lagrangian form of this equation can be obtained by making use of the transformation given by (1.20) to re-express (1.22) as

$$\frac{D\rho}{Dt} = -\text{div}(\rho \mathbf{v}) + (\mathbf{v} \cdot \mathbf{grad})\rho.$$

By making use of the standard vector relation,[12] this can be simplified to

(1.23) $$\boxed{\frac{D\rho}{Dt} + \rho \text{div } \mathbf{v} = 0.}$$ (Lagrange)

1.3.3 Equation of State

An equation of state is one that relates various thermodynamic variables such as pressure, density, and entropy, i.e., $p = p(r, s)$. For example, in the case of an

12. See Appendix D: $\text{div}(a\mathbf{A}) = (\mathbf{A} \cdot \mathbf{grad})a + a\text{div}\mathbf{A}$.

ideal gas under constant entropy conditions, this takes the form $p/p_o = (\rho/\rho_o)^\gamma$. However, rather than using the restrictions of a specific relation we shall proceed in a more general manner by first writing down the definition of the adiabatic compressibility in the form given by (1.2), viz:

(1.2)
$$\kappa = \frac{1}{\rho_o} \frac{\partial \rho}{\partial p}\bigg|_s .$$

This equation relates the change in density to the change in pressure of a given acoustic particle as it moves in the medium. Consequently, the rates of change of its pressure and density are related by:

(1.24)
$$\kappa\rho_o \frac{Dp}{Dt} = \frac{D\rho}{Dt},$$
(Lagrange)

which is the Lagrangian form. To transform this to the Eulerian form we again make use of (1.20) and obtain

(1.25)
$$\boxed{\frac{\partial \rho}{\partial t} + \mathbf{v} \cdot \mathbf{grad}\,\rho = \kappa\rho_o\left[\frac{\partial p}{\partial t} + \mathbf{v} \cdot \mathbf{grad}\,p\right]} .$$
(Euler)

1.3.4 Navier-Stokes Equation [6,18–20]

In deriving the Euler equation (see subsection 1.3.1), the assumption of an inviscid fluid enabled all the stress components acting tangentially to the surface of the moving fluid volume to be set to zero, leaving just the normal components. For a viscous fluid the presence of shear stresses can be accounted for through the addition of a viscous force term to the right-hand side of Euler's equation (1.19), yielding

(1.26)
$$\rho\frac{D\mathbf{v}}{Dt} = -\nabla p - \nabla \cdot \tau.$$

In this equation, τ is a second-rank tensor known as the *viscosity stress tensor*, which has nine (six independent) components that can be written in Cartesian coordinates as: $\tau_{xx}, \tau_{yy}, \tau_{zz}, \tau_{xy} = \tau_{yx}, \tau_{xz} = \tau_{yx}, \tau_{xy} = \tau_{yx}$. Moreover, $\nabla \cdot \tau$ represents a divergence operation on the second-rank tensor τ. It results in a vector whose components can be expressed in the matrix form:

$$[\nabla \cdot \tau] = \begin{bmatrix} \dfrac{\partial}{\partial x} & \dfrac{\partial}{\partial y} & \dfrac{\partial}{\partial z} \end{bmatrix} \begin{bmatrix} \tau_{xx} & \tau_{xy} & \tau_{xz} \\ \tau_{yx} & \tau_{yy} & \tau_{yz} \\ \tau_{zx} & \tau_{zy} & \tau_{zz} \end{bmatrix} .$$

It can be shown that these components can be expressed in terms of two coefficients that characterize the viscous properties of the fluid: the shear viscosity μ and the bulk viscosity μ_B. As its name suggests, the shear viscosity arises from velocity differences between adjacent fluid layers. The presence of velocity gradients in the fluid means that adjacent layers move at differing speeds, and as a result there is a frictional drag force that causes energy to be dissipated. The bulk viscosity accounts for the effects of energy loss during compression (see subsection 1.8.2) and enters into the stress tensor in a different manner to the shear viscosity. For an incompressible fluid, only the shear viscosity is present.

It can be shown that when the expressions for the stresses are determined and substituted into (1.19), the following compact form of the *Navier-Stokes equation* results:[13]

(1.27)
$$\rho\frac{D\mathbf{v}}{Dt} = -\nabla p + \left(\mu_B + \frac{4}{3}\mu\right)\nabla(\nabla\cdot\mathbf{v}) - \mu\nabla\times(\nabla\times\mathbf{v})$$
$$= -\nabla p + \left(\mu_B + \frac{1}{3}\mu\right)\nabla(\nabla\cdot\mathbf{v}) + \mu\nabla^2\mathbf{v},$$
(Lagrange)

where the second form follows through the use of a standard vector relation.[14] Conversion to the Eulerian form is again achieved through the use of (1.20):

(1.28)
$$\rho\left[\frac{\partial\mathbf{v}}{\partial t} + (\mathbf{v}\cdot\nabla)\mathbf{v}\right] = -\nabla p + \left(\mu_B + \frac{4}{3}\mu\right)\nabla(\nabla\cdot\mathbf{v}) - \mu\nabla\times(\nabla\times\mathbf{v})$$
$$= -\nabla p + \left(\mu_B + \frac{1}{3}\mu\right)\nabla(\nabla\cdot\mathbf{v}) + \mu\nabla^2\mathbf{v}.$$
(Euler)

1.3.5 Small-Signal Approximations

Obtaining linearized forms of the equation of state and the Navier-Stokes and continuity equations enables partial differential equations to be obtained that are much more amenable to analytic solution. To obtain these forms it is necessary to make some approximations concerning the relative magnitudes of the various terms appropriate to ultrasonic wave propagation. To do this we consider a homogeneous isotropic medium whose equilibrium density and pressure are ρ_o and p_o, respectively. As an acoustic field propagates, local changes occur in the density, pressure, and particle velocity of the medium. If these are denoted by $\rho_1(\mathbf{r}:t)$, $p_1(\mathbf{r}:t)$ and $\mathbf{v}(\mathbf{r}:t)$, and the equilibrium values of the density and pressure are ρ_o and p_o, the instantaneous values can be expressed as [21]:

(1.29)
$$\rho = \rho_o + \rho_1, \quad |\rho_1| \ll \rho_o$$
$$p = p_o + p_1, \quad |p_1| \ll \rho_o c_o^2$$
$$\mathbf{v} = 0 + \mathbf{v}, \quad |\mathbf{v}| \ll c_o.$$

As will be seen, the three inequalities are the conditions needed to ensure that ρ_1, p_1, and $\mathbf{v}$ are quantities of the first order of smallness.

---

13. In passing, it should be noted that for an incompressible fluid $\nabla(\nabla\cdot\mathbf{V}) = 0$, and consequently the middle terms on the right-hand side (1.27) and (1.28) are eliminated, making the equations independent of the bulk viscosity.

14. See Appendix D: $\nabla\times(\nabla\times\mathbf{A}) = \nabla(\nabla\cdot\mathbf{A}) - \nabla^2\mathbf{A}$.

Typically, the changes in density are small compared to ρ_o, i.e. $|\rho_1| \ll \rho_o$. For example, a 5 MHz plane wave in water with an intensity of 100 mW/cm^2 can be shown to result in a fractional density change of only 24×10^{-6}. However, for the same plane wave the corresponding pressure amplitude is 54 kPa, which is more than 50% of the equilibrium (atmospheric) pressure. It would therefore seem that for the small-signal condition to be valid the signal intensity should be much smaller. To investigate this further, it is helpful to examine the relation between the density and pressure in more detail.

For propagation under isentropic conditions in liquids and gases, a Taylor series expansion enables the relation between the excess pressure and excess density to be written as[15] [21]:

$$(1.30) \qquad p_1 = \rho_o c_o^2 \left[\frac{\rho_1}{\rho_o} + \frac{B}{2!A}\left(\frac{\rho_1}{\rho_o}\right)^2 + \frac{C}{3!A}\left(\frac{\rho_1}{\rho_o}\right)^3 + \cdots \right],$$

where B/A, and C/A are nonlinearity parameters. If the inequality $|\rho_1| \ll \rho_o$ is accepted, by rewriting (1.30) in the approximate form $p_1/(\rho_o c_o^2) \approx \rho_1/\rho_o$ it can be seen that the small-signal condition for the excess acoustic pressure is that $|p_1| \ll \rho_o c_o^2$. For propagation in water, this requires that $|p_1| \ll 1.5$ MPa, which is well satisfied for the above example.

Proper justification of the linearizing approximations, as used in obtaining the first-order equations given below, requires careful consideration of the magnitudes of the higher-order terms. Insana and Brown [22] have addressed this issue in detail and point out that when the above equations are substituted into Euler's equation, the continuity equation, and the equation of state, unlike ρ_o, p_o is absent. They provided details of the conditions required for discarding higher-order terms, a problem that appears to have been initially detailed by Eckart [23] in 1948.

By substituting (1.29) into the continuity equation (1.22) and ignoring higher-order terms, we find that

$$(1.31) \qquad \frac{\partial \rho_1}{\partial t} + \rho_o \nabla \cdot \mathbf{v} \approx 0.$$

Similarly, the equation of state can be approximated by substituting (1.29) into (1.25) and making use of (1.31):

$$(1.32) \qquad \kappa \frac{\partial p_1}{\partial t} + \nabla \cdot \mathbf{v} \approx 0,$$

and the linearized Navier-Stokes equation (1.28) is:

$$(1.33) \qquad \rho_o \frac{\partial \mathbf{v}}{\partial t} \approx -\nabla p_1 + \left(\mu_B + \frac{4}{3}\mu\right)\nabla(\nabla \cdot \mathbf{v}) - \mu \nabla \times \nabla \times \mathbf{v}.$$

Now any vector can be decomposed into the sum of two vectors, one of which has zero divergence and the other whose curl is zero, i.e., $\mathbf{v} = \mathbf{v_L} + \mathbf{v_T}$,

---

15. See subsection 4.4.2 for further details.

where $\nabla \times \mathbf{v_L} = 0$ and $\nabla \cdot \mathbf{v_T} = 0$. By substituting into (1.33), making use of the properties of $\mathbf{v_L}$ and $\mathbf{v_T}$, noting that $\nabla(\nabla \cdot \mathbf{v_L}) = \nabla^2 \mathbf{v_L}$, and dropping the subscript on p_1, two independent equations can be obtained that describe the behavior of the two velocity vectors, one of which is irrotational (**curl** $\mathbf{v_L} = 0$) and the other is divergenceless (div $\mathbf{v_T} = 0$):

$$\rho_o \frac{\partial \mathbf{v_L}}{\partial t} = -\nabla p + \left(\mu_B + \frac{4}{3}\mu \right) \nabla^2 \mathbf{v_L}, \tag{a}$$

(1.34)

$$\rho_o \frac{\partial \mathbf{v_T}}{\partial t} = -\mu \nabla \times \nabla \times \mathbf{v_T}. \tag{b}$$

The first equation describes the propagation of longitudinal wave waves, while the second corresponds to shear wave propagation involving no pressure or density changes. The pressure term in (1.34a) can be expressed in terms of the particle velocity by first differentiating, making use of (1.32), and noting the relation in footnote 14 and that $\nabla \times \mathbf{v_L} = 0$, yielding

$$(1.35) \qquad \kappa\rho_o \frac{\partial^2 \mathbf{v_L}}{\partial t^2} = \nabla^2 \mathbf{v_L} + \kappa\left(\mu_B + \frac{4}{3}\mu \right)\frac{\partial}{\partial t}(\nabla^2 \mathbf{v_L}).$$

Considerable simplification results if this can be expressed in a scalar form. Two such forms will be obtained: one in terms of the pressure, the second in terms of a scalar potential.

By taking the divergence of (1.34a) and then substituting for the velocity terms by using both (1.32) and its gradient, the scalar equation for the pressure is found to be identical in form to (1.35):

$$(1.36) \qquad \kappa\rho_o \frac{\partial^2 p}{\partial t^2} = \nabla^2 p + \kappa\left(\mu_B + \frac{4}{3}\mu \right)\frac{\partial}{\partial t}(\nabla^2 p).$$

It can be readily shown that the density equation also has the same form.

The form that we will frequently use can be obtained by using the fact that any irrotational vector can always be expressed as the gradient of a scalar potential. We shall define the *velocity potential* ϕ, by[16]

$$(1.37) \qquad \boxed{\mathbf{v_L} = -\mathbf{grad}\phi \equiv -\nabla\phi}\,,$$

which, when substituted into (1.35), gives

$$(1.38) \qquad \boxed{\kappa\rho_o \frac{\partial^2 \phi}{\partial t^2} = \nabla^2 \phi + \kappa\left(\mu_B + \frac{4}{3}\mu \right)\frac{\partial}{\partial t}(\nabla^2 \phi).}$$

A knowledge of the velocity potential enables the particle velocity vector to be found from (1.37), and hence the density and pressure can be obtained from (1.31) and (1.32). From this point onwards, unless ambiguity arises, the longitudinal particle velocity subscript $\mathbf{L}$ will be dropped. Of considerable value are

---

16. The sign chosen is consistent with electrical engineering practice. Some authors prefer to use the positive sign, resulting in equations that differ from some of those that follow, through a change in sign.

the relations between the pressure and velocity potential and between the pressure and particle velocity. For an *inviscid* fluid, these can be obtained by substituting (1.37) into (1.34a) and setting the viscosity coefficients to zero, yielding

(1.39)

$$p = \rho_o \frac{\partial \phi}{\partial t},$$

$$\nabla p = -\rho_o \frac{\partial \mathbf{v}}{\partial t}.$$

1.4 Propagation in Liquid and Solid Media

1.4.1 Phase and Group Speed[17]

In considering the effects of propagation of longitudinal waves in an attenuating medium, it may be necessary to take account of the fact that the propagation speed is frequency-dependent. As will be seen, the presence of dispersion in a medium is intimately related to its absorption via the Kramers-Kronig relations (see subsection 3.10.1). For a broadband ultrasound pulse propagating in a dispersive medium, the effect of changes in the propagation speed on the spectrum of frequencies present can, apart from the effects of attenuation, cause the waveform to become progressively distorted. As a result, the "center of gravity" of the pulse may propagate with a speed that differs from that of its frequency components.[18] It is therefore important to define carefully what we mean by the propagation speed. Sommerfeld and Brillouin contributed two fundamental papers on this topic in German that were published in 1914 and subsequently translated and published in a book by Brillouin [24].

As its name implies, the *phase speed* of a wave is the speed with which any given phase of the waveform propagates to a new spatial location. For a simple harmonic wave the phase speed can be determined from the time taken for a given point or phase of the waveform to propagate a specified distance. Let us consider the harmonic wave given by $\phi = \phi_o \cos(\omega t - kx)$ propagating in the x-direction, where k is the wave number and ω is the angular frequency. After a distance of Δx and a time interval of Δt, the wave will have the same phase if, $(\omega t - kx) = \omega(t + \Delta t) - k(x + \Delta x)$, i.e., when $\Delta x/\Delta t = \omega/k$, and consequently, the phase speed can be defined as the ratio of the angular frequency to the wave number, i.e.,

---

17. Generally referred to as group and phase velocity, but because our discussion is restricted to scalar quantities, footnote 3 applies.

18. This phenomena was well know in the 1800s, as evidenced by the remark by Lord Rayleigh in his classical paper of 1877 (*Proc. Lond. Math. Soc.*, **9**, 21, 1877): "It has often been remarked that, when a group of waves advances into still water, the velocity of the group is less than the velocity of the individual waves of which it is composed." It seems likely that the concept was first formulated in the field of optics by Hamilton (*Proc. Roy. Irish Acad.*, **1**, 267 & 341, 1839).

(1.40)   *Phase Speed*: $c_\phi = \omega/k$.

In a dispersive medium c_ϕ is a function of frequency, causing the shape of a pulse to change with the propagation distance. To characterize the pulse propagation speed a particular feature of the pulse must chosen, but changes to this feature may make it difficult to arrive at an appropriate definition. The presence of precursors (also called forerunners) whose amplitudes may be very small and that, by definition, arrive ahead of the signal creates some difficulties. The *wavefront* can be defined as the surface beyond which, at a given instant of time, the propagation medium is at rest [24, Chapter 1]. Alternatively, the wavefront speed can be taken as the speed with which the principal part of the signal starts to arrive; this speed is sometimes taken to be the high-frequency limit of the phase speed [25].

The *group speed* is used to describe the speed with which a representative characteristic of the pulse moves. Lamb [26, pp. 381–382], has provided a useful and fairly intuitive definition for the group speed. He noted that the wavelength could be considered as a function of space and time, i.e., $\lambda = \lambda(x, t)$. In the neighborhood of a point that travels with the group at a speed of c_g, the representative wavelength can be taken to be constant. To find this speed we make use of (1.20), which can be expressed as $D\lambda/Dt = \partial\lambda/\partial t + c_g \partial\lambda/\partial x = 0$. It follows that the group speed can be defined by

(1.41)   *Group Speed*: $c_g = -\dfrac{\partial\lambda}{\partial t} \Big/ \dfrac{\partial\lambda}{\partial x}$.   (a)

Using this definition, the speed with which the center of gravity of the pulse propagates can be written as

(1.41)
$$c_g = \left[\frac{dk}{d\omega}\right]^{-1}_{\omega=\omega_c},$$
(b)

where the derivative is evaluated at the angular frequency corresponding to the center frequency of the group. In the absence of dispersion, this equation reduces to the definition of the phase speed. Bearing in mind what the group speed represents, it is hardly surprising to find, as shown by Rayleigh [27], that it also corresponds to the speed with which the wave energy is propagated. In a medium whose group speed is always less than the phase speed, the medium is said to be *normally* dispersive. When the opposite is true, the medium said to exhibit *anomalous* dispersion. Soft tissue is anomalous, whereas bone appears to possess normal dispersion.

From the above definitions, the group speed can be expressed in terms of the phase speed by substituting (1.40) into (1.41) and evaluating the total derivative, yielding

(1.42)
$$c_g = c_c\left[1 - \frac{\omega_c}{c_c}\left(\frac{\partial c_\phi}{\partial\omega}\right)_{\omega_c}\right]^{-1},$$
(a)

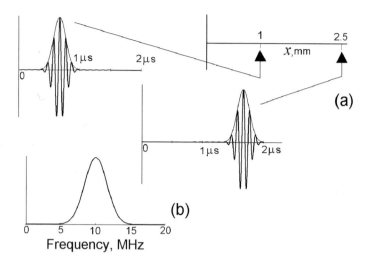

Figure 1.8 Gaussian modulated sinusoidal pulse in the absence of any dispersion and attenuation. The parameters of the pulse, whose equation is given by (1.43), are: $c_c = c_\phi = 1500$ m/s, $f_c = \omega_c/2\pi = 10$ MHz and $\sigma_\omega = 1 \times 10^7 s^{-1}$. (a) Illustrating the time domain waveform at two spatial locations as it propagates along the x-axis with the Gaussian envelopes shown as curves. (b) Normalized frequency spectrum of the pulse as calculated from the real part of (1.45).

where c_c is the phase speed at the center frequency. This equation, which is sometimes referred to as the Rayleigh formula, shows that if the phase speed increases with frequency (it usually does in ultrasound), the group speed is greater than the phase speed at the center frequency. An alternative form in terms of the wavelength λ is

(1.42)
$$c_g = c_c - \lambda \frac{dc_\phi}{d\lambda}.$$
(b)

An understanding of the group speed can be obtained considering the effect of dispersion on a plane wave pulse propagating in the x-direction. We assume that the wave consists of a Gaussian modulated sinusoidal pressure pulse that propagates without attenuation. The pulse is given by

(1.43)
$$p(x:t) = p_o e^{-\sigma_\omega^2\left(t-\frac{x}{c_\phi}\right)^2/2} \cos\left[\omega_c\left(t - \frac{x}{c_\phi}\right)\right]$$

where c_ϕ is the frequency dependent phase speed, $2\sqrt{2}/\sigma_\omega$ is approximately equal to the envelope full-width at half its maximum, ω_c is the center angular frequency, and $\sigma_\omega/(2.67f_c)$ is the −6 dB (0.5) fractional bandwidth.[19] This equation is plotted in Fig. 1.8 for the values given in the figure caption at two spatial

19. The more general equation is: Fractional Bandwidth = $\sigma_\omega 2 \sqrt{2\ln\left[10^{-r_{dB}/20}\right]}/\omega_c$, where r_{dB} is the level relative to the maximum in dB's.

locations. Moreover, a snapshot of the pulse at a given instant of time reveals its Gaussian spatial distribution.

Since the waveform can be represented by the real part of

$$(1.44) \qquad p(x{:}t) = p_o e^{-\sigma_\omega^2 \left(t - \frac{x}{c_\phi}\right)^2 / 2} e^{j\omega_c \left(t - \frac{x}{c_\phi}\right)},$$

the frequency spectrum can be found by evaluating its Fourier transform[20], i.e.,

$$\underline{p}(x{:}\omega) = p_o \int_{-\infty}^{\infty} e^{-\sigma_\omega^2 \left(t - \frac{x}{c_\phi}\right)^2 / 2} e^{j\omega_c \left(t - \frac{x}{c_\phi}\right)} e^{-j\omega t} dt$$

$$(1.45) \qquad \underline{p}(x{:}\omega) = p_o \frac{\sqrt{2\pi}}{\sigma_\omega} e^{-jx\omega/c_\phi} e^{-(\omega - \omega_c)^2 / 2\sigma_\omega^2},$$

which is also a Gaussian function. In the absence of dispersion ($c_\phi = c_o$), the frequency spectrum is unchanged as the wave progresses. If $c_\phi = c_\phi(\omega)$, then a Taylor series expansion about the center frequency ω_a can be used to express the wave number ($k_\phi = \omega/c_\phi$) as

$$\frac{\omega}{c_\phi} = \frac{\omega_c}{c_c} + (\omega - \omega_c)\left[\frac{d}{d\omega}\left(\frac{\omega}{c_\phi}\right)\right]_{\omega = \omega_c} + (\omega - \omega_c)^2 \left[\frac{d^2}{d\omega^2}\left(\frac{\omega}{c_\phi}\right)\right]_{\omega = \omega_c} \cdots$$

$$\approx \frac{\omega_c}{c_c} + \frac{(\omega - \omega_c)}{c_g} + b(\omega - \omega_c)^2,$$

where c_g is the group velocity as defined in (1.41) and $b = [d^2(\omega/c_\phi)/d\omega^2]_{\omega = \omega_c}$. By substituting this expression into (1.45), the frequency spectrum of the pulse is

$$\underline{p}(x{:}\omega) = p_o \frac{\sqrt{2\pi}}{\sigma_\omega} e^{-jx\left(\frac{\omega_c}{c_c} + \frac{\omega - \omega_c}{c_g}\right)} e^{-(\omega - \omega_c)^2 \left(\frac{1}{2\sigma_\omega^2} + jbx\right)}.$$

The time domain waveform can be obtained by taking the inverse Fourier transform of this, i.e., by evaluating, $p(x{:}t) = \frac{1}{2\pi} \int_{-\infty}^{\infty} \underline{p}(x{:}t) e^{j\omega t} d\omega$. By substituting the above expression for $\underline{p}(x{:}t)$ this integral can be written as

$$p(x{:}t) = \frac{p_o}{\sigma_\omega \sqrt{2\pi}} e^{j\omega_c \left(t - \frac{x}{c_c}\right)} \int_{-\infty}^{\infty} e^{j(\omega - \omega_c)\left(t - \frac{x}{c_g}\right)} e^{-(\omega - \omega_c)^2 \left(\frac{1}{2\sigma_\omega^2} + jbx\right)} d\omega,$$

which evaluates[20] to

---

20. See Appendix B for a summary of Fourier transforms. The integral can be evaluated with the help of the identity: $\int_{-\infty}^{\infty} \exp(Ax - Bx^2)dx = \sqrt{\pi/B}\exp(A^2/4B)$.

(1.46)
$$p(x{:}t) = \frac{p_o}{\sqrt{1+2jbx\sigma_\omega^2}}\, e^{j\omega_c\left(t-\frac{x}{c_c}\right)} e^{-\sigma_\omega^2\left(t-\frac{x}{c_g}\right)^2 \frac{1}{2}\left(\frac{1-jbx\sigma_\omega^2}{1+b^2x^2\sigma_\omega^4}\right)}.$$

If the wave number ($k_\phi = \omega/c_\phi$) varies *linearly* with frequency, i.e., $b = 0$, this reduces to

(1.47)
$$p(x{:}t) = p_o e^{j\omega_c\left(t-\frac{x}{c_c}\right)} e^{-\sigma_\omega^2\left(t-\frac{x}{c_g}\right)^2/2},$$

which has the same form as (1.44). For the case of $b = 0$, it can be seen from Fig. 1.9a that the Gaussian envelope moves at the group speed $c_g = 1{,}510$ m/s (assuming $c_g > c_c$) and, because the pulse width is determined by σ_ω, it retains the same shape as it propagates in the medium. But for $c_c \neq c_g$, the waveform (as opposed to the envelope) seen at various locations will differ.

On the other hand, if the wave number varies *nonlinearly* with frequency and $b \neq 0$, the real part of (1.46) must be evaluated to obtain the waveform. Examination of this expression shows that the pulse width increases with distance from the origin. It is caused by the differing phase speeds of the various frequency components so that they arrive at a specific x-location with differing phases from that at another location. The stretching of the original pulse shape caused by the effects of this form of dispersion can be seen in Fig. 1.9b.

As discussed in section 1.8 and more completely in section 3.9, absorption and dispersion are intimately connected: in the absence of any absorption,

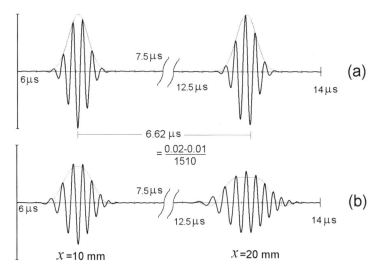

Figure 1.9 Effects of dispersion on a Gaussian modulated sinusoid: $f_c = \omega_c/2\pi = 10$ MHz, $\sigma_\omega = 1 \times 10^7$ s^{-1}, $c_g = 1510$ m/s, $c_c = 1500$ m/s. The waveform and envelope are shown for two spatial locations. (a) Calculated from (1.47) for no shape distortion, $b = 0$; (b) calculated from (1.46) for $b = 8 \times 10^{-13}$.

there should be no dispersion. At frequencies in the MHz region and below, the absorption of pure water is very small, and as a result the dispersion is either zero or too small to be of practical significance. On the other hand, over the diagnostic frequency range, the attenuation of soft tissue is considerably higher, and the increased effects of dispersion may have to be taken into account in predicting the propagation of wide-band pulses. For some media (Table 1.2) the phase speed depends logarithmically on frequency f, i.e., $c_p = c_{po} + k\ln(f)$, where k and c_{po} are constants, so that the change in speed with frequency is given by $dc_p/df = k/f$. It will also be noted in Table 1.2 that for bone, whose the attenuation can be an order of magnitude higher than that for soft tissue, the phase speed can decrease with increasing frequency. For example, Wear [28] reported that phase speed measurements on 24 human calcanei (heelbones) showed a decrease in speed as the frequency was increased from 0.2 to 0.7 MHz, with an average decrease of 9 m/s over this range.

1.4.2 Longitudinal Wave Speed in Fluids and Gases

Plane Waves in an Inviscid Fluid

For an inviscid medium, the velocity potential is given by solutions to the wave equation

(1.48a)
$$\nabla^2\phi - \kappa\rho_o\frac{\partial^2\phi}{\partial t^2} = 0$$

subject to the proper initial and boundary conditions.

In Cartesian coordinates and in the absence of losses, a plane longitudinal wave propagating in the direction of the unit vector $\tilde{\mathbf{k}}$ in an infinite medium and having an arbitrary time dependence can be written in the functional form

Table 1.2. Dispersion of Ultrasound Speed in Various Biological Media

Medium	$c_p(f)$, m/s	dc_p/df (m/s)/Hz	Freq. Range	Comments & Reference
Bone, human calcaneus	$= 1522 - 18 \times 10^{-6}f$	-18×10^{-6}	0.2–0.7 MHz	Average change measured on 24 autopsy samples [28]
Human hemoglobin	$= 1523.83 + 0.4013\ln(f)$	$= 0.4013/f$	0.3–10 MHz	Aqueous solution, 16.5 g/100 mL, measured 15°C [29]
Fresh canine lung tissue	644 @ 1 MHz 1472 @ 7 MHz	$= 138 \times 10^{-6}$	1–7 MHz	~60% air, 35°C: values given for specimen with $\rho_o = 0.4$ g/cm³ [30]

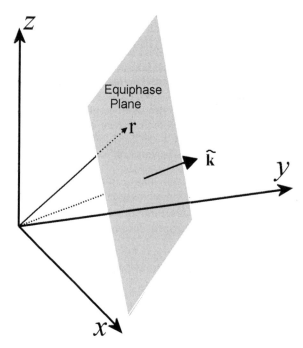

Figure 1.10 The wavefront for a plane wave is shown as it progresses in the direction of the unit vector $\hat{\mathbf{k}}$, which is normal to the surface. The distance of the surface from the origin is $\tilde{\mathbf{k}} \cdot \mathbf{r}$, where $\mathbf{r}$ is any point on the surface.

(1.49)
$$\phi(\mathbf{r}{:}t) = \phi(c_o t - \tilde{\mathbf{k}} \cdot \mathbf{r}),$$
(a)

where $\mathbf{r}$ is a position vector from the origin to any point. In addition, it can be readily verified[21] that c_o is the small-signal propagation speed. Now $\tilde{\mathbf{k}} \cdot \mathbf{r} =$ constant is the equation of a plane, i.e., all values of $\mathbf{r}$ that satisfy this equation must lie on this plane (Fig. 1.10). Consequently, a constant value for $\tilde{\mathbf{k}} \cdot \mathbf{r}$ in (1.49a), describes a planar surface upon which the velocity potential is constant at any fixed time. For the particular case of a simple harmonic wave, (1.49a) can be written in the complex form

(1.49)
$$\phi(\mathbf{r}{:}t) = \phi_o e^{jk(c_o t - \tilde{\mathbf{k}} \cdot \mathbf{r})},$$
(b)

where $k = \omega/c_o$.

By substituting (1.49a) into (1.48a), it can be shown [31, pp. 65–66] that this is a solution of the homogeneous wave equation and that the propagation speed is given by

(1.3)
$$\boxed{c_o = 1/\sqrt{\kappa\rho_o}},$$

---

21. The velocity potential will have the same value at a subsequent time $t + \Delta t$ if $c_o(t + \Delta t) - \tilde{\mathbf{k}} \cdot (\mathbf{r} + \Delta\mathbf{r}) = c_o t - \tilde{\mathbf{k}} \cdot \mathbf{r}$, i.e., if $c_o = \tilde{\mathbf{k}} \cdot \Delta\mathbf{r}/\Delta t$. But $\tilde{\mathbf{k}} \cdot \Delta\mathbf{r}$ is simply the distance moved by the wavefront in a time of Δt, and therefore c_o is the speed of propagation.

as previously noted. Consequently, (1.48a) can be written as

(1.48b)
$$\nabla^2\phi - \frac{1}{c_o^2}\frac{\partial^2\phi}{\partial t^2} = 0.$$

In Cartesian coordinates the 1-D form of this wave equation is

(1.50)
$$\frac{\partial^2\phi}{\partial x^2} - \frac{1}{c_o^2}\frac{\partial^2\phi}{\partial t^2} = 0,$$

whose solution for an arbitrary time dependence can be expressed as

(1.51)
$$\phi(x:t) = \phi_1(c_o t - x) + \phi_2(c_o t + x),$$

where the arbitrary functions ϕ_1 and ϕ_2 represent plane waves in the positive and negative x-directions, respectively. For example, the function ϕ_1 could consist of a pulse such as: $F_1(c_o t - x) = \mathcal{H}(c_o t - x)\mathcal{H}(c_o t - c_o\tau - x)$ where $\mathcal{H}$ is a Heaviside function[22] and τ is the pulse duration. To show that (1.50) is satisfied by both ϕ_1 and ϕ_2, we proceed as follows.

Suppose that only the positive going wave $\phi^+(x:t) = \phi_1(c_o t - x)$ is considered. Differentiating, first with respect to t and then with respect to x, yields

(1.52)
$$\frac{\partial\phi^+}{\partial t} = c_o\phi_1'(c_o t - x) \qquad \frac{\partial\phi^+}{\partial x} = -\phi_1'(c_o t - x),$$

where the prime indicates the derivative with respect to the argument. Eliminating ϕ_1' between these two equations yields the *reduced wave equation* given by

(1.53)
$$\frac{\partial\phi^+}{\partial t} = -c_o\frac{\partial\phi^+}{\partial x}.$$

Similarly, for the negative going wave, $\phi^-(x,t) = \phi_2(c_o t + x)$ the reduced wave equation

(1.54)
$$\frac{\partial\phi^-}{\partial t} = -c_o\frac{\partial\phi^-}{\partial x},$$

is obtained.[23] If both of the equations in (1.52) are again differentiated and the function is eliminated, (1.50) is obtained. Similarly, (1.50) is obtained if the same procedure is conducted for the negative going wave, i.e., both ϕ_1 and ϕ_2 satisfy the wave equation, as do the sum of these functions. But when just a unidirectional plane wave is considered, either of the reduced wave equations, (1.53) or (1.54), would suffice.

---

22. Defined by: $\mathcal{H}(t) = 1$ for $t > 0$, $\mathcal{H}(0) = 1/2$, and $\mathcal{H}(t) = 0$ for $t < 0$.

23. A much simpler way of obtaining the reduced equations is to re-write (1.50) in the operator form: $\left(\dfrac{\partial}{\partial t} - c_o\dfrac{\partial}{\partial x}\right)\left(\dfrac{\partial}{\partial t} + c_o\dfrac{\partial}{\partial x}\right)\phi = 0.$ Since either of the operator terms in parenthesis can be zero, (1.53) and (1.54) are obtained.

Harmonic Waves in a Viscous Fluid

If we consider a harmonic wave such that the velocity potential is given by

$$(1.55) \qquad \phi(\mathbf{r}{:}t) = \Phi(\mathbf{r}{:}\omega)e^{j\omega t},$$

then substitution into the wave equation for a viscous fluid (1.38) leads to the Helmholtz equation

$$(1.56) \qquad \boxed{\nabla^2 \Phi + \underline{k}^2 \Phi = 0}$$

where $\underline{k} = k / \sqrt{1 + j\omega\kappa(\mu_B + \frac{4}{3}\mu)}$ is a complex wave number in which $k = \omega/c_o$ is the wave number and $c_o = 1/\sqrt{\kappa\rho_o}$. If the harmonic wave propagates in a medium whose viscous loss is relatively small, the complex wave number can be expanded in a binomial and written as

$$\underline{k} \approx k\left[1 - \frac{j\omega\kappa}{2}\left(\mu_B + \frac{4}{3}\mu\right)\right] = k - j\alpha,$$

where $\alpha = \dfrac{\omega^2}{2\rho_o c_o^3}\left(\mu_B + \dfrac{4}{3}\mu\right)$ is the *amplitude attenuation coefficient* (see section 1.8 and subsection 3.10.5). If a sinusoidal source exists on the plane $x = 0$, a plane harmonic wave will be propagated in the positive and negative x-directions. For the positive x-wave the approximate steady-state velocity potential can be expressed as

$$\phi(x{:}t) = \phi_o e^{-\alpha x}\cos(\omega t - kx),$$

which describes an attenuated plane harmonic wave.

The pressure can be readily related to the velocity potential. By substituting $\nabla \cdot \mathbf{v} = -\nabla \cdot \nabla\phi$ and (1.55) into (1.31), we obtain $\kappa\dfrac{\partial p}{\partial t} = \nabla^2 \Phi e^{j\omega t}$ which, with the help of (1.56), yields $\kappa\dfrac{\partial p}{\partial t} = -\underline{k}^2 \Phi e^{j\omega t}$. But since p is also sinusoidal and can be written as $p = \underline{p}e^{j\omega t}$, where $\underline{p}$ is the pressure phasor, it follows that

$$(1.57) \qquad \underline{p} = j\underline{k}^2 \Phi \big/ (\omega\kappa).$$

It follows that in the absence of viscous loss, the pressure is exactly 90 degrees out of phase with the velocity potential, a relationship that is true for plane, spherical, and cylindrical waves.

By taking the gradient of (1.57) and noting the definition of the velocity potential, the particle velocity phasor can be expressed as

$$(1.58) \qquad \underline{\mathbf{v}} = j\omega\kappa\underline{p}\big/\underline{k}^2.$$

Both of the prior two equations demonstrate that the phase differences between p, $\mathbf{v}$, and ϕ depend on the viscous loss through the complex wave number $\underline{k}$. For spherical and cylindrical waves, in contrast to plane waves, the phase differences between p and $\mathbf{v}$ is position-dependent.

For an inviscid fluid medium, the relation between the particle velocity and pressure for a plane wave takes on a very simple form. If the pressure phasor is given by $\underline{p}(x{:}\omega) = p_o e^{-jkx}$, the velocity phasor can be found by substituting into (1.58), noting that $\underline{k} = k$ and that $c_o^2 = 1/(\kappa\rho_o)$, yielding

$$(1.59) \qquad\qquad \mathbf{v} = \tilde{\mathbf{x}}\underline{p}/(c_o\rho_o)$$

for a plane wave traveling in the x-direction. Consequently, for an inviscid medium the pressure and velocity are in phase.

Plane, Spherical, and Cylindrical Harmonic Waves in an Inviscid Fluid

In Cartesian coordinates the Helmholtz equation for an inviscid fluid is

$$(1.60) \qquad\qquad \frac{\partial^2\Phi}{\partial x^2} + \frac{\partial^2\Phi}{\partial y^2} + \frac{\partial^2\Phi}{\partial z^2} + k^2\Phi = 0.$$

A solution is $\Phi = \phi_o e^{-jkx}$, where ϕ_o is the velocity potential amplitude. Consequently, a solution to the wave equation is $\Phi = \phi_o e^{-jkx}$, which describes a plane harmonic wave traveling in the x-direction. Expressions for the pressure and velocity can be obtained from (1.39), the density from (1.31), and the particle displacement from $\partial\xi/\partial x = v_x$. Table 1.3 shows the various expressions expressed in real form.

In *spherical* coordinates (r,θ,φ), the Helmholtz equation is

$$(1.61) \quad \frac{1}{r^2}\frac{\partial}{\partial r}\left(r^2\frac{\partial\Phi}{\partial r}\right) + \frac{1}{r^2\sin\theta}\frac{\partial}{\partial\theta}\left(\sin\theta\frac{\partial\Phi}{\partial\theta}\right) + \frac{1}{r^2\sin^2\theta}\frac{\partial^2\Phi}{\partial\varphi^2} + k^2\Phi(r,\theta,\varphi{:}\omega)$$
$$= 0$$

If the wave is spherically symmetrical, i.e., $\Phi = \Phi(r)$, then (1.61) reduces to

$$(1.62) \qquad\qquad \frac{\partial^2\Phi}{\partial r^2} + \frac{2}{r}\frac{\partial\Phi}{\partial r} + k^2\Phi(r{:}\omega) = 0.$$

The simplest solution corresponds to a spherical wave traveling in the positive r-direction and is given by $\Phi = \dfrac{\phi_o'}{r}e^{-jkr}$, or $\phi = \dfrac{\phi_o'}{r}e^{j(\omega t - kr)}$. A sphere whose surface is vibrating sinusoidally in the radial direction can produce such a wave. Listed in Table 1.3 are the real parts of the velocity potential, together with expressions for the other quantities derived from it.

Finally, in *cylindrical* coordinates (r, θ, z), the Helmholtz equation is

$$(1.63) \qquad \frac{1}{r}\frac{\partial}{\partial r}\left(r\frac{\partial\Phi}{\partial r}\right) + \frac{1}{r^2}\frac{\partial^2\Phi}{\partial\theta^2} + \frac{\partial^2\Phi}{\partial z^2} + k^2\Phi(r,\theta,z{:}\omega) = 0.$$

Here again we shall assume that the wave is cylindrically symmetrical, i.e., $\Phi = \Phi(r)$, which enables (1.63) to be reduced to

$$(1.64) \qquad\qquad \frac{\partial^2\Phi}{\partial r^2} + \frac{1}{r}\frac{\partial\Phi}{\partial r} + k^2\Phi(r{:}\omega) = 0.$$

Table 1.3. Wave Quantities for 1-D Propagation in an Inviscid Fluid*

Quantity	Plane Wave	Spherical Wave	Cylindrical Wave (for $kr > 1$)
Velocity potential, ϕ	$\phi = \phi_o \cos(\omega t - kx)$	$\phi = \dfrac{\phi'_o}{r}\cos(\omega t - kr)$	$\phi \approx \dfrac{\phi''_o}{\sqrt{r}}\cos(\omega t - kr)$
Particle velocity, v	$v = k\phi_o \cos\left(\omega t - kx + \dfrac{\pi}{2}\right)$	$v = \dfrac{k\phi'_o}{r}\sqrt{1+(kr)^{-2}} \times \cos\left(\omega t - kr - \psi + \dfrac{\pi}{2}\right)$	$v = \dfrac{k\phi''_o}{\sqrt{r}}\sqrt{1+(2kr)^{-2}} \times \cos\left(\omega t - kr - \psi + \dfrac{\pi}{2}\right)$
Pressure, p	$p = kZ_o\phi_o \cos\left(\omega t - kx + \dfrac{\pi}{2}\right)$	$p = \dfrac{k\phi'_o Z_o}{r}\cos\left(\omega t - kx + \dfrac{\pi}{2}\right)$	$p \approx \dfrac{k\phi''_o Z_o}{\sqrt{r}}\cos\left(\omega t - kx + \dfrac{\pi}{2}\right)$
Density change, $\Delta\rho = \rho - \rho_o$	$\Delta\rho = \dfrac{k\rho_o\phi_o}{c_o}\cos\left(\omega t - kx + \dfrac{\pi}{2}\right)$	$\Delta\rho = \dfrac{k\rho_o\phi'_o}{c_o r}\cos\left(\omega t - kx + \dfrac{\pi}{2}\right)$	$\Delta\rho \approx \dfrac{k\rho_o\phi''_o}{c_o\sqrt{r}}\cos\left(\omega t - kx + \dfrac{\pi}{2}\right)$
Displacement, ξ	$\xi = \dfrac{\phi_o}{c_o}\cos(\omega t - kx)$	$\xi = \dfrac{\phi'_o}{c_o r}\sqrt{1+(kr)^{-2}} \times \cos(\omega t - kr - \psi)$	$\xi \approx \dfrac{\phi''_o}{c_o\sqrt{r}}\sqrt{1+(2kr)^{-2}} \times \cos(\omega t - kr - \psi)$
Specific acoustic impedance, $\underline{Z}$	$\underline{Z} = Z_o = \rho_o c_o$	$\underline{Z} = Z_o\dfrac{1+j/(kr)}{1+(kr)^{-2}}$	$\underline{Z} \approx Z_o\dfrac{1+j/(2kr)}{1+(2kr)^{-2}}$
Phase angle between p & v	$\psi = 0$	$\psi = \cot^{-1}(kr)$	$\psi \approx \cot^{-1}(2kr)$

*Based on a table given by Malecki [18].

34

It can be shown [6, pp. 356–357] that a solution to this equation for an outgoing wave of the lowest order is given by

$$\Phi(r{:}\omega) = \Phi_o[J_0(kr) - j\mathcal{N}_0(kr)]$$

where $J_0(.)$ is a cylindrical Bessel function of order zero, $\mathcal{N}_0(.)$ is a Neumann function of order zero, and Φ_o is a constant. As $kr \to 0$, $\mathcal{N}_0(kr) \to -\infty$ and $J_0(kr) \to 1$. On the other hand, it can also be shown [6] that if $kr > 1$, i.e., $r > \lambda/2\pi$, then a good approximation[24] to this equation is $\Phi \approx \sqrt{2/(\pi kr)}e^{-jkr}$, which enables the outgoing wave time-dependent velocity potential to be written as

$$\phi \approx \frac{\phi_o''}{\sqrt{r}}e^{j(\omega t - kr)},$$

where $\phi_o'' = \sqrt{2/(\pi k)}$. Such a wave can be produced by an infinitely long cylindrical shell whose surface is vibrating harmonically. Using this expression, the other related quantities can be readily obtained; these are also listed in Table 1.3.

Longitudinal Wave Speeds in Biological Media

Knowledge of the propagation speed in biological media is of considerable practical importance. A variety of methods are available for measuring samples, and these have been described and critically reviewed by Bamber [32]. Biological specimens are frequently far from ideal in terms of their shape, and achieving a good accuracy can require considerable care. One of the simplest techniques is the substitution method, based on observing the change in transit time of a short ultrasound pulse when the specimen is removed from the propagation path and is replaced by a fluid whose speed is known. Because the speed in pure water as a function of temperature has been accurately determined (see Fig. 1.5), it is often used as a reference.

Summaries of the results reported in the literature have been published from time to time [32,35–37]. These indicate that a relatively wide range of values can be obtained due to variations resulting from differences in preparation, differing mammals, temperature, and other factors. The results summarized in Fig. 1.11 clearly show this variability and also that the range of speeds for soft tissue is relatively narrow.

Speed measurements on extracted tissue samples could differ significantly from in vivo measurements [33]. Estimating the in vivo speed with sufficient accuracy so that the data could be used diagnostically is a much more difficult challenge. Such information could be of value for enabling corrections to be made for the distortions that arise from the inhomogeneous nature of the media as well as the possibility that the small differences in speed could enable tissue abnormalities to be detected. Work toward this end has been reviewed [33] and recent studies [34] using pulse-echo systems have indicated that

---

24. For $kr = 1$ the error is 3.6%: as kr increases the error rapidly reduces.

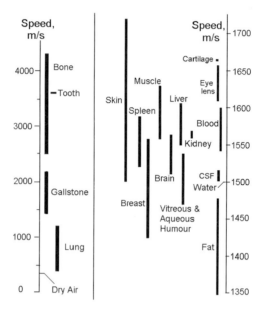

Figure 1.11 Summary of speed of sound measurements in various biological media generally made in the temperature range 20 to 37°C and over the frequency range 1 to 10 MHz. The original sources from which the data were obtained are given in [32]. (Reproduced, with permission, from Bamber, Ch. 5, in *Physical Principles of Medical Ultrasonics*, © 2004 John Wiley & Sons Limited.)

measurements could be achieved with an accuracy of around 0.5%, corresponding to an uncertainty in speed of approximately 7.5 m/s.

1.4.3 Compressional and Shear Wave Propagation in Solids [38,39]

Unbounded Propagation in Isotropic Solids

In describing wave propagation in an inviscid liquid, just a single elastic modulus was needed: the compressibility. For isotropic solids, shear stresses will be present that cause a deformation in shape, making the analysis rather more complex. It can be shown that for such a solid, the effects of these shear stresses on wave propagation can be accounted for by one additional elastic modulus. A much more complex situation arises with propagation in cancellous bone, whose network of bony plates and columns are filled with fat, bone marrow, and blood. In addition to a shear wave, two compressional components can exist: a fast wave associated with propagation in which the soft medium and rigid structures move in phase and a slow wave in which they are out of phase. Analysis [40] of propagation in cancellous bone is often based on a theory originally developed by Biot [41,42] in 1956 for predicting propagation in fluid-saturated porous rocks. Because of the complexities of this analysis we shall restrict our discussion to propagation in homogeneous isotropic solids.

Traditionally, the analysis of wave propagation in solids is generally conducted by introducing two elastic constants called the Lamé coefficients whose MKS units are Pascals. The *first Lamé constant* will be denoted by λ_ℓ, and the second by μ_ℓ. The latter is the coefficient (or modulus) of rigidity, often called the *shear modulus*, as defined in (1.12). An alternative pair of elastic constants is Young's modulus E and Poisson's ratio σ, as in (1.6) and (1.7), respectively. These are related to the Lamé constants by

(1.65) $$E = 2\mu_\ell(1+\sigma), \text{ and } 2\sigma = \lambda_\ell/(\lambda_\ell+\mu_\ell) \text{ for } \sigma \le 1/2.$$ (a)

Note that for a liquid, $\mu_\ell \to 0$, while for a perfectly rigid solid, $\mu_\ell \to \infty$. A further alternative pair of constants is Poisson's ratio σ and the compressibility κ (either the adiabatic or isothermal), and these are related to the Lamé constants [38]

(1.65) $$\kappa = 1/(\lambda_\ell + 2\mu_\ell/3), \text{ and } 2\sigma = \lambda_\ell/(\lambda_\ell+\mu_\ell) \text{ for } \sigma \le 1/2.$$ (b)

In terms of the Lamé coefficients, it can be shown that for an isotropic solid the equation describing the time and spatial variation of the particle displacement is given by

(1.66) $$\rho_o \frac{\partial^2 \xi}{\partial t^2} = \left(\mu_\ell + \mu\frac{\partial}{\partial t}\right)\nabla^2\xi + \left(\lambda_\ell + \mu_\ell + (\mu_B + \mu/3)\frac{\partial}{\partial t}\right)\nabla(\nabla \cdot \xi),$$ (a)

in which $\xi(\mathbf{r}{:}t)$ is the particle displacement vector and μ and μ_B are the shear and bulk viscosity coefficients (MKS units of Pa.s). In the absence of viscous loss this simplifies to

(1.66) $$\rho_o \frac{\partial^2 \xi}{\partial t^2} = \mu_\ell \nabla^2\xi + (\lambda_\ell + \mu_\ell)\nabla(\nabla \cdot \xi)$$ (b)

If this is written out in full for each of the three Cartesian components of the displacement vector ξ, we obtain

$$\rho_o \frac{\partial^2 \xi_x}{\partial t^2} = \mu_\ell\left\{\frac{\partial^2 \xi_x}{\partial x^2} + \frac{\partial^2 \xi_x}{\partial y^2} + \frac{\partial^2 \xi_x}{\partial z^2}\right\} + (\lambda_\ell+\mu_\ell)\left\{\frac{\partial^2 \xi_x}{\partial x^2} + \frac{\partial^2 \xi_y}{\partial x\partial y} + \frac{\partial^2 \xi_z}{\partial x\partial z}\right\}$$

$$\rho_o \frac{\partial^2 \xi_y}{\partial t^2} = \mu_\ell\left\{\frac{\partial^2 \xi_y}{\partial x^2} + \frac{\partial^2 \xi_y}{\partial y^2} + \frac{\partial^2 \xi_y}{\partial z^2}\right\} + (\lambda_\ell+\mu_\ell)\left\{\frac{\partial^2 \xi_x}{\partial y\partial x} + \frac{\partial^2 \xi_y}{\partial y^2} + \frac{\partial^2 \xi_z}{\partial y\partial z}\right\}$$

$$\rho_o \frac{\partial^2 \xi_z}{\partial t^2} = \mu_\ell\left\{\frac{\partial^2 \xi_z}{\partial x^2} + \frac{\partial^2 \xi_z}{\partial y^2} + \frac{\partial^2 \xi_z}{\partial z^2}\right\} + (\lambda_\ell+\mu_\ell)\left\{\frac{\partial^2 \xi_x}{\partial z\partial x} + \frac{\partial^2 \xi_y}{\partial z\partial y} + \frac{\partial^2 \xi_z}{\partial z^2}\right\}.$$

In the case of plane waves traveling in the z-direction, all the partial derivatives with respect to x and y vanish, leaving

$$\rho_o \frac{\partial^2 \xi_x}{\partial t^2} = \mu_\ell \frac{\partial^2 \xi_x}{\partial z^2}, \qquad \rho_o \frac{\partial^2 \xi_y}{\partial t^2} = \mu_\ell \frac{\partial^2 \xi_y}{\partial z^2}, \qquad \rho_o \frac{\partial^2 \xi_z}{\partial t^2} = (\lambda_\ell + 2\mu_\ell)\frac{\partial^2 \xi_z}{\partial z^2}.$$

The first two equations describe displacements at right angles to the propagation direction and correspond to two polarized transverse waves with propagation speeds of $c_T = \sqrt{\mu_\ell/\rho_o}$. The third equation describes a longitudinal wave with a speed of $c_L = \sqrt{(\lambda_\ell + 2\mu_\ell)/\rho_o}$.

An equation for the particle velocity vector $\mathbf{v}$ can be found by first differentiating (1.66a) with respect to time, substituting $\mathbf{v} = \partial\xi/\partial t$, and then using a standard vector relation.[14] These steps yield

(1.67)
$$\rho_o \frac{\partial^2 \mathbf{v}}{\partial t^2} =$$
$$\left[(\lambda_\ell + 2\mu_\ell) + \left(\mu_B + \frac{4}{3}\mu \right)\frac{\partial}{\partial t} \right]\nabla^2 \mathbf{v} + \left[(\lambda_\ell + \mu_\ell) + \left(\mu_B + \frac{1}{3}\mu \right)\frac{\partial}{\partial t} \right]\nabla \times \nabla \times \mathbf{v}.$$

The same procedure can now be used for transforming the linearized Navier-Stokes equation into two independent equations (see (1.33) and (1.34)). Because the velocity vector can be written as $\mathbf{v} = \mathbf{v_L} + \mathbf{v_T}$, in which $\nabla \times \mathbf{v_L} = 0$ and $\nabla \cdot \mathbf{v_T} = 0$, it can be readily be shown that (1.67) can be expressed as

(1.68)
$$\rho_o \frac{\partial^2 \mathbf{v_L}}{\partial t^2} = (\lambda_\ell + 2\mu_\ell)\nabla^2 \mathbf{v_L} + \left(\mu_B + \frac{4}{3}\mu \right)\frac{\partial}{\partial t}(\nabla^2 \mathbf{v_L})$$
(a)

(1.68)
$$\rho_o \frac{\partial^2 \mathbf{v_L}}{\partial t^2} = \mu_\ell \nabla^2 \mathbf{v_L} - \mu \frac{\partial}{\partial t}(\nabla^2 \mathbf{v_T}).$$
(b)

These two independent equations[25] describe the propagation of longitudinal and transverse (shear) waves in an isotropic viscous solid. For an inviscid medium these reduce to

(1.69)
$$\frac{\partial^2 \mathbf{v_L}}{\partial t^2} = c_L^2 \nabla^2 \mathbf{v_L} \quad \text{and} \quad \frac{\partial^2 \mathbf{v_T}}{\partial t^2} = c_T^2 \nabla^2 \mathbf{v_T},$$

in which the propagation speeds are

$$c_L = \sqrt{(\lambda_\ell + 2\mu_\ell)/\rho_o} \quad \text{and} \quad c_T = \sqrt{\mu_\ell/\rho_o}.$$

With the help of (1.65) the speeds can also be expressed in terms of Young's modulus and Poisson's ratio:

(1.70) $\quad c_L = \sqrt{(\lambda_\ell + 2\mu_\ell)/\rho_o} = \sqrt{\dfrac{E(1-\sigma)}{\rho_o(1-2\sigma)(1+\sigma)}} \quad \text{and} \quad c_T = \sqrt{\dfrac{\mu_\ell}{\rho_o}} = \sqrt{\dfrac{E}{2\rho_o(1+\sigma)}},$

so that the ratio of the two speeds can be written as

(1.71)
$$\frac{c_T}{c_L} = \sqrt{\frac{0.5-\sigma}{1-\sigma}}.$$

Fig. 1.12 shows how the ratio c_T/c_L varies with σ. For many solids Poisson's ratio is roughly $\sigma \sim 0.33$, and consequently $c_L/c_T \sim 2$, i.e., the shear wave speed

25. It should be noted that for a liquid, $\mu_\ell = 0$, so that $\kappa = 1/\lambda_\ell$ and as a result (1.68a) and (1.68b) reduce to (1.35) and (1.34b) respectively.

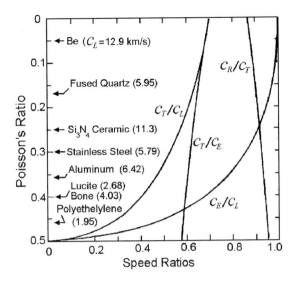

Figure 1.12 Propagation speed ratios shown as a function of Poisson's ratio. Values for typical solid materials are given with the longitudinal speed, in km/s, in parentheses. Subscript notation used: $R \equiv$ Rayleigh, $L \equiv$ Longitudinal, $T \equiv$ Transverse (shear), $E \equiv$ Extensional. Based on a similar figure by Kino [16].

is approximately half the compression wave speed. On the other hand, soft biological tissues can be considered to behave as a viscoelastic medium with a shear modulus (μ_ℓ) that is typically five or so orders of magnitude smaller than the bulk modulus ($1/\kappa$). As a result, Poisson's ratio approaches 0.5, so that from (1.65a) Young's modulus, $E \approx 3\mu_\ell$ and from (1.71) $c_L \gg c_T$. Whereas longitudinal speeds may be around 1500 m/s, the shear propagation speed may be in the order of a few meters per second. Thus, at frequencies in the MHz range the shear wavelengths are in the order of tens of microns, but at much lower frequencies (e.g., 100 Hz), they approach the dimensions of tissue organs. This is important in elastography, where shear wave propagation can be used to probe the characteristics of tissue (see subsection 8.8.3).

Propagation in a Bounded Solid Isotropic Medium:
Rayleigh Waves

If we consider a semi-infinite solid medium, three conditions exist for the medium on the other side of the boundary: (i) vacuum, (ii) liquid, or (iii) a different solid. The boundary conditions that must be satisfied for each case are (i) for a vacuum (free surface condition), all stresses at the interface must vanish; (ii) for a liquid–solid interface, the fluid pressure (stress) must be equal to the normal component of the stress just within the solid, the tangential stress in the solid must vanish, and the normal component of the velocity must be continuous; (iii) for another solid, all stress and velocity components on the boundary must be continuous.

For case (i), in which a vacuum (or a gas) exists above a solid surface, Rayleigh waves can be generated through the interaction of shear and longitudinal waves at the common boundary. Specifically, it can be shown that the solution of (1.69), with the condition that all stress components must vanish on the boundary, results in a secular equation for the speed c_R given by [5,44]

$$(1.72) \quad \left(\frac{c_R}{c_T}\right)^6 - 8\left(\frac{c_R}{c_T}\right)^4 + 8\left(\frac{c_R}{c_T}\right)^2\left[3 - 2\left(\frac{c_T}{c_L}\right)^2\right] - 16\left[1 - 2\left(\frac{c_T}{c_L}\right)^2\right] = 0.$$

It can be shown that there is only one real root, corresponding to the Rayleigh wave velocity, and for the range of Poisson's ratio from $0 < \sigma < 0.5$, this satisfies the condition $0.8743 < c_R/c_T < 0.9554$ (see Fig. 1.12). Such a wave consists of longitudinal and transverse waves that are coupled by the common boundary. If the solid extends from the plane $y = 0$ to $y = \infty$, and a Rayleigh wave propagates in the x-direction, then the particle displacement will have components in the x- and z-directions, corresponding to the longitudinal and transverse components. As a result the net particle motion is an ellipse and the displacement amplitudes of the two components decay with depth from the interface and their amplitudes become quite small at a depth of 1 (Rayleigh) wavelength λ_R. This behavior is illustrated in Fig. 1.13, where it can be seen that the direction of polarization reverses at about $0.2\lambda_R$.

A more complex situation exists if the medium above the solid is a liquid [44]. A pure surface wave (*Stoneley wave*) can always exist, and in addition, depending on the properties of the media, a complex *"leaky" Rayleigh wave* may also be present [45].

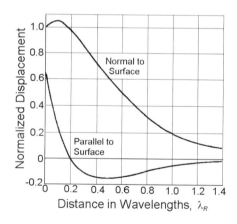

Figure 1.13 Particle displacement components parallel to and normal to a solid–gas interface as a function of the distance from the interface expressed in terms of the Rayleigh wavelength λ_R. Based on a similar figure by Dransfield and Salzmann [43].

Extensional Wave Propagation in a Thin Isotropic Semi-Infinite Rod

In considering acoustic wave propagation along a semi-infinitely long rod or wire, in general it is necessary to account for the presence of both shear and longitudinal components, which will be coupled through their interaction on the boundary. If the diameter is small compared to a wavelength, shear waves can be neglected. This situation corresponds to the thin waveguide [5, pp. 39 & 46; 18, pp. 427–430] approximation and, as previously noted, the wave is sometimes referred to as an *extensional wave* [16, pp. 14 & 89]. For this type of wave there will be no stress component perpendicular to the axis, just an axial component. Propagation of this wave causes changes in the wire diameter, which should be contrasted with the case of a plane wave in an infinite medium where no such changes are present. This suggests that the appropriate elastic constant is Young's modulus, so that the speed of propagation is given by

$$(1.8) \qquad c_E = \left(E/\rho \right)^{1/2},$$

which is less than the longitudinal speed c_L as given by (1.70). From (1.70) and (1.65) the ratio is given by:

$$(1.73) \qquad \frac{c_E}{c_L} = \left[\frac{(1+\sigma)(1-2\sigma)}{(1-\sigma)} \right]^{1/2},$$

from which it follows that for $0.5 > \sigma > 0$, (c_E/c_L) lies between 0 and 1. In addition, the ratio of the transverse to the extension speed can be found from (1.73) and (1.71) as

$$(1.74) \qquad \frac{c_T}{c_E} = \left[\frac{0.5-\sigma}{(1+\sigma)(1-2\sigma)} \right]^{1/2}.$$

Both (1.73) and (1.74) are plotted in Fig. 1.12.

1.5 Impedance, Energy Density, Intensity and Radiation Pressure

1.5.1 Specific Acoustic Impedance, Characteristic Impedance, and Acoustic Impedance

The concept of impedance is particularly valuable in characterizing wave propagation in the presence of boundaries between media with differing acoustical properties. For a harmonic wave of angular frequency ω at a spatial location $\mathbf{r}$, the specific acoustic impedance can be defined by

$$(1.75) \qquad \boxed{ \underline{Z}(\mathbf{r}, \omega) = \frac{p(\mathbf{r}, \omega)}{\underline{v}(\mathbf{r}, \omega)} }, \qquad \textit{Specific Acoustic Impedance}$$

where $\underline{p}(\omega)$ is the pressure phasor and $\underline{v}(\omega)$ is the particle velocity phasor. The term *specific* is used to draw attention to the fact that it involves the force per unit area rather than just the total force acting on a specified area, which is used for defining the acoustic impedance (see below). In general, the specific acoustic impedance is frequency- and position-dependent and, because the pressure and velocity can differ in phase, it is a complex quantity. The units for $\underline{Z}$ are Rayleighs (Rayl), where 1 Rayl = 1 Pa.s/m and the dimensions are $[ML^{-2}T^{-1}]$. Typical values are in the 10^6 Rayl range, i.e., in MRayl.

The simplest situation occurs with the propagation of a plane wave in an inviscid fluid medium. By substituting the pressure–velocity relation given by (1.59), into (1.75) we obtain

(1.76) $$\boxed{\underline{Z} = Z_o = \rho_o c_o}, \quad \textit{Characteristic (Acoustic) Impedance}$$

where Z_o is known as the characteristic (acoustic) impedance of the medium. The term characteristic is used because Z_o is the vital characteristic of the medium. In a viscous medium, it follows from (1.58) that there will be a phase difference between the pressure and velocity vector, and as a result $\underline{Z}$ is complex and $\underline{Z} \neq Z_o$. Typical values are given in Table 1.4.

Directly analogous to the electrical impedance, an acoustic impedance can be defined by

(1.77) $$\boxed{\underline{Z}_a(\mathbf{r}:\omega) = \frac{F(\mathbf{r}:\omega)}{\underline{v}(\mathbf{r}:\omega)}}, \quad \textit{Acoustic Impedance}$$

where $F(\mathbf{r}:\omega)$ is the total acoustic force acting on a specific area. The acoustic impedance has MKS units of Pa.s and dimensions of $[ML^{-1}T^{-1}]$.

For a spherical or cylindrical wave propagating in an inviscid medium, close to the origin a phase difference will exist between the pressure and velocity, and as a result the specific acoustic impedance is position-dependent. At large distances from the origin, where the wave becomes pseudo-plane, $\underline{Z} \approx Z_o$. Equations for the specific acoustic impedance for plane, spherical, and cylindrical waves are also given in Table 1.3.

1.5.2 Energy and Energy Density

Energy will be associated with wave propagation in a medium. If we consider an arbitrary volume V through which a wave is propagating, the total energy

Table 1.4. Characteristic Impedances of Selected Media

Medium	Z_o, MRayl	Medium	Z_o, MRayl
Aluminum	17.21	Dry air (1 atm)	0.000413
Steel (mild)	44.38	Water, 20°C	1.479
Tungsten	101.0	Blood, whole human 36°C, Hct = 40%	1.67
PZT-5A (ceramic)	33.7	Bone, fresh bovine phalanx	7.9

{$E(\mathbf{r}{:}t)$, Joules} of this volume will be increased due to the kinetic and potential energy of the acoustic particles within it. By determining the energy contained in a small element of volume within V, then the energy density {$\varepsilon(\mathbf{r}{:}t)$, Joules/m³} at this location can be obtained. Evidently, integrating the energy density over the entire volume V enables the total energy to be obtained. In general, both the energy density and total energy are time-dependent quantities. In what follows, a simplified approach is given for obtaining equations that describe these two quantities.

If we consider a small element of volume dV, the kinetic energy at a given instant of time t is given by

$$(1.78) \qquad \delta E_{KE} = \frac{1}{2}\rho_o |\mathbf{v}|^2 \, dV.$$

The potential energy δE_{PE}, can be determined by obtaining an expression for the work done by the pressure in changing the element of volume from its equilibrium value to the value that exists at the time t. To obtain this expression we proceed as follows.

Consider an equilibrium element of volume V_e. If the element changes to a volume $V_f = V_e + \Delta V$, then the work done to produce this change under adiabatic conditions by a pressure change from the equilibrium pressure p_o to $p_o + \Delta p$ at time t is given by $WD = \int_{V_e}^{V_e + \Delta V} p dV$. By using the definition for adiabatic compressibility as given by (1.1), this can be written as $WD = -\int_0^{\Delta p} \kappa p V dp$. For a small change in volume, $WD \approx -\kappa V \int_0^{\Delta p} p dp = -\kappa V \frac{\Delta p^2}{2}$. By applying this relation to the volume element dV, noting that Δp is the small-signal pressure p, that $\kappa = 1/(\rho_o c_o^2)$ and that $WD = -\delta E_{PE}$, we obtain

$$(1.79) \qquad \delta E_{KE} = \frac{p^2}{2\rho_o c_o^2} \, dV.$$

Consequently, the total energy stored at a given time t in the volume dV is the sum of (1.78) and (1.79), i.e.,

$$\delta E = \delta E_{KE} + \delta E_{PE} = \frac{1}{2}\left[\rho_o |\mathbf{v}|^2 + \frac{p^2}{2\rho_o c_o^2} \right] dV.$$

By integrating this over the total enclosed volume, the total instantaneous energy is given by

$$(1.80) \qquad E(t) = \iiint_V \frac{1}{2}\left[\rho_o |\mathbf{v}|^2 + \frac{p^2}{\rho_o c_o^2} \right] dV.$$

From this it can be seen that the instantaneous energy density $\varepsilon(\mathbf{r}{:}t)$ is

$$(1.81) \qquad \varepsilon(\mathbf{r}{:}t) = \frac{1}{2}\left[\rho_o |\mathbf{v}|^2 + \frac{p^2}{\rho_o c_o^2} \right].$$

As an example we shall consider a plane harmonic wave that is traveling in the x-direction and will obtain the *time-averaged* energy density. For a sinusoidal pressure given by $p(x{:}t) = p_o\cos(\omega t - kx)$, then $v(x{:}t) = (p_o/Z_o)\cos(\omega t - kx)$. Substituting these into (1.81) and averaging over the period $\mathcal{T}$ by using $\bar{\varepsilon} = \dfrac{1}{\mathcal{T}}\displaystyle\int_0^{\mathcal{T}} \varepsilon(x{:}t)dt$, it can be readily shown that

(1.82)
$$\bar{\varepsilon} = \bar{\varepsilon}_{PE} + \bar{\varepsilon}_{KE} = \frac{p_o^2}{2\rho_o c_o^2}.$$

1.5.3 Energy Flux and Intensity

By differentiating (1.80) with respect to time and making use of (1.3), (1.32), and (1.34a) and ignoring viscous damping, we find that the total energy flowing *out* of V is given by

$$W(t) = -\frac{\partial E}{\partial t} = \iiint_V (\mathbf{v}\cdot\nabla p + p\nabla\cdot\mathbf{v})dV = \iiint_V \nabla(p\mathbf{v})dV,$$

where use has been made of a standard vector relation.[12] Thus, $\nabla(p\mathbf{v})$ is the rate at which energy leaves an element of volume. Because the volume integral can be transformed to an integral over the surface S_o that bounds V, the energy flow can be expressed as

(1.83)
$$W(t) = \iint_{S_o} (p\mathbf{v})\cdot\tilde{\mathbf{n}}\, dS,$$

where $\tilde{\mathbf{n}}$ is a unit vector normal to the surface pointing in an outward direction. From this equation it can be seen that the vector quantity $(p\mathbf{v})$ is the instantaneous energy flow per unit area out from a surface element dS. This can be defined[26] to be the *instantaneous intensity* (watts/m²) vector $\mathbf{I}(\mathbf{r}{:}t)$, i.e.,

(1.84)
$$\boxed{\mathbf{I}(\mathbf{r}{:}t) = p\mathbf{v}}.$$

If a harmonic wave of period $\mathcal{T}$ is considered, then the *time-average intensity* vector $\bar{\mathbf{I}}$ (a real quantity) can be found from $\bar{\mathbf{I}}(\mathbf{r}{:}\omega) = \dfrac{1}{\mathcal{T}}\displaystyle\int_0^{\mathcal{T}} p\mathbf{v}dt$. By expressing p and $\mathbf{v}$ in the standard complex form and then evaluating the integral, it can be readily shown that

$$\bar{\mathbf{I}}(\mathbf{r}{:}\omega) = \overline{p\mathbf{v}} = \overline{\mathrm{Re}[\underline{p}(\mathbf{r})] \times \mathrm{Re}[\underline{\mathbf{v}}(\mathbf{r})] \times e^{2\,j\omega t}}$$

(1.85)
$$= \frac{1}{2}\mathrm{Re}[\underline{p}(\mathbf{r})\underline{\mathbf{v}}^*(\mathbf{r})],$$

where * indicates the complex conjugate, Re{.} denotes the real part, and the underlined quantities are phasors.

---

26. Many authors define the intensity as a time-averaged rather than an instantaneous quantity.

In the absence of any attenuation, time-averaged power from a source of ultrasound can be found by integrating the intensity vector over any surface that encloses the source, i.e.,

$$(1.86) \qquad \overline{W} = \oiint_{S_o} \overline{\mathbf{I}}(\mathbf{r}) \cdot \tilde{\mathbf{n}} \, dS.$$

In the presence of attenuation, the surface S_o must be sufficiently close to the source so that the intensity is not significantly reduced.

If we consider a plane harmonic wave traveling in an inviscid fluid in the direction $\tilde{\mathbf{n}}$, substituting (1.59), i.e., $\underline{\mathbf{v}} = \tilde{\mathbf{n}}\underline{p}/(c_o\rho_o)$ into (1.85) the time-averaged intensity can be written as [46]

$$(1.87) \qquad \overline{\mathbf{I}}(\mathbf{r}) = \frac{|p|^2}{2\rho_o c_o} \tilde{\mathbf{n}}, \quad \text{or as} \quad \overline{\mathbf{I}}(\mathbf{r}) = \frac{1}{2}\rho_o c_o |\underline{\mathbf{v}}|^2 \tilde{\mathbf{n}}.$$

We are now in a position to express the various physical quantities associated with the transmission of a plane harmonic wave in a fluid medium in terms of the average intensity $\overline{I}$, and these are shown in Table 1.5 for water at 37°C, an average intensity expressed in watts/cm² and for a frequency of f (expressed in MHz).

1.5.4 Radiation Pressure

When ultrasound is incident on a body consisting of medium that absorbs, scatters, or reflects the radiation, a force will be exerted that consists of two components. The first is an oscillatory component with a time-average of zero, arising from time-varying acoustic pressure acting on the body. The second is a steady component known as the *radiation pressure*. The presence of radiation pressure is an inherent property of the nonlinear relation between pressure and density in the propagation medium. Thus, for a medium that behaves in a perfectly linear manner, there would be no radiation pressure. Two types of radiation pressure are generally identified, depending on the measurement conditions: the *Langevin radiation pressure* and the *Rayleigh radiation pres-*

Table 1.5. Amplitudes for a Plane Harmonic Wave Propagating in Water at 37°C for a Time-Averaged Intensity $\overline{I}$ (W/m²) at a Frequency f (Hz)

Amplitude	Equation	@ 10 mW/cm², 5.0 MHz
Pressure, p_o	$p_o = 1.734 \times 10^3 \sqrt{\overline{I}}$ Pa	0.1734×10^5 Pa
Particle displacement, ξ_o	$\xi_o = 183.7 \times 10^{-6} f^{-1} \sqrt{\overline{I}}$ m	3.673×10^{-10} m
Particle velocity, v_o	$v_o = 1.154 \times 10^{-3} \sqrt{\overline{I}}$ m/s	1.154 cm/s
Acceleration, a_o	$a_o = 7.248 \times 10^{-3} f \sqrt{\overline{I}}$ m/s²	3.624×10^7 cm/s²
Fractional density change, $\Delta\rho/\rho_o$	$\Delta\rho/\rho_o = 7.646 \times 10^{-7} \sqrt{\overline{I}}$	7.646×10^{-6}

sure. Radiation pressure will also be present within a fluid medium and will cause the fluid to be displaced in the direction of the pressure gradient. This phenomenon, known as *acoustic streaming*, is a direct result of the radiation pressure: further details are contained in the reviews by Nyborg [47] and Duck [48].

It seems that Altberg [49] in 1903 was the first to report measurements of the radiation force produced by acoustic waves and to show how this could enable the absolute intensity of acoustic waves to be measured. For diagnostic ultrasound transducers, the radiation force can be quite small and errors can arise from this and a variety of other sources, making it difficult to achieve a high degree of accuracy. Nonetheless, absolute calibrations can be performed and the method is often used for routine checks of hospital equipment [50,51]. By measuring the radiation force acting on a small body such as a sphere, the intensity distribution of an ultrasound beam can also be determined. This requires that the characteristics of the body and the incident field profile be theoretically related to the force. Obtaining the necessary equations is far from trivial since, as mentioned earlier, the radiation force depends on second-order effects and therefore requires the use of second-order (nonlinear) acoustic theory.

Understanding the physics and obtaining equations that correctly describe the acoustic radiation pressure has been the subject of considerable controversy ever since the first publication in 1902 by Rayleigh [52]. Problems have arisen from improperly posed problems, confusion over definitions, and the difficulties associated with nonlinear phenomena. More recently, through a careful and rigorous analysis, many of the difficulties have been resolved. In this regard, the work reported by Lee and Wang [54,55] is particularly helpful and forms the basis of the description presented below.

To simplify the analysis we shall assume that the body being investigated is rigid so that the normal component of the particle velocity on its surface is zero. The total radiation force exerted on such a body is simply the vector sum of the forces acting on each elementary area of its surface[27] and therefore can be written as a surface integral of the force due to the time-averaged acoustic pressure acting on the element of area dS in an inward normal direction. Since the particle surface velocity is zero, the pressure at each point corresponds to that measured in a fixed (Eulerian) coordinate system. If $\tilde{\mathbf{n}}$ is a unit vector in the outward normal direction to dS, then the net radiation force is given by

(1.88)
$$\mathbf{F} = -\iint_{S_o} \overline{p_E}\,\tilde{\mathbf{n}}\,dS,$$

where $\overline{p_E}$ is the time-averaged Eulerian excess pressure, i.e., that due to the acoustic field. Lee and Wang [54,55] showed that $\overline{p_E}$ is given by

---

27. For the more general case where the body is not rigid, the surface velocity will be non-zero and the force components must then obtained by integrating the normal component of the radiation stress tensor over the surface. The radiation stress tensor is given by $\tau_{ij} = -\overline{p}\delta_{ij} - \rho_o\overline{v_i v_j}$ in which δ_{ij} is the Kronecker delta ($\delta_{ij} = 1$ for $i = j$, otherwise $\delta_{ij} = 0$), and the subscripts i and j are equal to x, y or z. For example: if $i = j = x$ then $\tau_{xx} = -\overline{p}$ or if $i = x$ and $j = y$, then $\tau_{xy} = -\rho_o\overline{v_x v_y}$.

$$(1.89) \qquad \overline{p_E} = \overline{\varepsilon}_{PE} - \overline{\varepsilon}_{KE} + C,$$

in which $\overline{\varepsilon}_{PE} - \overline{\varepsilon}_{KE} = \dfrac{1}{2}\left(\dfrac{\overline{p^2}}{\rho_o c_o^2} - \rho_o \overline{\mathbf{v} \cdot \mathbf{v}} \right)$ is the difference between the time-averaged potential and kinetic energy densities and C is a constant determined by a system constraint such as the conservation of mass in a closed system. Lee and Wang defined the *Langevin radiation pressure* to be present if it depends exclusively on the incident waves, i.e., no constraint needs to be satisfied ($C = 0$). This occurs when the system is in communication with fluid in equilibrium. On the other hand, a *Rayleigh radiation pressure* is present if the pressure depends on both the waves and a system constraint. This can occur when the system is enclosed so that the mass of fluid is conserved. The presence of a constraint requires that $C \neq 0$, but for most practical situations $C = 0$, so that the Langevin radiation pressure is present.

Ideal Reflecting Plane: Normal Incidence

Rayleigh [52,53] was the first to examine case of a plane harmonic wave incident on an ideal rigid plane reflector. In such a situation, the incident plane wave and the reflected wave add to form a standing wave whose amplitude is a function of the distance from the reflector. For an incident wave with a pressure waveform given by $p_o \cos(\omega t - kx)$ traveling in the positive x-direction that encounters a perfect reflector at $x = 0$, the total pressure of the standing wave is given by

$$(1.90) \qquad \begin{aligned} p(x\!:\!t) &= p_o \cos(\omega t - kx) + p_o \cos(\omega t + kx) \\ &= 2 p_o \cos(kx) \cos(\omega t). \end{aligned}$$

With the help of (1.39), the particle velocity of this standing wave can be expressed as

$$(1.91) \qquad v(x\!:\!t) = (2 p_o / Z_o) \sin(kx) \cos(\omega t - \pi/2),$$

where $Z_o = \rho_o c_o$ is the characteristic impedance of the medium. It should be noted that (1.91) satisfies the boundary condition for a rigid reflector which requires the velocity be zero on its surface at $x = 0$. It should also be noted that because the time-varying components of pressure and velocity are in phase quadrature, the specific acoustic impedance is then an imaginary quantity given by $\underline{Z}(x) = j Z_o \cot(kx)$. For this standing wave, normalized amplitudes of both the particle velocity and pressure are shown in Fig. 1.14.

By taking the time average of the square of (1.90) and (1.91), we find that the potential and kinetic energy densities are given by

$$\overline{\varepsilon}_{PE} = \rho_o (p_o / Z_o)^2 \cos^2(kx), \quad \overline{\varepsilon}_{KE} = \rho_o (p_o / Z_o)^2 \sin^2(kx).$$

Consequently

$$\overline{\varepsilon}_{PE} - \overline{\varepsilon}_{KE} = \rho_o (p_o / Z_o)^2 [\cos^2(kx) - \sin^2(kx)] = \rho_o (p_o / Z_o)^2 \cos(2kx),$$

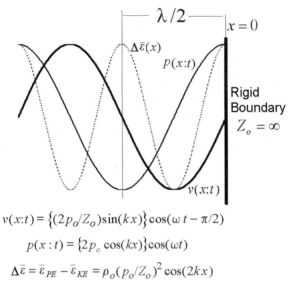

$$v(x{:}t) = \{(2p_o/Z_o)\sin(kx)\}\cos(\omega t - \pi/2)$$

$$p(x{:}t) = \{2p_o \cos(kx)\}\cos(\omega t)$$

$$\Delta\bar{\varepsilon} = \bar{\varepsilon}_{PE} - \bar{\varepsilon}_{KE} = \rho_o(p_o/Z_o)^2 \cos(2kx)$$

Figure 1.14 A standing wave is shown corresponding to that produced by the reflection of a harmonic plane wave by a perfectly reflecting plane rigid boundary $(Z_o = \infty)$. The normalized amplitudes of the pressure, particle velocity, and difference between the potential and kinetic energies of the standing wave are shown in the region $x \leq 0$. The amplitudes of the pressure and velocity correspond to the bracketed terms in the equations.

or

$$\Delta\bar{\varepsilon} = \bar{\varepsilon}_{PE} - \bar{\varepsilon}_{KE} = 2\bar{\varepsilon}_i \cos(2kx)$$

where $\bar{\varepsilon}_i$ is the time-averaged energy density of the incident wave as given by (1.82) (also shown in Fig. 1.14). By substituting this into (1.89) and assuming that there are no system constraints to satisfy $(C = 0)$, the time-averaged pressure on the reflecting plane $(x = 0)$ is given by[28]

(1.92) $$\boxed{\overline{p_E} = 2\bar{\varepsilon}_i}.$$ (a)

By using (1.82) and (1.87), this can be re-expressed in terms of the time-averaged intensity as

(1.92) $$\boxed{\overline{p_E} = 2\bar{I}/c_o}.$$ (b)

Ideal Absorbing Plane: Normal Incidence

As a second example, the somewhat controversial problem of a plane harmonic wave incident on a perfectly absorbing plane medium is considered.

---

28. If the system is closed then C can be evaluated by making use of the conservation of mass. When this is done it can be shown that $\overline{p_E} = (\gamma + 1)\bar{\varepsilon}_i$ for an ideal gas, which is the result originally obtained by Rayleigh [1.53].

Because the problem definition requires that there be no reflected wave, the characteristic impedance of the absorbing medium must be identical to that of the transmission medium. If it is temporarily assumed that we can proceed in the same manner as for the ideal reflecting plane, then the pressure and particle velocity are given by

$$p(x{:}t) = p_o \cos(\omega t - kx)$$
$$v(x{:}t) = (p_o/Z_o) \cos(\omega t - kx).$$

From these it can be readily shown that $\bar{\varepsilon}_{PE} = \bar{\varepsilon}_{KE} = \rho_o(p_o/2Z_o)^2 = \bar{\varepsilon}_i/2$, so that from (1.89) $\overline{p_E} = C$, which suggests that in the absence of any constraint, the average pressure due to the acoustic wave is zero. However, because the absorbing medium has been assumed to be perfectly matched to the transmission medium, it is inconsistent to assume that acoustic particles at the interface are stationary, and consequently the time-averaged Eulerian pressure as given by (1.89) is not appropriate. According to Lee and Wang [54,55], the time-averaged excess pressure experienced by the moving acoustic particles is given by

$$\overline{p}_L = \bar{\varepsilon} + C,$$

where the subscript L indicates that the pressure is measured in the Lagrangian coordinate system and $\bar{\varepsilon}$ is the total time-averaged energy density. In the absence of any constraints $C = 0$, and consequently the time-averaged pressure on the perfectly absorbing plane is

(1.93) $$\boxed{\overline{p}_L = \bar{\varepsilon}_i}\,,$$ (a)

or, from (1.82) and (1.87),

(1.93) $$\boxed{\overline{p}_L = \bar{I}/c_o}\,,$$ (b)

which is exactly half that of a perfectly reflecting plane.

   As an example, consider a plane wave with an intensity of $100\,\text{mW/cm}^2$ in water that is incident normally on a perfect absorbing interface with an area of $1.5\,\text{cm}^2$. The Langevin radiation force would be: $F = (\bar{I}/c_o) \times \text{Area} = (0.1 \times 10^4/1500) \times 1.5 \times 10^{-4} = 0.1\,\text{mN}$. If this force were balanced by a weight, the required mass would be: $0.1 \times 10^{-3}/9.81 = 10.2\,\text{mg}$.

1.6 Reflection and Refraction

Reflection and refraction of acoustic waves can be considered as a special case of scattering. To illustrate this concept we consider the field distribution illustrated by Fig. 1.15a in which waves from a circular source are incident on an object whose dimensions are large compared to a wavelength. The reflected waves can be considered as having originated from the surface of the object. If these are superimposed on the waves that occur in the absence of the object, then, except in the geometric shadow of the object, the actual field (that occurring in the presence of the object) will be correctly represented. But if the

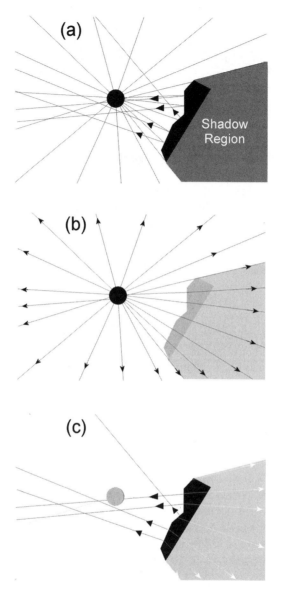

Figure 1.15 The scattered field plus the undisturbed illumination field equals the actual field. (a) The actual field from a circular source in the presence of a reflecting object. (b) Undisturbed field from circular source (the position of the object and the shadow region are indicated for the purpose of alignment with the other figures). (c) The scattered field. Note that in the "shadow" region, the scattered field cancels out the field in the same region of (b) when the two are added.

object is also considered to be a source of radiation into the shadow region, and provided the form of this radiation interferes destructively with the waves that occur in the absence of the object, then superposition will result in a correct representation of the entire actual field. As illustrated in Fig. 1.15c, the reflected and the interfering components originating from the object are the *scattered field*. It can also be seen from this figure that the scattered field consists of the sum of a classical geometrical optics reflected field and the shadow field. In summary, the scattered field is the difference between the field that occurs without the object and the actual field in the presence of the object. Thus, for example, the total pressure at a given location **r** can be written as

$$p(\mathbf{r};t) = p_i(\mathbf{r};t) + p_S(\mathbf{r};t),$$

where the subscripts i and s denote the incident and scattered field components. This way of treating the effect of a wave on an object will be particularly valuable in our detailed discussion of scattering in Chapter 5. But for the moment we shall treat the problem of reflection and refraction in a classical manner. Both the classical reflected and refracted fields, together with the shadow region field, are components of the scattered field.

1.6.1 Compressional Waves in Fluid Media

Consider a longitudinal plane harmonic wave incident on the boundary between two semi-infinite media, as illustrated in Fig. 1.16. The 3-D aspect of this problem can be reduced to 2-D by choosing the coordinate axes such that the y-axis is parallel to the plane of the incident wave. In general, if medium 2 is a solid, wave mode conversion can occur whereby a portion of the incident energy is converted into a shear wave, so that both the shear and longitudinal waves will propagate. If wave-mode conversion at the interface can be ignored, which is the case for liquid–gas or liquid–liquid junctions, then the velocity potentials of the incident, reflected, and transmitted waves can be obtained. We first note that a general expression for a plane wave

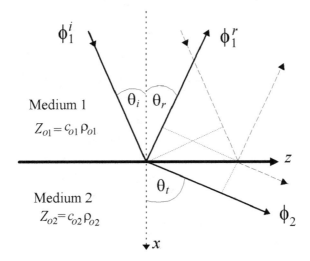

Figure 1.16 Reflection and refraction of an incident plane wave at a plane interface between two media in the absence of wave-mode conversion for $c_{o2} > c_{o1}$.

propagating in an inviscid fluid is $\phi(\mathbf{r}:t) = \phi_m \exp j\omega(t - \tilde{\mathbf{k}} \cdot \mathbf{r}/c_o)$, where the subscript m indicates the amplitude and $\tilde{\mathbf{k}}$ is a unit vector in the propagation direction. By expanding the dot product and expressing it in terms of the angles defined in Fig. 1.16, the velocity potentials for the three wave components can be expressed as the sum of two components along the x- and z-axes:

(1.94)
$$\begin{cases} \phi_1^i = \phi_{1m}^i e^{j\omega[t-(x/c_{o1})\cos\theta_i-(z/c_{o1})\sin\theta_i]} \\ \phi_1^r = \phi_{1m}^r e^{j\omega[t+(x/c_{o1})\cos\theta_r-(z/c_{o1})\sin\theta_r]}, \\ \phi_2 = \phi_{2m} e^{j\omega[t-(x/c_{o2})\cos\theta_t-(z/c_{o2})\sin\theta_t]} \end{cases}$$

in which the superscripts i and r denote the incident and reflected wave velocity potentials, respectively, and the subscripts 1 and 2 refer to the two media.

Boundary Conditions and Snell's Law

At the interface two conditions must be satisfied: (i) the pressure should be continuous and (ii) the particle velocity component normal to the interface should be continuous.

These two conditions follow from considering the physical implications of a discontinuity of either the pressure or velocity at the interface. For the pressure to be discontinuous, it would be necessary that a source of acoustic energy exist at the interface. Similarly, for the normal component of the velocity to be discontinuous (implying an infinitely large acceleration), there would need to be a dipole source layer at the boundary. Since neither is present, the above boundary conditions must be satisfied. Recalling from (1.39) that $p = -\rho_o \partial\phi/\partial t$ and $v_n = -\partial\phi/\partial x$, the boundary conditions can be expressed as

(1.95)
$$\rho_{o1}\left[\frac{\partial\phi_1^i}{\partial t} + \frac{\partial\phi_1^r}{\partial t}\right]_{x=0} = \rho_{o2}\left[\frac{\partial\phi_2}{\partial t}\right]_{x=0},$$

(1.96)
$$\left[\frac{\partial\phi_1^i}{\partial x} + \frac{\partial\phi_1^r}{\partial x}\right]_{x=0} = \left[\frac{\partial\phi_2}{\partial x}\right]_{x=0}.$$

Differentiating (1.94) with respect to time, substituting into (1.96), and putting $x = 0$ we obtain

(1.97)
$$\phi_{1m}^i \frac{\cos\theta_i}{c_{ol}} e^{-j\omega(z/c_{o1})\sin\theta_i} - \phi_{1m}^r \frac{\cos\theta_r}{c_{ol}} e^{-j\omega(z/c_{o1})\sin\theta_r} = \phi_{2m} \frac{\cos\theta_t}{c_{o2}} e^{-j\omega(z/c_{o2})\sin\theta_t}.$$

But this equation can be satisfied for all values of z only if

$$\frac{\sin\theta_i}{c_{ol}} = \frac{\sin\theta_r}{c_{ol}} = \frac{\sin\theta_t}{c_{o2}},$$

so that $\theta_i = \theta_r$ and

(1.98)
$$\boxed{\frac{\sin\theta_i}{\sin\theta_t} = \frac{c_{ol}}{c_{o2}},}$$

which is the acoustic form of *Snell's law*. Differentiating (1.94) with respect to time, substituting into (1.95), and putting $x = 0$ and $\theta_i = \theta_r$, we obtain

$$(1.99) \qquad \rho_{o1}\left[\phi_{1m}^i + \phi_{1m}^r\right] = \rho_{o2}\phi_{2m}e^{-j\omega z(\sin\theta_t/c_{o2} - \sin\theta_i/c_{o1})}.$$

Since the real portion can be equated to zero, it follows that

$$(1.100) \qquad \rho_{o1}\phi_{1m}^i + \rho_{o1}\phi_{1m}^r = \rho_{o2}\phi_{2m}.$$

Substituting Snell's law into (1.97) yields

$$(1.101) \qquad c_{o2}\left[\phi_{1m}^i - \phi_{1m}^r\right]\cos\theta_i = c_{o1}\phi_{2m}\cos\theta_t.$$

By eliminating ϕ_{2m} between (1.100) and (1.101) and expressing the characteristic impedances by $Z_{o1} = \rho_{o1}c_{o1}$, $Z_{o2} = \rho_{o2}c_{o2}$:

$$Z_{o2}\left[1 - \left(\phi_{1m}^r/\phi_{1m}^i\right)\right]\cos\theta_i = Z_{o1}\left[1 + \left(\phi_{1m}^r/\phi_{1m}^i\right)\right]\cos\theta_t.$$

or

$$(1.102) \qquad \frac{\phi_{1m}^r}{\phi_{1m}^i} = \frac{Z_{o2}\cos\theta_i - Z_{o1}\cos\theta_t}{Z_{o2}\cos\theta_i + Z_{o1}\cos\theta_t}$$
$$= p_m^r/p_m^i \equiv R_p,$$

where p_m^i and p_m^r are the pressure amplitudes of the incident and reflected waves and R_p is the pressure *amplitude reflection coefficient*. This can be expressed in terms of θ_i by means of

$$(1.103) \qquad \cos\theta_t = \sqrt{1 - \left[c_{o2}\sin\theta_i/c_{o1}\right]^2},$$

which was obtained from Snell's law. It should be noted from (1.102) that if $Z_{o2}\cos\theta_i < Z_{o1}\cos\theta_t$, then the reflected wave is 180 degrees out of phase with the incident wave; otherwise, it is in-phase.

Critical and Intromission Angles

If $c_{o2} \geq c_{o1}$ and the incident angle is given by $\theta_i \equiv \theta_c = \sin^{-1}(c_{o1}/c_{o2})$, then it follows from Snell's law that $\theta_t = 90$ degrees, i.e., the transmitted wave propagates along the surface. At the *critical angle* θ_c, it follows from (1.102) and (1.100) that $\phi_{1m}^i = \phi_{1m}^r$ and $\phi_{2m} = 2\phi_{1m}^i(\rho_{o1}/\rho_{o2})$. Thus, all the incident energy is reflected even though the transmitted beam amplitude remains non-zero. If $90° > \theta_i > \theta_c$, the transmitted angle becomes imaginary, and as a result (1.103) can be

can be written as $\cos\theta_t = -j\alpha$, in which $\alpha = \sqrt{\left[c_{o2}\sin\theta_i/c_{o1}\right]^2 - 1}$ and therefore $\sin\theta_t = \sqrt{1 - \cos^2\theta_t} = \sqrt{1 + \alpha^2}$. If these two expressions are substituted into (1.94), the velocity potential for the transmitted wave is found to have an exponent of $\left\{j\omega t - (\omega x\alpha/c_{o2}) - \left[(j\omega z/c_{o2})\sqrt{1 + \alpha^2}\right]\right\}$. Consequently, the x-component (normal to the interface) of the transmitted wave is attenuated exponentially with the distance from the interface, and therefore α is an attenuation factor. On the other hand, the z-component corresponds to the transmission of a wave along the interface. Waves with these characteristics are generally called *evanescent waves.* As an example we shall estimate the penetration depth for $\alpha = 1$, corresponding to $\theta_i = \sin^{-1}(\sqrt{2}\,c_{o1}/c_{o2})$. The ratio of the amplitude of the transmitted wave at a depth of one wavelength ($x = \lambda = 2\pi c_{o2}/\omega$) to that at the interface expressed as a percentage is: $100 \times \exp(-2\pi\alpha) = 0.187\%$, and as a result the wave is rapidly attenuated. If medium 2 is lossy, it can be shown that not all the incident energy is reflected: some is absorbed due to losses by the evanescent wave.

If the angle of incidence is such that $Z_{o2}\cos\theta_i = Z_{o1}\cos\theta_t$, then it follows from (1.102) that all the incident energy is transmitted and none is reflected. With the help of (1.98), this condition reduces to

$$(1.104) \qquad \sin\theta_I = \sqrt{\left[1-(Z_{o1}/Z_{o2})^2\right]\big/\left[1-(\rho_{o1}/\rho_{o2})^2\right]},$$

which is the *intromission angle* [31]. For this to exist the square root term must be ≥ 0 and ≤ 1, which sets certain requirements on the densities and impedances.

The phase of the reflected beam varies for incident angles greater than the critical angle; it also changes when the angle of intromission is reached. It can be readily shown from (1.102) that the phase angle of the reflected beam is given by

$$(1.105) \qquad \Theta = 2\tan^{-1}\left[\frac{\alpha Z_{o1}}{Z_{o2}\cos\theta_i}\right] \text{ for } \theta_c \leq \theta_i \leq 90°.$$

This variation is illustrated in the graph of Fig. 1.17, which shows both the magnitude and phase angle of the reflection coefficient versus the incident angle for two sets of density and speed ratios.

Reflection and Transmission Coefficients

We shall define the *intensity reflection coefficient*[29] R_I as the ratio of the time-averaged intensity magnitudes of the reflected and incident waves ($0 \leq R_I \leq 1$). Since the intensity for a plane wave is expressed in terms of pressure by (1.87), it follows that $R_I = (p_m^r/p_m^i)^2$, and consequently from (1.102) the reflection coefficient can be written as

$$(1.106) \qquad R_I = \left[\frac{Z_{o2}\cos\theta_i - Z_{o1}\cos\theta_t}{Z_{o2}\cos\theta_i + Z_{o1}\cos\theta_t}\right]^2,$$

in which θ_t can be expressed in terms of the incident angle by (1.103).

The *intensity transmission coefficient* T_I can be defined as the ratio of the time-averaged transmitted and incident intensities, so that from (1.87), $T_I = [(p_m^t)^2/2Z_{o2}]/[(p_m^i)^2/2Z_{o1}]$. While this can be evaluated using the equations given earlier, it is simpler to obtain the result by making use of the conservation of energy. From the geometry of Fig. 1.16 it is evident that the power incident on an area S of the interface is $SI_i\cos\theta_i$, and that leaving is $S(I_r\cos\theta_i +$

---

29. This should be distinguished from the pressure *amplitude* reflection and transmission coefficients (denoted by R_p and T_p, respectively), which are the ratios of the amplitudes of the reflected and transmitted waves to the incident wave.

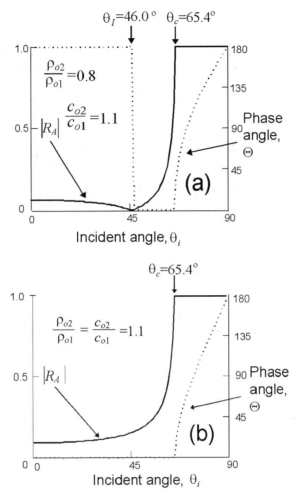

Figure 1.17 Graphs showing the pressure amplitude reflection coefficient and phase angle of the reflected beam versus angle of incidence for (a) $\rho_{o2}/\rho_{o1} = 0.8$, $c_{o2}/c_{o1} = 1.1$ and (b) $\rho_{o2}/\rho_{o1} = c_{o2}/c_{o1} = 1.1$. The critical and intromission angles are also indicated. The graphs were calculated from (1.102) and (1.105).

$I_t \cos \theta_t$). By equating these two components and noting the definitions of T_I and R_I, it follows that $T_I \cos \theta_t = (1 - R_I) \cos \theta_i$. Consequently, from (1.106) the intensity transmission coefficient is given by

(1.107)
$$T_I = \frac{4 Z_{o1} Z_{o2} \cos^2 \theta_i}{\left[Z_{o2} \cos \theta_i + Z_{o1} \cos \theta_t \right]^2}.$$

When the incident angle is equal to the intromission angle, i.e., $Z_{o2} \cos \theta_i = Z_{o1} \cos \theta_t$, then $R_I = 0$, and $T_I = Z_{o1}/Z_{o2}$. Because of the different transmitted beam cross-sectional area compared to the incident and reflected beams, the transmitted beam intensity differs from the incident beam intensity by the ratio of the impedances: nonetheless, all the incident power is transmitted.

The velocity potential, pressure, and time-averaged power reflection and transmission coefficients can all be calculated in a similar way [31,56], and these are summarized in Table 1.6 together with the relations between them. In particular, it should be noted that for the pressure, velocity potential, and intensity coefficients, in general $R + T \neq 1$. All of the equations clearly show that the characteristic impedance is of key importance in governing the energy transmitted through the interface between two differing media.

For the normal incidence condition ($\theta_i = \theta_t = 0$), (1.106) and (1.107) reduce to:

$$(1.108) \qquad R_I = \left[\frac{Z_{o2} - Z_{o1}}{Z_{o2} + Z_{o1}} \right]^2, \quad T_I = \frac{4 Z_{o1} Z_{o2}}{[Z_{o2} + Z_{o1}]^2},$$

and as a result, $T_I = 0$ and $R_I = 1$ for either $Z_{o2} = \infty$ or $Z_{o2} = 0$. The case corresponding to $Z_{o2} = \infty$ has been previously examined in subsection 1.5.3 (see Fig. 1.14), where it was shown that a standing wave is established whose velocity is zero at the boundary. For a soft boundary in which $Z_{o2} = 0$, a standing wave is also established, but in this case the pressure is zero on the boundary (hence the term pressure release) and the particle velocity is a maximum. Both of the above boundary conditions are examined for the more general case of an arbitrary angle of incidence in the next subsection.

Table 1.6. Equations for Plane Wave Reflection and Transmission Coefficients

Reflection Coefficient	Transmission Coefficient	Relationship
Velocity Potential		
$R_\phi = \dfrac{Z_{o2} \cos\theta_i - Z_{o1} \cos\theta_t}{Z_{o2} \cos\theta_i + Z_{o1} \cos\theta_t}$	$T_\phi = \dfrac{2 \rho_{o1} c_{o2} \cos\theta_i}{Z_{o2} \cos\theta_i + Z_{o1} \cos\theta_t}$	$R_\phi = \dfrac{\rho_{o2}}{\rho_{o1}} T_\Phi - 1$
Pressure		
$R_p = \dfrac{Z_{o2} \cos\theta_i - Z_{o1} \cos\theta_t}{Z_{o2} \cos\theta_i + Z_{o1} \cos\theta_t}$	$T_p = \dfrac{2 Z_{o2} \cos\theta_i}{Z_{o2} \cos\theta_i + Z_{o1} \cos\theta_t}$	$R_p = T_p - 1$
Intensity (Watts/m²)		
$R_I = \left[\dfrac{Z_{o2} \cos\theta_i - Z_{o1} \cos\theta_t}{Z_{o2} \cos\theta_i + Z_{o1} \cos\theta_t} \right]^2$	$T_I = \dfrac{4 Z_{o1} Z_{o2} \cos^2\theta_i}{[Z_{o2} \cos\theta_i + Z_{o1} \cos\theta_t]^2}$	$R_I + T_I \dfrac{\cos\theta_t}{\cos\theta_i} = 1$
Power (Watts)		
$R_w = \left[\dfrac{Z_{o2} \cos\theta_i - Z_{o1} \cos\theta_t}{Z_{o2} \cos\theta_i + Z_{o1} \cos\theta_t} \right]^2$	$T_w = \dfrac{4 Z_{o1} Z_{o2} \cos\theta_i \cos\theta_t}{[Z_{o2} \cos\theta_i + Z_{o1} \cos\theta_t]^2}$	$R_w + T_w = 1$

Rigid and Pressure-Release Boundaries

It can be seen from (1.106) and (1.107) that if $Z_{o2}/Z_{o1} \to \infty$, then region 2 behaves as an *ideal rigid boundary*, such that all the incident energy is reflected and none is transmitted, i.e., $R_I \to 1$ and $T_I \to 0$. On the interface at any given z-location the incident and reflected wave pressures are equal. This can be seen by first applying $p = -\rho_o \partial \phi/\partial t$ to (1.94) to obtain expressions for the incident and reflected wave pressures. Now (1.102) shows that when the velocity potential amplitudes are equal ($\phi^r_{1m} = \phi^i_{1m}$), $p^r_1(0,z{:}t) = p^i_1(0,z{:}t)$. Because the total acoustic pressure is the sum of the incident and reflected wave pressures, it follows that on a rigid boundary the pressure is twice that of the incident wave. Moreover, on such a boundary the normal component of the incident and reflected wave particle velocities must be equal and opposite so that their sum is zero. If $\tilde{\mathbf{x}}$ is a unit vector in the x-direction, these two boundary relations can be written as

$$(1.109) \qquad p(0, z{:}t) = 2p^i_1(0, z{:}t), \quad \tilde{\mathbf{x}} \cdot \mathbf{v}(0, z{:}t) = 0 \quad \text{(Rigid boundary)}.$$

An ideal *pressure-release boundary* corresponds to the situation in which $Z_{o2}/Z_{o1} \to 0$. From (1.106) and (1.107) it can be seen that $R_I \to 1$ and $T_I \to 0$, so that this boundary condition also causes perfect reflection. By following similar steps to those described for the rigid boundary, it can be readily shown that

$$(1.110) \quad p(0, z{:}t) = 0, \quad \mathbf{v}(0, z{:}t) = 2\tilde{\mathbf{x}} \cdot \mathbf{v}^i_1(0, z{:}t) \quad \text{(Pressure-release boundary)},$$

which shows that there is a doubling of the normal component of the incident particle velocity component.

Transmission Through a Layer for Normal Incidence

The case of a medium consisting of a layer of thickness ℓ separating two different media is of considerable practical importance. As will be seen, proper choice of the thickness and acoustic properties of the layer provides a means of impedance matching such that a plane wave can be transmitted from one medium to another without any loss of intensity. For the geometry shown in Fig. 1.18a and a harmonic plane wave at normal incidence, it can be shown that the intensity (and power) transmission coefficient is given by [56, p. 128]

$$(1.111) \qquad T_I = \frac{4 Z_{o3} Z_{o1}}{\left(Z_{o1} + Z_{o3}\right)^2 \cos^2 \theta_2 + \left(Z_{o2} + Z_{o1} Z_{o3}/Z_{o2}\right)^2 \sin^2 \theta_2}$$

where Z_{o1}, Z_{o2}, Z_{o3} are the characteristic impedances of the three regions, $\theta_2 = 2\pi\ell/\lambda_2$, and λ_2 is the wavelength in the layer. Since normal incidence has been assumed, the media in all three layers can be either liquid or solid. If the angle of incidence is non-zero a more complex situation exists, particularly if the layer is solid. As described in the next subsection, wave-mode conversion can occur in which the transmission of both a longitudinal and transverse wave

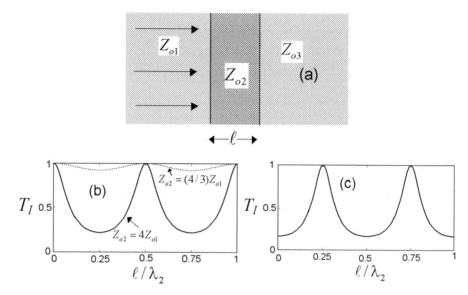

Figure 1.18 Transmission through a layer at normal incidence for various values of the thickness to wavelength ratio (ℓ/λ_2), as calculated from (1.111). (a) The assumed scheme and notation. (b) Transmission from water ($Z_{o1} = 1.5\,$MRayl) through to water ($Z_{o3} = Z_{o1}$) for a layer with $Z_{o2} = 4Z_{o1}$ and $Z_{o2} = (4/3)Z_{o1}$. (c) Transmission coefficient from a ceramic (PZT, $Z_o = 34.0\,$MRayl) through to water for the condition $Z_{o2} = \sqrt{Z_{o1}Z_{o3}} = 7.141\,$MRayl.

must be accounted for. Two conditions for normal incidence are of particular importance in (1.111). They are $\cos^2\theta_2 = 1$ and $\sin^2\theta_2 = 1$, which will now be examined.

The condition $\cos^2\theta_2 = 1$ corresponds to $\ell = n\lambda_2/2$ ($n = 0,1,2\ldots$) and if $Z_{o1} = Z_{o3}$ then $T_I = 1$. This is illustrated in Fig. 1.18b for two values of the layer characteristic impedance. It will be noted that if the slab is sufficiently thin compared to a wavelength, i.e., $\ell \ll \lambda_2$, then the layer appears transparent. Even for a fairly wideband pulse a sufficiently thin layer is nearly transparent, and consequently a thin plastic protective layer can be used without seriously affecting the transmission properties of an ultrasound transducer.

The second condition of $\sin^2\theta_2 = 1$ is satisfied when the layer thickness is given by $\ell = n\lambda_2/4$, where $n = 1,2\ldots$ The smallest slab thickness that satisfies this condition is one whose thickness is a quarter wavelength ($\ell = \lambda_2/4$). If, in addition, the characteristic impedance of layer 2 is given by $Z_{o2} = \sqrt{Z_{o1}Z_{o3}}$, then it can be readily shown from (1.111) that the transmission coefficient will be unity, corresponding to perfect matching between media 1 and 3. For the case of a PZT ceramic matched to water through a layer having a characteristic impedance of 7.141 Mrayl, Fig. 1.18c illustrates how the transmission coefficient varies with frequency ($\propto 1/\lambda$). It can be seen that for a fixed layer thickness the transmission coefficient falls off fairly rapidly as the frequency is changed from the $T_I = 1$ condition, and consequently the layer acts as a narrowband filter distorting a wideband pulse as it is transmitted through the layer.

1.6.2 Wave-Mode Conversion

Wave-mode conversion refers to a phenomenon whereby a wave incident on a boundary between two media can result in waves that propagate with a different vibrational mode than that incident. For example, a longitudinal wave propagating in a fluid toward a solid plane boundary can result in both a transmitted longitudinal and transverse wave, as illustrated in Fig. 1.19a. At the lower boundary, both the incident longitudinal and transverse waves give rise to both reflected longitudinal and transverse waves as well as a transmitted longitudinal wave. Wave-mode conversion results from the boundary conditions that must be satisfied when the incident wave interacts with the boundary.

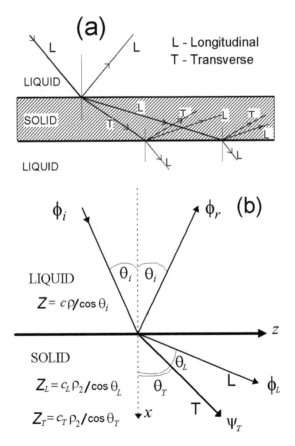

Figure 1.19 Wave-mode conversion for an incident longitudinal wave from fluid that does not support transverse wave propagation. (a) A solid slab immersed in a fluid. (b) A semi-infinite liquid bounded by a semi-infinite solid, showing the simplified notation used for analysis.

Using the simplified notation given in Fig. 1.19b, we shall outline the derivation [5,57] and results for the case of a plane harmonic longitudinal wave incident from the liquid onto a solid–liquid boundary. Both media are assumed to be lossless and the coordinate axes are chosen so that the y-axis is parallel to the plane of the incident wave, resulting in no particle displacement component normal to the plane of the figure. The particle velocities in the liquid can be written in terms of the velocity potential ($\mathbf{v} = -\nabla\phi$), and both ϕ_i and ϕ_r must satisfy the Helmholtz equation. In the solid the longitudinal and transverse particle velocities are given by $\mathbf{v_L} = -\nabla\phi_L$, and $\mathbf{v_T} = \nabla \times \psi_\mathbf{T}$, where $\psi_\mathbf{T}$ is a vector potential with zero divergence, which is also governed by Helmholtz's equation. Because the incident wave contains no displacement component parallel to the y-axis, the only transverse wave that can exist is one whose polarization is parallel to the plane $y = 0$.

Expressions for the three longitudinal plane-wave velocity potentials are the same as in (1.94), while the only transverse wave that can be present is represented by the velocity potential $\psi_T = \psi_{Tm}\exp\{j\omega[t - (x/c_T)\cos\theta_T - (z/c_T)\sin\theta_T]\}$. The normal components of the velocity and the stresses, and the tangential components of the velocity and stresses must be continuous across the boundary at $x = 0$. By imposing these conditions on the velocity potential equations, it can be shown that

$$(1.112) \qquad \frac{\sin\theta_i}{c} = \frac{\sin\theta_L}{c_L} = \frac{\sin\theta_T}{c_T},$$

which is the interface refraction law. This equation shows that if $c_L \geq c$ and $c_T \geq c$, there can be two incident angles for which one of the transmitted components is extinguished. The first critical angle corresponds to $\theta_L = 90°$ and the second to the transverse wave angle $\theta_T = 90°$. For $c_L \geq c$ and $c_T \geq c$, these two angles can be expressed as:

$$(1.113) \qquad \theta_{icL} = \sin^{-1}(c/c_L), \quad \theta_{icT} = \sin^{-1}(c/c_T).$$

In addition to obtaining the refraction law, application of the boundary conditions also enables the velocity potentials for the reflected wave and the transmitted longitudinal and transverse waves to be obtained. If these expressions are divided by the incident wave velocity potential, the reflection (R_ϕ) and transmission (T_ϕ) velocity potential amplitude ratios can be obtained as:

$$R_\phi = \frac{Z_L \cos^2(2\theta_T) + Z_T \sin^2(2\theta_T) - Z}{Z_L \cos^2(2\theta_T) + Z_T \sin^2(2\theta_T) + Z}, \qquad (a)$$

$$(1.114) \qquad T_\phi^L = \frac{(2\rho/\rho_2) \times Z_L \cos(2\theta_T)}{Z_L \cos^2(2\theta_T) + Z_T \sin^2(2\theta_T) + Z}, \qquad (b)$$

$$T_\phi^T = \frac{(-2\rho/\rho_2) \times Z_T \sin(2\theta_T)}{Z_L \cos^2(2\theta_T) + Z_T \sin^2(2\theta_T) + Z}, \qquad (c)$$

where the following impedances have been defined

(1.115) $Z = \rho c / \cos \theta_i$, $Z_L = \rho_2 c_L / \cos \theta_L$, $Z_T = \rho_2 c_T / \cos \theta_T$.

With the help of (1.112), the reflection and transmission coefficients can be evaluated for a given angle of incidence. It should be noted that beyond the first critical angle, θ_L becomes complex, and as a result the amplitude ratios also become complex.

Because energy conservation requires that the sum of the time-averaged power incident on the boundary should be equal to that leaving the boundary, it makes sense to express the contribution of each component in terms of the ratio of its power to that of the incident power. These reflection (R_W) and transmission (T_W) power ratios can be found with the help of (1.87) and (1.112) as

$$\text{(1.116)} \quad R_W = |R_\phi|^2, \quad T_W^T = |T_\phi^T|^2 \left(\frac{\rho_2 \tan \theta_i}{\rho \tan \theta_T} \right), \quad T_W^L = |T_\phi^L|^2 \left(\frac{\rho_2 \tan \theta_i}{\rho \tan \theta_L} \right),$$

which can then be evaluated by using (1.112) to (1.115).

As an example of wave-mode conversion, we consider a longitudinal wave incident at various angles from tissue onto bone. As a rough approximation, tissue properties are represented by water. Taking the values listed in Table 1.1 and using (1.112) to (1.116), the results are presented in Fig. 1.20. It will be noted that beyond the first critical angle of 21.85 degrees, the longitudinal wave is extinguished, and the conversion efficiency to transverse waves becomes greater than that for longitudinal waves prior to the critical angle. This is because the transverse wave impedance is closer to that of water. At and beyond the second critical angle of 64.64 degrees, according to the

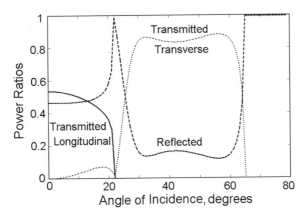

Figure 1.20 Example of wave-mode conversion for a plane wave incident from water onto a water–bone boundary. The power ratios are shown versus angle of incidence for the reflected and two transmitted components. The two critical angles are 21.85° and 64.64° for $c_o = 1500\,\text{m/s}$, $c_L = 4030\,\text{m/s}$, $c_T = 1660\,\text{m/s}$, $\rho = 1000\,\text{kg/m}^3$, and $\rho_2 = 1960\,\text{kg/m}^3$.

simplified theory given above all the incident energy is reflected. However, as noted earlier (see subsection 1.3.1), just beyond this angle, Rayleigh surface waves are excited, and as a result some of the incident energy will not be reflected but will propagate along the bone surface.

1.7 Elements of Diffraction

1.7.1 Historical Background: Huygens' Principle

Diffraction is a phenomenon that affects all types of wave propagation in bounded space; optical waves, microwaves, and acoustic waves are all affected. While several definitions of diffraction have been proposed, one of the most concise is that given by Sommerfeld. In his classical book on optics [58, p. 179] he states, "Any deviation of light rays from rectilinear paths which cannot be interpreted as reflection or refraction is called diffraction."

In geometrical optics or acoustics the radiation field is treated in terms of rays that obey simple geometric laws, as illustrated in Fig. 1.21a. The first clear experimental demonstration that optical rays when confined by boundaries did not obey the laws of geometric optics was reported in a book by Grimaldi published in 1665.[30] Huygens, who was apparently unaware of Grimaldi's work, proposed in his treatise published in 1690 that light was a wave phenomenon whose propagation could be regarded as a sequence of spherical disturbances. In essence, the Huygens' principle [60] provides a means for constructing subsequent wavefronts given an initial wavefront such as that illustrated in Fig. 1.21b. This principle has been elegantly stated in Born and Wolf [59, p. 132] as "each element of a wave-front may be regarded as the centre of a secondary disturbance which gives rise to spherical wavelets; and moreover that the position of the wave-front at any later time is the envelope of all such wavelets." It was not until early in the 19th century that the wave nature of light became widely accepted.[30] Based on the work of Huygens and the concept of wave interference proposed by Thomas Young, Fresnel in 1816 provided an initial mathematical and physical explanation of diffraction effects. But it was not until the second half of the 19th century, with the realization that optical waves were governed by Maxwell's equations, that the diffraction of light was placed on a sound theoretical basis.

Except in a limiting case, geometrical acoustics, like geometric optics, cannot correctly account for the potential field near a boundary. In the limit as the wavelength approaches zero, the behavior of acoustical fields predicted from diffraction theory approaches that governed by geometrical acoustics. In acoustics, as with optics, is convenient to refer to those regions that lie outside the direct illuminated regions predicted by geometric optics as the "geometrical shadow regions."

---

30. See, for example, the historical introduction in [59]; a very readable account of the early 19th-century developments is given in [61].

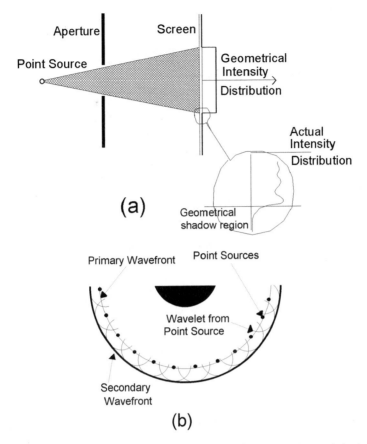

Figure 1.21 The effects of diffraction are illustrated. (a) Comparison of the intensity distributions produced by a point source through an aperture according to geometrical acoustics and in practice. (b) Use of Huygens' principle for constructing a secondary wavefront from a primary wavefront created by a spherical source.

For a small number of properly posed diffraction problems, rigorous analytical solutions have been obtained. Among these, the earliest rigorous solution is that described by Sommerfeld in 1896 [58] for a plane optical wave incident on a perfectly conducting infinite half-plane. But because of the difficulty in obtaining exact solutions of properly posed problems, approximate methods are often used. One of the simplest is that based on the Huygens-Fresnel approach, and this will now be illustrated.

1.7.2 Approximate Analysis of Diffraction by a Half-Plane

As illustrated in Fig. 1.22, a plane harmonic wave is assumed to be incident on an infinite half-plane aperture that consists of a perfectly rigid membrane of negligible thickness. Of course, such an aperture cannot be realized in practice, since an appreciable thickness is required to make the aperture rigid.

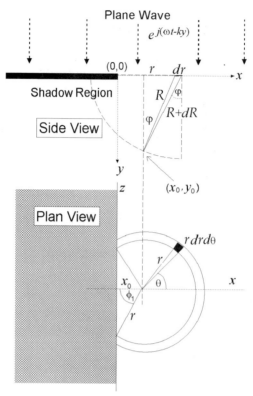

Figure 1.22 Geometry assumed for calculating the diffraction of a plane wave by an infinite half-plane sheet by using the Huygens' method of constructing secondary wavefronts and Fresnel's assumptions. The aperture is assumed to be a very thin perfect rigid reflector. Both side and plan views are shown.

In accordance with Huygens' principle, we assume that on the transparent portion of aperture there exist an infinite number of point sources. By calculating the contribution each such source makes at the observation point $(x_0, y_0, 0)$, the total pressure amplitude can be obtained. From Table 1.3, the pressure due to an elementary area $dx\,dz$ located at $(x, 0, z)$ whose strength is $A\,dx\,dz$ is given by

$$dp = \frac{A}{R} e^{j(\omega t - kR)} dx\,dz,$$

where R is the distance of the observation point to the element. It seems reasonable to expect that the contribution such a source makes at the observation point should depend on the angle φ (see Fig. 1.22) through an inclination factor $f(\varphi)$, which should be a maximum in the forward direction and drop to zero as $\varphi \to 0$ or $\pi/2$. If we make the ad hoc assumption that this inclination factor is equal to $\cos\varphi$ and convert to cylindrical coordinates (r, θ), with the origin of coordinates at $(x_0, 0, 0)$, then the pressure phasor can be expressed as

(1.117)
$$dp = \frac{e^{-jkR}}{R}\cos(\varphi)r\,dr\,d\theta,$$

in which it has been assumed that $A = 1$. It follows from Fig. 1.22 that $r^2 = R^2 - y_0^2$ and $\cos\varphi = y_0/R$, so that the total pressure is given by[31]

(1.118)
$$\underline{p}(x_0, y_0) = 2\int_{y_0}^{\infty}\int_0^{\phi} e^{-jkR}(y_0/R)d\theta dR = 2\pi\int_{y_0}^{\sqrt{x_0^2+y_0^2}} e^{-jkR}(y_0/R)dR$$

$$+ 2\int_{\sqrt{x_0^2+y_0^2}}^{\infty}\int_0^{\pi-\phi_1} e^{-jkR}(y_0/R)d\theta dR,$$

where $\phi_1 = \cos^{-1}\left(x_0/\sqrt{R^2-y_0^2}\right)$. Letting $X_0 = x_0/\lambda$, $Y_0 = y_0/\lambda$, and $R_0 = R/\lambda$ in (1.118) then, depending on the x-position of the observation point, the pressure is given by:

(i)   for $x_0 > 0$, (a complete circle can be formed)

(1.119)
$$\frac{\underline{p}}{\lambda Y_0} = 2\pi\int_{Y_0}^{\sqrt{X_0^2+Y_0^2}}\frac{e^{-j2\pi R_0}}{R_0}dR_0 + 2\int_{\sqrt{X_0^2+Y_0^2}}^{\infty}\frac{e^{-j2\pi R_0}}{R_0}\left[\pi - \cos^{-1}\left(X_0/\sqrt{R_0^2-Y_0^2}\right)\right]dR_0: \quad \text{(a)}$$

(ii)   for $x_0 = 0$, (a semicircle is formed)

(1.119)[32]
$$\frac{\underline{p}}{\lambda Y_0} = \pi\int_{Y_0}^{\infty} e^{-j2\pi R_0}(1/R_0)dR_0: \quad \text{(b)}$$

(iii)   for $x_0 < 0$, (a complete circle cannot be formed)

(1.119)
$$\frac{\underline{p}}{\lambda Y_0} = 2\int_{\sqrt{X_0^2+Y_0^2}}^{\infty} e^{-j2\pi R_0}(1/R_0)\cos^{-1}\left(|X_0|/\sqrt{R_0^2-Y_0^2}\right)dR_0. \quad \text{(c)}$$

The normalized pressure amplitude at the observation point is shown in Fig. 1.23 for three different observation planes. It will be noted that for all three cases the normalized pressure magnitude is very close to 0.5 at $x = 0$. In fact, numerical evaluation of (1.119a) shows that provided $Y_0 \geq 2$, then, to within an accuracy of $\pm 2\%$, $|\underline{p}|/\lambda = 0.5$. As the observation plane distance increases, the interference fringes become more widely spaced and the pressure amplitude in the shadow region increases. The above equations can be

31. If the inclination factor had been assumed to be zero, the $1/R$ term would be absent from the integrand and as a result the integral would not converge.
32. This integral, known as the exponential integral, can be expressed as [62]

$$\int_y^{\infty}\frac{e^{-j2\pi r}}{r}dr = -\text{Ci}(2\pi y) - j\left\{\frac{\pi}{2} + \text{Si}(2\pi y)\right\},$$

where $\text{Si}(x) = \int_0^x\frac{\sin r}{r}dr$, $\text{Ci}(x) = \gamma + \ln x + \int_0^x\frac{\cos(r)-1}{r}dr$ and $\gamma = $ Euler's constant $= 0.5772156649$. It can be readily shown that as $y\to\infty$ $I(y)\to\pi$.

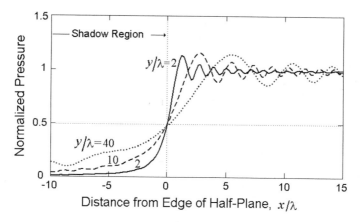

Figure 1.23 Approximate diffraction pattern due to a plane harmonic wave incident normal to a half-plane rigid baffle that lies on the plane $y = 0$. The observation points are expressed in terms of the wavelength λ and are shown for three different planes. The pressure axis shows the value of $|p|/\lambda$ as calculated from (1.119).

readily modified for a plane wave incident on the half-plane at any arbitrary angle.

1.7.3 Sommerfeld's Exact Analysis of Diffraction by a Half-Plane

It was mentioned earlier that Sommerfeld's analysis [58] for diffraction by a half-plane is an exact solution of the wave equation. It is therefore of some interest to examine the difference in the predicted results between the exact method and the approximate Huygen-Fresnel approach given in the previous subsection. Sommerfeld's result has been re-derived by several authors, including Born and Wolf [59, Chapter 11] using an angular spectrum approach (see Chapter 2) and by Skudrzyk [63]. We make use of the equations derived by Skudrzyk for a harmonic plane wave incident at an arbitrary angle φ on a half-plane as shown in Fig. 1.24a. For an incident plane wave of unit pressure amplitude, they can be written as

(1.120)
$$p(r{:}t) = e^{\left[j\left(\omega t - kr\cos\left(\frac{3\pi}{2} - \theta - \varphi\right)\right)\right]}\left\{\frac{1}{2} \pm \frac{j+1}{2}\int_0^{|\zeta|} e^{-j\pi s^2/2}\,ds\right\},$$ (a)

where

(1.120)
$$\zeta(r, \theta) = 2\sqrt{kr/\pi}\,\cos\left[\frac{3\pi}{4} - \frac{\theta + \varphi}{2}\right],$$ (b)

and the positive sign corresponds to the region where $\zeta > 0$ and the negative sign for $\zeta < 0$. These expressions can be put in terms of the normalized Cartesian coordinates for the observation point $(X_0 = x_0/\lambda, Y_0 = y_0/\lambda)$ by means of $r = \sqrt{x_0^2 + y_0^2}$ and $\varphi = \tan^{-1}(x_0/y_0)$. For normal incidence,

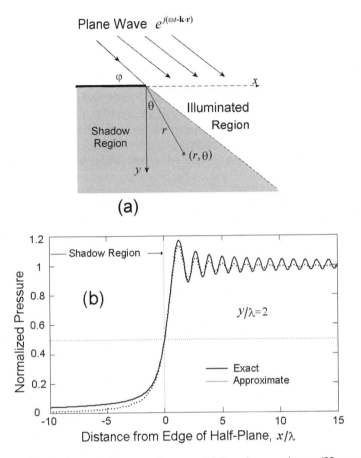

Figure 1.24 Comparison of the exact (Sommerfeld) and approximate (Huygens-Fresnel) analysis of diffraction by a half-plane. (a) Analysis geometry. (b) For normal incidence and observation points on the plane $y = 2\lambda$, the pressure magnitude was calculated from (1.119) for the approximate pattern and from (1.120) for the exact result.

$$\zeta(X_0, Y_0) = 2\sqrt{2}\left(X_0^2 + Y_0^2\right)^{1/4} \cos\left[\frac{\pi}{2} - \frac{\tan^{-1}(X_0/Y_0)}{2}\right],$$

so that on the shadow boundary where $X_0 = 0$, $\zeta = 0$, and consequently from (1.120a) the pressure is exactly half of the incident pressure. Moreover, for the illuminated region where $\zeta > 0$, by writing (1.120a) as

$$p(r{:}t) = e^{j\left[\omega t - kr\cos\left(\frac{3\pi}{2} - \theta - \varphi\right)\right]}\left\{1 + \left[-\frac{1}{2} + \frac{j+1}{2}\int_0^{|\zeta|} e^{-j\pi s^2/2}ds\right]\right\} = p_i + p_{d1},$$

it can be seen that the total field is the sum of the incident field plus the diffracted field, the latter being given by

$$p_{d1} = -e^{i\left[\omega t - kr\cos\left(\frac{3\pi}{2} - \theta - \varphi\right)\right]} \left[\frac{1}{2} - \frac{j+1}{2} \int_0^{|\zeta|} e^{-j\pi s^2/2} ds \right].$$

On the other hand, the only component that exists in the shadow region ($\zeta < 0$) is a diffracted field, and this is given by

$$p_{d2} = -e^{i\left[\omega t - kr\cos\left(\frac{3\pi}{2} - \theta - \varphi\right)\right]} \left[\frac{1}{2} - \frac{j+1}{2} \int_0^{|\zeta|} e^{-j\pi s^2/2} ds \right] = -p_{d1}.$$

Hence, for a rigid half-plane of negligible thickness, the field due to an incident plane wave can be treated as the superposition of a geometrical optics field and a diffraction field.

Fig. 1.24b compares the predictions of the above exact theory with that of the approximate Huygens-Fresnel theory for normal incidence and for observation points that are 2λ below the plane. While the general pattern is very similar, there are some differences in the detailed nature of the predicted fields.

1.7.4 Babinet's Principle

A principle that is attributed to a publication by Babinet in 1837 [59,60] concerns the field resulting from diffraction by apertures in a screen and its relation to that resulting from a complementary screen. A complementary screen is one with the same geometry but with the apertures replaced by opaque screens and the screens replaced by transparent apertures. For the arrangement illustrated in Fig. 1.25a, the plane screen has an arbitrary-shaped transparent aperture and is illuminated by a source of radiation. In the absence of the screen the velocity potential at any point is $\Phi_i(x,y,z)$. In the presence of the screen the velocity potential is denoted by $\Phi_t(x,y,z)$. For the complementary screen and aperture shown in Fig. 1.25b and the same radiation source as in Fig. 1.25a, the velocity potential field is denoted by $\Phi_o(x,y,z)$. Now Φ_t and Φ_o can be expressed as surface integrals[33] over the transparent regions, and because the entire surface area of the screen is exactly the sum of these two regions, it follows that $\Phi_t + \Phi_o = \Phi_i$, i.e., the sum of the two fields is exactly equal to the field in the absence of any screen.

Another form of Babinet's principle [60,63] is illustrated in Fig. 1.25 for an arbitrary aperture in a plane rigid screen that lies on the plane $x = 0$. Since the screen is assumed to be rigid, it acts as a perfect reflector and the normal component of the particle velocity on its surface will be zero. The screen is assumed to be insonated by a harmonic acoustic source that, in the absence of the screen, produces a velocity potential of $\Phi_i(x,y,z)$. At any location the total velocity potential can be expressed as the sum of the incident field and a diffracted field Φ_d, i.e.,

(1.121) $$\Phi(x, y, z) = \Phi_i(x, y, z) + \Phi_d(x, y, z).$$

---

33. The Huygens-Fresnel surface integral, as discussed in section 1.7.2, is an approximate form; more exact surface integrals are discussed in Chapter 2.

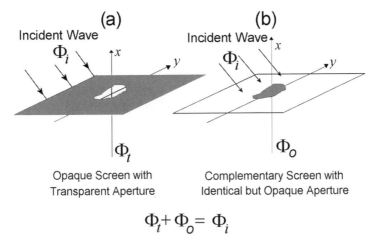

$$\Phi_t + \Phi_o = \Phi_i$$

Figure 1.25 Sketches used to illustrate Babinet's principle. (a) A plane opaque screen with a transparent aperture illuminated by a source. (b) A screen and aperture that is the complement of (a). The sum of the fields at the same location for the two cases is equal to the field in the absence of any screen.

For a point $(0,y,z)$ that lies within the area of the aperture area, it is evident that the diffracted field contribution will be zero $(\Phi_d(0,y,z) = 0)$, so that the velocity potential is simply that due to the source, i.e., $\Phi(0,y,z) = \Phi_i(0,y,z)$. Because the acoustic pressure for an inviscid medium is proportional to the velocity potential potential $(p = j\omega\Phi)$, this is equivalent to stating that the pressure at a point in the aperture area is equal to the incident pressure at that point. On the areas of the rigid opaque screen $\partial\Phi/\partial x = 0$, so that from (1.121) $\partial\Phi_i/\partial x = -\partial\Phi_d/\partial x$ on both the upper and lower faces of the screen. If we now consider a rigid screen with a plane source replacing the aperture shown in Fig. 1.26a (see Fig. 1.26b), and if the source and screen have identical boundary conditions to that of (a), then the field produced by the pressure source shown in (b) should be identical to that of (a). An equivalent result is obtained for the case in which the baffle in (a) is a soft baffle and the source in (b) is a rigid, and this is proven in [63].

1.8 Attenuation, Absorption, Scattering, and Dispersion

During its passage through a medium, an ideal plane wave will be subject to energy loss through absorption and a redirection of some of its energy by scattering due to changes in compressibility and density. Absorption is the process whereby ultrasound energy is converted into other energy forms such as heat, chemical energy, or light: it also includes the effects of heat conduction, which is discussed further in subsection 1.8.3. On the other hand, scattering represents ultrasound wave energy that has been redirected, much of which will be

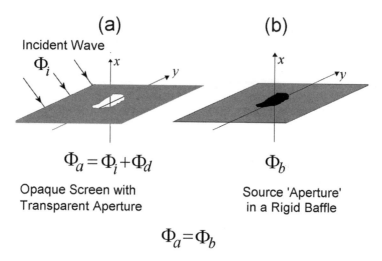

(a)

Incident Wave

Φ_i

x

y

$\Phi_a = \Phi_i + \Phi_d$

Opaque Screen with
Transparent Aperture

(b)

x

y

Φ_b

Source 'Aperture'
in a Rigid Baffle

$$\Phi_a = \Phi_b$$

Figure 1.26 Two plane rigid screens are shown that produce the same field for $x < 0$. (a) An incident wave results in a velocity potential that is given by (1.121). (b) A plane source of the same shape replaces the aperture. This source has the same pressure distribution as that produced by the incident wave within the aperture region of (a).

along paths that differ from the incident wave. The scattered energy can be subsequently absorbed and multiple scattering can occur. As discussed in section 1.6, it is convenient to consider the processes of reflection and refraction as special cases of scattering in which some of the incident radiation energy is redirected in an organized manner and the shadow region is a result of interference between the scattered wave and the incident wave in the absence of the scatterer (see Fig. 1.15). Attenuation accounts for the effects of both absorption and scattering (which includes reflection and refraction) and is most simply treated by considering its effects on a plane incident wave.

Consider the simple arrangement shown in Fig. 1.27a, in which a plane wave is incident on a specimen. If we assume that the coupling medium is perfectly matched to the specimen, then the energy that exits from the specimen in the direction of the incident wave can be calculated by considering the incremental cross-section of unit area shown in Fig. 1.27b. Over the incremental distance dx, the scattered power will be proportional to the time-averaged incident intensity $\bar{I}$ and dx, and similarly for the absorbed power. Consequently, each of these two components contributes to a loss of the transmitted beam intensity of

$$d\bar{I}_s = -2\alpha_s \bar{I}(x)dx, \quad d\bar{I}_a = -2\alpha_a \bar{I}(x)dx,$$

where α_s, α_a are coefficients that characterize the two processes. Thus, over the thickness of the slab the intensity changes by

$$d\bar{I} = d\bar{I}_s + d\bar{I}_a = -2(\alpha_s + \alpha_a)\bar{I}(x)dx \quad or \quad \frac{d\bar{I}}{\bar{I}(x)} = -2(\alpha_s + \alpha_a)dx$$

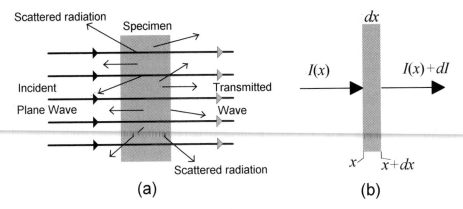

Figure 1.27 Absorption and attenuation. (a) Distinguishing between the absorbed, scattered, and attenuated waves for a simple plane specimen. (b) Change in intensity for the passage of a plane wave through an incremental distance dx.

If the incident intensity at $x = 0$ is $\bar{I}(0)$, then the intensity at a location x in the specimen can be found by integration as

(1.122)
$$\bar{I}(x) = \bar{I}(0)e^{-2(\alpha_s + \alpha_a)x} = \bar{I}(0)e^{-2\alpha x}$$

where α is the *amplitude attenuation coefficient*, which is simply the sum of the scattering and absorption amplitude attenuation coefficients ($\alpha = \alpha_s = \alpha_a$). The attenuation coefficient is dependent on frequency, temperature, and pressure.

From (1.122) it will be noted that the units for α are m^{-1}, but in practice the units are generally expressed as nepers/centimeter, or simply Np/cm. To expedite "back of the envelope" calculations, it is helpful to deal with a logarithmic scale. By taking the logarithm to the base 10 of both sides of (1.122) and multiplying by 10 we find that

$$10\log\{\bar{I}(0)/\bar{I}(x)\} = 20\alpha x \log(e) = 8.686\,\alpha x.$$

If we define $\alpha_{dB} = 8.686\alpha$, then the attenuation coefficient can be written in terms of either the intensity or pressure and is generally expressed in dB/cm (deciBels/cm) as

(1.123)
$$\boxed{\alpha_{dB} = \frac{10}{x}\log\{\bar{I}(0)/\bar{I}(x)\}}.$$
(a)

The presence of attenuation results in a phase difference between the pressure and the particle velocity, causing the specific acoustic impedance to contain both real and imaginary parts. Nonetheless, for attenuation coefficients that are not too large, the pressure amplitude $p_o^2(x) \propto \bar{I}(x)$, so that

(1.123)
$$\boxed{\alpha_{dB} = \frac{20}{x}\log[p_o(0)/p_o(x)]}.$$
(b)

It is convenient to note that the conversion of dB/cm to Np/cm and vice versa can be achieved through:

$$(1.124) \qquad \alpha_{dB} = 8.686\,\alpha_{Np}$$
$$\alpha_{Np} = 0.1151\,\alpha_{dB}.$$

An important advantage of the dB scale is that in calculating the total attenuation over a path involving several different attenuation coefficients and interface reflections and transmissions, the total intensity loss can be quickly estimated though a simple addition of the various contributions.

1.8.1 Absorption and Scattering Attenuation Coefficients

The attenuation coefficient expressed above was defined in terms of the effects of absorption and scattering on an incident *plane* wave. Ideally, measurements should be made using a wave that closely approximates a plane wave; if this is not possible, corrections must be applied to account for the nonplanar characteristics of the field.[34] Many additional difficulties are encountered in accurately measuring the attenuation coefficient, and even more are encountered in attempting to determine the relative contributions of scattering and absorption. Even with an ideal incident plane wave and perfect impedance matching to the specimen, the transmitted wave amplitude will always include a portion of the scattered field. A small receiving transducer aperture placed far away enables the forward scattered field contribution to be reduced. In practice, either a long pulse that is nearly monochromatic or a wide bandwidth pulse can be used. For the broadband pulse the frequency spectra of both the incident and transmitted pulse waveforms are determined, and from these the attenuation coefficient can be determined over a range of frequencies. Bamber [64–66] has reviewed the merits and problems associated with different measurement techniques and provided an assessment of the sources of error.

Initially it was widely thought that attenuation in tissue was caused entirely by absorption, and consequently many of the early results were reported as absorption rather than attenuation measurements. By the mid-1970s it was realized [76,77] that tissue scattering could form an appreciable contribution to attenuation, and subsequently a number of papers were published showing the relative contributions for a variety of tissues. Table 1.7 summarizes some of the results published by Nassiri and Hill [78]. Additional results have been summarized by Bamber [65]. They point out that for some biological fluids (amniotic fluid, aqueous humor, and vitreous humour), scattering has not been observed at diagnostic ultrasound frequencies, while for lung tissue and trabecular bone, with their porous-like structure and very high attenuation coefficients, scattering appears to predominate. However, Wear [79] has reported that over the range 300 to 700 kHz, the frequency dependence of the backscattering from the calcaneus (heelbone) is proportional to the cube of the fre-

---

34. The effects of diffraction will always be present for a finite-size radiation source, and errors as high as 30% can result if corrections are not applied [64].

Table 1.7. Contributions of Scattering to the Attenuation Coefficient*

Medium	$2\alpha_s$, cm^{-1}	2α, cm^{-1}	α_s/α	Freq.
Fresh human liver	0.09	0.72	12%	4 MHz
Fresh human liver	0.32	1.4	23%	7 MHz
Human blood, Hct = 40%	0.28×10^{-3}	0.17	0.1%	4 MHz
Human blood, Hct = 40%	1.8×10^{-3}	0.37	0.5%	7 MHz
Fresh skeletal muscle	0.16	0.94	17%	4 MHz
Fresh skeletal muscle	0.32	1.8	18%	7 MHz

*Data from Nassari and Hill [78].

quency, whereas the attenuation is proportional to the frequency. Based on this difference he concluded that absorption is a greater component of attenuation than scattering.

Frequency Dependence of the Attenuation Coefficient

Our primary purpose in this subsection is to provide an empirical description of the frequency dependence of the attenuation coefficient. Since attenuation is a combination of the effects of absorption and scattering, its frequency dependence combines the frequency dependence of both phenomena. A theoretical account of scattering, including the frequency dependence, together with a summary of experimental observations on biological media is given in Chapter 5. For pure fluids there will be no scattering, and as a result the attenuation and absorption characteristics are identical. For many pure fluids, primarily the effects of viscous govern the attenuation and relaxation losses, and these are accounted for by the shear and bulk viscosity coefficients μ and μ_B. The theoretical analysis presented in Chapter 3 shows that the effects of both coefficients give rise to an attenuation frequency dependence that, to a first order, varies as the square of the frequency. Thus $\alpha = \alpha_o f^2$, where α_o is a temperature-dependent factor with units that can be expressed in Np/(cm.MHz^2) or dB/(cm.MHz^2), where f is in MHz. Because pure water is frequently used as a reference medium for speed and attenuation measurements, accurate measurement of the speed (see Fig. 1.5) and attenuation is particularly important. The experimental results reported by Pinkerton [80] are frequently used as a standard. He measured the dependence of the attenuation coefficient both on frequency and temperature and showed that over a very wide range of temperatures, the square law frequency dependence is accurately obeyed. In fact, subsequent measurements [81] showed that a quadratic frequency dependence holds to at least 3 GHz. Pinkerton's results are summarized in Fig. 1.28, where the attenuation values shown on the vertical axis are those for 1 MHz, and the values at any other frequency can be obtained by multiplying by the square of the frequency in MHz.

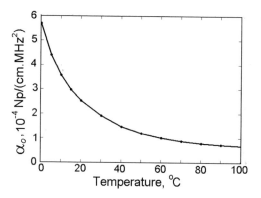

Figure 1.28 Experimental results showing the temperature dependence of the attenuation factor for water. The points are those given by Pinkerton [see Table I in reference 80]. The vertical axis is the value of the attenuation factor $\alpha_o = \alpha/f^2$, where f is expressed in MHz. For example, at 5 MHz and 20°C, the attenuation is $2.53 \times 10^{-4} \times 5^2 = 0.00633$ Np/cm ($\equiv 0.055$ dB/cm).

Attenuation of Biological Tissues

A variety of experimental methods have been used for determining the attenuation-versus-frequency characteristics of biological specimens, many of which have been reviewed by Bamber [64]. It has also been demonstrated that in vivo measurements can be made through the extraction and processing of data from ultrasonic diagnostic measurement systems. A compilation [64–66] of the results from many different sources under a variety of experimental conditions is shown in Fig. 1.29. Most of the results have been obtained on excised specimens For some media there may be appreciable differences between the characteristics measured from an extracted specimen and those measured in vivo, perhaps due to the presence of blood flow, though variations can also be expected to arise from the conditions under which the specimen is stored. It can be seen that a good approximation for the frequency dependence for most soft tissue is given by[35]

(1.125)
$$\alpha = \alpha_o f^n,$$

where n lies in the range from 1 to 2. For bone, although the attenuation is generally much higher than soft tissue, it also exhibits a power law dependence, though over a more limited frequency range. A great deal of effort has been devoted to developing methods that make use of the attenuation-versus-frequency characteristics as a means of identifying abnormal tissue. The initial expectations for the diagnostic uses of tissue characterization were arguably not fulfilled, except perhaps in one area: that of osteoporosis assessment, as described in the next subsection.

---

35. Sometimes this equation is written in terms of the angular frequency, i.e., $\alpha = \alpha_o' \omega^n$, so that $\alpha_o = \alpha_o'(2\pi)^n$.

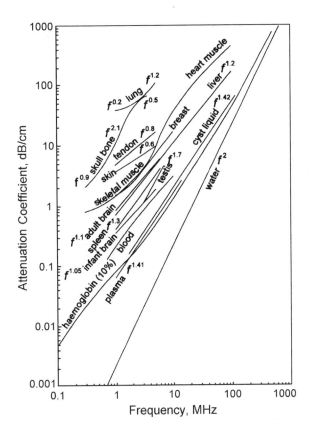

Figure 1.29 Summary of published experimental results for the attenuation-versus-frequency characteristics of various biological media and water. The approximate value of the power-law dependence on frequency is also indicated. References to the data sources are given in Bamber [64]. (Reproduced, with permission of IOP Publishing Ltd., from Bamber [65], Ch. 4 in *Ultrasound in Medicine*, © 1998 Institute of Physics.)

A useful compilation of measured values for soft human tissue of the speed of sound, density, attenuation, and parameter of nonlinearity (see Chapter 4) is that that given in Table 1.8. The values are those used by Mast [67] in his investigation of the correlation between various acoustic parameters. For example, he showed that the density and speed of sound values for a wide range of tissue types are quite strongly correlated (corr. coeft. = 0.917).

Because of the importance of measuring the backscattering by blood and because these generally require substantial corrections for the effects of attenuation, considerable effort has been made to determine the attenuation characteristics of blood over a range of frequencies and hematocrits. For example, Wang and Shung [68] have measured the attenuation of porcine red blood cell suspensions and found that the attenuation increases with frequency and to a first order increases linearly with hematocrit. This is illustrated in Fig. 1.30.

Table 1.8. Properties of Certain Soft Human Tissue at 37°C*

Human Tissue Type	c_o m/s	ρ_o kg/m^3	α_{dB}, @1 MHz dB/cm	B/A Parameter of Nonlinearity
Connective	1613	1120	1.57	—
Muscle	1547	1050	1.09	—
Fat	1478	950	0.48	—
Adipose	1450	950	0.29	10.0
Blood	1584	1060	0.20	6.1
Brain	1560	1040	0.60	7.1
Breast	1510	1020	0.75	—
Eye: lens	1645	1070	0.80	—
Eye: vitreous	1528	1010	0.1	—
Kidney	1560	1050	1.0	7.4
Liver	1595	1060	0.50	6.6
Muscle, cardiac	1576	1060	0.52	7.1
Muscle, skeletal	1580	1050	0.74	6.6
Skin	1615	1090	0.35	7.9
Fatty	1465	0985	0.40	8.5
Non-fatty	1575	1055	0.60	7.0
Blood cells	1627	1093	0.28	—
Blood plasma	1543	1027	0.069	—
Eye: cornea	1586	1076	—	—
Spinal cord	1542	1038	—	—
Spleen	1567	1054	0.4	7.8
Testis	1595	1044	0.17	—

*Reproduced, with permission, from Mast [67], *Acoustics Res. Lett.*, 1, 37–42, © 2000 Acoustical Society of America.

Osteoporosis Assessment Using Attenuation and Speed

Cancellous (trabecular or spongy) bone, unlike compact (cortical) bone, is a 3-D network of bony plates and columns: fat and bone marrow fills the spaces between them. Osteoporosis is a metabolic bone disease characterized by low bone mass density and microarchitectural deterioration of bone tissue, causing increased bone fragility that leads to a greater susceptibility to fractures, especially of the wrist, spine, and hip. The economic cost associated with the resulting treatment and hospitalizations is enormous, and as a result a great deal of effort has been expended on developing noninvasive methods for detecting those at risk and for monitoring the effects of treatment. Such methods use a variety of approaches, including attenuation measurements of photons emitted from radionuclide source (e.g., single photon absorptiometry), dual photon X-ray absorptiometry, quantitative CT, and quantitative ultrasound [69,70].

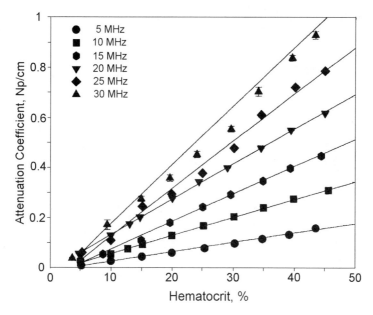

Figure 1.30 Measured results for the attenuation of porcine red blood cell suspensions in a buffered saline solution. To a first order, the attenuation varies linearly with hematocrit. (Reproduced, with permission, from Wang and Shung [68], *IEEE Trans. Biomed. Eng.*, 44, 549–554, © 1997 IEEE.)

Ultrasound methods have focused on two variables, the speed of sound and broadband attenuation, both of which can be measured noninvasively using relatively inexpensive systems. The broadband ultrasonic attenuation (BUA) is the slope of the attenuation-frequency characteristics measured in dB/(MHz.cm), which is found by linearly fitting the attenuation values over a fairly broad frequency range. Both the speed and BUA are related to the bone density, and evidence has been presented that this relationship appears to be linear [71]. Following publication of the seminal work by Langton et al. [72,73] in 1984, much effort has been devoted toward developing measurement systems that could be used clinically, and a number of such systems became commercially available by the mid-1990s. Many of the clinical studies measured the speed and attenuation of the calcaneus (heelbone) by transmission. The calcaneus, which is 90% cancellous bone, is readily accessible and has reasonably flat surfaces. An important advantage of measuring cancellous bone is that its attenuation has a frequency dependence that is close to unity over a broad frequency range (e.g., 0.2–1 MHz). For example, measurements made [74] on 1-cm-thick specimens of trabecular bone taken from the calcaneus of 14 human cadavers yielded $\alpha \approx 14f^{1.09}$ over the frequency range from 0.2 to 1.7 MHz. However, the range of values for α_o was from 2 to 40 (dB/cm) and that for n was 0.4 to 2.2. Nonetheless, it was found that α_o was strongly correlated to the bone mineral density, which contributes in an important way to the bone strength.

Some ultrasonic measurement schemes are illustrated in Fig. 1.31. In (a) the transmitting and receiving transducers are gel coupled to the skin and are at a fixed distance apart. Generally, a speed measurement is made by the time of flight of a broadband pulse from transmitter to receiver. The bone thickness, which does affect the time of flight, may not be easily measured, and as a result the speed is sometimes calculated based on an assumed thickness that can be based on normal values for a particular age, size, and sex. A further difficulty in speed measurements arise from the large frequency-dependent attenuation and phase speed that can cause distortion of the received waveform, making it difficult to determine the time of flight [75]. As illustrated in (b), the time of flight can be measured with and without the heel: the difference enables the speed to be determined. Measurement of the BUA is best made by the substitution method, in which a medium with a known frequency-dependent attenuation is used as a reference. If degassed water is used, then, over the frequency range normally employed (0.2–0.5 MHz), the reference medium can

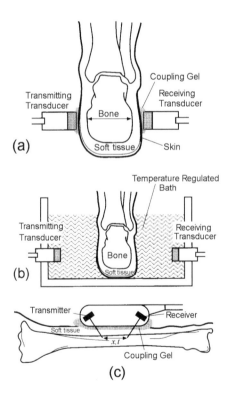

Figure 1.31 Methods for measuring speed of sound in bone. (a) Gel-coupled system. (b) Water bath system. (c) Axial transmission system. (Reprinted by permission of Elsevier from Njeh et al. [69], Ch. 4, in *Quantative Ultrasound: Assessment of Osteoporosis and Bone Status*, Martin Dunitz Ltd, © 1999 Elsevier.)

be assumed to be non-attenuating. The frequency-dependent attenuation can be calculated by taking the Fourier transform of the received signals with and without the reference. Because the bone thickness may not be known, and the variation between subjects in a given disease category is small, the BUA is generally expressed as $x\alpha_{dB}$ (dB/MHz) and might be in the range 40 to 70 dB/MHz.

Absorption Mechanism

Absorption occurs when a phase difference occurs between the pressure and density, and this can be caused by classical viscous friction or by relaxation processes. Various types of relaxational processes have been proposed and theoretically developed. As pointed out by Markham et al. [82], the theories fit into four groups: (i) kinetic theory, (ii) irreversible thermodynamics, (iii) statistical thermodynamics, and (iv) phenomenological approach. As noted earlier, absorption and dispersion are intimately related. Based on causality, relations known as the Kramers-Kronig equations can be derived, and these enable the phase speed to be expressed in terms of the absorption coefficient (see section 3.9).

For soft tissue, it is generally believed that relaxation mechanisms play a dominant role. During the passage of an ultrasound wave through a medium that perhaps consists of large molecules of different types, there will be many degrees of freedom. The ultrasound energy at a given location at a specific time can be redistributed as the molecular translational and vibrational energy and the "lattice" energy. The distribution of energy at any given instant depends on the coupling of the various modes. Since the rate at which the energy from the acoustic wave is redistributed is finite, energy that was redistributed may be returned out of phase with the acoustic wave, constituting energy loss. If the frequency is sufficiently low so that the rate of energy redistribution is not a limiting factor, the absorption will be small. Similarly, at very high frequencies, there will be insufficient time for significant energy coupling, and the loss can be expected to decrease as the frequency is raised. In the intermediate range, when the frequency is close to the characteristic relaxation frequencies of the processes, the absorption will be high. In a complex medium, there would be a wide distribution of relaxation frequencies present such that the distribution can be regarded as quasi-continuous. If this is the case, the absorption characteristics might be expected to increase with frequency in a simple monotonic manner.

A second type of relaxation—*structural relaxation*—is associated with changes in the short-term order. For water, Hall [83] presented good evidence that this could account for the difference between the calculated frequency-dependent absorption coefficient and that measured (see subsection 1.8.3).

Our understanding of the mechanism of absorption in biological tissue is far from complete. Accounting for and measuring the absorption characteristics of gases, fluids, and tissue has been an area of considerable scientific effort over the past 150 years, and much of this has been summarized in books and journal articles [64,82,84,85].

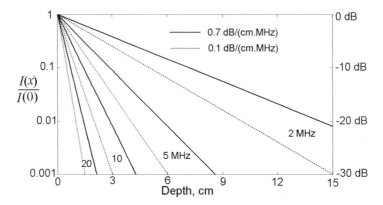

Figure 1.32 Intensity of a harmonic plane wave as it propagates in a tissue-like medium at frequencies in the range 2 to 20 MHz. Two typical values have been assumed for the frequency-dependent attenuation factor.

Some Effects of Frequency Dependent-Attenuation and Scattering

The effect of attenuation in the propagation of harmonic plane waves is illustrated in Fig. 1.32. This shows the one-way intensity ratio for various frequencies and two different values of the attenuation factor (α_o) assuming a power law frequency dependence with an exponent $n = 1.0$. If a perfect reflector were placed at a given depth parallel to the plane of the wave, the signal returned to the surface would be attenuated twice, and as a result the intensity reduction expressed in dB's would be doubled.

An important effect of frequency-dependent attenuation concerns its effects on a wide bandwidth transmitted pulse. For $n > 0$, the center frequency of such a pulse will be down-shifted as it progresses, causing the pulse duration to be increased. As an example we consider the plane-wave Gaussian modulated sinusoidal pressure pulse, as expressed by (1.43) and (1.44), with a center frequency of f_c and a -6 dB fractional bandwidth of $\sigma_\omega/(2.66 f_c)$. This was used in our earlier discussion of the effects of dispersion. By multiplying the frequency domain representation of this pulse, as given by (1.45), by the amplitude exponential attenuation factor of $e^{-x\alpha_o f^n}$, the attenuated amplitude spectrum is given by

$$(1.126) \qquad \underline{p}(x\!:\!y) = p_o \frac{\sqrt{2\pi}}{\sigma_\omega} e^{-jx(2\pi f/c_o)} e^{-2\pi^2(f-f_c)^2/\sigma_\omega^2} e^{-x\alpha_o f^n},$$

in which it has been assumed that the effects of velocity dispersion are negligible ($c_\phi = c_o$). By differentiating with respect to f and equating to zero, the following equation can be obtained:

$$f_{max} - f_c + \frac{n f_{max}^{n-1} \alpha_o x \sigma_\omega^2}{4\pi^2} = 0,$$

where f_{max} is the peak frequency. For $n = 1$ and 2, the roots of this equation can be obtained analytically, enabling the change in peak frequency to be expressed as[36]

(1.127)
$$\Delta f_1 = f_{max} - f_c = \frac{-\alpha_o x \sigma_\omega^2}{4\pi^2}, \qquad n = 1$$

$$\Delta f_2 = f_{max} - f_c = \frac{-f_c 2\alpha_o x \sigma_\omega^2}{2\alpha_o x \sigma_\omega^2 + 4\pi^2}, \qquad n = 2.$$

Thus, it can be seen that the center frequency is down-shifted by an amount that increases with depth. In the case $n = 1$, it can be seen that the change in peak frequency is directly proportional to the depth, and increases as the square of the incident pulse bandwidth. For both cases it can be shown that the spectrum is Gaussian [86] and that for $n = 1$ the variance remains unchanged, while for $n = 2$ it is reduced.

To illustrate these changes, (1.126) and (1.127) have been evaluated at a depth of 6.0 cm for a center frequency (f_c) of 5.0 MHz, a –6 dB fractional bandwidth of ~0.376, corresponding to $\sigma_\omega = 5.0 \times 10^6 s^{-1}$, $n = 1$, and α_o values of 0, 1, and 2 dB/(cm.MHz). The normalized frequency spectra calculated from the magnitude of (1.126) are plotted in Fig. 1.33a. In addition, Fig. 1.33b shows the change in center frequency as a function of depth for $n = 1$ and 2 for two values of the attenuation factor.

As discussed in Chapter 5, backscattering is also a frequency-dependent process that can be approximately represented by a power law ($\propto f^m$), especially for scatterers whose dimensions are small compared to a wavelength. Specifically, for small spherical scatterers, $m = 4$, while for infinite cylinders whose radii are small compared to a wavelength, $m = 9/4$. Soft tissue measurements indicate that m is typically in the range from 3 to 4. Round and Bates [87] studied the influence of scattering on the spectrum when the incident pulse is Gaussian and obtained approximate expressions for the center frequency and bandwidth. They also investigated the combined effect of scattering and attenuation on the spectrum. More recently, Wear [88] performed experimental and theoretical studies of the combined effect. As can be seen in Fig. 1.34a, while the center frequency increases with m, the bandwidth diminishes. When the effects of both frequency-dependent scattering and attenuation are included, the center frequency can either decrease or increase, depending on the depth and other parameters. An example is shown in Fig. 1.34b, in which the pulse-echo signal spectrum is shown for a scatterer at a depth of 6 cm.

1.8.2 Heat Generation

The process of ultrasound absorption generally involves conversion of virtually all the absorbed energy into heat rather than into other energy forms. A

---

36. If the intensity had been assumed to be Gaussian (rather than the amplitude) with a frequency standard deviation of σ_f, the values for Δf_1 and Δf_2 would be the same as those given by (1.127), but with σ_f replacing σ_ω and $\frac{1}{2}$ replacing $(2\pi)^2$, in agreement with the equations (11) and (13) given by Narayana and Ophir in [86].

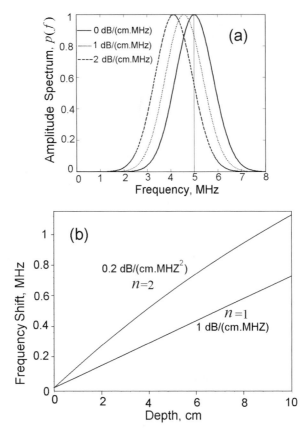

Figure 1.33 The spectrum of a Gaussian modulated sinusoidal pressure pulse, in the form of a plane wave, is down-shifted by the effect of attenuation. The pulse was assumed to be characterized by $f_c = 5.0\,\text{MHz}$ and $\sigma_\omega = 5.0 \times 10^6\,\text{s}^{-1}$. (a) Spectrum at a depth of 6.0 cm for $n = 1$ and three different values of α_o. The spectra have been normalized to the center frequency of each. Specifically, at the center frequencies of the three spectra the amplitudes are attenuated by: 0, −28.7, and −54.7 dB, respectively. (b) The change in center frequency as a function of depth for $n = 1$ and 2, as calculated from (1.127).

variety of ultrasound devices for treatment [89–91] and surgery [92] make use of the fact that when the incident intensity is sufficiently high and well focused, fairly localized heating of tissue can be achieved in a zone remote from the skin surface. Since the 1930s ultrasound has been used in physiotherapy for localized tissue heating. In more recent years ultrasound has been used for hyperthermia. Hyperthermia is the process of heating a volume to sufficiently high temperatures (42 to 46°C) for a sufficient length of time (minutes to several hours) to cause cell destruction. As a therapeutic modality for tumor destruction, ultrasound hyperthermia can be used alone. However, it is more frequently used in combination with other therapeutic modalities such as

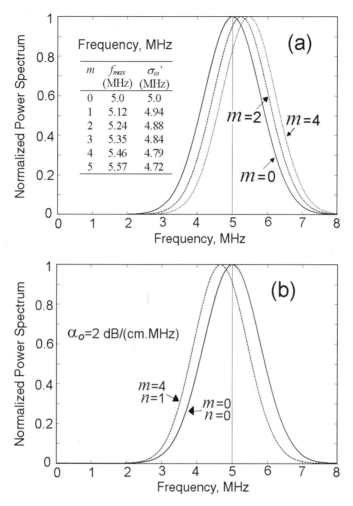

Figure 1.34 Changes in the spectra due to frequency-dependent scattering and attenuation for a Gaussian modulated incident pulse ($f_c = 5.0\,\text{MHz}$, $\sigma_\omega = 5.0 \times 10^6 \text{s}^{-1}$). (a) Due to frequency-dependent backscattering in the absence of attenuation. (b) Due to attenuation and backscattering at a depth of 6 cm.

chemotherapy or radiation therapy. The objective is to induce cell death in a localized volume without causing damage to the surrounding tissue. This proves to be a rather challenging task, because such factors as heat transport by blood, thermal conduction, and the temperature dependence of the attenuation coefficient make it difficult to accurately predict the temperature distribution. Clearly, though, the ability to predict the rate of heat production per unit volume for a given incident field is of major importance.

We shall assume that scattering can be ignored and that all the absorbed energy is converted into heat. For simplicity, the incident energy will be assumed to be in the form of a plane harmonic wave. If the medium has an amplitude absorption coefficient of α_a, the rate of heat production per unit volume can be found by differentiating (1.122),

$$(1.128) \qquad \overline{q_v} = -\frac{d\overline{I}(x)}{dx} = 2\alpha_a \overline{I}(x).$$

For a plane harmonic wave, the time-averaged intensity was expressed in terms of either the pressure (p_o) or velocity (v_o) amplitudes by means of (1.87). By using this expression, two alternative forms for the average heat production rate are given by

$$(1.129) \qquad \overline{q_v} = \frac{\alpha_a p_o^2}{\rho_o c_o} \qquad \qquad (a)$$

$$= \rho_o c_o \alpha_a v_o^2. \qquad \qquad (b)$$

If the absorption coefficient has a power-law frequency dependence of $\alpha_a = \alpha_{ao} f^n$, then from (1.122) and (1.128)

$$\overline{q_v} = 2\alpha_{ao} f^n \overline{I}(0) e^{-2\alpha_{ao} f^n x}.$$

By differentiation with respect to f, it can be readily shown that for the same incident intensity the heat production rate at a given depth is a maximum when the frequency is given by $f_{opt} = 1/(2\alpha_{ao}x)^{1/n}$. As illustrated in Fig. 1.35, for media whose absorption coefficient varies either linearly with frequency or as $f^{1.5}$, the optimal frequency diminishes with increasing depth and decreasing n. These and other practical aspects related to ultrasound surgery have been discussed by Hill [93].

Although (1.129a), expressing the rate of heat production in terms of the incident pressure amplitude, assumed an incident plane wave, Nyborg has shown [94] that the same expression is obtained for an arbitrary incident wave provided the shear viscosity (μ) is negligible.[37] This assumption implies that absorption must arise from mechanisms other than viscous shear losses. Nonetheless, for a plane wave (1.129a) remains true even in the presence of viscous losses.

1.8.3 Absorption and the Bulk (Volume) Viscosity of Fluids

In 1845 Stokes first noted the possibility that liquids could possess a bulk viscosity. By assuming that the propagation process for a compressional wave was purely adiabatic, and that the effects of bulk viscosity could be ignored, he obtained the following classical equation for the absorption coefficient of ultrasound in fluids[38]

$$(1.130) \qquad \alpha_c \approx \frac{2\omega^2 \kappa \mu}{3c_o},$$

37. This assumption makes the stress tensor isotropic. Note that that bulk viscosity can still have a non-zero value.

38. See subsection 3.10.3 for a derivation.

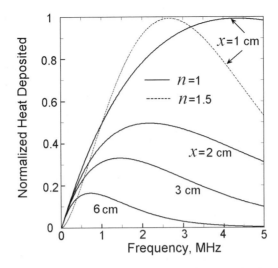

Figure 1.35 Dependence of the normalized average heat production rate per unit volume on frequency at various depths for incident plane waves. The medium was assumed to have a frequency-dependent absorption coefficient of either $1\,dB/(cm.MHz)$ or $1\,dB/(cm.MHz^{1.5})$ and the same incident intensity.

where κ is the adiabatic compressibility and μ is the shear viscosity. Subsequently, in 1868 Kirchhoff described how thermal conduction could affect the absorption coefficient and showed that

$$(1.131) \qquad \alpha_c = \frac{\omega^2 \kappa}{2c_o}\left[\frac{4}{3}\mu + (\gamma - 1)\frac{\mathcal{K}}{C_p}\right],$$

where $\gamma = C_p/C_v$ is the ratio of specific heats and $\mathcal{K}$ is the thermal conductivity of the medium. For water, the thermal contribution is less than 0.1%, but for other liquids it can be considerably higher (~8% for acetone), while for gases the two contributions are of similar magnitude (~40% for oxygen at NTP) [18, p. 267].

As previously explained, thermal conduction affects α because heat will flow from the crests of the pressure wave towards the valleys, which tends to smooth out the temperature fluctuations. Compressed regions on re-expanding do less work than was expended on compression, and as a result energy is lost. Also, as previously noted, a longitudinal wave behaves more adiabatically at lower frequencies because the ω^2 dependence of thermal conduction more than compensates for the increased time interval ($1/\omega$) over which conduction can occur [6, p. 275; 7, p. 45].

In practice, the measured absorption coefficients are significantly higher than those predicted by (1.130) or (1.131). For example, in water at 20°C, α is approximately 3.1 times greater [80]. Good evidence has been presented that structural relaxation [83,95] processes can play an important role in the passage of a compressional wave. For instance, in water the short-range molecular structure will be changed during compression, and these structural changes will generally be out of phase with the pressure, leading to energy loss. Other loss mechanisms, such as *thermal relaxation*, can also be important [96]. Specifically, associated with the passage of a compressional wave, there will be very rapid changes in temperature due to the adiabatic nature of the propagation process. For example, these temperature changes can cause the equilibrium of molecular reaction to be perturbed, or perhaps redistribute energy between the vibrational and rotational modes of molecules, all of which can result in energy loss.

To account for these energy loss mechanisms as well as the classical viscous shear loss and thermal conduction, an additional bulk (volume) viscous term is often introduced whose value, when added to the shear viscosity, gives the correct value for α. Inclusion of a bulk viscosity μ_B in the Navier-Stokes equation results in:

$$(1.132) \qquad \alpha_t = \frac{\omega^2 \kappa}{2c_o}\left[\frac{4}{3}\mu + \mu_B + (\gamma - 1)\frac{\mathcal{K}}{C_p}\right]$$

If the measured value of the absorption coefficient is denoted by α_m, then for this to be equal to α_t, the ratio of the two viscous components, in the absence of thermal loss, can be found from (1.131) and (1.132) as

$$(1.133) \qquad \frac{\mu_B}{\mu} = \frac{4}{3}\frac{(\alpha_m - \alpha_c)}{\alpha_c},$$

which forms the basis of the method for determining μ_B. For example, Pinkerton [80] has found that for water at 15°C, $\mu_B = 2.81\mu = 0.0031$ kg/m.s, and Litovitz and Davis [95] have listed values for μ_B for a wide variety of fluids.

1.8.4 Shear Wave Absorption in Fluids and Tissue

As previously noted, the differential equation describing the particle velocity in a fluid medium can be separated into two equations. One describes the longitudinal component $\mathbf{v_L}$ which curl$\mathbf{v_L}$ = 0, the other describing $\mathbf{v_T}$ for which div($\mathbf{v_T}$) = 0, where the total velocity is given by $\mathbf{v} = \mathbf{v_L} + \mathbf{v_T}$. The latter is rewritten here as

$$(1.134) \qquad \rho_o \frac{\partial \mathbf{v_T}}{\partial t} = -\mu \nabla \times \nabla \times \mathbf{v_T},$$

where μ is the shear viscosity.

If we consider a plane transverse (shear) y-polarized wave propagating in the x-direction with an attenuation constant α, then, to a first order, there will be no pressure or density variations due to such a wave. The particle velocity in the y-direction for such a wave can be represented by

$$(1.135) \qquad v_{Ty} = v_o e^{j(\omega t - kx)} e^{-\alpha x},$$

where the wave number $k = \omega/c_T$ and c_T is the transverse wave speed. By substituting (1.34) into (1.135), and by noting that v_{Ty} is independent of y and z, the curl term can be evaluated and we find that $j\omega\rho_o = \mu(jk + \alpha)^2$. But since

$$\sqrt{j} = (1+j)/\sqrt{2}, \quad \text{this results in} \quad k = \sqrt{\frac{\omega \rho_o}{2\mu}}, \quad \text{and} \quad \alpha = \sqrt{\frac{\omega \rho_o}{2\mu}}.$$

Hence, $c_T = \sqrt{2\omega\mu/\rho_o}$, and $\alpha = \omega/c_T = 2\pi/\lambda_T$, where λ_T is the wavelength. Thus, over a distance of one wavelength, the amplitude decreases decreases by $e^{-2\pi}$ = 535. For example, let us calculate the wavelength of a shear wave in water at 20°C and 1.0 MHz. From Table 1.1 $\mu = 0.001$ kg/m.s and $\rho_o = 1000$ kg/m³, yielding $\lambda_T = 3.7\,\mu$m. Consequently, high-frequency shear waves in most fluids are very rapidly attenuated and it is a good approximation to assume that only longitudinal waves are propagated at such frequencies.

On the other hand, soft biological tissue and tissue-like media have a non-zero shear modulus (second Lamé constant, μ_ℓ) that results in wave-mode conversion at abrupt interfaces. By measuring the complex reflection coefficient between the sample and an optically flat fused silica surface, Madsen et al. [97] have determined the transverse wave speed and attenuation coefficient of a number of biological media over a frequency range from 2 to 14 MHz. Some of the results from this study are summarized in Table 1.9. It will be noted that the transverse wave speeds are a small fraction of the longitudinal speeds. Moreover, the attenuation coefficients result in penetration depths on the order of 1 μm.

Problems

P1. A 4-MHz CW ultrasound plane wave whose intensity is 3 mW/cm² is propagated from a planar source into caster oil (a good tissue-mimicking fluid) at 28°C. At this temperature and frequency, $\rho_o = 946$ kg/m³, $c_o = 1452$ m/s, and $\alpha = 0.7$ dB/cm.
At distances: (a) Close to the source and (b) 2.0 cm from the source, determine: (i) Particle displacement amplitude, (ii) Particle velocity amplitude, (iii) Acoustic density amplitude, and (iv) Pressure amplitude.

P2. A small-signal plane wave consisting of a symmetric square waveform whose fundamental frequency is 10 MHz is launched into a water-like medium whose attenuation constant is 0.5 dB/cm at 1.0 MHz and that varies with frequency to the power of 1.5. Assuming $c_o = 1600$ m/s and

Table 1.9. Transverse Wave Speed and Attenuation in Various Biological Media*

Medium	~Speed, m/s	~Attenuation, Np/cm	Comments
Bovine striated muscle	20–50	4000–18000	From 3 to 14 MHz: both increase with frequency
Bovine cardiac muscle	16–54	5000–20000	From 3 to 14 MHz: both increase with frequency
Bovine liver	10–75	10000–22000	From 3 to 14 MHz: both increase with frequency

*Values listed are those reported by Madsen et al. [97].

$Z_o = 1.7\,\text{MRay}$, determine the distance at which the beam intensity is reduced to 15% of the value at the launching site, and plot graphs to show the waveform at that distance and the power spectrum (in dBs).

P3. Consider the propagation of a plane sinusoidal wave into carbon tetrachloride. This fluid exhibits classical viscous loss over a very wide frequency range. Assuming that the attenuation factor is given by $\alpha_o = 0.535\,\text{Np/[m.(MHz)}^2]$, and $c_o = 926\,\text{m/s}$ at $10.0\,\text{MHz}$, determine the frequency at which the imaginary part of the specific acoustic impedance is 10% of the real part.

P4. A sphere of radius a is pulsates harmonically with a velocity amplitude of v_o and radiates into an inviscid medium whose characteristic impedance is Z_o. The velocity potential for $r \geq a$ is given by

$$\phi(r:t) = \frac{\phi_0 e^{j(\omega t - kr)}}{r}.$$

a. Show that the particle velocity for $r \geq a$ is given by

$$v(r:t) = v_o \frac{a^2}{r^2} \frac{1 + jka}{1 + jkr} e^{-jk(r-a)} e^{j\omega t}, \text{ and that the acoustic radiation}$$

impedance seen by the sphere is $\underline{Z} = Z_o \dfrac{(ka)^2 + jka}{1 + (ka)^2}$.

Note that as $ka \to 0$ the pressure and velocity will be 90 degrees out of phase and that as $ka \to \infty$ the impedance becomes identical to the plane-wave impedance.

b. Show that the real power radiated from the sphere is given by

$$\overline{W_{Re}} = 2\pi a^2 v_o^2 Z_o \frac{(ka)^2}{1 + (ka)^2}.$$

This shows that the real power radiated for a given surface velocity falls off to zero as $ka \to 0$, and reaches a constant value if $ka \gg 1$.

P5. A plane harmonic wave originating from a semi-infinite medium of specific impedance $\underline{Z}_1$ is normally incident on a semi-infinite medium of specific impedance $\underline{Z}_2$. Show that the impedance seen by the incident wave at a distance ℓ from the interface is given by

$$Z_{in}(\ell) = Z_1 \frac{\underline{Z}_2 + j\underline{Z}_1 \tan(2\pi\ell/\lambda_1)}{\underline{Z}_1 + j\underline{Z}_2 \tan(2\pi\ell/\lambda_1)}.$$

P6. A plane harmonic wave is incident at normal incidence on a plane parallel-sided layer of thickness ℓ and impedance Z_2 that separates a semi-infinite incident medium of specific impedance Z_1 from a semi-infinite medium of specific impedance Z_3. The intensity ratio is given by equation (1.111), namely

$$T_I = \frac{4Z_3 Z_1}{(Z_1 + Z_3)^2 \cos^2\varphi + (Z_2 + Z_1 Z_3/Z_2)^2 \sin^2\varphi}, \text{ where } \varphi = 2\pi\ell/\lambda_2 \text{ and } \lambda_2$$

is the wavelength in the middle layer.

a. Comment on the use of this expression in relation to impedance matching between two media.

b. Two liquid media, water and carbon tetrachloride, both have impedances of 1.48 MRayl. To separate them acoustically, a thin sheet of Mylar is used ($Z_o = 3.00$ MRayl, $c_o = 2540$ m/s). If the thickness is less than a quarter wavelength so that attenuation can be ignored, determine the maximum thickness that can be used so that the transmitted intensity is reduced by no more than 5% at 10 MHz.

c. In transmitting from a piezoelectric ceramic transducer (PZT, 34 MRayl) into water at 5 MHz, what medium would you choose (give the thickness, impedance, and type of material) to achieve nearly perfect matching?

P7. In problem P6, suppose that the load impedance is complex such that $\underline{Z}_3 = R_3 + jX_3$. Show that if middle layer impedance is real and equal to the magnitude of $\underline{Z}_3$, i.e., $\underline{Z}_2 = |\underline{Z}_3|$, and its thickness is given by $\ell = \lambda_2/8$, the impedance seen by the incident wave is also real and is given by

$$Z_{in} = \frac{R_3 \sqrt{R_3^2 + X_3^2}}{\sqrt{R_3^2 + X_3^2} - X_3}.$$

P8. A plane ultrasound wave in water has an intensity of 50 mW/cm^2 and is incident at an angle of 12 degrees to the normal on a plane semi-infinite glass slab. Determine the intensity of the reflected and transmitted beams if the effects of attenuation can be neglected, but accounting for wave-mode conversion. Assume that: c_o(water) = 1480 m/s, c_L(glass) = 5570 m/s, c_T(glass) = 3520 m/s and ρ_o(glass) = 2.6 g/cm^3.

P9. If a region has a monotonic change of impedance with no discontinuities, it is possible to calculate the response to a plane incident wave of arbitrary waveform by convolving it with the pressure impulse response. This figure illustrates a monotonic impedance change from Z_o to Z_n over a distance z. Such a change can be approximated by steps of impedance change such that the reflection coefficients at each step are identical. For this to be the case, the z-dimension of each step will generally differ. Let us consider a unit impulse pressure wave incident from a region of impedance Z_o in the z-direction. When this wave encounters boundary 1, there will be a transmitted and reflected component.

a. If the pressure reflection coefficient is denoted by R (omitting the subscript to simplify the notation), show that if multiple reflections are ignored, then the total reflected pressure due to reflections at all n interfaces of the incident δ-function, i.e., the impulse response, is given by

$$h(t) = R \sum_{k=1}^{n} (1 - R^2)^{k-1} \delta(t - 2t_k)$$

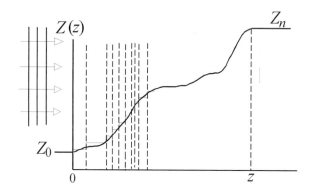

where the impulse has been assumed to be incident on the first interface at $t = 0$, and $2t_1, 2t_2, \ldots 2t_n$ are the total transit times, i.e., $2t_n$ is the transit time from the first interface to the last interface and back again.

b. Show that by integrating this equation,

$$\int_0^{2t_n} h(t)dt = nR - (nR)^3 \frac{(n-1)}{2n^2} + (nR)^5 \frac{(n-1)(n-2)}{6n^4} - \ldots\ldots$$

c. The impulse is assumed to come from a half-space region of impedance Z_o and ends up in a half-space region of impedance Z_n after crossing the region of varying impedance. Noting that $\frac{Z_n}{Z_0} = [(1+R)/(1-R)]^n$ show that in the limit that:

$$\lim_{n \to \infty} \int_0^{2t_n} h(t)dt = 0.5\ln(Z_n/Z_0), \text{ i.e., } \int_0^{2t} h(t)dt = 0.5\ln[Z(t)/Z_0], \text{ which}$$

is the first-order impediography equation. The identity $2\tanh^{-1}R = \ln[(1 + R)/(1 - R)]$ may be helpful.

d. From the above result show that that pressure impulse response is given by $h(2t) = \dfrac{dZ(t)/dt}{4Z(t)}$, when multiple reflections are ignored and the impedance change is monotonic.

References

1. Rayleigh, J.W.S., *The Theory of Sound*, Vols. I and II, McMillan Co., London, 1877 and 1878. (A second revised edition was republished by Dover Publications, New York, 1945. Vol. I contains an interesting biographical sketch of Lord Rayleigh and a historical account of the development of acoustics.)
2. Langevin, P., *Oeuvres Scientifiques de Paul Langevin*, Centre National de la Recherche Scientifique, Paris, 1950.
3. Wood, R.W., and Loomis, A.L., The physical and biological effects of high frequency sound waves of great intensity, *Phil. Mag.*, 4, 417–436, 1927.

4. Graff, K.E., A history of ultrasonics, Ch.1, pp. 1–97 in: *Physical Acoustics*, Vol. 25, W.P. Mason, and R.N. Thurston (Eds.), Academic Press, New York, 1981.

5. Ristic, V.M., *Principles of Acoustic Devices*, Wiley, New York, 1983.

6. Morse, P.M., and Ingard, K.U., *Theoretical Acoustics*, McGraw-Hill, New York, 1968.

7. Hertzfield, K.F., and Litovitz, T.A., *Absorption and Dispersion of Ultrasonic Waves*, Academic Press, New York, 1959.

8. Hassan, W., and Nagy, P.B., Simplified expressions for the displacements and stresses produced by the Rayleigh wave, *J. Acoust. Soc. Am.*, 104, 3107–3110, 1998.

9. Kuttruff, H., *Ultrasonics: Fundamentals and Applications*, Elsevier, New York, 1991.

10. Zemansky, M.W., and Dittman, R.H., *Heat and Thermodynamics*, 7th Edn., McGraw-Hill, New York, 1997.

11. Wang, S.H., Lee, L.P., and Lee, J.S., A linear relation between the compressibility and density of blood, *J. Acoust. Soc. Am.*, 109, 390–396, 2001.

12. Del Grosso, V.A., and Mader, C.W., Speed of sound in pure water, *J. Acoust. Soc. Am.*, 52, 1442–1446, 1972.

13. Bilaniuk, N., and Wong, G.S.K., Speed of sound in pure water as a function of temperature, *J. Acoust. Soc. Am.*, 93, 1609–1612, 1993.

14. Temkin, S., *Elements of Acoustics*, Wiley, New York, 1981.

15. Lubbers, J., and Graaff, R., A simple and accurate formula for the sound velocity in water, *Ultrasound Med. Biol.*, 24, 1065–1068, 1998.

16. Kino, S., *Acoustic Waves: Devices, Imaging and Analog Signal Processing*, Prentice-Hall, Englewood Cliffs, NJ, 1986.

17. Truesdell, C., Mechanical foundation of elasticity and fluid dynamics, *J. Rational Mechanics and Analysis*, 1, 125–171, 1952.

18. Malecki, I., *Physical Foundations of Technical Acoustics*, Pergamon Press, Oxford, 1969.

19. Landau, L.D., and Lifshitz, E.M., *Fluid Mechanics*, 2nd Edn. Pergamon Press, Oxford, 1987.

20. Currie, I.G., *Fundamental Mechanics of Fluids*, 2nd Edn., McGraw-Hill, New York, 1993.

21. Blackstock, D.T., *Fundamentals of Physical Acoustics*, Wiley, New York, 2000.

22. Insana, M.F., and Brown, D.G., Acoustic scattering theory applied to soft biological tissues, Ch. 4, pp. 75–124 in: *Ultrasonic Scattering in Biological Tissues*, K.K. Shung, and G.A. Thieme (Eds.), CRC Press, Boca Raton, FL, 1993.

23. Eckart, C., Vortices and streams caused by sound waves, *Phys. Rev.*, 73, 68–76, 1948.

24. Brillouin, L., *Wave Propagation and Group Velocity*, Academic Press, New York, 1960.

25. Leander, J.L., On the relation between the wavefront speed and the group velocity concept, *J. Acoust. Soc. Am.*, 100, 3503–3507, 1996.

26. Lamb, H., *Hydrodynamics*, 6th Edn., Cambridge University Press, Cambridge, 1932.

27. Rayleigh, J.W.S., *The Theory of Sound* (see Appendix in Vol. 1), 2nd Edn., 1894; republished by Dover Publications, New York, 1945.

28. Wear, K.A., Measurement of phase velocity and group velocity in human calcaneus, *Ultrasound Med. Biol.*, 26, 641–646, 2000.

29. Carstensen, E.L., and Schwan, H.P., Acoustic properties of hemoglobin solutions, *J. Acoust. Soc. Am.*, 31, 305–311, 1959.

30. Dunn, F., Attenuation and speed of ultrasound in lung: dependence on frequency and inflation, *J. Acoust. Soc. Am.*, 80, 1248–1250, 1986.

31. Ziomek, L.J., *Fundamentals of Acoustic Field Theory and Space-Time Signal Processing*, CRC Press, Boca Raton, FL, 1995.
32. Bamber, J.C., Speed of sound, Ch. 5 in: *Physical Principles of Medical Diagnosis*, 2nd Edn., C.R. Hill, J.C. Bamber, and G.R. ter Haar (Eds.), Wiley, Chichester, U.K., 2004.
33. Robinson, D.E., Ophir, J., Wilson, L.S., and Chen, C.F., Pulse-echo sound speed measurements: progress and prospects. *Ultrasound Med. Biol.*, 17, 633–646, 1991.
34. Anderson, M., and Trahey, G.E., The direct estimation of sound speed using pulse-echo ultrasound. *J. Acoust. Soc. Am.*, 104, 3099–3106, 1986.
35. Duck, F.A., *Physical Properties of Tissue: A Comprehensive Reference Book*, Ch. 4, Academic Press, London, 1990.
36. Gross, S.A., Johnston, R.L., and Dunn, F., Comprehensive compilation of empirical ultrasonic properties of mammalian tissues, *J. Acoust. Soc. Am.*, 64, 423–457, 1978.
37. Gross, S.A., Johnston, R.L., and Dunn, F., Comprehensive compilation of empirical ultrasonic properties of mammalian tissues II, *J. Acoust. Soc. Am.*, 68, 93–108, 1980.
38. Auld, B.A., *Acoustic Fields and Waves in Solids*, Vol. 1, 2nd Edn., Krieger, Malabar, FL, 1990.
39. Rose, J.L., *Ultrasonic Waves in Solid Media*, Cambridge Univ. Press, Cambridge, 1999.
40. Fellah, Z.E.A., Chapelon, J.Y., Berger, S., Launks, W., and Depollier, C., Ultrasonic wave propagation in human cancellous bone: application of Biot theory, *J. Acoust. Soc. Am.*, 116, 61–71, 2004.
41. Biot, M.A. Theory of propagation of elastic waves in a fluid saturated solid. I. Low frequency range, *J. Acoust. Soc. Am.*, 28, 168–178, 1956.
42. Biot, M.A. Theory of propagation of elastic waves in a fluid saturated solid. II. High frequency range, *J. Acoust. Soc. Am.*, 28, 179–191, 1956.
43. Dransfield, K., and Salzmann, E., Excitation, detection, and attenuation of high-frequency elastic surface waves, Ch. 4, pp. 219–272 in: *Physical Acoustics*, Vol. 7, W.P. Mason, and R.N. Thurston (Eds.), Academic Press, New York, 1970.
44. Uberall, H., Surface Waves in Acoustics, Ch. 1, pp 1–60 in: *Physical Acoustics*, Vol. 10, W.P. Mason, and R.N. Thurston (Eds.), Academic Press, New York, 1973.
45. Brower, N.G., Himberger, D.L., and Mayer, W.G., Restrictions on the existance of leaky surface waves, *IEEE Trans. on Sonics and Ultrasonics*, SU-26, 306–308, 1979.
46. Beissner, K., On the plane-wave approximation of acoustic intensity, *J. Acoust. Soc. Am.*, 56, 1043–1048, 1974.
47. Nyborg, W.L., Acoustic streaming, Ch. 7, pp. 207–231 in: *Nonlinear Acoustics*, M.F. Hamilton, and D.T. Blackstock (Eds.), Academic Press, New York, 1998.
48. Duck, F.A., Radiation pressure and acoustic streaming, Ch. 3, pp. 39–56 in: *Ultrasound in Medicine*, F.A. Duck, A.C. Baker, and H.C. Starritt (Eds.), Inst. of Physics Pub., Bristol, England, 1998.
49. Altberg, W., Uber die Druckkrafte der Schallwellen und die absolute Messung der Schallintensitat (On the force due to sound waves and the absolute measurement of sound intensity), *Annalen der Physik*, 11, 405–420, 1903.
50. Whittingham, T.A., The purpose and techniques of acoustic output measurement, Ch. 7, pp. 129–148 in: *Ultrasound in Medicine*, F.A. Duck, A.C. Baker, and H.C. Starritt (Eds.), Inst. of Physics Pub., Bristol, England, 1998.
51. Perkins, M.A., A versatile force balance for ultrasound power measurement, *Phys. Med. Biol.*, 34, 1635–1651, 1989.

52. Rayleigh, Lord, On the pressure of vibrations, *Phil. Mag.*, 3, 338–346, 1902.

53. Rayleigh, Lord, On the momentum and pressure of gaseous vibrations, and on the connection with the virial theorem, *Phil. Mag.*, 10, 364–374, 1905.

54. Lee, C.P., and Wang, T.G., Acoustic radiation pressure, *J. Acoust. Soc. Am.*, 94, 1099–1109, 1993.

55. Wang, T.G., and Lee, C.P., Radiation pressure and acoustic levitation, Ch. 6, pp. 177–205 in: *Nonlinear Acoustics*, M.F. Hamilton, and D.T. Blackstock (Eds.), Academic Press, New York, 1998.

56. Kinsler, L.E., Frey, A.R., Coppens, A.B., and Sanders, J.V., *Fundamentals of Acoustics*, 3rd Edn., Wiley, New York, 1982.

57. Brekhovskikh, L.M., *Waves in Layered Media*, 2nd Edn., Academic Press, New York, 1980.

58. Sommerfeld, A., *Optics: Lectures on Theoretical Physics*, Vol. IV, Academic Press, New York, 1954.

59. Born, M., and Wolf, E., *Principles of Optics*. 6th Edn., Pergamon Press, New York, 1980.

60. Baker, B.B., and Copson, E.T., *The Mathematical Theory of Huygens' Principle*, 2nd Edn., Clarendon Press, Oxford, 1950.

61. Buchwald, J.Z., *The Rise of the Wave Theory of Light: Optical Theory and Experiment in the Early Nineteenth Century*, Univ. of Chicago Press, Chicago, 1989.

62. Abramowitz, M, and Stegun, I.A. (Eds.), *Handbook of Mathematical Functions*, Dover, New York, 1965.

63. Skudrzyk, E., *The Foundations of Acoustics*, Springer-Verlag, New York, 1971.

64. Bamber, J.C., Attenuation and absorption, Ch. 4, pp. 118–199 in: *Physical Principles of Medical Ultrasonics*, 2nd Edn., C.R. Hill, J.C. Bamber, and G.R. ter Haar (Eds.), Wiley, Chichester, U.K., 2004.

65. Bamber, J.C., Ultrasonic properties of tissues, Ch. 4, pp. 57–88 in: *Ultrasound in Medicine*, F.A. Duck, A.C. Baker, and H.C. Starritt (Eds.), Inst. of Physics Pub., Bristol, England, 1998.

66. Bamber, J.C., Acoustical characteristics of biological media, Ch. 141, pp. 1703–1726 in: *Encyclopedia of Acoustics*, M.J. Crocker (Ed.), Wiley, New York, 1997.

67. Mast, T.D., Empirical relationships between acoustic parameters in human soft tissues, *Acoustics Res. Lett.*, 1, 37–42, 2000.

68. Wang, S-H., and Shung, K.K., An approach for measuring ultrasonic backscattering from biological tissues with focused transducers, *IEEE Trans. Biomed. Eng.*, 44, 549–554, 1997.

69. Njeh, C.F., Nicholson, P.H.F., and Langton, C.M., The physics of ultrasound applied to bone, Ch. 4, pp. 67–75 in: *Quantative Ultrasound: Assessment of Osteoporosis and Bone Status*, C.F. Njeh, H.D. Fuerst, C-C. Gluer, and H.K. Genant (Eds.), Martin Dunitz, London, 1999.

70. Langton, C.M., and Njeh, C.F., Acoustic and ultrasonic tissue characterization: assessment of osteoporosis, *Proc. Inst. Mech. Eng.: Part H: J. Eng. Med.*, 213, 261–269, 1999.

71. Avecilla, L.S., and Miller, P.D., Normal reference data, Ch. 13, pp. 221–243 in: *Quantative Ultrasound: Assessment of Osteoporosis and Bone Status*, C.F. Njeh, H.D. Fuerst, C-C. Gluer, and H.K. Genant (Eds.), Martin Dunitz, London, 1999.

72. Langton, C.F., Palmer, S.B., and Porter, R.W., Measurement of broadbamd ultrasonic attenuation in cancellous bone, *Engineering in Med.*, 13, 89–91, 1984.

73. Langton, C.F., Ali, A.V., Riggs, C.M., Evans, G.P., and Barfield, W.A., A contact method for the assessment of ultrasonic velocity and broadband attenuation in cortical and cancellous bone, *Clin. Phys. Physiol. Meas.*, 11, 243–249, 1990.

74. Chaffai, S., Padilla, F., Berger, G., Laugier, P., In vitro measurement of the frequency-dependent attenuation in cancellous bone between 0.2 and 2 MHz, *J. Acoust. Soc. Am.*, 108, 1281–1289, 2000.

75. Wear, K.A., A numerical method to predict the effects of frequency-dependent attenuation and dispersion on speed of sound estimates in cancellous bone, *J. Acoust. Soc. Am.*, 109, 1213–1218, 2001.

76. Chivers, R.C., and Hill, C.R., Ultrasonic attenuation in human tissue, *Ultrasound Med. Biol.*, 2, 25–29, 1975.

77. Wells, P.N.T., Absorption and dispersion of ultrasound in biological tissue, *Ultrasound Med. Biol.*, 1, 369–376, 1975.

78. Nassiri, D.K., and Hill, C.R., The differential and total bulk acoustic scattering cross sections of some human and animal tissues, *J. Acoust. Soc. Am.*, 79, 2034–2047, 1986.

79. Wear, K.A., Fundamental mechanisms underlaying broadband ultrasonic attenuation in calcaneus, pp. 427–429 in: *Ultrasonic Imaging and Signal Processing*, M.F. Insana, and K.K. Shung (Eds.), Vol. 4325 (Proc. SPIE), 2001.

80. Pinkerton, J.M.M., The absorption of ultrasonic waves in liquids and its relation to molecular constitution, *Proc. Phys. Soc.* B62, 129–141, 1949.

81. Davidovich, L.A., Makhkamov, S., Pulatova, L., Khabibullaev, P.K., and Khaliulin, M.G., Acoustic properties of certain organic liquids at frequencies 0.3 to 3 GHz, *Soviet Physics: Acoustics*, 18, 264–266, 1972.

82. Markham, J.J., Beyer, R.T., and Lindsay, R.B., Absorption of sound in fluids, *Rev. Mod. Phys.*, 23, 353–411, 1951.

83. Hall, L. The origin of ultrasonic absorption in water, *Phys. Rev.*, 73, 773–781, 1948.

84. Herzfeld, K., and Litovitz, T.A., *Absorption and Dispersion of Ultrasonic Waves*, Academic Press, New York, 1959.

85. Matheson, A.J., *Molecular Acoustics*, Wiley, New York, 1971.

86. Narayana, P.A., and Ophir, J., A closed form method for the measurement of attenuation in nonlinearly dispersive media, *Ultrasonic Imaging*, 5, 17–21, 1983.

87. Round, W.H., and Bates, R.H.T., Modification of spectra of pulses from ultrasonic transducers by scatterers in non-attenuating and attenuating media, *Ultrasonic Imaging*, 9, 18–28, 1987.

88. Wear, K.A., A Gaussian framework for modeling effects of frequency-dependent attenuation, frequency-dependent scattering, and gating, *IEEE Trans. Ultrason. Ferroelect. Freq. Contr*, 49, 1572–1582, 2002.

89. Hand, J.W., Ultrasound hyperthermia and the prediction of heating, Ch. 8, pp. 151–176 in: *Ultrasound in Medicine*, F.A. Duck, A.C. Baker, and H.C. Starritt (Eds.), Inst. of Physics Pub., Bristol, England, 1998.

90. Hunt, J.W., Principles of ultrasound for generating localized hyperthermia, pp. 371–422 in: *Practical Aspects of Clinical Hyperthermia*, S.B. Field, and J.W. Hand, (Eds.), Taylor and Francis, London, 1990.

91. Diederich, C.J., and Hynynen, K., Ultrasound technology for hyperthermia, *Ultrasound in Med. Biol.*, 25, 871–887, 1999.

92. ter Harr, G.R., Focused ultrasound surgery, Ch. 9, pp. 177–187 in: *Ultrasound in Medicine*, F.A. Duck, A.C. Baker, and H.C. Starritt (Eds.), Inst. of Physics Pub., Bristol, England, 1998.

93. Hill, C.R., Optimum acoustic frequency for focused ultrasound surgery, *Ultrasound Med. Biol.*, 20, 271–277, 1995.

94. Nyborg, W.L., Heat generation by ultrasound in a relaxing medium, *J. Acoust. Soc. Am.*, 70, 310–312, 1981.

95. Litovitz, T.A., and Davis, C.M., Structural and shear relaxation in liquids, Ch. 5, pp. 281–349 in: *Physical Acoustics*, Vol. 2A, W.P. Mason (Ed.), Academic Press, New York, 1965.

96. Lamb, J., Thermal relaxation in liquids, Ch. 4, pp. 203–280 in: *Physical Acoustics*, Vol. 2A, W.P. Mason (Ed.), Academic Press, New York, 1965.

97. Madsen, E.L., Sathoff, H.J., and Zagzebski, J.A., Ultrasonic shear wave properties of soft tissues and tissuelike matherials, *J. Acoust. Soc. Am.*, 74, 1346–1355, 1983.

2

Theoretical Basis for
Field Calculations

Of considerable practical importance is the ability to accurately predict the field caused by an acoustic source of given dimensions. The changes in pressure, particle velocity, and density can be determined by solving the appropriate wave equation subject to the prescribed boundary and initial conditions. An appropriate wave equation could be one that accounts for the properties of the transmission medium, including nonlinearities, absorption, and dispersion, as well as any anisotropic and inhomogeneities present. Solving such an equation is often very difficult, and as a result several assumptions and approximations are generally made.

In the classical approach for linear propagation, a homogeneous, isotropic inviscid fluid is assumed and simplifying assumptions are made in regard to the boundary conditions. Two different conditions are considered, leading to two equations that describe the field distribution in terms of surface integrals over the prescribed boundary. They are commonly referred to as the Rayleigh-Sommerfeld *diffraction equations*. One of these leads to the Rayleigh integral, which we use to solve for the on-axis field distribution of a circular-symmetric source. An alternative approach, of more recent origin, is based on the *angular spectrum* technique. It makes use of the 2-D Fourier transform to represent the field on any given plane. Given this field distribution, it provides a relatively simple approach for calculating the field on an adjacent plane. As will be shown, it is equivalent to the Rayleigh integral method. Examples of both methods will be presented in the next chapter. Finally, although not described in this chapter, it should be noted that if the field region is divided into a grid of sufficiently fine resolution, *numerical* methods provide a flexible means for determining the field. Such methods are particularly appropriate when the source and boundary conditions are complex.

For soft biological tissue, it is often assumed that ultrasonic wave propagation is well approximated by assuming that the medium behaves as a fluid and that any shear wave propagation can be ignored. However, tissue is an elastic medium that can also support low-frequency shear wave propagation. For example, the radiation pressure created by ultrasound propagation in a viscoelastic medium such as tissue can result in shear wave generation (see section 8.8). To predict the manner in which such waves propagate, it is necessary to use a wave equation that accounts for the elastic nature of the medium. Such an equation is discussed in section 1.4.3, where the particle displacement field (see (1.66)) is expressed in terms of the Lamé constants and viscous loss parameters. Even if the medium is assumed to be unbounded and inviscid, solving such an equation is a fairly complex task and beyond the scope of this book. Nonetheless, it is interesting to note that Stokes [1], in 1849, published a general solution (see his eqn. (36)) for the lossless displacement field generated by an arbitrary forcing function (in essence, a Green's function solution). The solution contained three terms, two of which depend inversely on the distance from the source, and these describe far-field longitudinal and shear propagation. The final term, which decays rapidly with distance, accounts for longitudinal and shear wave propagation in the near field. In his paper Stokes acknowledged that Poisson [2] had previously derived a solution but indicated that the assumptions used were not entirely satisfactory.

The much simpler case of longitudinal propagation in an inviscid medium, as described by the Rayleigh-Sommerfeld diffraction equations, forms the staring point of this chapter. These are then applied to determine the axial field distribution due to a simple piston source for sinusoidal and pulse excitations. The final section contains a description of the theory underlying the angular spectrum approach, practical examples of which are given in the next chapter.

2.1 Rayleigh-Sommerfeld Diffraction Equations

To determine the pressure or velocity field produced by a vibrating source excited by an arbitrary waveform, we must solve the appropriate wave equation that characterizes the manner in which the wave is propagated and must constrain the solution to meet the boundary conditions defined by the problem. Much of what follows is based on the classical works of Goodman [4, Chapter 3], Morse and Ingard [6], and Skudrzyk [7].

As in Chapter 1, we write our equations in terms of a scalar velocity potential $\phi(\mathbf{r}:t)$ defined by

$$(2.1) \qquad\qquad \mathbf{v}(\mathbf{r}:t) = -\nabla\phi(\mathbf{r}:t),$$

in which ∇ is the gradient operator and $\mathbf{v}$ is the "particle" velocity at the position $\mathbf{r}$. For small-amplitude compressional waves propagating in a homogeneous medium of adiabatic compressibility κ, shear viscosity μ, and bulk viscosity μ_B, the equation describing the spatial and time dependence of ϕ was derived in Chapter 1 (1.38), and is

(2.2)
$$\kappa\rho_o \frac{\partial^2 \phi}{\partial t^2} = \nabla^2\phi + \kappa\left(\mu_B + \frac{4}{3}\mu\right)\frac{\partial}{\partial t}(\nabla^2\phi).$$

In a homogeneous inviscid ($\mu = \mu_B = 0$) medium, the velocity potential ϕ at **r** for an arbitrary distribution of sources must satisfy the wave equation with an extra term to account for the source distribution [12], i.e.,

(2.3)
$$\frac{1}{c_o^2}\frac{\partial^2 \phi}{\partial t^2} - \nabla^2\phi = -f(\mathbf{r}{:}t),$$

where $c_o = 1/\sqrt{\kappa\rho_o}$ is the small-signal wave propagation speed and $f(\mathbf{r}{:}t)$ describes the strength of the source distribution. To solve this inhomogeneous equation for a given set of boundary conditions, it is simpler to transform (2.3) to the frequency domain. The transformation can be accomplished by using the *Fourier transform*, defined by[1]:

(2.4)
$$Q(\omega) = \int_{-\infty}^{\infty} q(t)e^{-j\omega t}\,dt.$$

Once the solution is obtained, then the *inverse Fourier transform*,

(2.5)
$$q(t) = \frac{1}{2\pi}\int_{-\infty}^{\infty} Q(\omega)e^{j\omega t}\,d\omega$$

enables $\phi(\mathbf{r}{:}t)$ to be obtained. Transforming (2.3) by using (2.4) yields the inhomogeneous form of the Helmholtz equation

(2.6)
$$(\nabla^2 + k^2)\Phi = -F(\mathbf{r}{:}\omega),$$

in which $k = \omega/c_o$ is the wave number and $\Phi(\mathbf{r}{:}\omega)$ and $F(\mathbf{r}{:}\omega)$ are the Fourier transforms of ϕ and f, respectively.

The problem of determining the field distribution due to an arbitrary source distribution $f(\mathbf{r}{:}t)$ enclosed by a surface S_o reduces to solving the Helmholtz equation subject to the boundary conditions on S_o. A convenient method is based on the use of a *Green's function* [3,8]. Such a function[2] $G(\mathbf{r}|\mathbf{r_o})$ is a particular solution of (2.6) for a point source located at $\mathbf{r_o}$, i.e., it satisfies

(2.7)
$$(\nabla^2 + k^2)G(\mathbf{r}|\mathbf{r_o}) = -\delta(\mathbf{r} - \mathbf{r_o}),$$

---

1. See Appendix B. A variety of other definitions for the Fourier transform are possible and are in use. The choice of a negative-signed exponent for the forward and a positive sign for the inverse Fourier transforms should be noted. Definitions with the signs reversed are frequently used. The Fourier transform pair $q(t)$ and $Q(\omega)$, as with subsequent pairs, are distinguished by lower- and upper-case letters.

2. The notation $G(\mathbf{r}|\mathbf{r_o})$ is a shorthand for the value of the function G at **r** for a source at $\mathbf{r_o}$.

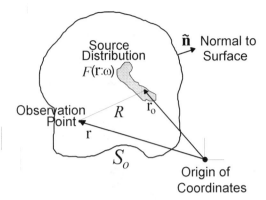

Figure 2.1 Method for determining the velocity potential at **r** due a distributed source vibrating at an angular frequency ω enclosed by a surface S_o. The source is assumed to have the same propagation characteristics as the surrounding medium.

where $\delta(\mathbf{r} - \mathbf{r_o})$ is the Dirac delta function,[3] whose value is zero for all values of **r** except for $\mathbf{r} = \mathbf{r_o}$. Fundamentally, the idea is to represent an arbitrary source by an infinite collection of point sources. By obtaining the velocity potential for each point source, the velocity potential for the entire source can be obtained by summation. Evidently, for $G(\mathbf{r}|\mathbf{r_o})$ to be a Green's function of the problem under study, it must satisfy the same boundary conditions as imposed on the original problem.

The transformed source surrounded by the surface S_o and a unit vector $\tilde{\mathbf{n}}$ pointing in an outward direction are shown in Fig. 2.1. To obtain an integral expression for the velocity potential at an observation point **r** that lies within S_o, we multiply (2.6) by $G(\mathbf{r}|\mathbf{r_o})$ and (2.7) by $\Phi(\mathbf{r}{:}\omega)$ and subtract the two equations, yielding

(2.8) $G(\mathbf{r}|\mathbf{r_o})\nabla^2\Phi - \Phi\nabla^2 G(\mathbf{r}|\mathbf{r_o}) = \Phi\delta(\mathbf{r} - \mathbf{r_o}) - G(\mathbf{r}|\mathbf{r_o})F(\mathbf{r}{:}\omega).$ (a)

Noting the reciprocal properties, i.e., $G(\mathbf{r}|\mathbf{r_o}) = G(\mathbf{r_o}|\mathbf{r})$, and $\delta(\mathbf{r} - \mathbf{r_o}) = \delta(\mathbf{r_o} - \mathbf{r})$, then **r** and $\mathbf{r_o}$ can be exchanged. The form of (2.8) remains the same, though $\Phi(\mathbf{r})$ transforms to $\Phi(\mathbf{r_o})$ and $F(\mathbf{r}{:}\omega)$ to $F(\mathbf{r_o}{:}\omega)$, i.e., they are expressed in terms of the source coordinates, so that (2.8a) becomes

(2.8) $G(\mathbf{r_o}|\mathbf{r})\nabla^2\Phi(\mathbf{r_o}) - \Phi(\mathbf{r_o})\nabla^2 G(\mathbf{r_o}|\mathbf{r}) = \Phi(\mathbf{r_o})\delta(\mathbf{r_o} - \mathbf{r}) - G(\mathbf{r_o}|\mathbf{r})F(\mathbf{r_o}{:}\omega).$ (b)

To determine the velocity potential both within the enclosed volume and on the surface S_o, we first integrate (2.8) over the entire enclosed volume V_o

3. Definition: if $f(x)$ is any well-behaved function, then

$$\int_{x_2}^{x_1} f(x)\delta(x)dx = \begin{cases} f(0) & \text{if integration range includes } x = 0 \\ 0 & \text{if integration range includes } x = 0 \end{cases}$$

This definition of $\delta(x)$ is adopted from [3, Chapter 1]; its properties are also discussed in [38, Chapter 5]. In dimensional analysis it is helpful to remember that the δ-function has dimensions that are the inverse of its argument. Thus, for example, the dimension of $\delta(\mathbf{r})$ is $[L^{-3}]$.

enclosed by S_o. Then, by using Green's theorem (Appendix D), the left-hand side of the equation can be converted to a surface integral over S_o. Noting that the volume integral of $\Phi\delta(\mathbf{r} - \mathbf{r_o})$ is simply $\Phi(\mathbf{r})$, we find

$$(2.9) \quad \iint_{S_o}\left[G(\mathbf{r}|\mathbf{r_o})\frac{\partial\Phi}{\partial n} - \Phi\frac{\partial G(\mathbf{r}|\mathbf{r_o})}{\partial n}\right]dS_o = \Phi(\mathbf{r}) - \iiint_{V_o} G(\mathbf{r}|\mathbf{r_o})F(\mathbf{r_o}:\omega)dV_o,$$

where $\partial/\partial n$ denotes a partial derivative in the outward normal direction for a given point on the surface S_o. This equation can be rewritten to express in integral form the velocity potential at $\mathbf{r}$ as

$$(2.10) \quad \Phi(\mathbf{r}:\omega) = \iint_{S_o}\left[G\frac{\partial\Phi}{\partial n} - \Phi\frac{\partial G}{\partial n}\right]dS_o + \iiint_{V_o} G(\mathbf{r}|\mathbf{r_o})F(\mathbf{r_o}:\omega)\,dV_o.$$

Thus, given a particular source distribution, the velocity potential can be found, provided the boundary conditions for the velocity potential and the Green's function are known. In the next three subsections three special cases will be examined.

2.1.1 Volume Source in an Unbounded Medium

Perhaps the simplest case to consider is one in which the source radiates into a medium unimpeded by any boundaries. The absence of an external boundary implies that there will be no reflected waves, i.e., all waves are outgoing. The Green's function for this unbounded case corresponds to a point source radiating into space, and consequently

$$(2.11) \quad G_p(\mathbf{r}|\mathbf{r_o}) = G_p(|\mathbf{r} - \mathbf{r_o}|) = e^{-j\omega R/c_o}/4\pi R,$$

where $R = |\mathbf{r} - \mathbf{r_o}|$ is the magnitude of the distance of the observation point from a point in the source distribution. Thus (2.11) corresponds to a harmonic point source located at $\mathbf{r_o}$ that generates a wave whose amplitude falls off as $1/R$. By substituting (2.11) into (2.6) and letting $S_o \to \infty$, it can be shown that this Green's function is an unbounded solution to the Helmholtz equation [6,12].

The inverse transform of (2.11) yields the time-dependent free-space Green's function, i.e.,

$$(2.12) \quad g_p(R:t) = \frac{1}{4\pi R}\delta\left(t - \frac{R}{c_o}\right).$$

It should be noted that $g_p(R:t)$ is also called the *free-space impulse response* of the medium, h_f. For an impulse at a time t_0 at the position $\mathbf{r_o}$, the impulse response can be expressed in a more general form as

$$(2.13) \quad h_f(\mathbf{r}|\mathbf{r_o}:t|t_0) = g_p(\mathbf{r}|\mathbf{r_o}:t|t_0) = \frac{1}{4\pi|\mathbf{r} - \mathbf{r_o}|}\delta[t - (t_0 + |\mathbf{r} - \mathbf{r_o}|/c_o)].$$

This equation makes it clear that the response at $\mathbf{r}$ due to an impulse at $\mathbf{r_o}$ is identical to the response at $\mathbf{r_o}$ due to an impulse at $\mathbf{r}$, which is consistent with the principle of reciprocity.[4] It should also be noted that (2.13) is the solution to

(2.14)
$$\frac{1}{c_o^2}\frac{\partial^2 h_f}{\partial t^2} - \nabla^2 h_f = -\delta(\mathbf{r}-\mathbf{r_o})\delta(t-t_0),$$

i.e., the inhomogeneous wave equation with a δ-function source at the point $\mathbf{r} = \mathbf{r_0}$.

Noting that[5] $G_p(\mathbf{r}|\mathbf{r_o}) \to 0$ and that $\Phi(\mathbf{r}) \to 0$ as $\mathbf{r} \to \infty$, the velocity potential in the frequency domain, as expressed by (2.10), simplifies to

$$\Phi(\mathbf{r}:\omega) = \iiint_{V_o} G_p(\mathbf{r}|\mathbf{r_o})F(\mathbf{r_o}:\omega)dV_o,$$

whose inverse Fourier transform is

(2.15)
$$\phi(\mathbf{r}:t) = \frac{1}{2\pi}\iiint_{V_o}\int_{-\infty}^{\infty} G_p(\mathbf{r}|\mathbf{r_o})F(\mathbf{r_o}:\omega)e^{j\omega t}d\omega dV_o.$$

By making use of the superposition integral as given in Appendix A as (A.6) and knowing that the impulse response is given by (2.14), the velocity potential can be written as the convolution integral

(2.16)
$$\phi(\mathbf{r}:t) = \frac{1}{4\pi}\iiint_{V_o}\frac{f\left(\mathbf{r_o}:t-\dfrac{|\mathbf{r}-\mathbf{r_0}|}{c_o}\right)}{|\mathbf{r}-\mathbf{r_0}|}dV_o,$$

where $f(.)$ is the time-dependent source distribution.

An alternative way of obtaining this equation is to use the convolution theorem enabling the inner portion of the integral in (2.15) to be expressed as

$$\frac{1}{2\pi}\int_{-\infty}^{\infty} G_p(\mathbf{r}|\mathbf{r_o})F(\mathbf{r_o}:\omega)e^{j\omega t}d\omega = g_p(R:t)*f(\mathbf{r}:t) = \int_{-\infty}^{\infty}\frac{\delta\left(t-\dfrac{R}{c_o}-\tau\right)}{4\pi R}f(\mathbf{r_o}:t)d\tau$$

$$= f\left(\mathbf{r_o}:t-\frac{R}{c_o}\right)$$

and consequently the time-dependent velocity potential to be written as

(2.16)
$$\phi(\mathbf{r}:t) = \frac{1}{4\pi}\iiint_{V_o}\frac{f\left(\mathbf{r_o}:t-\dfrac{R}{c_o}\right)}{R}dV_o.$$

4. In his classical treatise, Lord Rayleigh [13, Vol. 2, p. 145] provided the following statement of the principle of reciprocity attributed to Helmholtz: "If in a space filled with air which is partly bounded by finitely extended fixed bodies and is partially unbounded, sound waves be excited at any point A, the resulting velocity-potential at a second point B is the same both in magnitude and phase, as it would have been at A, had B been the source of sound."

5. The Sommerfeld radiation condition [7, section 23.2.3] implies that regions at infinity do not contribute to the radiation field.

In this equation, $(t - R/c_o)$ is generally referred to as the *retarded time*: it represents the time taken for a signal transmitted from a source at $\mathbf{r_o}$ to arrive at the observation point $\mathbf{r}$. Thus, it expresses the fact that the velocity potential at the observation point can be found by summing the contributions of each elementary volume of the source distribution in a time-retarded sense and weighting each by $1/4\pi R$.

An alternative form for the time-dependent velocity potential can also obtained from (2.15). From Appendix B, the inner integral to be written as $2\pi g(\mathbf{r}{:}t)*f(\mathbf{r}{:}t)$, enabling (2.15) to be expressed as

$$(2.17) \qquad \phi(\mathbf{r}{:}t) = \iiint_{V_o} \int_{-\infty}^{\infty} g_p(\mathbf{r}|\mathbf{r_o}{:}t|t_0) f(\mathbf{r}|\mathbf{r_o}{:}t|t_o) dt_0 dV_o,$$

where the Green's function (impulse response) is given by (2.13).

2.1.2 Source Distribution Enclosed by a Surface in an Infinite Medium

As a second example we consider the case illustrated in Fig. 2.2, where a surface S_i encloses all sources and where no external boundary exists. The velocity potential at any point exterior to S_i is determined by the boundary conditions on S_i. Since the derivation leading to (2.10) is also valid when the observation point lies outside the enclosing surface, the velocity potential is given by

$$(2.18) \qquad \Phi_K(\mathbf{r}{:}\omega) = \iint_{S_i} \left[G \frac{\partial \Phi}{\partial n} - \Phi \frac{\partial G}{\partial n} \right] dS_i$$

If the bounding surface is of a simple form such that no reflections are produced, then it is appropriate to use the free-space Green's function as given by (2.11). The derivative of this with respect to the normal is given by

$$\frac{\partial G_p}{\partial n} = -\cos(\tilde{\mathbf{n}}, \tilde{\mathbf{R}})\left(jk + \frac{1}{R} \right) G_p,$$

where $(\tilde{\mathbf{n}}, \tilde{\mathbf{R}})$ denotes the angle between the outward normal unit vector $\tilde{\mathbf{n}}$ and the unit vector $\tilde{\mathbf{R}} = (\mathbf{r} - \mathbf{r}_i)/|\mathbf{r} - \mathbf{r}_i|$. When these two expressions are substituted into (2.18), the velocity potential at the observation point is given by

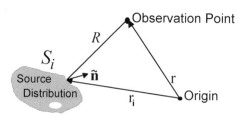

Figure 2.2 A source distribution enclosed by a surface S_i in an infinite medium. Each point on the surface contributes to the potential at the observation point.

$$(2.19) \qquad \Phi_K(\mathbf{r}:\omega) = \frac{1}{4\pi} \iint_{S_i} \frac{e^{-jkR}}{R} \left[\frac{\partial \Phi}{\partial n} + \Phi \left(jk + \frac{1}{R} \right) \cos(\tilde{\mathbf{n}}, \tilde{\mathbf{R}}) \right] dS_i,$$

which is sometimes referred to as *Helmholtz's formula*.

For the particular situation where the surface is quasi-planar, further simplification is possible. If it is assumed that each elementary area dS_i is locally plane [14, p. 160], then very close to each area the emitted wave will also be plane. Now, for a plane wave moving in the direction $\tilde{\mathbf{n}}$, $\partial \Phi / \partial n = -jk\Phi$; consequently, (2.19) can be expressed as

$$(2.20) \qquad \Phi_K(\mathbf{r}:\omega) = \frac{-jk}{4\pi} \iint_{S_i} \Phi \frac{e^{-jkR}}{R} \left[1 - (1 + 1/jkR) \cos(\tilde{\mathbf{n}}, \tilde{\mathbf{R}}) \right] dS_i.$$

This equation expresses the velocity potential due to a quasi-planar source in an infinite medium, and the boundary conditions are commonly referred to as Kirchhoff or free-field conditions [15–17]. As will be seen, this expression is the geometric mean of the velocity potentials for two other boundary conditions commonly considered.

2.1.3 Bounded Region With No Internal Sources

Of particular practical importance is the case in which no sources exist within a closed surface S_o. If a non-zero velocity potential exists within S_o, portions of the boundary must be acting as a source. For example, a piezoelectric transducer whose surface forms part of the boundary could produce surface velocity vibrations. As will be seen, exact expressions for the velocity potential within and on S_o can be obtained for certain geometric configurations under specific boundary conditions. With the help of Fig. 2.3 we will sketch the derivation of an integral expression for the velocity potential in the time domain. Although this expression can be obtained in a much simpler way by an inverse Fourier transform, it is perhaps instructive to seek an appropriate solution of

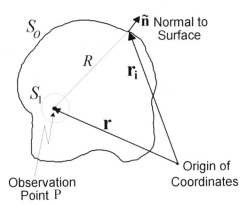

Figure 2.3 Obtaining Kirchhoff's integral theorem relating the potential at the observation point P to the conditions on the surrounding surface.

the homogeneous wave equation given by (2.3). This derivation assumes the Huygens' principle and embodies the wave interference ideas of Fresnel, both of which were considered in section 1.7.

Integral Theorem of Kirchhoff

In 1882 Kirchhoff obtained a general integral expression for the time-dependent velocity potential at any point on or within a closed surface S_o in terms of the conditions on that surface. This formulation is a generalization of the earlier contributions by Helmholtz and Poisson in formulating Huygens' principle for acoustic waves. The outline of the proof that follows is based on that given in [7, p. 506; 18, p. 38].

Each elementary surface area acts like a Huygens source, emitting radiation consisting of spherical wavelets. Thus, at the observation point P (see Fig. 2.3), the wave due to a Huygens point source at $\mathbf{r_i}$ can be written as

$$\varphi(\mathbf{r}|\mathbf{r_i}:t) = \vartheta\phi = \frac{1}{R}\phi\left(\mathbf{r}|\mathbf{r_i}:\frac{t-R}{c_o}\right),$$

where R is the distance of the observation point from the source. It should be noted that while ϕ satisfies the wave equation $1/R$ does not, though it does satisfy the Laplace equation, i.e., $\nabla^2(1/r) = 0$. The functional form of ϕ expresses the fact that the wave arriving at $\mathbf{r}$ is due to what happened at $\mathbf{r_i}$ at an earlier time equal to the time taken for the disturbance to travel the distance R. To find the potential at P due to S_o, we can surround P with a sphere of radius a_1 and surface area S_1 and determine the surface potential that must exist on it to give the same potential at P.

A relation between the functions ϕ and ϑ can be obtained by applying Green's theorem (Appendix D) to the region within S_o that is exterior to S_1. Both functions are well behaved (first and second partial derivatives are continuous) over this volume and on the surfaces. Recalling that $\nabla^2(1/R) = 0$, Green's theorem gives

$$\iint_{S_o+S_1}\left[\frac{1}{R}\frac{\partial\phi}{\partial n} - \phi\frac{\partial(1/R)}{\partial n}\right]dS = \iiint_{V_o-V_1}\frac{1}{R}\nabla^2\phi\,dV,$$

where V_o is the volume enclosed by S_o and V_1 that enclosed by S_1. In the limit as $a_1 \to 0$, the volume integral over V_1 goes to zero and the surface integral over S_1 can be shown to contribute $-4\pi\phi(\mathbf{r}:t)$. Consequently, the Green's theorem expression reduces to:

$$\phi(\mathbf{r}:t) = \frac{-1}{4\pi}\left[\iint_{S_o}\left[\phi\frac{\partial(1/R)}{\partial n} - \frac{1}{R}\frac{\partial\phi}{\partial n}\right]dS + \iiint_{V_o}\frac{1}{R}\nabla^2\phi\,dV\right].$$

The final steps are to convert the volume integral to a surface integral and to express the results in terms of retarded time. Since these are somewhat lengthy, we shall proceed directly to the final form, in which *Kirchhoff's integral theorem* can be expressed as

(2.21) $$\phi(\mathbf{r}{:}t) = \frac{-1}{4\pi} \iint_{S_o} \left\{ \langle\phi\rangle \frac{\partial(1/R)}{\partial n} - \frac{1}{R} \left\langle \frac{\partial\phi}{\partial n} \right\rangle - \frac{1}{c_o R} \frac{\partial R}{\partial n} \left\langle \frac{\partial\phi}{\partial t} \right\rangle \right\} dS,$$

and where time-retarded quantities are denoted by $\langle . \rangle$, i.e., $\langle\phi(\mathbf{r}|\mathbf{r}_i{:}t)\rangle = \phi(\mathbf{r}|\mathbf{r}_i{:}t - R/c_o)$.

A much simpler approach for deriving (2.21) starts with the frequency domain expression for the velocity potential as given by (2.10) and assumes that the free-space Green's function (2.11) is appropriate. Because there are no sources within the surface S_o, the second term in (2.10) is zero, and after taking appropriate steps to avoid the discontinuity at the observation point, it can be shown [4, pp. 40–42; 14, pp. 150–153] that

(2.22) $$\Phi(\mathbf{r}{:}\omega) = \frac{1}{4\pi} \iint_{S_o} \left[\frac{e^{-jkR}}{R} \frac{\partial\Phi}{\partial n} - \Phi \frac{\partial}{\partial n} \left(\frac{e^{-jkR}}{R} \right) \right] dS_o$$

By taking the inverse Fourier transform of (2.22), it can be shown that (2.21) is obtained.

Both methods of deriving Kirchhoff's integral theorem assume that the effects of wave reflections from the boundary surface can be ignored, and consequently the assumed boundary conditions may not be recovered by the solution. In essence, the free-space Green's function, which characterizes outgoing spherical waves, is an inappropriate choice.

Specifying the Green's Function

Let us consider the expression for the frequency domain velocity potential at an observation point $\mathbf{r}$ within S_o. In the absence of any sources inside S_o, (2.10) simplifies to

(2.23) $$\Phi(\mathbf{r}{:}\omega) = \iint_{S_o} \left[G \frac{\partial\Phi}{\partial n} - \Phi \frac{\partial G}{\partial n} \right] dS_o .$$

As noted earlier, a suitable Green's function must satisfy the Helmholtz equation as well as the boundary conditions. These requirements make it difficult, if not impossible, to obtain an analytic form of the field distribution without making any approximations. However, for some simple geometric shapes, expressions can be obtained. From (2.23) it can be seen that if either G or $\partial G/\partial n$ is zero over the bounding surface, then either Φ or $\partial\Phi/\partial n$ needs to be specified; in other words, it avoids the need for specifying both quantities, which can lead to overspecification difficulties. As will be seen, these two types of boundary conditions, as summarized in Table 2.1, are good approximations for the conditions that occur in practice.

We shall first consider the homogeneous Dirichlet condition in which $G = 0$ and $\partial G/\partial n \neq 0$ on the surface S_o. This means that the velocity potential Φ must be specified throughout S_o. But because the pressure phasor is propor-

Table 2.1. Dirichlet and Neumann boundary conditions

Boundary Condition	Required Green's Function & Partial Derivative	To Be Specified:
Dirichlet (D)	$G_D(\mathbf{r}\text{:}\omega)]_{S_o} = 0$	$\Phi_D(\mathbf{r}\text{:}\omega)]_{S_o}$
	$\dfrac{\partial G_D(\mathbf{r}\text{:}\omega)}{\partial n}\bigg]_{S_o} \neq 0$	i.e., $p(\mathbf{r}\text{:}\omega)]_{S_o}$
Neumann (N)	$G_N(\mathbf{r}\text{:}\omega)]_{S_o} \neq 0$	$\dfrac{\partial \Phi_N(\mathbf{r}\text{:}\omega)}{\partial n}\bigg]_{S_o}$
	$\dfrac{\partial G_N(\mathbf{r}\text{:}\omega)}{\partial n}\bigg]_{S_o} = 0$	i.e., $v_n(\mathbf{r}\text{:}\omega)_{S_o}$

tional to Φ, this corresponds to prescribing the pressure distribution. In the second type of boundary condition $\Phi = 0$ and $\partial\Phi/\partial n \neq 0$, which is the homogeneous Neumann condition. But $\partial\Phi/\partial n$ is equal to the particle velocity phasor normal to the surface pointing inward, i.e., in the opposite direction to $\tilde{\mathbf{n}}$. Consequently, the Neumann condition corresponds to specifying the normal component of the particle velocity on the surface. Boundary conditions intermediate between these two extremes may also be present. For example, the mixed inhomogeneous boundary condition $a\Phi(\mathbf{r}\text{:}\omega) + b[\partial\Phi(\mathbf{r}\text{:}\omega)/\partial n]_o = s(\mathbf{r}\text{:}\omega)$ could be more appropriate.

Green's Functions for a Plane Surface

The appropriate Green's functions for both Neumann and Dirichlet conditions can be found if the closed surface containing the observation point is flat over a large area and is capped by a semispherical surface of infinite radius. The plane boundary causes reflections, and consequently the field produced by a point source can be treated as the sum of two components: one from the free-space wave and the other from the reflected wave. This suggests that the method of images often used in electrical engineering to determine the field distribution [see, for example, Chapter 5 in reference 19] could be helpful in obtaining the Green's functions [8, pp. 812–813; 9, pp. 199–201].

Consider the two point sources P and P′ shown in Fig. 2.4. If their magnitudes and distances from the boundary are identical but they are on opposite sides of the surface S_o, the source at P′ will be an image of that at P. If the field on the boundary ($z = 0$) created by both sources satisfies the boundary conditions, then the boundary can be removed and the field in the region $z > 0$ will be the same as that produced by the original source and the boundary.

Consider the free-space Green's function source $e^{-jkR}/(4\pi R)$ and its image of $-e^{-jkR'}/(4\pi R')$, both of which are solutions to the Helmholtz equation. The sum and difference of the two will also be solutions. From (2.11), the two resulting functions can be written as

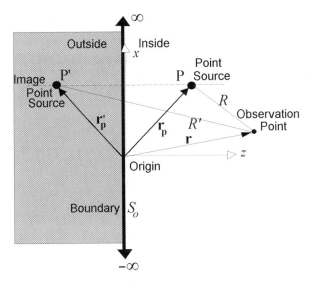

Figure 2.4 Portion of a flat surface showing a point source and its image on the opposite side. The presence of these two sources enables the boundary conditions given in Table 2.1 to be met.

(2.24)
$$G_D(\mathbf{r}) = G_p(\mathbf{r}|\mathbf{r_p}) - G_p(\mathbf{r}|\mathbf{r'_p}) = \frac{1}{4\pi}\left[e^{-jkR}/R - e^{-jkR'}/R'\right]$$

$$G_N(\mathbf{r}) = G_p(\mathbf{r}|\mathbf{r_p}) + G_p(\mathbf{r}|\mathbf{r'_p}) = \frac{1}{4\pi}\left[e^{-jkR}/R + e^{-jkR'}/R'\right],$$

where $R = |\mathbf{r} - \mathbf{r_p}|$ and $R' = |\mathbf{r} - \mathbf{r'_p}|$. Thus, if the observation point $\mathbf{r}$ lies on the plane surface, because $R = R'$, then

(2.25)
$$G_D(\mathbf{r})\big]_{S_o} = 0, \quad G_N(\mathbf{r})\big]_{S_o} = \frac{e^{-jkR}}{2\pi R}.$$

By taking the normal derivatives of both of the equations given in (2.24), it can be readily shown that on the plane surface,

(2.26)
$$\left[\frac{\partial G_D(\mathbf{r})}{\partial n}\right]_{S_o} = \frac{\cos(\tilde{\mathbf{n}}, \tilde{\mathbf{R}})}{2\pi}\left[\frac{\partial}{\partial R}\left(e^{-jkR}/R\right)\right]_{S_o}, \quad \left[\frac{\partial G_N(\mathbf{r})}{\partial n}\right]_{S_o} = 0,$$

in which the angle $(\tilde{\mathbf{n}}, \tilde{\mathbf{R}})$ is between the outward normal unit vector $\tilde{\mathbf{n}}$ and the unit vector $\tilde{\mathbf{R}} = (\mathbf{r} - \mathbf{r_p})/|\mathbf{r} - \mathbf{r_p}|$. Since (2.25) and (2.26) correspond to the conditions for the two sets of boundary conditions listed in Table 2.1, the two sets of Green's functions given by (2.24) are suitable for solving problems in which either the pressure or the normal component of the velocity is specified on the boundary.

2.1.4 Diffraction Equations

The derivation of the diffraction integral given by (2.21) was based on the assumption that the free-space Green's function was appropriate for solving the Helmholtz equation for any specific boundary conditions. However, as noted earlier, depending on the specified conditions, this solution does not necessarily recover the assigned boundary conditions, and consequently when the observation point is within a few wavelengths of the boundary, the solution may be in error. A self-consistent approach, based on using the Green's functions of (2.24), was used by Rayleigh [5] and Sommerfeld [9]. When the dimensions of the aperture(s) (excitation region) and distance of the observations points from the aperture(s) are many wavelengths, the results predicted by the Kirchhoff and Rayleigh-Sommerfeld are in close agreement for moderate angles of diffraction [10]. For acoustical wavelengths, where the aperture size and observation distances may be no more than few wavelengths, most researchers have tended to use the Rayleigh-Sommerfeld approach. A fuller account of the historical and scientific development of these concepts is provided in [4, Chapter 3; 11].

By substituting (2.25) and (2.26) into (2.23), the velocity potentials for the two sets of boundary conditions can be written as

(2.27)

$$\Phi_D(\mathbf{r}{:}\omega) = \frac{-1}{2\pi} \iint_{S_o} \Phi \cos(\tilde{\mathbf{n}}, \tilde{\mathbf{R}}) \frac{\partial}{\partial R}\left(\frac{e^{-jkR}}{R} \right) dS_o$$

$$= \frac{1}{2\pi} \iint_{S_o} \Phi \cos(\tilde{\mathbf{n}}, \tilde{\mathbf{R}}) \frac{e^{-jkR}}{R}\left[jk + \frac{1}{R} \right] dS_o$$

$$\Phi_N(\mathbf{r}{:}\omega) = \frac{1}{2\pi} \iint_{S_o} \frac{e^{-jkR}}{R} \frac{\partial \Phi}{\partial n} dS_o,$$

which are commonly referred to as the Rayleigh-Sommerfeld diffraction equations. It should be noted that the geometric mean of the two velocity potentials is

(2.28) $$\frac{\Phi_D(\mathbf{r}{:}\omega) + \Phi_N(\mathbf{r}{:}\omega)}{2} = \frac{1}{4\pi} \iint_{S_i} \frac{e^{-jkR}}{R}\left[\frac{\partial \Phi}{\partial n} + \Phi \cos(\tilde{\mathbf{n}}, \tilde{\mathbf{R}})\left(1 + \frac{1}{jkR} \right) \right] dS_i.$$

This equation, which is identical to (2.19), simplifies to the Kirchhoff free-field solution [15–17] as expressed by (2.20) when the source is quasi-planar.

The time-dependent form of the Rayleigh-Sommerfeld diffraction equations can be found by taking the inverse Fourier transform of (2.27). After changing the order of integration and putting $k = \omega/c$, these become:

(2.29)

$$\phi_D(\mathbf{r}{:}t) = \left(\frac{1}{2\pi} \right)^2 \iint_{S_o} \int_{-\infty}^{\infty} \cos(\tilde{\mathbf{n}}, \tilde{\mathbf{R}}) \frac{\Phi}{R}\left[\frac{j\omega}{c_o} + \frac{1}{R} \right] e^{j\omega\left(t - \frac{R}{c_o} \right)} d\omega dS_o$$

$$\approx \left(\frac{1}{2\pi} \right)^2 \iint_{S_o} \int_{-\infty}^{\infty} \cos(\tilde{\mathbf{n}}, \tilde{\mathbf{R}}) \frac{j\omega\Phi}{c_o R} e^{j\omega\left(t - \frac{R}{c_o} \right)} d\omega dS_o$$

$$\phi_N(\mathbf{r}{:}t) = \left(\frac{1}{2\pi} \right)^2 \iint_{S_o} \int_{-\infty}^{\infty} \frac{1}{R} \frac{\partial \Phi}{\partial n} e^{j\omega\left(t - \frac{R}{c_o} \right)} d\omega dS_o,$$

in which $(t - R/c_o)$ is retarded time and the approximation assumes the observation point is such that $R \gg \lambda/2\pi$. Denoting retarded time quantities by $\langle . \rangle$, the following inverse Fourier transform identities can be obtained:

$$\langle \phi \rangle = \frac{1}{2\pi} \int_{\infty}^{\infty} \Phi(\mathbf{r}{:}\omega) e^{j\omega\left(t - \frac{R}{c_o}\right)} d\omega$$

$$\langle \partial\phi/\partial t \rangle = \frac{1}{2\pi} \int_{\infty}^{\infty} j\omega \Phi(\mathbf{r}{:}\omega) e^{j\omega\left(t - \frac{R}{c_o}\right)} d\omega$$

$$\langle \partial\phi/\partial n \rangle = \frac{1}{2\pi} \int_{\infty}^{\infty} \frac{\partial\Phi(\mathbf{r}{:}\omega)}{\partial n} e^{j\omega\left(t - \frac{R}{c_o}\right)} d\omega.$$

By substituting these into (2.29), we obtain

(2.30)

$$\phi_D(\mathbf{r}{:}t) \approx \frac{1}{2\pi} \iint_{S_o} \frac{\cos(\tilde{\mathbf{n}}, \tilde{\mathbf{R}})}{c_o R} \left\langle \frac{\partial\phi_D}{\partial t} \right\rangle dS_o$$

$$\phi_N(\mathbf{r}{:}t) = \frac{1}{2\pi} \iint_{S_o} \frac{1}{R} \left\langle \frac{\partial\phi_N}{\partial n} \right\rangle dS_o.$$

The final step consists of expressing the two partial derivative terms in terms of the boundary pressure and velocity. Since $p(\mathbf{r}{:}t) = \rho_o \partial\phi/\partial t$, the first equation becomes:

(2.31)

$$\boxed{\phi_D(\mathbf{r}{:}t) \approx \frac{1}{2\pi} \iint_{S_o} \frac{p\left(t - \frac{R}{c_o}\right)}{\rho c_o R} \cos(\tilde{\mathbf{n}}, \tilde{\mathbf{R}}) \, dS_o,}$$

for $R \gg \lambda/2\pi$.

The assumptions underlying this equation are that the observation point is several wavelengths from the surface, that the surface is plane, and that the pressure distribution is specified. This is sometimes referred to as the "pressure release surface problem."

For the second equation of (2.30), since the normal outward surface velocity component is $-\partial\phi_N/\partial n$, the inner directed component will be: $v_n = \partial\phi_N/\partial n$, and hence

(2.32)

$$\boxed{\phi_N(\mathbf{r}{:}t) = \frac{1}{2\pi} \iint_{S_o} \frac{v_n\left(t - \frac{R}{c_o}\right)}{R} \, dS_o.}$$

This equation, generally referred to as the Rayleigh integral, assumes a flat boundary on which the normal component of the velocity is defined. It also assumes propagation in an inviscid medium and sufficiently small fluctuations so that nonlinear effects can be ignored. It states that the velocity potential at the observation point can be found by integrating the normal component of the velocity over the entire surface. Evidently, regions where the velocity is zero make no contribution. In essence, this integral is a restatement of Huygens' principle as developed by Fresnel (see section 1.7.1). Specifically, the source can be considered to consist of an array of elementary point sources that emit spherical waves whose superposition gives rise to the signal at the observation point. The use of a different form of Rayleigh's integral for calculating the field distribution for a disk transducer is studied in the next section.

2.2 The Rayleigh Integral

It will be shown that the Rayleigh integral can be transformed into a convolution of the normal component of the surface velocity and the velocity potential impulse response. This provides a powerful method for calculating the field distribution due to either pulse or continuous wave excitation of a transducer.

2.2.1 Impulse Response

For simplicity we assume that the transducer surface coincides with the plane $z = 0$, and that elsewhere on this plane, the normal component of the surface velocity is zero. In addition, it is assumed that everywhere on this plane the normal component of the velocity waveform has the same time variation, i.e., $v_z(x, y, 0{:}t) = \xi_o(x, y)v_{no}(t)$, where $\xi_o(x, y)$ denotes the spatial variation, called the *apodization* function. Thus, the Rayleigh integral can be written as

$$(2.33) \qquad \phi_N(\mathbf{r}{:}t) = \iint_{S_o} \frac{v_{no}\left(t - \dfrac{R}{c_o}\right)\xi_o(x, y)}{2\pi R}\, dS_o.$$

But v_{no} can be written as the convolution integral:

$$v_{no}\left(t - \frac{R}{c_o}\right) = \int_{-\infty}^{\infty} v_{no}(\tau)\delta\left(t - \frac{R}{c_o} - \tau\right) d\tau,$$

which, when substituted into (2.33) and after changing the order of integration, enables the velocity potential to be written as

$$(2.34) \qquad \phi_N(\mathbf{r}{:}t) = \int_{-\infty}^{\infty} v_{no}(\tau)\iint_{S_o} \frac{\xi_o(x, y)\delta\left(t - \dfrac{R}{c_o} - \tau\right)}{2\pi R}\, dS_o\, d\tau.$$

We now let

$$(2.35) \qquad \boxed{\, h(\mathbf{r}{:}t) = \iint_{S_o} \frac{\xi_o(x, y)\delta\left(t - \dfrac{R}{c_o}\right)}{2\pi R}\, dS_o \,},$$

which is simply the velocity potential at the observation point due to a δ-function of velocity at each point on the surface, i.e., it is the impulse response. This expression for the impulse response can be interpreted with the help of

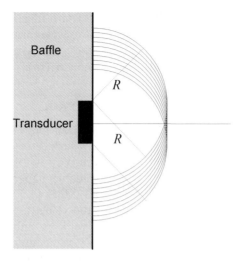

Figure 2.5 The spherical waves emitted from all points on the cross-sectional surface from a simple planar transducer at a particular instant of time $t = R/c_o$, when the transducer is excited with a δ-function. The total contribution at a given observation point and specific time is the sum of all wavelets originating from points on the transducer surface that are at a distance of tc_o from the observation point.

Fig. 2.5, which shows a cross-sectional view of a simple planar transducer excited by a δ-function. Each point on the surface can be considered as an elementary source of a spherical wave, and the impulse response at a given time and location is simply the sum of the contributions weighed by the apodization function.

By making use of (2.35), (2.34) can be expressed in the compact form

(2.36) $$\boxed{\phi_N(\mathbf{r}{:}t) = v_{no}(t) * h(\mathbf{r}{:}t)},$$

which is simply the convolution of the velocity waveform and the impulse response.[6] From this the pressure and velocity waveforms can be readily obtained. Noting that $p = \rho_o \partial \phi_N / \partial t$ and that $\mathbf{v}(\mathbf{r}{:}t) = -\nabla \phi_N$:

$$p(\mathbf{r}{:}t) = \rho_o v_{no}(t) * \frac{\partial h(\mathbf{r}{:}t)}{\partial t}, \qquad \text{(a)}$$

(2.37)[7]   or $$= \rho_o h(\mathbf{r}{:}t) * \frac{\partial v_{no}(t)}{\partial t}, \qquad \text{(b)}$$

and $$\mathbf{v}(\mathbf{r}{:}t) = -v_{no}(t) * \nabla h(\mathbf{r}{:}t). \qquad \text{(c)}$$

6. If the pressure release surface condition had been assumed, then (31) would have formed the starting point rather than the Rayleigh integral. The resulting equation for the pressure impulse response would be the same as (35) but the integrand would now include a $\cos(\tilde{\mathbf{n}},\tilde{\mathbf{R}})$ term. The velocity potential would then be expressed as $\phi_D(\mathbf{r}{:}t) = p_o(t) * h_D(\mathbf{r}{;}t)$, where $h_D(\mathbf{r},t)$ is the pressure impulse response.

7. These follow from: $\dfrac{d}{dx}\{f(x) * g(x)\} = f(x) * \dfrac{dg(x)}{dx} = \dfrac{df(x)}{dx} * g(x)$, [38, p. 122].

For example, if the velocity waveform is a δ-function, i.e., $v_{no} = A\delta(t)$, then $p_\delta(\mathbf{r}{:}t) = A\rho_o \partial h(\mathbf{r}{:}t)/\partial t$. Alternatively, if the waveform is a Heaviside unit step function[8], i.e., $v_{no} = A\mathcal{H}(t)$, then, since the derivative of a step function is a δ-function, the pressure response is given by $p_\mathcal{H}(\mathbf{r}{:}t) = A\rho_o h(\mathbf{r}{:}t)$.

2.2.2 The Piston Transducer: On-Axis

Many papers have been devoted to the transient response of a circular disk embedded in an ideal baffle having zero surface velocity. Freedman [39] provided a useful review of the contributions up to 1959; these and subsequent developments are reviewed in the valuable paper by Harris [40] and the chapter by Hutchins and Hayward [41]. Miles [42] was the first to derive an expression for the time derivative of the velocity potential in response to a step function change in the surface velocity. Subsequently Oberhettinger [43,44] and Chadwick and Tuphlome [45], using integral transform techniques, obtained expressions for the velocity potential in response to a δ-function movement. A much more elegant and powerful approach is that based on linear systems theory, namely the impulse response method first described by Tupholme [46], and independently by Stepanishen [47,48]. Using this technique, more complex geometries have been analyzed: for example, wedges and infinite strips by Tupholme [46], rectangles by Lockwood and Willette [49], concave and convex surfaces by Ohtsuki [50] and by Penttinen and Luukkala [51], and triangles by Jensen [52].

Impulse Response: On-Axis

We first consider the straightforward problem of determining the on-axis transient response of a piston transducer. Such a problem avoids some of the complexities of a more general approach and will allow us to focus on obtaining physical insight. Calculation of the field distribution (e.g., pressure) for the circular disk illustrated in Fig. 2.6 requires that the impulse response be calculated at each point $\mathbf{r}$.

The on-axis impulse response can be found by converting to cylindrical coordinates (r, z), so that (2.35) becomes

$$h(0, z{:}t) = \int_0^a \frac{\delta(t - R/c_o)}{2\pi R} 2\pi r \, dr.$$

Since $R^2 = r^2 + z^2$, the integral can be transformed to

$$h(0, z{:}t) = \int_z^{\sqrt{a^2 + z^2}} \delta\left(t - \frac{R}{c_o}\right) dR = c_o \left[\mathcal{H}\left(t - \frac{z}{c_o}\right) - \mathcal{H}\left(t - \frac{\sqrt{a^2 + z^2}}{c_o}\right)\right]$$

(2.38)
$$= c_o \mathcal{H}\left(t - \frac{z}{c_o}\right) \mathcal{H}\left(\frac{\sqrt{a^2 + z^2}}{c_o} - t\right).$$

---

8. Defined by: $\mathcal{H}(t) = 1$ for $t > 0$, $\mathcal{H}(0) = 1/2$, and $\mathcal{H}(t) = 0$ for $t < 0$.

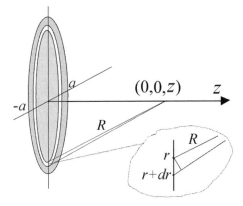

Figure 2.6 Piston transducer of radius a embedded in a perfect baffle. The on-axis impulse response at $(0,0,z)$ can be found by calculating the contributions from elementary annular rings of radius r and width dr.

As illustrated in Fig. 2.7a, the first form of this equation consists of two Heaviside step functions: the first occurs when the pulse from the transducer center arrives at z, and the second starts when the pulse from the edge arrives. In the second form, the second step function finishes when the edge pulse arrives. It is evident that as the observation point moves further away, the duration of the impulse response diminishes, approaching a δ-function as $z \rightarrow \infty$.

If the transducer surface velocity is a δ-function of unit strength, $\left(\int_{-\infty}^{\infty} v_{no}(t)dt = 1 \right)$, i.e., $v_{no} = \delta(t)$, then it follows from (2.37) that the pressure waveform consists of the two δ-functions shown in Fig. 2.7b and c, and is given by:[9]

$$p_\delta(z{:}t) = \rho_o c_o \delta\left(t - \frac{z}{c_o} \right) - \rho_o c_o \delta\left(t - \frac{\sqrt{a^2 + z^2}}{c_o} \right),$$

(2.39)   **Direct Wave**   **Edge Wave**

the second being an inverted replica of the first. The more general case of an arbitrary waveform can be solved by convolving this with the velocity waveform, yielding

$$p(z{:}t) = \rho_o c_o \left[v_{no}\left(t - \frac{z}{c_o} \right) - v_{no}\left(t - \frac{\sqrt{a^2 + z^2}}{c_o} \right) \right].$$

(2.40)   **Direct Wave**   **Edge Wave**

9. At first sight the dimensions may appear to be incorrect, since the dimensions of a δ-function are 1/argument. However, we are considering a unit strength δ-function, in which the "1" has dimensions [L].

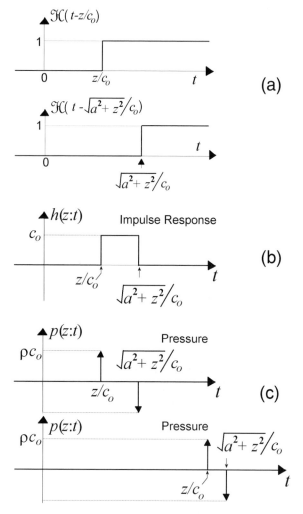

Figure 2.7 On-axis waveforms for a simple piston transducer. (a) Interpretation of the impulse response function (2.38). (b) Impulse response and pressure response for a δ-function transducer velocity at a z-position fairly close to the transducer (c) Pressure waveform further away.

Thus, the pressure field can be considered to consist of two components: the first is always present, while the second (the edge wave) will occur only if the transducer is non-infinite. If a pulse excites the transducer, then an on-axis observer will see a plane wave arriving at a time z/c_o and will know that the transducer has finite dimensions only when the edge wave arrives at a subsequent time. It is the interference between the two components emanating from

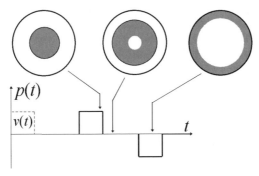

Figure 2.8 On-axis pressure response close to a disk transducer for a rectangular velocity excitation. The shaded areas correspond to those regions of the transducer that contribute to the pressure at the times indicated.

the center and periphery of the disk[10] that gives rise to the resulting waveform. Although the above analysis was restricted to on-axis locations, this concept is also valuable in understanding and describing the off-axis transient response [41,53]. Kozina and Makarov [54], in their development and discussion of equations for the step function response of a plane transducer, recognized and properly interpreted the existence of these two components. Subsequently, Tupholme [55], in his study of the transient radiation from a spherical cap, introduced the direct and edge wave terminology and later made use of this in a study of the transient radiation characteristics of other transducer geometries [46].

Visualizing the Response

A useful means of visualizing the contribution to the pressure at a given instant of time is based on the work of Beaver [56]. In calculating the pressure waveform, he summed the contributions made by each elementary area of the transducer surface at each instant of time. Though this technique is more complex than the impulse response method, it has the advantage of providing additional insight into the process by which the response is generated. The sketch of Fig. 2.8 illustrates this for a rectangular velocity pulse and an observation point close to the transducer. The shaded areas of the transducer surface indicate the region that contributed to the pressure waveform at the indicated time. Because the velocity pulse duration was assumed to be roughly two times less than that of the velocity potential impulse pulse response (see Fig. 2.7b), the times when there is no pressure response can be seen to correspond to the times at which the shaded annular ring is entirely within the disk. Thus, a pressure response is seen to occur only when the center or the periphery of the transducer is contributing.

---

10. Sometimes the component from the center is simply referred to as the *plane* or *center* wave. See also the discussion associated with eqn. (3.19).

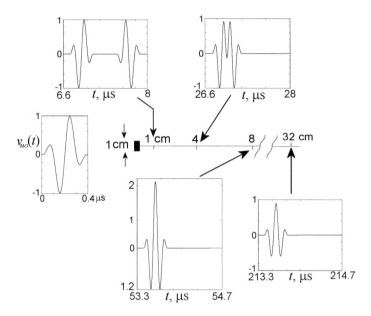

Figure 2.9 On-axis pressure response for a disk transducer ($a = 5$ mm) transmitting into water and excited to give the velocity waveform shown near the left margin, and described by (2.41). The velocity and pressure waveform amplitudes have been normalized: all time scales have been retained.

An Example

We shall consider a 5.0 MHz (center frequency) velocity pulse produced by a 1.0 cm diameter disk transducer and determine the pressure pulse at various on-axis locations. If the pulse is given by

$$(2.41) \qquad v_{no}(t) = v_o \sin^2(0.25\omega t)\sin(\omega t),$$

for $0 < t < 0.4$ μs and $v_{no}(t) = 0$ elsewhere, then its derivative is:

$$dv_{no}/dt = 0.125 v_o \omega [4\cos(\omega t) - 3\cos(1.5\omega t) - \cos(0.5\omega t)].$$

As indicated in Fig. 2.9, this velocity pulse is much like that used for B-mode ultrasound imaging. By convolving it with the pressure response impulse, as given by (2.39), the responses at various on-axis positions were calculated, and these are shown in Fig. 2.9. It will be noted that close to the transducer, the pulses from the center and edge are distinct, the second being an inverted replica of the first. At $z = 4$ cm interference is present, while at $z = 8$ cm ($\sim a^2/\lambda$) the interference is constructive, resulting a doubling of the positive peak amplitude. At 32 cm, the amplitude is reduced due to destructive interference between the direct and edge waves.

The on-axis peak pressure magnitude presented in Fig. 2.10 clearly shows the effect of interference. Also shown in this figure is the on-axis energy delivered per unit area $\left(\propto \int_0^\infty p^2(0{:}t)dt\right)$. This also has a maximum at the

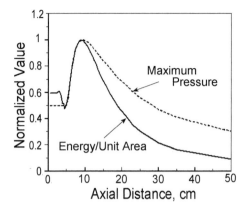

Figure 2.10 Normalized on-axis peak pressure magnitude and energy delivered per unit area for the same transducer and excitation waveform given in Fig. 2.9. The peak occurs close to $a^2/\lambda = 8.33$ cm.

near-field/far-field transition point. In the near-field region, the shape of both plots depends on the excitation waveform.

Limiting Conditions

Let us suppose that the piston radius $a \to \infty$. As the observation point approaches the transducer, $\partial h/\partial t \to c_o\delta(t)$, so that from (2.37a) the pressure is given by $p(t) = \rho_o c_o v_{no}(t)$, i.e., the Pressure waveform = Characteristic impedance × Velocity, which is the classical relation for a plane wave.

A second condition of interest occurs when the observation point is far removed ($z \gg a$). Under this circumstance, as noted earlier, the impulse response approaches a δ-function and is given by [58]:

$$h(z{:}t) \approx z\left[\sqrt{1+\frac{a^2}{z^2}}-1\right]\delta\left(t-\frac{z}{c_o}\right) \approx \frac{a^2}{2z}\delta\left(t-\frac{z}{c_o}\right), \text{ for } z \gg a.$$

Consequently, from (2.37b) the pressure can be expressed as

$$(2.42) \qquad\qquad p(z{:}t) = \frac{\rho_o a^2}{2z}\frac{\partial v_{no}(t)}{\partial t}\bigg|_{t-z/c_o}.$$

As expected, this shows that the pressure falls off inversely with the distance: a result that is identical to the limiting result (2.46) obtained in the next subsection for sinusoidal excitation.

Sinusoidal Response

Pressure and Velocity The response to a sinusoidal transducer velocity waveform of angular frequency ω_o is a straightforward extension of the results just obtained. If we assume that $v_{no}(t) = v_o e^{j\omega_o t}$, where v_o is the velocity amplitude, then the pressure response given by (2.37a), or by (2.40), can be expressed as

(2.43)
$$p(z{:}t) = \rho_o v_o c_o \left[e^{j\omega_o t} * \frac{\partial h(z{:}t)}{\partial t} \right]$$
$$= \rho_o v_o c_o \left[e^{j\omega_o(t-z/c_o)} - e^{j\omega_o\left(t-\sqrt{z^2+a^2}/c_o\right)} \right].$$

The frequency domain response can be found by rewriting this as

$$p(z{:}t) = \rho_o v_o c_o \left[e^{-j\omega_o z/c_o} - e^{-j(\omega_o/c_o)\sqrt{z^2+a^2}} \right] e^{j\omega_o t},$$

from which it is immediately evident that the pressure phasor (denoted by an underscore) is given by

(2.44)
$$\underline{p}(z{:}\omega_o) = \rho_o v_o c_o \left[e^{-j\omega_o z/c_o} - e^{-j(\omega_o/c_o)\sqrt{z^2+a^2}} \right].$$

Dropping the subscript on ω_o, this can be written in either of the following two forms:

(2.45)
$$\underline{p}(z{:}\omega) = \rho_o v_o c_o \left(1 - e^{-j(\omega/c_o)\sqrt{a^2+z^2}-z} \right) e^{-j\omega z/c_o} \tag{a}$$

$$\underline{p}(z{:}\omega) = 2j\rho_o c_o v_o \sin\left[(\omega/2c_o)\left(\sqrt{a^2+z^2}-z\right) \right] e^{-j(\omega/2c_o)\left(z+\sqrt{a^2+z^2}\right)}. \tag{b}$$

When the z-location is such that argument of the sine function is an odd multiple of $\pi/2$, the pressure will have a maximum value given by $|p|_{max} = 2\rho_o c_o v_o$. The variation of the pressure magnitude squared with z is shown in the graph of Fig. 2.11a, and this will be discussed shortly. For far distant points such that $z \gg a$, (2.45) reduces to

(2.46)
$$\underline{p}(z{:}\omega) \approx \frac{\rho_o v_o \omega a^2}{2z} e^{-j\left(\frac{\omega z}{c_o}-\frac{\pi}{2}\right)},$$

which states that the pressure varies inversely with the axial distance and as the square of the disk radius.

To calculate the particle velocity vector, we first note that on the axis the radial component of $\mathbf{v}$ is zero. Since $\mathbf{v} = -\text{grad}\phi_N$, and because $\phi_N = p/(j\omega\rho_o)$, the velocity phasor is given by $\underline{v}(z) = -(\partial p/\partial z)/(j\omega\rho_o)$. By substituting (2.45a) into this expression and evaluating, we find that the particle velocity phasor is

(2.47)
$$\underline{v}(z{:}\omega) = v_o \left(1 - \frac{z}{\sqrt{a^2+z^2}} e^{-j(\omega/c_o)\left(\sqrt{a^2+z^2}-z\right)} \right) e^{-j\omega z/c_o}.$$

Intensity   In Chapter 1 (subsection 1.5.3) it was pointed out that the intensity $\mathbf{I}(\mathbf{r}{:}t)$ is a vector quantity that represents the magnitude and direction of energy flow. For a sinusoidal field the time average of the intensity was written in (1.85) as

(2.48)
$$\bar{\mathbf{I}}(\mathbf{r}) = \frac{1}{2}\text{Re}\{\underline{p}\underline{v}^*\},$$

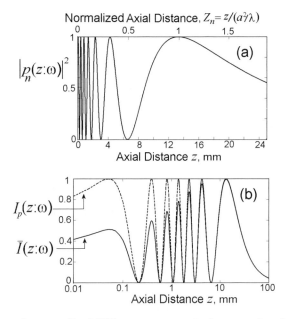

Figure 2.11 On-axis, normalized CW pressure magnitude squared and time-averaged intensity profiles for a 5.0 MHz circular transducer of 4 mm diameter ($a = 6.67 \lambda$) transmitting into water ($c_o = 1500$ m/s, $\rho_o = 1000$ kg/m^3), as calculated from (2.45), (2.48), and (2.50). (a) Square of the normalized pressure magnitude $\left\{ |p_n|^2 = \left[|\underline{p}| / (\rho_o c_o v_o) \right]^2 \right\}$ versus the axial distance (linear scale). (b) Log scale showing both the true intensity (solid line) and the plane-wave assumption value (broken line). Both $\bar{I}(z,\omega)$ and $\bar{I}_p(z,\omega)$ have been normalized by dividing by $2\rho_o c_o v_o^2$. For example, if the maximum intensity is 50 mW/cm^2, the velocity and displacement amplitudes at the transducer surface are: $v_o = 1.29$ cm/s, $\xi_o = 4.11 \times 10^{-10}$ m, respectively, and the maximum pressure amplitude is $p_{max} = 19.36$ kPa.

where the superscript * denotes the complex conjugate, Re{.} denotes the real part of the argument, and the overscore denotes a time-averaged value. For an elementary surface area of dS, the dot product $\bar{\mathbf{I}}(\mathbf{r}) \cdot \mathbf{dS}$ is equal to the power (in Watts) that flows through it in the direction of $\mathbf{dS}$.

For a plane harmonic wave propagating in a lossless medium $\underline{p} = \rho_o c_o |\underline{\mathbf{v}}|$, i.e., $\underline{\mathbf{v}}$ and $\underline{p}$ are in phase, and consequently, by substitution into (2.48), the plane-wave intensity is given by

$$(2.49) \qquad \bar{I}_p = |\underline{p}|^2 / (2\rho_o c_o).$$

In regions reasonably far from a source such that the wavefront is approximately plane, this is a good approximation [57]. For other situations, one must take care to properly account for any phase difference; this becomes particularly important in the near-field region [41].

To illustrate the above point we consider the on-axis intensity of a piston transducer. On the axis of symmetry the plane-wave intensity can be obtained by substituting (2.45b) into (2.49), yielding

(2.50) $\bar{I}_p(z{:}\omega) = 2\rho_o c_o v_o^2 \sin^2\left[(\omega/2c_o)(\sqrt{a^2 + z^2} - z)\right],$

which is plotted in Fig. 2.11b for a 5.0 MHz transducer with a radius of 2.0 mm. On the other hand, noting that the velocity vector is directed along the z-axis, then the intensity can be evaluated from (2.48) by using (2.45a) and (2.47), and this is also shown in Fig. 2.11b. It can be seen that the difference between the true axial intensity profile (solid line) and that calculated using the plane-wave approximation (dashed line) becomes large very close to the transducer.

Maxima and Minima   The log and linear graphs of Fig. 2.11 illustrate some important features of this simple transducer, providing a useful framework for understanding the behavior of transducers with more complex geometry. The presence of seven maxima and six minima (excluding that at $z = \infty$) is caused by the effects of constructive and destructive interference of the wavelets arriving from different annuli on the transducer. These maxima and minima correspond to path differences of about 7λ, which is approximately equal to the transducer radius expressed in terms of λ ($a = 6.77\lambda$). Thus, with increasing radius, the number of maxima and minima increase proportionately. A second observation is that the z-positions of the intensity maxima and minima correspond closely to the pressure maxima and exactly to the minima, and these can be found by equating the argument of the sine function in (2.45b) to odd or even multiples of $\pi/2$, respectively. As a result we find:

$$\text{Maxima Condition: } Z_n^{\max} = \frac{z^{\max}}{a^2/\lambda} = \frac{1}{n} - n\left(\frac{\lambda}{2a}\right)^2, n = 1, 3, 5, \ldots$$

(2.51)

$$\text{Minima Condition: } Z_n^{\min} = \frac{z^{\min}}{a^2/\lambda} = \frac{1}{n} - n\left(\frac{\lambda}{2a}\right)^2, n = 2, 4, 6, \ldots,$$

where Z_n is the normalized axial distance. Beyond the last maximum at $Z_n = 1 - (\lambda/2a)^2 \approx 1$ (for $a \gg \lambda$), the intensity begins to diminish and approaches a rate $\propto 1/z^2$. A third observation is that very close to the transducer surface, the effects of interference are also very evident. If the transducer radius is exactly equal to an even integer multiple of $\lambda/2$, the intensity will approach zero at the center, while if it is an odd multiple, it will be a maximum. For the values given in Fig. 2.11, the intensity at the center is $\bar{I}(0) = 18.75 \text{ mW/cm}^2$, corresponding to a normalized value of 0.375.

Additional insight into the process that gives rise to the maxima and minima can be gained by writing the surface velocity as $v_{no} = v_o \sin(\omega t)$. With the help of (2.39) the on-axis pressure can be expressed as

$$p(z{:}t) = v_o \rho_o c_o \left[\delta\left(t - \frac{z}{c_o}\right) - \delta\left(t - \frac{\sqrt{a^2 + z^2}}{c_o}\right)\right] * \sin(\omega t).$$

Now the interval of time between these two δ-functions is

$$\Delta t = \left(\sqrt{z^2 + a^2} - z\right)/c_o,$$

so that when this interval is exactly equal to 1, 2..n periods, i.e., when $n\lambda = \sqrt{z^2 + a^2} - z$, the pressure will be zero. Similarly, maxima occur when the interval is exactly 1,3,5 . . . m half periods, i.e., when $m\lambda/2 = \sqrt{z^2 + a^2} - z$. This is illustrated in Fig. 2.12 for the last maximum and the last minimum.

2.3 Angular Spectrum Method

It is well known that a 2-D aperture distribution of a field quantity, such as the velocity potential or pressure, can be represented by its spatial frequency components in that plane. Booker and Clemmow [20,21], in seeking to obtain a better understanding of the Fourier transform of an antenna aperture, observed that the propagation from a 2-D aperture can be exactly represented by an infinite set of plane waves whose angular directions encompass the entire 2π solid angle associated with the propagation half-space. The distribution of such a set is their angular spectrum, and the technique is called the plane-wave angular spectrum method [4, pp. 55–61]. In acoustics, the plane-wave spectrum has been used to calculate the radiation from transducers [22–24] and to calculate the transmit–receive response [28]. The equivalence of the angular spectrum and the Rayleigh integral representations for both monochromatic [23] and time-dependent [25] velocity sources has also been established. Liu and Waag [29] have presented a comparison of the angular spectrum approach with other methods, together with a discussion of the limitations.

If the harmonic field pattern on a given plane is known, then the field distribution on a parallel plane can be calculated by using the angular spectrum approach. Williams and Maynard [35] showed that by making use of a highly efficient 2-D FFT algorithm, the computation time needed for calculating the harmonic field profile could be reduced by several orders of magnitude as

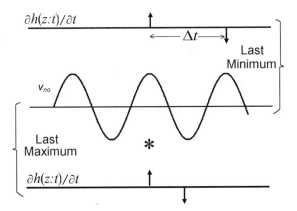

Figure 2.12 The convolution of a sinusoidal signal with the derivative of the velocity potential impulse response at two on-axis locations: the last minimum and the last maximum ($z \approx a^2/\lambda$).

compared to a numerical evaluation using the 2-D Rayleigh integral. The plane to be determined can be either behind (closer to the source) or in front of the known plane. If it is behind, then the problem is one of back-projection; otherwise it is a forward projection problem. One application of this technique is to determine the field distribution on the surface of an ultrasound source from measurements made on a more convenient plane away from the source. Schafer and Lewin [30] have used this method to determine the surface velocity patterns of transducers having both simple and complex geometries. Moreover, by measuring the spatial and temporal field distribution on a given plane, the method can be extended to wide-band excitation conditions. More recently, Wu and Stepinski [31] have proposed extensions to the angular spectrum approach that enable the spectrum to be obtained for curved radiation sources.

2.3.1 Basic Principles

The arbitrary monochromatic source illustrated in Fig. 2.13 with a wave number $k = \omega/c$ will give rise to a certain field distribution on the plane $z = 0$. Let us assume that the spatial frequencies in the x- and y-directions are denoted by k_x and k_y, respectively. Then the velocity potential on this plane can be expressed in terms of the spatial frequency spectral density function $S(k_x, k_y)$ by using the 2-D inverse Fourier transform relation.

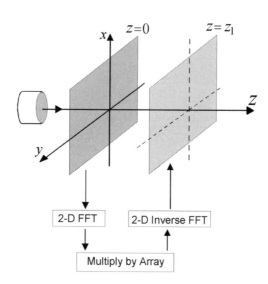

Figure 2.13 An arbitrary harmonic source gives rise to a field pattern on the plane $z = 0$. By taking a 2-D Fourier transform of this field, the 2-D spatial angular spectrum is obtained. By multiplying by an array and then taking the inverse transform, the field pattern in the plane $z = z_1$ can be obtained. Based in Vecchio et al. [34].

$$(2.52) \qquad \Phi(x, y, z) = \frac{1}{4\pi^2} \int\!\!\!\int_{-\infty}^{\infty} S(k_x, k_y : z) e^{j(k_x x + k_y y)} dk_x dk_y,$$

and the spectral density function is given by the 2-D Fourier transform definition:

$$(2.53) \qquad S(k_x, k_y : z) = \int\!\!\!\int_{-\infty}^{\infty} \Phi(x, y, z) e^{-j(k_x x + k_y y)} dx dy.$$

To obtain a physical interpretation of (2.52), we first note that a unit amplitude plane harmonic wave propagating in the direction of the wave vector $\mathbf{k} = \tilde{\mathbf{k}}k = \tilde{\mathbf{x}}k_x + \tilde{\mathbf{y}}k_y + \tilde{\mathbf{z}}k_z$ can be expressed as

$$\psi = e^{j(\omega t - \mathbf{k} \cdot \mathbf{r})} = e^{j\omega t} e^{-jk(\alpha x + \beta y + \gamma z)},$$

in which the direction cosines of the plane wave are α, β, and γ, e.g., $\alpha = \cos\theta = \tilde{\mathbf{k}} \cdot \tilde{\mathbf{x}}$, and unit vectors are indicated by the overscore ~. Since only two angles are needed to define the direction of a plane wave, it follows that $\gamma = \sqrt{1 - (\alpha^2 + \beta^2)}$. By comparing the above plane-wave expression with (2.52), it can be seen that on the plane $z = 0$ the terms under the integral sign represent a complex plane-wave component that has an amplitude of $S(k_x, k_y) dk_x dk_y$ and direction cosines of $\alpha = -k_x/k$, $\beta = -k_y/k$, $\gamma = -k_z/k$, where

$$(2.54) \qquad k_z = -k\sqrt{1 - (\alpha^2 + \beta^2)} = -k\gamma.$$

Hence, on this plane (2.53) can be written as

$$(2.55) \qquad S(\alpha, \beta : 0) = \int\!\!\!\int_{-\infty}^{\infty} \Phi(x, y, 0) e^{+jk(\alpha x + \beta y)} dx dy,$$

which is the *angular spectrum* of $\Phi(x,y,0)$. Thus, the velocity potential can be represented by plane waves whose directions have an angular distribution over a solid angle of 2π steradians.

2.3.2 Angular Spectrum of the Velocity Potential and its Relation to the Velocity

To determine the velocity potential on any plane $z =$ const., in terms of that on the plane $z = 0$, we note that both $\Phi(x,y,0)$ and $\Phi(x,y,z)$ must both satisfy the homogeneous Helmholtz equation given by (1.56). From (2.52), the velocity potential can be expressed in terms of the angular spectrum on the plane z:

$$(2.56) \qquad \Phi(x, y, z) = \frac{k^2}{4\pi^2} \int\!\!\!\int S(\alpha, \beta : z) e^{-jk(\alpha x + \beta y)} d\alpha d\beta.$$

By substituting this into the Helmholtz equation and making use of (2.54), a differential equation results:

$$(2.57) \qquad \frac{d^2}{dz^2} \{ S(\alpha, \beta : z) \} + \gamma^2 k^2 S(\alpha, \beta : z) = 0,$$

the elementary solution to which gives the angular spectrum on the plane z as

$$(2.58) \qquad S(\alpha, \beta\!:\!z) = C_1 e^{-jk\gamma z} + C_2 e^{+jk\gamma z},$$

where the two constants depend on k_x and k_y only.

Two conditions governing γ are important. First, suppose γ is real, i.e., $\alpha^2 + \beta^2 < 1$, then the two exponents in (2.58) represent waves in the $+z$ and $-z$ directions, respectively. Since there is no wave in the negative z-direction, $C_2 = 0$, and therefore $C_1 = S(\alpha,\beta\!:\!0)$. Consequently, the angular spectra on the planes $z = \text{const.}$ and $z = 0$ are related by

$$(2.59) \qquad S(\alpha, \beta\!:\!z) = S(\alpha, \beta\!:\!0) e^{-jk\gamma z}.$$

By substituting this into (2.52) and recalling that $\gamma = -k_z/k$, we obtain

$$(2.60) \qquad \Phi(x, y, z) = \frac{1}{4\pi^2} \int\!\!\int_{-\infty}^{\infty} S(k_x, k_y\!:\!0) e^{j(k_x x + k_y y + k_z z)} dk_x dk_y.$$

On the other hand, if γ is imaginary, i.e. $\alpha^2 + \beta^2 > 1$, then, letting $\bar{\gamma} = j\gamma = \sqrt{\alpha^2 + \beta^2 - 1}$, (2.58) becomes

$$(2.61) \qquad S(\alpha, \beta\!:\!z) = C_1 e^{-k\bar{\gamma} z} + C_2 e^{+k\bar{\gamma} z} = S(\alpha, \beta\!:\!0) e^{-k\bar{\gamma} z},$$

since $C_2 = 0$ and $C_1 = S(\alpha,\beta\!:\!0)$. Thus, for imaginary values of γ the angular spectrum consists of exponentially decaying waves that are generally referred to as *evanescent* waves. Since the maximum value of $k\bar{\gamma}$ is equal to $k(= 2\pi/\lambda)$, it can be seen that these waves decay rapidly with distance, becoming negligible a few wavelengths away from the plane $z = 0$. By substituting (2.61) into (2.52) and noting that $k\bar{\gamma} = -jk_z$, the velocity potential due to these evanescent waves is also given by (2.60). Thus, on the plane $z = \text{const.}$ the total velocity potential, as given by (2.60), is the sum of the contributions due to the homogeneous and evanescent components. The evanescent waves carry no net energy[11] and can be regarded as a nonphysical outcome of the method. In the forward direction their influence can often be disregarded, but for backprojecting the field they give rise to exponentially increasing terms that can create computational difficulties. These problems have been considered by Leeman and Healey [33], who showed that through appropriate pivoted angle projections of the field, the evanescent components can be eliminated.

Since the normal component of the velocity distribution on the surface of a transducer is related to the driving waveform, it is useful to express the angular spectrum on the plane $z = 0$ in terms of the normal component of the velocity in that plane, i.e. $v_z(x,y,0)$. This can be achieved by differentiating both (2.59) and (2.53), equating, noting that $v_z = -\partial\Phi/\partial z$, and evaluating at $z = 0$.

---

11. Evanescent means "quickly fading." Bracewell [32, p. 225] has given a helpful discussion and has pointed out that such waves are present in a hollow microwave rectangular waveguide. When excited at a wavelength such that the lateral dimensions are too small to support propagation, the field decays exponentially from the plane of excitation and all the incident power is reflected.

Thus, on the plane $z = 0$, the velocity potential angular spectrum and the normal velocity distribution can be expressed as

$$(2.62) \qquad S(k_x, k_y : 0) = \frac{1}{-jk_z} \iint\limits_{-\infty}^{\infty} v_z(x, y, 0) e^{-j(k_x x + k_y y)} dx dy.$$

Similarly, by differentiating (2.60), the z-component of the particle velocity on the plane z can be expressed in terms of the angular spectrum on the plane $z = 0$ by

$$(2.63) \qquad v_z(x, y, z) = \frac{-jk_z}{4\pi^2} \iint\limits_{-\infty}^{\infty} S(k_x, k_y : 0) e^{j(k_x x + k_y y + k_z z)} dk_x dk_y.$$

It should be noted that $S(k_x, k_y : z)$ is the angular spectrum of the *velocity potential*, so that the angular spectrum of the *normal component of the velocity* is $-jk_z$ times that of the velocity potential.

A difficulty with evaluating (2.62) arises from the singularity produced by k_z on the circle $k_x^2 + k_y^2 = k^2$, which, as shown by Williams and Maynard [35], can cause serious numerical errors in the case of a rectangular transducer. Since (2.63) is valid for negative values of z, it can also be used to determine the velocity field needed to produce a specified field on the plane $z = 0$. This is referred to as the backward projection problem. For example, if we know the field distribution needed to achieve a certain imaging task, then, by back projection, the field at the source can be determined.

2.3.3 Transfer and Point Spread Function Representations

Transfer Function

Now the angular spectrum of a 2-D field at any arbitrary z-position can be written in terms of that on the plane $z = 0$, or, for that matter, any other plane. Equations (2.59) and (2.61) expressing these relationships for the homogeneous and evanescent waves can be rewritten in terms of the angular spectra at a plane $z = z_1$ with respect to that at a plane $z = z_0$, i.e.,

$$(2.64) \qquad \begin{aligned} S(k_x, k_y : z_1) &= S(k_x, k_y : z_0) e^{-j|k_z|(z_1 - z_0)}, \text{ for } k_z^2 > 0 \\ S(k_x, k_y : z_1) &= S(k_x, k_y : z_0) e^{-|k_z|(z_1 - z_0)}, \text{ for } k_z^2 < 0. \end{aligned}$$

We define the ratio of the spectra on the two planes as the *spatial frequency transfer function* (also called the propagation function). Consequently, the spectrum on the plane $z = z_1$ can be written as

$$(2.65) \qquad S(k_x, k_y : z_1) = H(k_x, k_y : z_1 | z_0) S(k_x, k_y : z_0).$$

As noted earlier, if the observation plane is several wavelengths distant from the plane at z_0, the evanescent component can be neglected, and consequently, using just the first equation in (2.64), the spatial frequency transfer function is approximately given by

$$(2.66) \qquad H(k_x, k_y : z_1 | z_0) \approx e^{-j|k_z|(z_1 - z_0)} = e^{-j(z_1 - z_0)\sqrt{k^2 - (k_x^2 + k_y^2)}}, \qquad \text{(a)}$$

whose magnitude is unity and that varies only in phase. Thus, the angular spectrum on the plane z_1 is related to that on the plane z_0 by the phase changes that take place to each spatial frequency component. As a result, the steps that must taken to determine the field on z_1, given the field pattern on the plane z_0, are those illustrated in Fig. 2.13.

It should be noted that the transfer function between planes z_0 and z_1 for both the pressure and normal component of velocity is also given (2.66). In addition, the normal component of the velocity to pressure transfer function can be found from:

$$(2.66) \qquad H_{p|v}(k_x, k_y : z_1|z_0) = \frac{\omega \rho_o}{\sqrt{k^2 - (k_x^2 + k_y^2)}} e^{-j(z_1 - z_0)\sqrt{k^2 - (k_x^2 + k_y^2)}}. \qquad (b)$$

The derivative of phase angle with respect to the spatial frequency magnitude $(k_x^2 + k_y^2)^{1/2}$ is known as the *phase dispersion*. By taking the derivative of the exponent in (2.66), it can be seen that the system phase dispersion increases with the spatial frequency magnitude: it approaches infinity as $(k_x^2 + k_y^2)^{1/2} \to k$ and vanishes as $(k_x^2 + k_y^2)^{1/2} \to 0$.

Point Spread Function

An alternative way of representing the relation between the two angular spectra is through the *point spread function* (PSF, also called the *impulse response function*) $h_p(x,y,z)$ of the propagation process. The PSF describes the manner in which the field at a given point on the plane $z = z_0$ is mapped into the field on the plane $z = z_1$. If we take the inverse Fourier transform of (2.65) and make use of the convolution theorem, the velocity potential can be written as the 2-D convolution:

$$(2.67) \qquad \Phi(x, y, z_1) = \iint_{-\infty}^{\infty} \Phi(x, y, z_0) h_p(x - x', y - y'; z_1|z_0) dx' dy'$$

$$= \Phi(x, y, z_0) * h_p(x, y; z_1|z_0),$$

where the impulse response function is simply the inverse Fourier transform of the transfer function, i.e.,

$$(2.68) \qquad h_p(x, y; z_1|z_0) = \frac{1}{4\pi^2} \iint_{-\infty}^{\infty} H(k_x, k_y : z_1|z_0) e^{j(k_x x + k_y y)} dk_x dk_y.$$

Thus, a knowledge of the PSF throughout the plane $z = z_0$ enables the potential distribution to be found on the plane $z = z_1$.

An expression for the PSF can be obtained by first finding the angular spectrum for the free-space Green's function by making use of (2.55) and (2.11). Apart from a dimensioned constant (which subsequently cancels out), the spectral density function is given by

$$(2.69) \qquad S(k_x, k_y : z) = \iint_{-\infty}^{\infty} \frac{e^{-jkR}}{4\pi R} e^{-j(k_x x + k_y y)} dx dy,$$

where $R = \sqrt{x^2 + y^2 + z^2}$. If the field is cylindrically symmetrical, then, by means of a transformation[12] to cylindrical coordinates, the above 2-D integral can be shown to reduce to

$$S(k_x, k_y : z) = \int_0^\infty \frac{e^{-jk\sqrt{r^2+z^2}}}{2\sqrt{r^2+z^2}} J_0(r\sigma) r dr,$$

where $\sigma = \sqrt{k_x^2 + k_y^2}$ and $r = \sqrt{x^2 + y^2}$. With reference to Appendix B, this can be recognized as a zero-order Hankel transform of $\left[e^{-jk\sqrt{r^2+z^2}} \big/ (2\sqrt{r^2+z^2}) \right]$. By means of standard transform tables [36, p. 9, eqn. 25] this can be evaluated as

(2.70)
$$S(k_x, k_y : z) = \frac{-je^{-jz\sqrt{k^2-\left(k_x^2+k_y^2\right)}}}{2\sqrt{k^2-\left(k_x^2+k_y^2\right)}}.$$

In view of the self-reciprocal nature of the Hankel transform, the inverse Hankel transform of $S(k_x, k_y : z)$ is equal to the free-field Green's function, i.e.,

(2.71)
$$\frac{e^{-jkR}}{4\pi R} = \int_0^\infty \frac{-je^{-jz\sqrt{k^2-\sigma^2}}}{2\sqrt{k^2-\sigma^2}} J_0(\sigma r) \sigma d\sigma.$$

Taking the partial derivative of this with respect to z gives

(2.72)
$$\frac{\partial}{\partial z} \left\{ \frac{e^{-jkR}}{4\pi R} \right\} = \int_0^\infty \frac{-e^{-jz\sqrt{k^2-\sigma^2}}}{2} J_0(\sigma r) \sigma d\sigma$$

If we now substitute (2.66) into the PSF definition given by (2.68) and transform the coordinates [4, pp. 11–12] to put it in the form of an inverse Hankel transform, the following equation results:

(2.73)
$$h_p(x, y, z) = \int_0^\infty e^{-jz\sqrt{k^2-\sigma^2}} J_0(\sigma r) \sigma d\sigma.$$

Comparison of this equation with the right hand side of (2.72) shows that the PSF is given by

(2.74)
$$h_p(x, y, z) = -2 \frac{\partial}{\partial z} \left\{ \frac{e^{-jkR}}{4\pi R} \right\} = \frac{ze^{-jkR}}{2\pi R^2} \left[\frac{1}{R} + jk \right].$$

This result was originally obtained by Waag et al. [37] and subsequently re-derived by Liu and Waag [29] using a slightly different approach. At distances large compared to λ, the $1/R$ term can be neglected.

Let us suppose that an aperture Ω is present on the plane $z = 0$, such that the aperture transmission function $u = 1$ for (x,y) on Ω, and $u = 0$ elsewhere, and that the aperture is irradiated by monochromatic sources. Then the velocity potential on the plane $z = \Delta z$, just beyond the aperture, can be expressed

12. Proof of this transformation is given in subsection 3.1.1, as well as in [4, pp. 11–12].

in terms of that incident by $\Phi(x,y,\Delta z) = \Phi(x,y,0)u(x,y)$. Using the convolution theorem, the angular spectrum just beyond the aperture is given by

(2.75) $$S(k_x, k_y:\Delta z) = S(k_x, k_y:0) * U(k_x, k_y),$$

where

$$U(k_x, k_y) = \iint_{-\infty}^{\infty} u(x, y)e^{-j(k_x x + k_y y)}dxdy.$$

For the special case where a plane wave is incident normal to the aperture, the incident angular spectrum is given by $S(k_x,k_y:0) = \delta(k_x,k_y)$, so that the transmitted angular spectrum is simply the Fourier transform of the aperture function.

2.3.4 Relation to the Rayleigh Integral

That the angular spectrum method for determining the velocity field is related to the Rayleigh integral can be established by showing their equivalence in the frequency domain [23,25]. By substituting (2.62) into (2.60) and changing the order of integration, the velocity potential can be expressed as

(2.76)
$$\Phi(x, y, z) = \iint_{-\infty}^{\infty} v_z(x_0, y_0, 0)\left[\frac{j}{4\pi^2}\iint_{-\infty}^{\infty}\frac{1}{k_z}e^{-j[k_x(x-x_0)+k_y(y-y_0)+k_z z]}dk_x dk_y\right]dx_0 dy_0.$$

To evaluate the term in square brackets we make use of an expression for the point source Green's function that was originally obtained by Sommerfeld [26] and subsequently quoted by Weyl [27].

$$\frac{e^{-jkR}}{R} = \frac{-j}{2\pi}\int_0^{2\pi}\int_0^{\pi}k\sin\beta e^{-jk[x\cos\alpha\sin\beta+y\sin\alpha\sin\beta+z\cos\beta]}d\alpha d\beta$$

By using the transform relations: $k_x = k\cos\alpha\sin\beta$, $k_y = k\sin\alpha\sin\beta$, $k_z = k\cos\beta$ and noting that

$$\iint F(\alpha, \beta)d\alpha d\beta = \iint F(\alpha(k_x, k_y), \beta(k_x, k_y))|J(k_x, k_y)|dk_x dk_y,$$

where the Jacobian is given by $|J(k_x, k_y)| = \begin{vmatrix}\dfrac{\partial\alpha}{\partial k_x} & \dfrac{\partial\alpha}{\partial k_y} \\ \dfrac{\partial\beta}{\partial k_x} & \dfrac{\alpha\beta}{\partial k_y}\end{vmatrix}$, the expression for the

Green's function at $R = \sqrt{(x-x_0)^2 + (y-y_0)^2 + z^2}$ can be expressed as

$$\frac{e^{-jkR}}{4\pi R} = \frac{j}{8\pi^2}\iint_{-\infty}^{\infty}\frac{1}{k_z}e^{-j[k_x(x-x_0)+k_y(y-y_0)+k_z z]}dk_x dk_y.$$

But this equation is of the same form as the inner integral in (2.76), so that by substitution, (2.76) can be written as

(2.77)
$$\Phi(\mathbf{r}:\omega) = \int\!\!\int_{-\infty}^{\infty} v_z(x_0, y_0, 0)\frac{e^{-jkR}}{2\pi R}\,dx_0dy_0$$

Now $v_z(x_0,y_0,0)$ is the velocity in the direction of $-\mathbf{n}$, i.e., $v_z = +\partial\Phi/\partial n$, and because $dx_0dy_0 \equiv dS_o$, it follows that (2.27) and (2.77) are identical. But since the Rayleigh integral, as expressed by (2.32), was obtained by taking the inverse Fourier transform of (2.27), it follows that the angular spectrum approach and that expressed by the Rayleigh integral are identical.

Problems

P1. A simple and useful form for the time-dependent transducer surface velocity is the Gaussian modulated cosine given by

$$v_n(t) = v_o e^{-t^2/(4\sigma^2)}\cos(\omega_o t),$$

in which ω_o is the center angular frequency and σ is a constant.
  a. Prove that the frequency spectrum is given by

$$V_n(\omega) = v_o\sigma\sqrt{\pi}\left[e^{-\sigma^2(\omega-\omega_o)^2} + e^{-\sigma^2(\omega+\omega_o)^2}\right],$$

  and find an expression for the fractional $-6\,\mathrm{dB}$ bandwidth.
  b. For a 5.0 mm diameter transducer, the pulse defined in part (a) has a $-6\,\mathrm{dB}$ bandwidth of 5 MHz and center frequency of 10 MHz. For a medium with $\rho_o = 1000\,\mathrm{kg/m^3}$, $c_o = 1500\,\mathrm{m/s}$, and for $v_o = 1.0\,\mathrm{cm/s}$, compute the on-axis pressure waveform at $z = 5\,\mathrm{mm}$ and $z = 50\,\mathrm{mm}$
    (i) by convolution of the derivative of velocity impulse response with $v_n(t)$;
    (ii) by determining the spectrum and taking the inverse Fourier transform.

P2. If a disk of radius a on the x-y plane centered at $z = 0$ is excited such that its normal velocity component is a circularly symmetric sinusoidal function $\xi_o(r)v_o e^{j\omega t}$ prove that the velocity potential on the z-axis is given by

$$\phi(0, z:t) = v_o e^{j\omega t}\int_z^{\sqrt{z^2+a^2}} \xi_o\left(\sqrt{R^2 - z^2}\right)e^{-jkR}dR$$

Check this by evaluating the case in which the disk is uniformly excited, obtaining an expression for the pressure phasor response and comparing it with (2.45a).
(The above equation is used in Chapter 3, (see 3.74), for obtaining the axial response when the apodization is a Gaussian function.)

P3. The suface velocity of a disk of radius a is given by $v(r,0:t) = v_o(1 - r^2/a^2)e^{j\omega t}$ for $r \le a$.

a. Using the result of P2, prove that the on-axis pressure response phasor is given by

$$p(0, z{:}\omega) = \frac{\rho_o c_o v_o}{a^2 k^2} \left\{ e^{-jkz} \left[a^2 k^2 + 2 + 2jkz \right] - 2e^{-jk\sqrt{z^2 + a^2}} \left[1 + jk\sqrt{z^2 + a^2} \right] \right\}$$

b. Plot a normalized graph for $a = 15\lambda/\pi$, showing $|p|/(\rho_o v_o c_o)$ versus $Z = kz$ from $Z = 0$ to 500, and determine the value of Z at which the last maximum occurs.

c. Determine the on-axis velocity impulse response if the apodization function is $\xi_o(r) = (1 - r^2/a^2)$ for $r \leq a$, and from this obtain the equation derived in part (a) for the on-axis sinusoidal velocity pressure response.

P4 a. Prove that the Rayleigh integral (2.32) can be expressed in the form of the following 3-D convolution:

$$\phi(x.y, z{:}t) = v_n(x, y, 0{:}t) \underset{x\,y\,t}{***} c_o \delta(c_o t - R)/(2\pi R),$$

where the source is on the plane $z = 0$, R is the distance of the field point from the origin, and $v_n(x,y,0{:}t)$ is the normal component of the velocity on the boundary.

b. If v_n is separable, i.e., $v_n(x,y,0{:}t) = \xi_o(x,y,0)v_{no}(t)$, show that the velocity potential can be expressed as

$$\phi(x.y, z{:}t) = v_{no}(t) \underset{t}{*} h(\mathbf{r}{:}t),$$

where $h(\mathbf{r}{:}t) = \xi_o(x, y, 0) \underset{x\,y}{**} c_o \delta(c_o t - R)/(2\pi R)$ is the impulse response.

c. If the source velocity is axially symmetric, show that the spatial Fourier transform of $h(\mathbf{r}{:}t)$ is given by

$$\bar{h}(\rho, z{:}t) = c_o \bar{\xi}_o(\rho) J_0 \left\{ \rho\sqrt{(c_o^2 t^2 - z^2)} \right\}, \text{ for } c_o t > z,$$

where $\rho^2 = f_y^2 + f_y^2$, f_x and f_y are the spatial frequencies, $J_0\{.\}$ is a cylindrical Bessel function of the first kind of zero order, and the bar denotes the spatial transform.

Hint: First make use of a property of the δ function given in Appendix B to transform the right hand side of the x-y convolution in part (b) to a form whose Hankel transform (as defined in Appendix B) can be readily evaluated.

P5. Derive (2.57) from (2.56) with the help of the Helmholtz equation.

P6. a. Obtain the Fresnel approximation for the PSF from the angular spectrum transfer function by assuming that the distribution of angles for the plane-wave spectrum is fairly narrow. Specifically, expand the exponent in (2.66), which expresses the transfer function for the angular spectrum at z_1 in terms of that at z_0, and show that the resulting PSF for a plane z with respect to the plane $z = 0$ is given by:

$$h_p\left(x, y; z_1\big|z_0\right) \approx \frac{jke^{-jkz}}{2\pi z} e^{-jk\left(x^2+y^2\right)/2z}$$

b. Obtain an approximate expression (the Fraunhofer approximation) for the velocity potential that is valid for locations far from an aperture on the plane $z = 0$ and not far off axis. Specifically, by starting with (2.65) and (2.66), assuming $z^2 \gg (x^2 + y^2)/2$ and that the dimensions of the aperture are small compared to the observation plane distance {more severe restrictions than those assumed in part (a)}, show that

$$\Phi(x, y, z) \approx \frac{jke^{-jkz}}{2\pi z} \Im\{\Phi(x, y, 0)\}_{k_x, k_y},$$

where the transform is evaluated at $k_x = -xk/z$, $k_y = -yk/z$.

The Fresnel and Fraunhofer approximations, which provide a valuable means for calculating the approximate field distributions on planes not too close to a transducer, will be discussed more fully in section 3.4.

P7. By using the 2-D form of the convolution theorem, show that the velocity potential angular spectrum formula given by (2.60) can be derived from the Rayleigh-Sommerfeld diffraction equation (2.29),

specifically: $\Phi(\mathbf{r}:\omega) = \dfrac{1}{2\pi} \displaystyle\iint_{S_o} \dfrac{e^{-jkR}}{R} v_z(x_0, y_0, 0)dS_o.$ In   evaluating   a

Fourier transform, the following relation should prove useful:

$$\frac{e^{js\sqrt{a^2+b^2+c^2}}}{\sqrt{a^2+b^2+c^2}} = \frac{j}{2\pi} \iint_{-\infty}^{\infty} \frac{e^{j\left[ax+by+c\sqrt{s^2-\left(x^2+y^2\right)}\right]}}{\sqrt{s^2-\left(x^2+y^2\right)}} dxdy, \quad \text{for } c \geq 0.$$

In addition, (2.62) should also be noted (see: Sherman, G.C., Application of the convolution theorem to Rayleigh's integral formulas, *J. Opt. Soc. Am.*, **57**, 546–547, 1967).

References

1. Stokes, G.G., On the dynamical theory of diffraction, *Camb. Phil. Soc., Trans.*, 9, 1–62, 1849.
2. Poisson, Memoire sur le movement des deux fluides elastiques superposes, *Memoires de L'Academie Royale des Sciences de L'Institut de France*, 10, 317–404, 1831.
3. Barton, G., *Elements of Green's Functions and Propagation*, Oxford Univ. Press, Oxford, 1989.
4. Goodman, J.W., *Introduction to Fourier Optics*, 2nd Edn., McGraw-Hill, New York, 1996.
5. Lord Rayleigh, On the passage of waves through apertures in plane screens and allied problems, *Phil. Mag.* 43, 259–272, 1897.
6. Morse, P.M., and Ingard, K.U., *Theoretical Acoustics* (Ch. 7), McGraw-Hill, New York, 1968.

7. Skudrzyk, E., *The Foundations of Acoustics*, Springer-Verlag, New York, 1971.

8. Morse, P.M., and Feshbach, H., *Methods of Theoretical Physics* (Ch. 7), McGraw-Hill, New York, 1953.

9. Sommerfeld, A., *Optics: Lectures on Theoretical Physics*, Vol. IV, pp. 197–207, Academic Press, New York, 1954.

10. Wolfe, E., and Marchand, E.W., Comparison of the Kirchhoff and the Rayleigh-Sommerfeld theories of diffraction at an aperture, *J. Opt. Soc. Am.*, 54, 587–594, 1964.

11. Born, M., and Wolf, E., *Principles of Optics*. 6th Edn., pp. 375–382, Pergamon Press, New York, 1980.

12. Temkin, S., *Elements of Acoustics*, Sect. 5.2, Wiley, New York, 1981.

13. Rayleigh, J.W.S., *The Theory of Sound* (in two vols., 2nd Edn., 1894), republished, Dover Publications, New York, 1945.

14. Malecki, I., *Physical Foundations of Technical Acoustics*, Pergamon Press, New York, 1969.

15. Delannoy, B., Lasota, H., Bruneel, C., Torguet, R., and Bridoux, E., The infinite planar baffles problem in acoustic radiation and its experimental verification, *J. Appl. Phys.*, 50, 5189–5195, 1979.

16. Archer-Hall, J.A., and Gee, D., A single integral computer method for axisymmetric transducers with various boundary conditions, *NDT International*, 13, 95–101, 1980.

17. Markiewicz, A., and Chivers, R.C., Effects of baffle conditions on the near-field of piston disk radiators, *Acustica*, 60, 289–294, 1986.

18. Baker, B.B., and Copson, E.T., *The Mathematical Theory of Huygens' Principle*, 2nd Edn., Clarendon Press, Oxford, 1950.

19. Bewley, L.V., *Two-Dimensional Fields in Electrical Engineering*, Dover Pub., New York, 1963.

20. Booker, H., and Clemmow, P., The concept of an angular spectrum of plane waves and its relation to that of polar diagram and aperture distribution, *Proc. IEE*, 97, 11–17, 1950.

21. Clemmow, P., *Plane Wave Representation of Electromagnetic Fields*, Pergamon Press, New York, 1966.

22. Stepanishen, P.R., and Benjamin, K.C., Forward and backward projection of acoustic fields using FFT methods, *J. Acoust. Soc. Am.*, 71, 803–812, 1982.

23. Williams, E.G., Numerical evaluation of the radiation from unbaffled finite planes using the FFT, *J. Acoust. Soc. Am.*, 74, 343–347, 1983.

24. Guyomar, D., and Powers, J., A Fourier approach to diffraction of pulsed ultrasonic waves in a lossless medium, *J. Acoust. Soc. Am.*, 92, 354–359, 1987.

25. Stepanishen, P.R., Forbes, M., and Letcher, S., The relationship between the impulse response and angular spectrum methods to evaluate acoustic transient fields, *J. Acoust. Soc. Am.*, 90, 2794–2798, 1991.

26. Sommerfeld, A., Uber die Ausbreitung der Wellen in der drahtlosen Telegraphie, *Annalen der Physik*, 28, 665–736, 1909.

27. Weyl, H., Ausbreitung electromagnetischer Wellen uber einen ebenen Leiter, *Annalen der Physik*, 60, 481–500, 1919.

28. Fung, C.C.W., Cobbold, R.S.C., and Bascom, P.A.J., Radiation coupling of a transducer-target system using the angular spectrum method, *J. Acoust. Soc. Am.*, 92, 2239–2247, 1992.

29. Liu, D-L., and Waag, R.C., Propagation and backpropagation for ultrasonic wavefront design, *IEEE Trans. Ultrson. Ferroelect., Freq. Contr.*, 44, 1–13, 1997.

30. Schafer, M.E., and Lewin, P.A., Transducer characterization using the angular spectrum method, *J. Acoust. Soc. Am.*, 85, 2202–2214, 1989.

31. Wu, P., and Stepinski, T., Extension of the angular spectrum approach to curved radiators, *J. Acoust. Scoc. Am.*, 105, 2618–2627, 1999.

32. Bracewell, R.N., *Two-Dimensional Imaging*, Prentice-Hall, Englewood Cliffs, NJ, 1995.

33. Leeman, S., and Healey, A.J., Field propagation via the angular spectrum method, pp. 363–368 in: *Acoustical Imaging*, Vol. 23, S. Lees, and L.A. Ferrari, (Eds.), Plenum Press, New York, 1997.

34. Vecchio, C.J., Schafer, M.E., and Lewin, P.A., Prediction of ultrasonic field propagation through layered media using the extended angular spectrum method, *Ultrasound in Med, Biol.*, 20, 611–622, 1994.

35. Williams, E.G., and Maynard, J.D., Numerical evaluation of the Rayleigh integral for planar radiators using the FFT, *J. Acoust. Soc. Am.*, 72, 2020–2030, 1982.

36. Erdelyi, A. (Ed.), *Table of Integral Transforms*, Vol. 2, McGraw-Hill, New York, 1954.

37. Waag, R.C., Campbell, J.A., Ridder, J., and Mesdag, P., Cross-sectional measurements and extrapolations of ultrasonic fields, *IEEE Trans. Sonics and Ultrasonics*, 32, 26–35, 1985.

38. Bracewell, R.N., *The Fourier Transform and its Applications*, 2nd Edn., McGraw-Hill, New York, 1978.

39. Freedman, A., Transient fields of acoustic radiators, *J. Acoust. Soc. Am.*, 48, 135–138, 1970.

40. Harris, G.R., Review of transient field theory for a baffled planar piston, *J. Acoust. Soc. Am.*, 70, 10–20, 1981.

41. Hutchins, D.A., and Hayward, G., Radiated Fields of Ultrasonic Transducers, Ch. 1, pp. 1–80 in: *Physical Acoustics: Ultrasonic Measurement Methods*, Vol. 19, R.N. Thurston, and A.D. Pierce (Eds)., Academic Press, New York, 1990.

42. Miles, J.W., Transient loading of a baffled piston, *J. Acoust. Soc. Am.*, 25, 200–203, 1955.

43. Oberhettinger, F., On transient solutions to the baffled piston problem, *J. Research NBS*, 65B, 1–6, 1961.

44. Oberhettinger, F., Note on the baffled piston problem, *J. Research NBS*, 65B, 203–204, 1961.

45. Chadwick, P., and Tupholme, G.E., Generation of an acoustic pulse by a baffled circular piston, *Proc. Edinburgh Math. Soc.*, 15, 263–277, 1967.

46. Tupholme, G.E., Generation of acoustic pulses by baffled plane pistons, *Mathematika*, 16, 209–224, 1969.

47. Stepanishen, P.R., Transient radiation from pistons in an infinite baffle, *J. Acoust. Soc. Am.*, 49, 1629–1638, 1971.

48. Stepanishen, P.R., The time-dependent force and radiation impedance on a piston in a rigid infinite baffle, *J. Acoust. Soc. Am.*, 49, 841–849, 1971.

49. Lockwood, J.C., and Willette, J.G., High speed method for computing the exact solution for the pressure variations in the nearfield of a bafflled piston, *J. Acoust. Soc. Am.*, 53, 735–741, 1973.

50. Ohtsuki, S., Ring function method for calculating nearfield of sound source, *Bull. Tokyo Inst. Tech.*, No. 123, 23–27, 1974. Also published in Japanese as: Calculation method for the nearfield of a sound source with ring function, *J. Acoust. Soc. Japan*, 30, 76–81, 1974.

51. Penttinen, A., and Luukkala, M., The impulse response and pressure nearfield of a curved ultrasonic radiator, *J. Phys. D*, 9, 1547–1557, 1976.

52. Jensen, J.A., Ultrasound fields from triangular apertures, *J. Acoust. Soc. Am.*, 100, 2049–2056, 1996.

53. Kramer, S.M., McBride, S.L., Mair, H.D., and Hutchins, D.A., Characteristics of wide-band planar transducer using plane and edge wave contributions, *IEEE Trans. Ultrason. Ferroelec. Freq. Contr.*, 35, 253–263, 1988.

54. Kozina, O.G., and Makarov, G.I., Transient proceses in the acoustic fields generated by a piston membrane of arbitrary shape, *Soviet Physics—Acoustics*, 7, 39–43, 1961.

55. Tupholme, G.E., Generation of an axisymmetrical acoustic pulse by a deformable sphere, *Proc. Cambridge Phil. Soc.*, 63, 1285–1308, 1967.

56. Beaver, W.L., Sonic nearfields of a pulsed piston radiator, *J. Acoust. Soc. Am.*, 71, 1406–11411, 1982.

57. Beissner, K., On the plane-wave approximation of acoustic intensity, *J. Acoust. Soc. Am.*, 56, 1043–1048, 1974.

58. Stepanishen, P.R., Acoustic transients in the far field of a baffled circular piston using the impulse response approach, *J. Sound Vib.*, 32, 295–310, 1974.

3

Field Profile Analysis

This chapter primarily focuses on the application of the methods developed in the previous chapter for analyzing the field distribution produced by a variety of single acoustic sources, ranging from piston transducers to those with more complex geometries. For an inviscid propagation medium, exact and approximate methods are examined, including the Fresnel and Fraunhofer approximations. The Fraunhofer approximation allows a greatly simplified approach to calculating the far-field response. On the other hand, the Fresnel approximation is fairly accurate much closer to the source, though it generally results in more complex expressions. An account of the use of apodization as a means for reducing the effects of diffraction is presented, and this leads to a description of diffractionless and minimally diffracting sources. The important practical issue of the effects of attenuation and the accompanying dispersion is then addressed, dealing first with classical viscous losses, and then addressing the question as to how the effects of attenuation and dispersion in soft tissue can be accounted for.

3.1 Angular Spectrum Method

The angular spectrum technique is particularly important from a computational perspective, since modern algorithms allow 2-D Fourier transforms to be performed very efficiently. Even though it is essentially a frequency domain method, transient problems can also be efficiently solved.

The fundamental aspects of the angular spectrum method were described in Chapter 2, where it was shown that the field on a given plane can be expressed in terms of an angular distribution of plane waves. We shall first illustrate this technique by evaluating the continuous wave (CW) field of a circular piston transducer. Although such an approach for this particular problem is more complex than the integral method described in section 3.2, it is important to note that problems such as determining the scattering from a sphere or infinite cylinder are most simply solved in terms of an incident plane wave. Thus, by describing the radiation pattern of a transducer in terms of an angular distribution of plane waves, the overall problem of determining the scattered field arising from the presence of a sphere or cylinder can be solved. For instance, the method has been used for describing the CW transmit–receive response for a baffled piston transducer and various targets with circular geometry [6]. It has also been used for studying the sample volume sensitivity for ultrasound beams incident on a cylindrical vessel [7]. A second example illustrates the use of a 2-D Fast Fourier Transform (FFT) to calculate the angular spectrum of the velocity on the plane of a disk transducer and then, following the scheme shown in Fig. 2.13, to obtain the field on a distal plane.

3.1.1 Spatial Spectrum of a Piston

We shall assume a piston transducer of radius a that lies on the plane $z = 0$. Moreover, the amplitude of the normal component of the surface velocity will be assumed to be constant over the piston surface and to be denoted by v_o: elsewhere on this plane the velocity is zero. Such a cylindrically symmetric distribution can be described by $v_z(r,0) = v_o \text{circ}(r/a)$, where $\text{circ}(\varsigma) = 1$ for $\varsigma \leq 1$ and is zero elsewhere.

An expression for the velocity potential angular spectrum of the piston can be obtained by first recalling (2.62):

$$S(k_x, k_y:0) = \frac{j}{k_z} \iint_{-\infty}^{\infty} v_z(x, y, 0) e^{-j(k_x x + k_y y)} dx dy,$$

in which $k_z = -\sqrt{k^2 - (k_x^2 + k_y^2)}$. Now the cylindrical symmetry of the geometry enables the following coordinate transform relations to be used:

(3.1)
$$r^2 = x^2 + y^2, \quad x = r\cos\theta, \quad y = r\sin\theta, \quad dxdy = rdrd\theta$$
$$k_r^2 = k_x^2 + k_y^2, \quad k_x = k_r\cos\varphi, \quad k_y = k_r\sin\varphi,$$

so that the angular spectrum can be written as

$$S(k_r:0) = \frac{-j}{\sqrt{k^2 - k_r^2}} \int_0^{2\pi}\int_0^{\infty} v_z(r,0) e^{-jrk_r(\cos\varphi\cos\theta + \sin\varphi\sin\theta)} rdrd\theta$$

$$= \frac{-j}{\sqrt{k^2 - k_r^2}} \int_0^{2\pi}\int_0^{\infty} v_z(r,0) e^{-jrk_r\cos(\theta - \varphi)} rdrd\theta.$$

By means of the Bessel identity $J_0(\varsigma) = \frac{1}{2\pi}\int_0^{2\pi} e^{-j\varsigma\cos(\theta - \varphi)} d\theta$, this reduces to

$$S(k_r:0) = \frac{-2\pi j}{\sqrt{k^2 - k_r^2}} \int_0^\infty v_z(r,0) J_0(rk_r) r dr,$$

where $J_0(.)$ is a cylindrical Bessel function of order zero. This can be recognized as the zero-order Hankel transform of $v_z(r,0)$. For a uniformly excited disk of radius a, the spectrum is therefore given by

$$(3.2)\ S(k_r:0) = \frac{-2\pi j}{\sqrt{k^2 - k_r^2}} \int_0^\infty v_o \mathrm{circ}(r/a) J_0(rk_r) r dr = \frac{-2\pi j}{\sqrt{k^2 - k_r^2}} \int_0^a v_o J_0(rk_r) r dr.$$

By letting $\zeta = rk_r$, this can be written as

$$S_v(k_r:0) = \frac{-2\pi j}{k_r^2 \sqrt{k^2 - k_r^2}} \int_0^{ak_r} v_o J_0(\zeta) \zeta d\zeta,$$

which, by using the Bessel function identity $\zeta J_1(\zeta) = \int_0^\zeta J_0(\chi) \chi d\chi$ enables the spatial spectrum can be expressed as

$$(3.3) \qquad S(k_r:0) = \frac{-\pi j a^2 v_o}{\sqrt{k^2 - k_r^2}} \left\{ \frac{2J_1(ak_r)}{ak_r} \right\}.$$

This expresses the spectrum in a cylindrical spatial frequency coordinate system, and the term in braces, which is the Fourier transform of $\mathrm{circ}(r/a)$, is sometimes referred to as a jinc function. At $x = y = 0$ it has a value of 1. Alternatively, by using (3.1), (3.3) can be expressed in Cartesian coordinates as

$$(3.4) \qquad S(k_x, k_y:0) = \frac{-\pi j a^2 v_o}{\sqrt{k^2 - (k_x^2 + k_y^2)}} \left\{ \frac{2J_1\left(a\sqrt{k_x^2 + k_y^2}\right)}{a\sqrt{k_x^2 + k_y^2}} \right\}.$$

The Cartesian form of the jinc function (the term in braces) is plotted in Fig. 3.1.

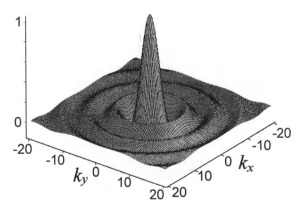

Figure 3.1 The 2-D Fourier transform of the $\mathrm{circ}(r/a)$ function yields the jinc function, which is plotted for $a = 1$ in Cartesian spatial frequency coordinates.

3.1.2 Angular Spectrum in Spherical Coordinates

To obtain an expression for the angular spectrum it is helpful to convert to a spherical coordinate system (k,θ,φ) by using the transform relations:

(3.5)
$$k_x = k\sin\theta\cos\varphi, \quad k_y = k\sin\theta\sin\varphi, \quad k_z = k\cos\theta,$$
$$dk_x dk_y = k^2\cos\theta\sin\theta d\theta d\varphi.$$

It should be noted that because k_z becomes imaginary when $k_x^2 + k_y^2 < k^2$ (corresponding to the evanescent component in the plane-wave spectrum), the angle θ also becomes complex. With this consideration it can be shown that (2.60) transforms to [6]

(3.6)
$$\Phi(\mathbf{r}) = \int_0^{\frac{\pi}{2}-j\infty} \int_{-\pi}^{\pi} \hat{S}(\theta,\varphi)e^{j\mathbf{k}\cdot\mathbf{r}}d\varphi d\theta,$$

in which the angular spectral density function is

(3.7)
$$\hat{S}(\theta,\varphi) = \frac{1}{4\pi^2}k^2\cos\theta\sin\theta \times S(k\sin\theta\cos\varphi, k\sin\theta\sin\varphi),$$

and where $\mathbf{k} = (k_x,k_y,k_z)$ and $\mathbf{r} = (x,y,z)$. The integration contour on the complex θ plane, which was chosen by using Cauchy's integral theorem, is from 0 to $\pi/2$ along the real axis and from 0 to $-j\infty$ along the imaginary axis. By substituting (3.4) into (3.7) and noting that $k_z = k\cos\theta$, the angular spectrum is given by

(3.8)
$$\hat{S}(\theta) = \frac{jav_o}{2\pi}J_1(ka\sin\theta),$$

which is plotted in Fig. 3.2 for real values of θ, i.e., for the homogeneous component.

3.1.3 Field Profile

The pressure field profile can be found by first noting that $\hat{S}(.)$ is cylindrically symmetric, so that in cylindrical coordinates (r,z), the pressure can be written as $p(r,z) = p(x,0,z)$. By substituting (3.8) into (3.6) and noting that the phasor pressure $\underline{p} = j\rho_o c_o k\Phi$ we obtain

$$\underline{p}(r,z) = \frac{-a\rho_o c_o k v_o}{2\pi}\int_0^{\frac{\pi}{2}-j\infty} \int_{-\pi}^{+\pi} J_1(ka\sin\theta)e^{jk(r\sin\theta\cos\varphi + z\cos\theta)}d\varphi d\theta.$$

Using the standard Bessel function relation $J_0(\varsigma) = \frac{1}{\pi}\int_0^{\pi} e^{j\varsigma\cos\varphi}d\varphi$, this can be rewritten as

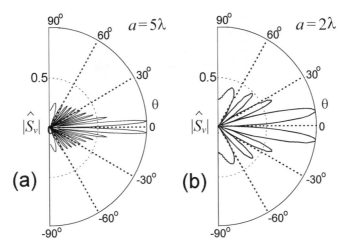

Figure 3.2 Homogeneous component of the angular spectra for a disk transducer with two different disk radii: (a) $a = 5\lambda$, (b) $a = 2\lambda$. The magnitudes are normalized to $av_o/2\pi$.

$$\underline{p}(r,z) = -a\rho_o c_o k v_o \int_0^{\frac{\pi}{2}-j\infty} J_0(kr\sin\theta)J_1(ka\sin\theta)e^{jkz\cos\theta}d\theta.$$

Noting that $\sin(\pi/2 + j\theta_i) = \cosh\theta_i$, and $\cos(\pi/2 + j\theta_i) = -j\sinh\theta_i$, where θ_i is the imaginary part of θ, the above equation can be written as:

(3.9)
$$\underline{p}(r,z) = -a\rho_o c_o k v_o\left[\int_0^{\pi/2} J_0(kr\sin\theta)J_1(ka\sin\theta)e^{jkz\cos\theta}d\theta\right.$$
$$\left. -j\int_0^{\infty} J_0(kr\cosh\theta_i)J_1(ka\cosh\theta_i)e^{-kz\sinh\theta_i}d\theta_i\right],$$

where the first and second terms correspond to the homogeneous and evanescent components, respectively. Evaluation of this equation[1] shows that the evanescent component has a significant influence on the field profile close to the transducer but becomes negligible further away. This is illustrated in Fig. 3.3 for a transducer of radius $a = 2.5\lambda$.

3.1.4 Fourier Transform Method

Of considerable significance is the ability to calculate the field profile on a given plane given the field on another plane. This will be illustrated with two examples for a uniformly excited circular disk transducer. In the first, we make

---

1. An alternative form that is more suitable for numerical computation is given in [6].

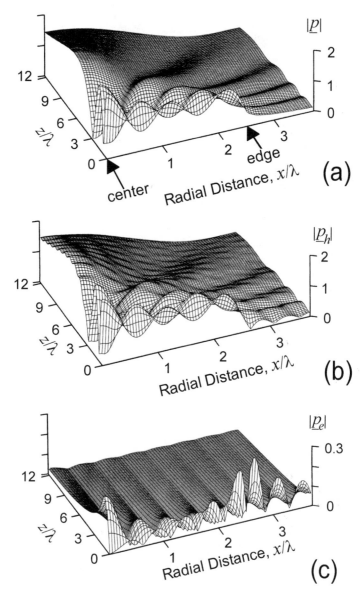

Figure 3.3 3-D representation of the normalized pressure magnitude from a uniformly vibrating piston with a radius of 2.5λ, as calculated from (3.9). The normalization constant is $\rho_o c_o v_o$. (a) Sum of the two components. (b) Homogeneous component. (c) Evanescent component (note the change in scale). (Reproduced, with permission, from Fung et al. [6], *J. Acoust. Soc. Am.*, 92, 2239–2247, © 1992 Acoustical Society of America.)

use of the cylindrical symmetry to analytically perform an inverse Fourier transform; in the second, the 2-D Fourier transform and its inverse are performed numerically.

Analytical Approach

If the field to be determined is several wavelengths distal to the known plane, the evanescent component can be ignored, and the calculation requires multiplication of the angular spectrum on the known plane by the spatial frequency transfer function as given by (2.66), and then recovery of the field pattern by an inverse transform. This process will first be illustrated by using the equation for the spatial frequency transfer function of a piston transducer derived in the last chapter.

Now (2.65) and (2.66) can be rewritten as

$$(3.10) \qquad S(k_x,k_y:z) = H(k_x,k_y:z|0)S(k_x,k_y:0)$$

$$(3.11) \qquad H(k_x,k_y:z|0) \approx e^{-jz\sqrt{k^2-\left(k_x^2+k_y^2\right)}},$$

where S is the angular spectrum and H is the spatial frequency transfer function from the plane $z = 0$ to the plane z, which is assumed to be several wavelengths beyond $z = 0$. For a uniformly excited disk of radius a, the angular spectrum on the z-plane can be obtained by substituting (3.3) and (3.10) into (3.11), yielding

$$(3.12) \qquad S(k_r) = \frac{-2\pi j a^2 v_o}{\sqrt{k^2-k_r^2}} \frac{J_1(ak_r)}{ak_r} e^{-jz\sqrt{k^2-k_r^2}}.$$

Now the 2-D inverse Fourier transform of this angular spectrum can be found by first applying the coordinate transformation equations given by (3.1) to the 2-D inverse Fourier transform expression for the velocity potential given by (2.52). Then, following the same steps outlined in section 3.1.1, and noting that $J_0(\varsigma) = \dfrac{1}{2\pi}\displaystyle\int_0^{2\pi} e^{j\varsigma\cos(\varphi-\theta)}d\varphi$, the velocity potential simplifies to[2]

$$(3.13) \qquad \Phi(r,z) = jav_o \int_0^{k^-} \frac{J_1(ak_r)}{\sqrt{k^2-k_r^2}} e^{-jz\sqrt{k^2-k_r^2}} J_0(rk_r)dk_r,$$

in which the integral upper limit has been chosen to exclude the evanescent component. This enables the pressure to be expressed as

$$(3.14) \qquad \underline{p}(r,z) = j\omega\rho_o\Phi = \omega\rho_o av_o \int_0^{k^-} \frac{J_1(ak_r)}{\sqrt{k^2-k_r^2}} e^{-jz\sqrt{k^2-k_r^2}} J_0(rk_r)dk_r.$$

On-axis, this reduces to

---

2. This equation, but with an upper limit of ∞, can be obtained from King's integral (3.70). See subsection 3.8.1 and footnote 20.

(3.15)
$$\underline{p}(0,z) = \omega \rho_o a v_o \int_0^{k^-} \frac{J_1(ak_r)}{\sqrt{k^2 - k_r^2}} e^{-jz\sqrt{k^2 - k_r^2}} \, dk_r$$

for $z > 3\lambda$, which is plotted in Fig. 3.4a together with the exact expression given by (2.45). The agreement between the two is excellent provided $z > \sim 2\lambda$, where the evanescent component starts to become significant. In Fig. 3.4b the radial pressure field calculated from (3.14) is shown for two axial distances corresponding to the last maximum and the last but one minimum.

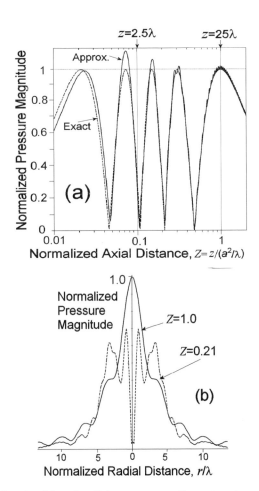

Figure 3.4 Calculated axial and radial pressure profiles using the angular spectrum method for a piston transducer with $a = 5\lambda$. The pressure magnitude scale has been normalized by dividing by $2\rho_o c_o v_o$, which is the pressure magnitude at the last maximum (i.e., at $z = a^2/\lambda$). Because the evanescent wave has been ignored, the results become inaccurate for $z < \sim 3\lambda$. (a) Exact and approximate profiles as calculated from (2.45) and (3.15), respectively. (b) Radial profiles at the last maximum and the last but one minimum as calculated from (3.14).

Numerical 2-D FFT

In the above example, the cylindrical symmetry of the disk transducer allowed the field profile to be numerically evaluated from a single integral. For a more complex transducer geometry that lacks symmetry, the angular spectrum approach can also be used but now requires the evaluation of a 2-D FFT. As described in section 2.3.3, the velocity on a plane z for a given velocity distribution on the plane $z = 0$ can be found by means of the following steps:

1. Perform a 2-D FFT of the velocity on the source plane.
2. Multiply this by the transfer function H from the source plane to the plane of interest.
3. Take the inverse 2D-FFT of the product.

These steps are summarized in

$$(3.16) \qquad v_z(x,y,z) = \Im^{-1}\left\{ e^{-jz\sqrt{k^2 - (k_x^2 + k_y^2)}} \Im\{v_o(x,y,0)\} \right\},$$

where $\Im\{.\}$ and $\Im^{-1}\{.\}$ stand for a 2-D Fourier transform and its inverse. For a circular piston transducer, the steps in this process are described in the caption to Fig. 3.5. Because of the large axial distance step $(\Delta z = a^2/\lambda)$, the effects of the evanescent component could be neglected.

3.2 Integral Methods

Direct use of the Rayleigh integral requires the numerical evaluation of a double integral over the transducer surface area [1]. A more economical approach is to make use of the approach described in 1941 by Schoch [19] in which he transformed the Rayleigh surface integral into a line integral over the transducer rim. For CW excitation and a plane transducer of arbitrary shape in a rigid baffle, he obtained expressions for the pressure field distribution both within and outside the transducer geometrical shadow. Part of this work and extensions from it are described in this section.

3.2.1 Rigid Baffle Boundary Condition

In Fig. 3.6 we consider a field point that lies within the geometric shadow of a plane transducer of arbitrary shape in a rigid baffle, and we assume uniform excitation by a sinusoidal waveform such that the normal component of the surface velocity is given by $v_{no}(t) = v_o e^{j\omega t}$. Substituting this into (2.32) and noting that the pressure is given by $p = \rho_o \partial\phi/\partial t$, the pressure phasor at the field point is given by

$$(3.17) \qquad \underline{p}(r, z{:}\omega) = \frac{j\omega\rho_o v_o}{2\pi} \iint_S \frac{e^{-jkR}}{R}\,dS.$$

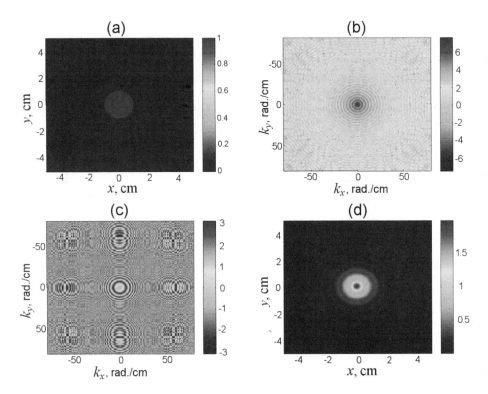

Figure 3.5 Field computation with the angular spectrum method using a 2-D FFT for a piston transducer with a radius $a = 1$ cm, excited at 5 MHz with a normal velocity $v_o = 1$ cm/s. The axial component of the particle velocity was computed on a plane at $z = a^2/\lambda (= 33.3$ cm). (a) Normal particle velocity profile on the transducer plane at $z = 0$. Sampling out to ±5 cm using 256 × 256 samples over the entire plane, i.e., $\Delta x = \Delta y = 0.39$ mm per sample. (See color insert.) (b) Angular spectrum of the source obtained by taking the 2-D Fourier transform of the source. The source plane was zero padded to ±10 cm and the scale is the logarithmic magnitude of the 2-D FFT. The maximum spatial frequencies represent $\pi/\Delta x$ and $\pi/\Delta y$ and have 512 × 512 samples across the domain. (c) Complex argument of the transfer function $H(k_x,k_y$: $a^2/\lambda)$, plotted in the spatial frequency domain using 512 × 512 points. The map range is from $-\pi$ to π. (d) Normal component of the particle velocity (cm/s) field on the plane $z = a^2/\lambda$. This was obtained by taking the 2-D inverse discrete Fourier transform of the product of the transfer function H and the source angular spectrum. Results are shown out to ±5 cm using 256 × 256 points. Note that the distribution peaks at 2.0 cm/s (twice the normal particle velocity), as expected.

Since the element of area $dS = r\,dr\,d\theta$,

(3.18)
$$\underline{p}(r, z{:}\omega) = \frac{j\omega\rho_o v_o}{2\pi} \int_0^{2\pi} \int_0^{r_1(\theta)} \frac{e^{-jkR}}{R} r\,dr\,d\theta.$$

where $r_1(\theta)$ denotes the boundary location and the other quantities are defined in Fig. 3.6. Now $r^2 + z^2 = R^2$, so that (3.18) transforms to

(3.19)
$$\underline{p}(r, z{:}\omega) = \frac{j\omega\rho_o v_o}{2\pi} \int_0^{2\pi} \int_z^{R_1(\theta)} e^{-jkR}\,dR\,d\theta$$

$$= \rho_o c_o v_o e^{-jkz} - \frac{\rho_o c_o v_o}{2\pi} \int_0^{2\pi} e^{-jkR_1(\theta)}\,d\theta.$$

Schoch [19] originally obtained this expression for the pressure at field points that lie within the geometric shadow. The two terms that make up the total pressure response consist of a plane wave $\rho_o c_o v_o e^{j(\omega t - kz)}$ and a diffraction term that originates from the periphery (the edge wave). An expression for the pressure outside the geometric shadow [2, p. 522; 19] shows that the plane wave is absent in this region and the contributions are only from the periphery. Wright and Berry [28] subsequently used a similar approach in analyzing the field response of a circular plane transducer in a rigid baffle. Moreover, their analysis treated the more general case of an arbitrary transducer displacement waveform $\xi(t)$. For the geometry illustrated in Fig. 3.7, they showed that the velocity potential for a disk of radius a is given by

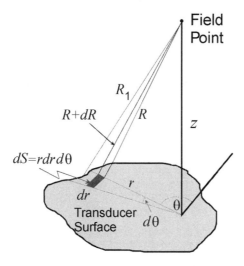

Figure 3.6 Geometry used for calculating the CW pressure response due to a plane transducer of arbitrary shape in a rigid baffle. The field point is assumed to lie within the geometric shadow.

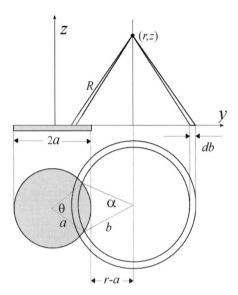

Figure 3.7 Geometry for calculating the response for a piston transducer of radius a at an off-axis position. Cylindrical polar coordinates are used, and the case of $r > a$ is illustrated. Both a cross-sectional (top) and a plane view (bottom) are shown.

$$(3.20) \quad \phi(r,z{:}t) = c\mathcal{H}(a-r)\xi\left(t - \frac{z}{c_o}\right) + \frac{c_o}{\pi}\int_0^\pi \frac{ar\cos\theta - a^2}{a^2 + r^2 - 2ar\cos\theta}\xi\left(t - \frac{R}{c_o}\right)d\theta,$$

where $\mathcal{H}(.)$ is the Heaviside step function, and $R^2 = z^2 + b^2 = z^2 + a^2 + r^2 - 2ar\cos\theta$.

Based on the work by Schoch [19], the more general case of a plane transducer of arbitrary shape excited by an arbitrary waveform to produce the same velocity $v_{no}(t)$ over the transducer surface (no apodization) was described in 1961 by Kozina and Makarov [17]. Cathignol et al. [20] have derived their results in a simpler and more general manner so that they can also be applied to concave and convex radiators. For an observation point lying in the geometric shadow of the transducer shown in Fig. 3.6, the pressure is given by

$$(3.21a) \qquad p(r,z{:}t) = \rho_o c_o v_{no}\left(t - \frac{z}{c_o}\right) - \frac{\rho_o c_o}{2\pi}\int_0^{2\pi} v_{no}\left(t - \frac{R_{max}(\theta)}{c_o}\right)d\theta,$$

where R_{max} corresponds to the maximum distance of the observation point to the transducer surface for a given value of θ. For points lying outside the geometric shadow, the pressure is given by the contour integral:

$$(3.21b) \qquad p(r,z{:}t) = \frac{\rho_o c_o}{2\pi}\oint v_{no}\left(t - \frac{R_{max}(\theta)}{c_o}\right)d\theta.$$

These two equations enable the response to be calculated by means of line integrals, which as shown by Cathignol et al. [20] imposes a much smaller computational burden than evaluating the Rayleigh surface integral.

3.2.2 Three Sets of Boundary Conditions

In this subsection we shall examine how the three sets of boundary conditions described in the last chapter affect the field response for uniform CW excitation. For a disk transducer surrounded by an infinite ideal baffle, the velocity was taken to be zero on the baffle. Specifically, if the ratio of specific acoustic impedance of the baffle to that of the propagation medium is very large, i.e., $Z_B \gg Z_M$, then the velocity will be small, corresponding to the conditions for the validity of the Rayleigh integral (Case i). The second condition previously examined was that in which the pressure is specified throughout the transducer plane (see (2.31)). If the medium surrounding the transducer is acoustically soft, i.e., $Z_B \to 0$, the pressure will be approximately zero on this boundary (Case ii). Finally, if a transducer that produces no radiation from its back surface is suspended in a uniform infinite medium, i.e., $Z_B = Z_M$, the Kirchhoff or free-field conditions (see (2.20)) are present (Case iii).

For all three conditions, Archer-Hall and Gee [4] have shown that at any arbitrary point the double surface integrals for the CW response of a uniformly excited disk can be reduced to single integral expressions. Specifically, for the geometry shown in Fig. 3.7, they have shown that if the normal component of the transducer surface velocity amplitude is v_o, the pressure phasors for the three cases are given by:

$$(3.22) \quad p(r,z{:}t) = \rho_o c_o v_o \left[\mathcal{H}(a-r)e^{-jkz} + \frac{1}{\pi}\int_0^\pi e^{-jkR}\frac{ar\cos\theta - a^2}{a^2 + r^2 - 2ar\cos\theta}f_r(z,R)d\theta \right],$$

where $R^2 = z^2 + b^2 = z^2 + a^2 + r^2 - 2ar\cos\theta$ and $f_r(z,R)$ is given in Table 3.1. In fact, for Case i this expression can be obtained from (3.20) by putting $\xi(t) = \xi_a e^{j\omega t}$, noting that $v_o = j\omega\xi_a$, $p = \rho_o \partial\phi/\partial t$, and differentiating. Equation (3.22) clearly shows that for all three cases the pressure wave consists of two components: a plane wave $\rho_o c_o v_o e^{j(\omega t-kz)}$ that is present only when the observation point $r < a$, and an edge-wave component that is present everywhere [10]. For on-axis observation points $(r = 0)$, the square of the pressure amplitude magnitudes can be obtained from (3.22) as

$$(3.23) \quad \begin{cases} \text{Case i} & |p_N(0,z)|^2 = 2(\rho_o c_o v_o)^2\{1 - \cos[k(z_a - z)]\} \\ \text{Case ii} & |p_D(0,z)|^2 = (\rho_o c_o v_o)^2\left\{1 + \dfrac{z}{z_a}[1 - 2\cos[k(z_a - z)]]\right\}, \\[2ex] \text{Case iii} & |p_K(0,z)|^2 = (\rho_o c_o v_o)^2\left\{1 - \left(1 + \dfrac{z}{z_a}\right)\cos[k(z_a - z)] \right. \\ & \left. \qquad\qquad -0.25\left(1 + \dfrac{z}{z_a}\right)^2\right\} \end{cases}$$

where $z_a = \sqrt{z^2 + a^2}$. These equations were used to calculate the normalized pressure amplitudes $\{P = p/(\rho_o c_o v_o)\}$ shown in Fig. 3.8 for a disk of radius

Table 3.1. Effect of the Assumed Boundary Condition on $f_r(z,R)$

Case	Boundary Condition	$f_r(z,R)$
(i)	Rayleigh: Rigid Baffle	1
(ii)	Pressure Release Surface	z/R
(iii)	Kirchhoff: Free Field	$(1 + z/R)/2$

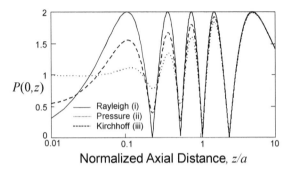

Figure 3.8 On-axis CW normalized pressure amplitudes for the three sets of boundary conditions given in Table 3.1 and a transducer whose radius $a = 5\lambda$. Note the log scale for the axial distance.

$a = 5\lambda$. It will be noted that the differences become significant only well into the near-field region. A more detailed examination of both the amplitude and phase variations for all three cases has been presented by Markiewicz and Chivers [5], who point out that while the far-field amplitude differences are small, the phases can differ appreciably, especially in the near-field.

3.2.3 Pressure Distribution On- and Off-Axis

In Fig. 3.9 the radial variations of the pressure amplitudes are shown for three different z-axis locations. Close to the transducer ($z/a = 0.2$) the beam is roughly cylindrical in shape extending to the edge of the disk. At the near-field/far-field transition point ($z/a = 5$) the beam is significantly narrower, beyond which ($z/a = 10$) the amplitude reduces and the beam spreads out.

Finally, in Fig. 3.10 we show the computed CW contours for a disk whose radius is also equal to 5λ. These clearly show that close to the near-field/far-field transition position, the beam width is a minimum and that beyond this point the contours display a more disciplined nature.

3.3 Impulse Response Method

To obtain the velocity potential impulse response for any arbitrary location from a plane transducer, we shall follow the method of Ohtsuki [14] and start

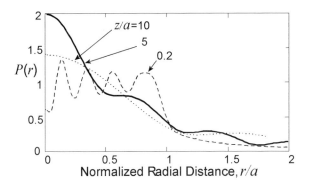

Figure 3.9 Normalized CW pressure amplitude variation in the radial direction for $a = 5\lambda$ and Rayleigh (i) boundary conditions at three different distances along the axis. Equation (3.22) was used for the calculations.

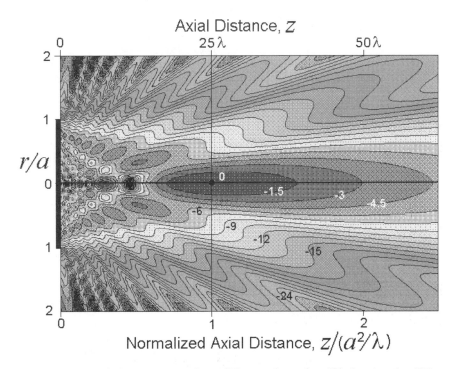

Figure 3.10 Encoded contour map for a disk transducer ($a = 5\lambda$) showing the CW spatial pressure distribution for Rayleigh (i) boundary conditions. Both the axial and radial distances are normalized to the disk radius. The contour lines are expressed in dB's relative to the value at $(0,5a)$. (See also color insert.)

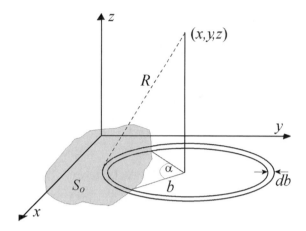

Figure 3.11 Calculating the velocity impulse response at (x,y,z) for a plane transducer S_o that lies on the plane $z = 0$. At an instant of time t, the shaded area subtending an angle α contributes to the signal at the observation point. Note that R is a function of time, as is the angle α.

with the defining equation for the impulse function, namely (2.35), which we repeat here for convenience:

$$(3.24) \qquad h(\mathbf{r}{:}t) = \iint\limits_{S_o} \frac{\xi_o(x,y)\delta\left(t - \dfrac{R}{c_o}\right)}{2\pi R}\, dS_o.$$

The more general case in which the apodization function $\xi_o(x,y)$ is not constant over the transducer surface has been considered by several authors [21,22]. Since this somewhat complicates matters, for the present[3] we shall consider the simpler case in which the normal component of the transducer surface velocity is constant over the transducer surface, i.e., $\xi_o(x,y) = 1$. As illustrated in Fig. 3.11, the contribution at a time t comes from the portion of the annular ring that subtends an angle α from the projection of the observation point on the plane $z = 0$. For the field point illustrated, $0 < \alpha < 2\pi$. If the annular ring lies entirely within S_o, i.e., $\alpha = 2\pi$ from $t = z/c_o$ up to t_1, then $h(x,y,z{:}t) = c_o$. Also, if the ring lies outside of S_o, i.e., $\alpha = 0$ from a time t_2 up to ∞, then $h(x,y,z{:}t) = 0$. In the more general case there will be several regions of intersection, and consequently several angles will be subtended, $\alpha_1, \alpha_2, \ldots\ldots$.

Now $R dR = b\,db$, so that $dS_o = \alpha R dR$, and consequently for the case illustrated, (3.24) can be expressed as

$$h(x, y, z{:}t) = \frac{1}{2\pi} \int\limits_{R_{\min}}^{R_{\max}} \alpha\left(\frac{R}{c_o}\right)\delta\left(t - \frac{R}{c_o}\right) dR$$

---

3. The more general case is considered in problem P1, following the treatment given by Tjøtta and Tjøtta [22].

$$(3.25) \qquad h(x,y,z:t) = \frac{c_o}{2\pi}\alpha(t),$$

for $R_{min} < c_o t < R_{max}$, i.e., $t_1 < t < t_2$, where R_{min} and R_{max} denote the initial and final (minimum and maximum) values of R that occur at times $t_1 = R_{min}/c_o$ and $t_2 = R_{max}/c_o$, respectively. For the case where there are multiple values of α, a similar result holds, except that if the times overlap then the impulse response of each during the overlap times must be added to obtain the total response during this interval.

3.3.1 Piston Transducer

The problem of determining general impulse response for the piston transducer, whose on-axis impulse response was obtained in Chapter 2, reduces to the problem of finding an expression for the angle α. With the help of Fig. 3.7, straightforward geometric analysis enables $\alpha(t)$ to be expressed as [14]

$$(3.26) \qquad \alpha(t) = 2\cos^{-1}\left[\frac{r^2 - a^2 - z^2 + c_o^2 t^2}{2r\sqrt{c_o^2 t^2 - z^2}}\right]$$

for $r > a$ and $t_1 < t < t_2$, in which

$$t_1 = R_{min}/c_o = \sqrt{z^2 + (r-a)^2}/c_o$$

$$t_2 = R_{max}/c_o = \sqrt{z^2 + (r+a)^2}/c_o$$

For the entire range of possible radial positions r, the impulse response can be expressed as [12]:

$$(3.27) \qquad \begin{cases} h(r,z:t) = c_o, & \text{if } r < a \quad \text{and} \quad t_0 < t < t_1 \\[2mm] h(r,z:t) = \dfrac{c_o}{\pi}\cos^{-1}\left[\dfrac{r^2 - a^2 - z^2 + c_o^2 t^2}{2r\sqrt{c_o^2 t^2 - z^2}}\right], & \text{if } t_1 < t < t_2, \\[2mm] h(r,z:t) = 0, & \text{elsewhere.} \end{cases}$$

where $t_0 = z/c_o$, and t_1 and t_2 are defined above. Fig. 3.12 shows the impulse response for a 0.5 cm radius transducer at various radial locations and at $z = 8$ cm (corresponding to the last maximum for a 5 MHz transducer). It should be noted that a rapid reduction in the maximum value of the response occurs when the radial position exceeds the transducer radius, and that at that location, the delay to the first appearance of the pulse starts to increase.

Examination of the pressure response for different burst lengths having the same center frequency shows that the effects of interference in the near-field region is diminished as the number of cycles in the pulse is reduced. As shown in Fig. 3.13, the far-field response remains virtually unchanged, while the near-field exhibits a much smoother response. If the number of cycles in the excitation waveform is greater than approximately six, it is reasonable to assume that the field response can be approximated by the CW response. Interpretation of these results is aided by considering both the direct and edge-wave

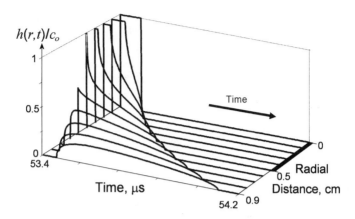

$h(r,t)/c_o$

Time

Time, μs

Radial Distance, cm

Figure 3.12 Off-axis velocity impulse response of a 5.0 mm radius disk transducer for $z = 8.0$ cm at radial distance increments of 1.0 mm.

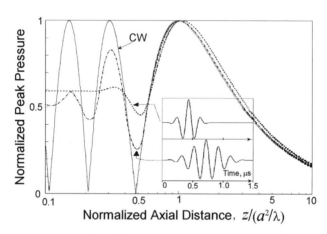

Normalized Peak Pressure

CW

Time, μs

Normalized Axial Distance, $z/(a^2/\lambda)$

Figure 3.13 Comparison of the CW on-axis pressure response with that obtained using two different pulse waveforms whose center frequencies were 5 MHz. The transducer radius was assumed to be given by $a = 5\lambda$. For the pulsed excitation, the peak value of the pressure has been plotted normalized to the maximum on-axis value.

components. On the axis, close to the transducer the edge and direct waves are sufficiently separated in time so that no interference occurs, and as a result the peak pressure magnitude is determined by either the direct or edge wave in this region. Further along the axis, a point is reached where the transit times are sufficiently close that the edge and direct waves overlap.

3.3.2 Experimental and Theoretical Results

In general, good agreement has been observed with theory for both transient and CW excitation, and these have been described in a number of papers.

However, significant discrepancies have been observed due to the excitation of transducer vibration modes that are not normal to the surface. Specifically, Delannoy et al. [23] studied the CW radiation behavior of transducers with small lateral dimensions and found parasitic side lobes, which they properly attributed to parasitic Lamb waves propagation in the transducer medium and radiating into the fluid. An important contribution in comparing theoretical and experimental results was the work of Weight [24]. Using a 19 mm diameter piston transducer with no apodization, the transmit and transmit–receive profiles were measured and compared using both single-cycle pulse and 2.0-MHz CW excitation. Some of the measured and predicted results for the lateral peak pressure profiles are shown in Fig. 3.14. For pulse excitation, the response exhibits a smoothly varying characteristic both in the near and far field.

Experimental observations of the transient response, especially with very brief pulses and observation points in the near field, have shown significant discrepancies with theoretical predictions based on the simple piston model. Hayman and Weight [25], in their experimental and theoretical studies of direct and edge waves from thin circular and square piezoceramic transducers, reported the presence of a *head* wave whose arrival time could precede that of the edge wave, provided the observation point was sufficiently close to the transducer. They proposed that this wave was caused by the presence of laterally propagating plate waves that originate from the rim of the transducer and that radiate into the surrounding fluid medium. By means of stroboscopic Schliern photographs, together with hydrophone pressure measurements and transit time calculations, they showed that the head wave arrival time was consistent with plate waves originating at the rim, propagating in the piezoceramic, and radiating compressional waves into the surrounding fluid medium.

To understand this effect we shall follow the approach used by Baboux et al. [26] and suppose that the disk transducer shown in Fig. 3.15 is excited by a pulse of very short duration. We wish to determine the path that corresponds to the minimum transit time of the pulse from the rim to a given axial location z. The simplest way of doing this is to make use of Fermat's principle, which states that the geometric path taken by a ray is that with the smallest transit time. Let us denote the group speed of a radial wave in or on the surface of the ceramic by c_g and that in the surrounding liquid medium by c_o. If $c_g > c_o$, then this wave will radiate a leaky wave into the medium as it progresses from the rim. With the aid of Fig. 3.15, the transit time from the rim to the observation point can then be written as

$$t_r = \frac{a - z\tan\theta}{c_g} + \frac{z}{c_o\cos\theta}, \quad \text{for} \quad z \le a\cot\theta.$$

By differentiating with respect to θ and equating to 0, the minimum time is found to occur when

(3.28)
$$\theta = \theta_c = \sin^{-1}(c_o/c_g),$$

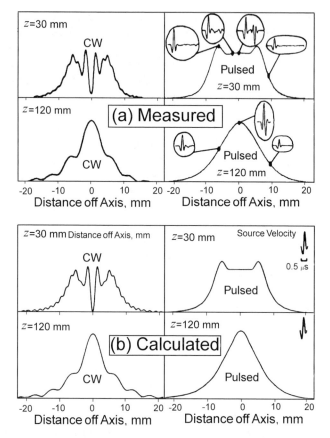

Figure 3.14 (a) Measured and (b) calculated CW (2.0 MHz) and pulsed pressure profiles for a 1.9 cm diameter piston transducer in water. The lateral profiles are shown at a point in the near-field region ($z = 30$ mm) and at the last axial maximum ($z = a^2/\lambda = 120$ mm). Using a miniature hydrophone, the pulsed waveforms were measured for a single cycle of excitation, and several of these are shown. The calculated pulsed profiles were obtained using the source velocity indicated. For both the measured and calculated pulse response, the peak value of the pressure magnitude is plotted. (Modified version reproduced, with permission, from Weight [24], *J. Acoust. Soc. Am.*, 76, 1184–1191, © 1984 Acoustical Society of America.)

which is the well-known equation for the critical angle, i.e., Snell's law, when the angle of refraction is 90 degrees. Thus, the path taken by those leaky waves that reach on-axis observation points ahead of the edge wave lie on the surface of a cone whose half-angle is given by (3.28) and whose apex lies at the observation point. It is also evident from Fig. 3.15 that for observation points $z \geq a \cot \theta$, the radiation produced by the radial waves can no longer arrive earlier than the edge wave.

In the case of a thick piezoceramic disk as studied by Baboux et al. [26], it is likely that the radial wave consists of a Rayleigh-type surface wave;

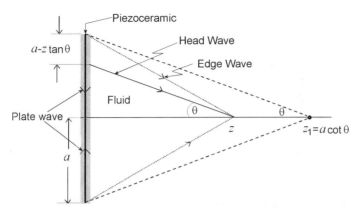

Figure 3.15 The manner in which head waves are produced from a piezoceramic disk immersed in a fluid medium. At and beyond $z = z_1$ the head wave no longer precedes the edge wave.

however, for a disk that is thin compared to the radius, there is good evidence that the waves responsible for generating the head wave consist of Lamb waves. By an optical interference measurement technique Jia et al. [27] recorded the transient displacement at the center of a thin (1 mm), large-diameter (20 mm) piezoceramic disk that was excited by a very brief pulse. They also measured the pressure pulse by means of a small hydrophone. Comparison of these experiments with the known properties of Lamb waves provided good evidence that the radiation produced by these waves was responsible for the head wave phenomenon in thin disks.[4]

3.4 Approximate Methods

3.4.1 Fresnel and Fraunhofer Approximations

Approximate methods for quickly predicting the behavior of transducers, especially when the observation point is beyond the near-field zone, have traditionally played an important role in design. Such methods can often provide a clearer insight into the parameters that govern the field distribution than the computationally more complex "exact" methods. Two approximations that have been widely used for sinusoidal excitation are based on the Fraunhofer (far-field) and Fresnel (mid- and far-field) approximations.

With reference to the geometry illustrated in Fig. 3.16, we first write down the velocity potential at (x_o, y_o, z) due to the transducer of area S that is excited over its entire area, but not necessarily in a uniform manner. If the excitation is sinusoidal, then the normal component of its velocity will be given by

---

4. See also the discussion in subsection 3.5.7 and the evidence for Lamb wave effects in thin concave transducers.

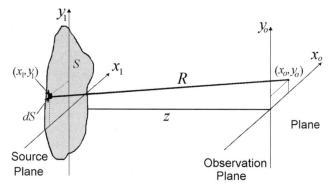

Figure 3.16 An arbitrary plane radiating surface S that lies on the plane $(x_1, y_1, 0)$, an element of area dS at $(x_1, y_1, 0)$, which is at a distance of R from an observation point that lies on the plane (x_o, y_o, z).

$v_{no}(t) = \xi_o(x_1, y_1) v_o e^{j\omega_o t}$, in which $\xi_o(.)$ denotes the spatial variation, i.e., the apodization function. Consequently, from the Rayleigh integral given by (2.33), the velocity potential is

$$(3.29) \qquad \phi_N(x_o, y_o, z:t) = \iint_S \frac{\xi_o v_o e^{j\omega\left(t - \frac{R}{c_o}\right)}}{2\pi R} dS \approx \frac{v_o e^{j\omega t}}{2\pi R} \iint_S \xi_o e^{-j\omega \frac{R}{c_o}} dS,$$

provided that the observation point is sufficiently distant in comparison to the dimensions of S so that the variation of R for the surface integration process can be ignored.[5]

Using the coordinate system shown in Fig. 3.16, the distance R can be written as

$$R = \sqrt{z^2 + (x_o - x_1)^2 + (y_o - y_1)^2} = z\left[1 + \left(\frac{x_o - x_1}{z}\right)^2 + \left(\frac{y_o - y_1}{z}\right)^2\right]^{1/2},$$

which can be expanded as

$$(3.30) \qquad R = z\left\{1 + \frac{1}{2z^2}\left[(x_o^2 + y_o^2) - 2(x_o x_1 + y_o y_1) + (x_1^2 + y_1^2)\right] + \ldots\ldots\right\}.$$

If terms of order higher than those shown above are ignored, then we have the *Fresnel* approximation. If it is also is assumed that $\dfrac{\pi(x_1^2 + y_1^2)_{\text{max.}}}{\lambda} \ll z$, where the subscript indicates the maximum value, then the $(x_1^2 + y_1^2)$ term can be neglected and we have the *Fraunhofer* approximation.

5. Simply taking the R outside the integral may not be consistent with the Fresnel approximation over the z-range for which it is valid; this is considered in [29].

3.4.2 Fraunhofer Approximation

Neglecting the $(x_1^2 + y_1^2)$ term in (3.30), noting that $k = \omega/c_o$, $dS = dx_1 dy_1$, and substituting into (3.29) yields

$$\phi_N(x_o, y_o, z{:}t) \approx \frac{v_o e^{j\omega t}}{2\pi R} e^{-jk\left[z + \frac{x_o^2 + y_o^2}{2z}\right]} \iint_S \xi_o(x_1, y_1) e^{j\frac{k}{z}(x_o x_1 + y_o y_1)} dx_1 dy_1.$$

In this equation, integration is over the surface area of the source. To express the integral in terms of an integral over all space, it is necessary that either ξ_o be defined over all space or that the kernel be multiplied by an aperture function $\Omega(x_1, y_1)$ that is zero outside S and unity inside. Using the latter approach, the velocity potential is given by

$$\phi_N(x_o, y_o, z{:}t) \approx \frac{v_o e^{j\omega t}}{2\pi R} e^{-jk\left[z + \frac{x_o^2 + y_o^2}{2z}\right]} \int_{-\infty}^{\infty} \int_{-\infty}^{\infty} \Omega(x_1, y_1) \xi_o(x_1, y_1) e^{j\frac{k}{z}(x_o x_1 + y_o y_1)} dx_1 dy_1$$

If we define the spatial frequencies in the x- and y-directions by $k_x = -kx_o/z$ and $k_y = -ky_o/z$ and note that pressure phasor is related to the velocity potential phasor by $\underline{p} = j\omega\rho_o\underline{\phi}_N$, then the pressure at the observation point can be expressed as

$$\underline{p}(x_o, y_o, z{:}\omega) \approx \frac{j\omega\rho_o v_o}{2\pi R} e^{-jk\left[z + \frac{x_o^2 + y_o^2}{2z}\right]} \int_{-\infty}^{\infty} \int_{-\infty}^{\infty} \Omega(x_1, y_1) \xi_o(x_1, y_1) e^{-j(k_x x_1 + k_y y_1)} dx_1 dy_1.$$

By comparison with the definition of the 2-D Fourier transform given by (2.53), the integral portion of this equation can be recognized as the 2-D Fourier transform of the product of the aperture and apodization functions, evaluated at the spatial frequencies k_x and k_y. Consequently the pressure phasor can be written as

$$(3.31) \qquad \underline{p}(x_o, y_o, z{:}\omega) \approx \frac{j\omega\rho_o v_o}{2\pi R} e^{-jk\left[z + \frac{x_o^2 + y_o^2}{2z}\right]} \Im[\xi_o(x_1, y_1)\Omega(x_1, y_1)],$$

where $\Im(.)$ denotes the 2-D Fourier transform.

That the far-field response for a uniformly excited transducer surface can be obtained by taking the Fourier transform of the product of the aperture and apodization functions is a particularly valuable result. It enables the response of a variety of geometries to be very simply determined, especially when $\xi_o = 1$. Some simple examples will be considered in the next two subsections.

3.4.3 Fraunhofer Approximation for a Piston Transducer: Directivity Function

For a uniformly excited ($\xi_o = 1$) piston transducer of radius a, the use of cylindrical coordinates (r,z) enables the aperture function to be written as $\Omega(r_1) =$

circ(r_1/a), where the circ function was defined in section 3.1.1. In the same section it was also shown that for a cylindrically symmetric function the 2-D Fourier transform reduces to a zero-order Hankel transform that can be denoted by $\mathcal{H}_0(.)$, i.e.,

$$\Im[\Omega(r_1)] = 2\pi \int_0^\infty r_1 \Omega(r_1) J_0(r_1 k_r) dr_1 = 2\pi \mathcal{H}_0\{\Omega(r_1)\}.$$

Thus, from (3.31) the pressure phasor can be written as

$$\underline{p}(r,z{:}\omega) \approx \frac{j\omega\rho_o v_o}{R} e^{-jk[z+r^2/(2z)]} \mathcal{H}_0\{\text{circ}(r_1/a)\}.$$

Evaluating this transform at the spatial frequency of $k_r = kr/z$ yields[6]

$$\mathcal{H}_0[\text{circ}(r_1/a)] = a^2 \frac{J_1(kar/z)}{kar/z},$$

which enables the pressure phasor to be written as

(3.32)
$$\underline{p}(r,z{:}\omega) \approx \frac{j\omega\rho_o v_o a^2}{2R} \left[\frac{2J_1(kar/z)}{kar/z} \right] e^{-jk[z+r^2/(2z)]}.$$

Noting that $[2J_1(\varsigma)/\varsigma]_{\lim \varsigma \to 0} = 1$, it can be seen that for on-axis points ($r = 0$), this expression reduces to (2.46), which is the approximate expression previously derived for distant axial points. The question as the accuracy of the Fraunhofer approximation can be estimated by determining the pressure magnitude at the location of the last maximum, which occurs at $z \approx a^2/\lambda$. At this point the pressure predicted by (3.32) is a factor of $\pi/2$ greater than that obtained from (2.45), corresponding to an error of 57%. As is illustrated in Fig. 3.17, for a distance such that $z > 2.3a^2/\lambda$, the error is less than 5%.

It should be noted that (3.32) represents the far-field pressure distribution in a cylindrical coordinate system. A particularly useful way of representing the far-field pattern is to use the polar coordinate system (R_o, θ) illustrated in Fig. 3.18. To obtain an approximate expression for the Rayleigh integral for harmonic excitation, consider the geometry illustrated in Fig. 3.19. Because of the cylindrical symmetry it will be noted that the field for the general polar coordinate observation point (R_o, θ, φ) will be identical to that at $(R_o, \theta, 0)$. If the observation point is such that the disk radius $a \ll R_o$, then neglecting the second- and higher-order terms in the binomial expansion, we find

$$R = R_o \sqrt{1 + (r_1/R_o)^2 - 2(r_1/R_o)\cos\varphi_1 \sin\theta}$$
$$\approx R_o\{1 - (r_1/R_o)\cos\varphi_1 \sin\theta\},$$

which corresponds to the Fraunhofer approximation. From (3.29) and $\underline{p} = j\omega\rho_o\phi_N$, the pressure phasor is given by

6. See Appendix B.

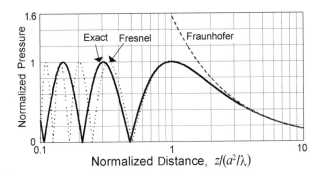

Figure 3.17 The accuracy of the Fraunhofer and Fresnel approximations for on-axis locations, CW excitation, and $a = 5\lambda$, in comparison with the exact expression. For the Fresnel approximation, the accuracy at a given normalized distance increases with a/λ. At the normalized distance of 3.0, the pressure is 50% of the maximum pressure. Note the use of a logarithmic normalized distance axis.

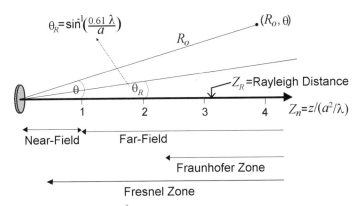

Figure 3.18 The various zones for a simple piston transducer, and the polar coordinate system (R_o, θ) used for obtaining a far-field expression based on the Fraunhofer approximation. The angle θ_R is beam divergence half-angle, and the Rayleigh distance $(z_R = \pi a^2/\lambda)$ is approximately the location where the pressure has decreased by nearly 50% from the maximum value.

$$
\begin{aligned}
\underline{p}(R, \theta : \omega) &= j\omega\rho_o v_o \iint_S \underline{\xi}_o \frac{e^{-jkR}}{2\pi R} dS \\
&\approx \frac{j\omega\rho_o v_o}{2\pi R_o} \int_0^a r_1 dr_1 \int_0^{2\pi} \underline{\xi}_o(r_1) e^{-jk[R_o - r_1 \cos\varphi_1 \sin\theta]} d\varphi_1 \\
&= \frac{j\omega\rho_o v_o}{R_o} e^{-jkR_o} \int_0^a \underline{\xi}_o(r_1) J_0(kr_1 \sin\theta) r_1 dr_1,
\end{aligned}
$$

where the integral was evaluated with the help of Appendix C. For no apodization $\underline{\xi}_o(r_1) = 1$, and also with the help of Appendix C,

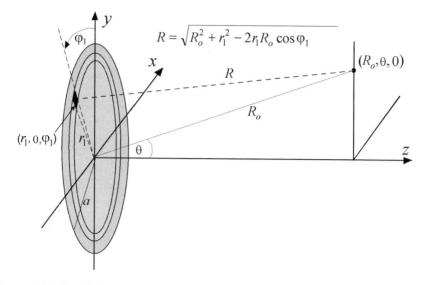

Figure 3.19 Sketch showing the geometry used in obtaining an expression for the far-field profile of a disk transducer of radius a.

$$\underline{p}(R_o,\theta:\omega) \approx \frac{j\omega\rho_o v_o a^2}{2R_o} e^{-jkR_o}\left[\frac{2J_1(kR_o\sin\theta)}{kR_o\sin\theta}\right].$$

This can be rewritten as

(3.33)
$$\underline{p}(R_o,\theta:\omega) \approx \frac{j\omega\rho_o v_o a^2}{2R_o} D(\theta)e^{-jkR_o},$$
(a)

where
$$D(\theta) = \frac{2J_1(ka\sin\theta)}{ka\sin\theta},$$
(b)

is the *directivity* function. It should be noted that the factor of 2 has been incorporated in the definition so that $D(\theta)$ will be unity when $\theta = 0$. The far-field pressure response can be written in the form

(3.34)
$$|\underline{p}(R_o,\theta:\omega)| \propto \frac{D(\theta)}{R_o},$$

which expresses the fact that the directivity function determines the angular pressure distribution for any radial location, and that the magnitude diminishes inversely with the radial distance. This useful result was obtained by King [68] in 1934 as a special case ($\xi_o(r_1) = 1$) in his treatment of an arbitrary circularly symmetric apodization function.

The directivity function is plotted in Fig. 3.20a, b, and c for three different values of ka. It shows that as the transducer radius diminishes, the main lobe response becomes dominant and approaches a constant value over 180

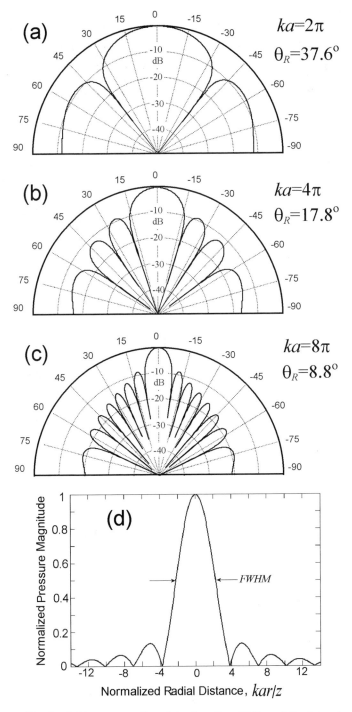

Figure 3.20 The far-field pressure directivity function $D(\theta)$ and the lateral profile for a disk transducer. Polar graphs obtained from (3.33) for (a) $a = \lambda$, (b) $a = 2\lambda$, and (c) $a = 4\lambda$. The value of $-10\log_{10}[D(\theta)]$ is plotted and the beam divergence angle θ_R is given. (d) Pressure magnitude profile in the lateral direction obtained from (3.32).

degrees. For larger radii the main lobe narrows and the number of side lobes increases. Fig. 3.20d shows the pressure response in the lateral direction as calculated from (3.32). A useful measure of the lateral resolution is the *full width at half maximum* (*FWHM*) of the central lobe, and this can be expressed as

$$(3.35) \qquad FWHM = 4.41\frac{z}{ka} = 1.4\frac{z\lambda}{2a}.$$

Note that the *FWHM* in the Fraunhofer zone increases linearly with the axial distance z. For example, if $ka = 8\pi$ ($a = 4\lambda$), and $z = 15\,cm$ (which is in the far field if $\lambda < 1\,mm$), then $FWHM = 2.6\,cm$.

The directivity function is of importance in the design of hydrophones used for measuring field profiles. Accurate measurements in the near field of a source require that the effective dimensions (as opposed to the physical dimensions) be much smaller than a wavelength, a goal that may be difficult to achieve in practice. As pointed out by Harris [30], two of the problematic characteristics of hydrophones are the frequency response and the effective dimensions. For a disk hydrophone, the effective radius can be determined by comparing the measured angular response to that predicted by theory. However, for a very-small-diameter transducer, the boundary and mounting conditions become very important factors in determining the response. For a disk with a diameter equal to the wavelength ($ka = \pi$), the theoretical responses for three different boundary conditions previously discussed (see Table 3.1) are shown in Fig. 3.21. For larger values of ka the three response curves approach one another, while for smaller values they diverge. Measurements of the angular response for small hydrophones frequently show angular characteristics that differ significantly from the theoretical response [31].

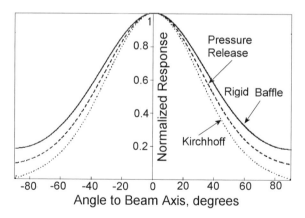

Figure 3.21 Directivity pattern for a disk transducer whose diameter is equal to the wavelength $ka = \pi$ for three different boundary conditions corresponding to (i) a rigid baffle (3.33b), (ii) a pressure release surface (3.33b) $\times \cos\theta$, and (iii) Kirchhoff (free-field) condition (3.33b) $\times [(1 + \cos\theta)/2]$.

The various zones frequently referred to in the literature [39] are those shown in Fig. 3.18. Generally, the near- and far-field boundary is taken as the position of the last maximum, which in the case of a piston transducer is at $z = a^2/\lambda$. The zone where the Fraunhofer approximation is reasonably accurate extends from around $z \approx 2a^2/\lambda$, and the Fresnel approximation, as discussed below, provides sufficient accuracy for predicting the response well into the near-field zone. In addition, $\theta_R = \sin^{-1}(0.61\lambda/a)$ is the angle at which the beam diverges in the far-field as measured from the center of the transducer and corresponds to the first minimum of the directivity function, i.e., when $J_1(ka\sin\theta)$ first becomes zero. Finally, the *Rayleigh distance* ($z_R = \pi a^2/\lambda$), is approximately the location beyond the last maximum where the amplitude has reduced by 50%.

3.4.4 Fresnel Approximation for a Piston Transducer

The relative accuracy of the Fresnel approximation can be determined by comparison of the on-axis response. This can be achieved by substituting all the terms given in (3.30) into (3.29), assuming that $\xi_o = 1$ and noting that $p = j\omega\rho_o\phi_N$, yielding

$$(3.31) \qquad \underline{p}(x_o,y_o,z{:}\omega) \approx \frac{j\omega\rho_o v_o}{2\pi R} e^{-jk\left[z+\frac{x_o^2+y_o^2}{2z}\right]} \iint\limits_S e^{j\frac{k}{z}\left(x_ox_1+y_oy_1-x_1^2-y_1^2\right)} dx_1 dy_1.$$

On the axis, $x_o = y_o = 0$, and by letting $r_1^2 = x_1^2 + y_1^2$ so that $dx_1 dy_1 = 2\pi r_1 dr_1$, the integral can be evaluated as

$$(3.34) \qquad \underline{p}(0,z{:}\omega) = c_o\rho_o v_o e^{-jkz}\left(1 - e^{-jka^2/2z}\right),$$

which is also plotted in Fig. 3.17. It can be clearly seen that for the assumed disk radius of $a = 5\lambda$, this equation is an excellent approximation to the exact equation as expressed by (2.45) for normalized axial distances of greater than 0.5. However, it should be noted that the agreement depends on the a/λ ratio: as it increases the agreement improves, and vice versa.

3.5 Concave and Convex Transducers

It has been long recognized that transducers with a concave geometry are particularly efficient in concentrating much of their radiated energy in a highly localized focal zone. They have found many uses in medical diagnostic and therapeutic systems, and substantial efforts have been made to develop efficient methods for predicting their behavior for both sinusoidal and transient excitations [34]. For concave transducers, the field distribution for sinusoidal excitation was explored analytically by Williams [32] in 1946. However, O'Neil [33], in his classic paper of 1949, presented a much more extensive analysis.

3.5.1 Fundamental Approximations

In considering the response of a nonplanar transducer, it is important to recall that the Rayleigh integral was derived under the assumption that the transducer and the medium in which it is imbedded was a flat surface. Thus, the question arises as to how close to flat the surface must be in order that the Rayleigh integral approach gives a good approximation to the actual response. The possible influence of the effects of a curved surface can be appreciated by noting that other portions of the surface will diffract a wavelet emitted from an elementary area of a concave surface. This secondary diffraction is not accounted for by the Rayleigh integral, which assumes that the source lies on an infinite planar surface and that each incremental area acts as a hemispherical source that contributes in a simple time-retarded sense to the velocity potential at the observation point. O'Neil [33] and Penttinen and Luukkala [15] have discussed these limitations and point out that if the aperture is large compared to the acoustic wavelength, and for gently curved sources, the Rayleigh integral should be a good approximation. Nonetheless, because of this approximation it should not be surprising to find that the assumed boundary conditions are not recovered by the solution. For example, O'Neil [33] showed that for a sinusoidal surface velocity, the expression for the axial particle velocity does not reduce to the assumed velocity magnitude and phase at the transducer surface.

Using the above assumptions, a number of different methods have been described for calculating the CW and the transient response for concave and convex radiators [14,15,20,33–37]. In the formulation presented by de Hoop et al. [37] and Schmerr et al. [38] for a concave radiator, the pressure field was expressed in terms of the sum of a spherically convergent or divergent *direct* wave and an *edge* wave[7], similar to that originally discussed by Tupholme [18] for transient radiation from a spherical cap.

3.5.2 Impulse Response Using the Ring Function Method

With the assumptions noted above, we can make use of the ring function method of Ohtsuki [14] that was described in section 3.3. The ring function $\alpha(t)$ is equal to the fractional arc length of a circle that lies on the transducer surface. For a transducer surface that forms part of the spherical surface, the ring function can be determined by making use of spherical geometry. We shall initially consider the simpler case of the convex spherical radiator shown in Fig. 3.22 that has a radius of curvature a and that suspends a half-angle of θ_T at the center of curvature. The observation point is specified by the radial coordinate R and the angle θ, using the center of curvature as the origin of coordinates. As will be seen, the results for a concave radiator can be obtained by using the same equations, though additional considerations are needed depending on the angular position of the field point.

---

7. This approach is similar to that described in sections 2.2.2 and 3.2 for a piston transducer.

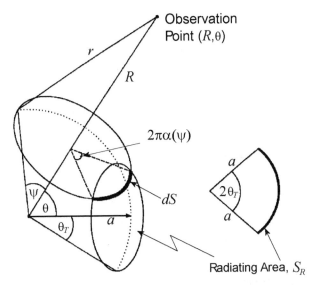

Figure 3.22 A convex radiator of area S_R with a half-angle of θ_T and radius of curvature a. The origin of coordinates is the center of curvature. All points on the elementary area dS are equidistant from the observation point (R,θ). The contribution from dS at time t arrives at the observation point at a time $(t + r/c_o)$.

With reference to Fig. 3.22, the element of area that contributes to the signal at the observation point at a given instant of time is shown as arising from the area dS. To find an expression for dS, we first obtain an expression for the area of the semispherical cap formed by the intersection of the periphery of the base of the cone that suspends a half-angle of ψ at the center of curvature. This is given by $S_c = \pi(a/R)\left[r^2 - (R - a)^2\right]$. By differentiating this with respect to r, and noting that $dS = \alpha(t)dS_c$, the elementary area is given by

$$(3.38) \qquad dS = 2\pi a\alpha(\psi)rdr/R.$$

The velocity impulse response for a uniformly excited transducer ($\xi(R,\theta) = 1$) is therefore given by substituting (3.38) into (2.37):

$$(3.39) \qquad h(R,\theta{:}t) = \iint_S \frac{\delta\left(t - \dfrac{r}{c_o}\right)}{2\pi r}\,dS = \frac{a}{R}\int_{R_{min}}^{R_{max}} \alpha(\psi)\delta\left(t - \frac{r}{c_o}\right)dr = c_o\frac{a}{R}\alpha(R,\theta{:}t),$$

where R_{max} and R_{min} are the maximum and minimum distances, respectively, from the observation point to the transducer surface. To determine $\alpha(R,\theta{:}t)$ it is necessary to make use of spherical triangle geometry, which yields

$$(3.40) \qquad \alpha(R,\theta{:}t) = \frac{1}{\pi}\cos^{-1}\left(\frac{\cos\theta_T - \cos\psi\cos\theta}{\sin\psi\sin\theta}\right), \qquad (a)$$

where

$$\cos \psi = \frac{R^2 + a^2 - t^2 c_o^2}{2aR} = \frac{R^2 + a^2 - r^2}{2aR}. \quad \text{(b)}$$

These equations are valid *provided* the arc area dS does *not* form a complete circle. When a complete circle is formed, corresponding either to the condition $0 \leq \psi \leq \theta_T - \theta$ and $\theta \leq \theta_T$, or the condition $(2\pi - \theta_T - \theta) \leq \psi \leq \pi$ and $(\pi - \theta_T) \leq \theta \leq \pi$, then $\alpha(R, \theta : t) = 1$. Consequently, the velocity impulse response for the entire range of angles is given by:

(3.41)
$$h(R, \theta : t) = \begin{cases} c_o(a/R), & 0 \leq \psi \leq (\theta_T - \theta) \text{ and } \theta \leq \theta_T, \text{ or} \\ & (2\pi - \theta_T - \theta) \leq \psi \leq \pi \text{ and} \\ & (\pi - \theta_T) \leq \theta \leq \pi, \\ c_o(a/R)\alpha(R, \theta : t), & |\theta_T - \theta| < \psi \leq (\theta_T + \theta), \\ 0, & \text{otherwise.} \end{cases}$$

For *on-axis* locations, where $\theta = 0$, the impulse response is the rectangular function

(3.42)
$$h(R, 0 : t) = c_o(a/R)\text{rect}\left[\frac{t - (t_{max} + t_{min})/2}{t_{max} - t_{min}}\right], \quad \text{(a)}$$

in which

$$t_{min} c_o = R_{min}(\theta = 0) = R - a, \quad \text{and} \quad t_{max} c_o = R_{max}(\theta = 0)$$
$$= \sqrt{R^2 + a^2 - 2aR\cos\theta_T}, \quad \text{(b)}$$

and where the equations for R_{max} and R_{min}, as given in Fig. 3.23d, have been used.

For the case of a *concave* radiator, R remains as the distance from the center of curvature, and the equations for the impulse response are also given by (3.40) and (3.41). Three cases can be identified depending on θ, and these are illustrated in Fig. 3.23a, b, and c, together with the equations for R_{max} and R_{min}. For on-axis cases ($\theta = 0$ or π), the equations for R_{max} and R_{min} given in Fig. 3.23a and c must be used in (3.42b). It is evident that for $R = 0$, $t_{min} = t_{max}$, and as expected the impulse response at the geometrical focus is a δ-function.

3.5.3 Sinusoidal Response

If the transducer excitation is given by $v_{no}(t) = v_o e^{j\omega t}$, where v_o is the velocity amplitude, then the velocity potential response can be obtained by direct substitution of (3.38) into (2.32), yielding

(3.43)
$$\phi_N(R, \theta : \omega) = \frac{av_o e^{j\omega t}}{R} \int_{R_{min}}^{R_{max}} \alpha(\psi) e^{-j\omega r/c_o} dr \quad \text{(a)}$$

where $\alpha(\psi)$ is given by

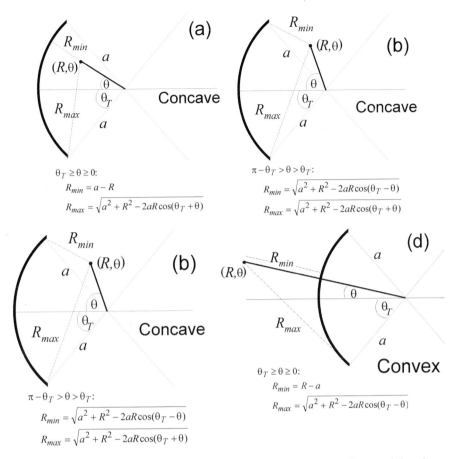

Figure 3.23 Geometry for (a), (b), (c) concave and (d) convex radiators, giving the minimum and maximum distances from the observation point (R,θ) to the radiator surface. The origin of coordinates is the center of curvature.

$$
(3.43) \quad \alpha(R,\theta:\psi) = \begin{cases} 1, & 0 \le \psi \le (\theta_T - \theta) \text{ and } \theta \le \theta_T, \text{ or} \\ & (2\pi - \theta_T - \theta) \le \psi \le \pi \text{ and} \\ & (\pi - \theta_T) \le \theta \le \pi, \\ \text{Equation (3.40)}, & |\theta_T - \theta| < \psi \le (\theta_T + \theta), \\ 0, & \text{otherwise.} \end{cases} \quad (b)
$$

In addition, R_{max} and R_{min} are the maximum and minimum distances, respectively, from the observation point to the transducer surface, and equations for these are given in Fig. 3.23 for both concave and convex geometries.

For the particular case of axial observation points ($\theta = 0$ or π), (3.43) can be simplified to

$$
(3.44) \quad \phi_N(R, 0 \text{ or } \pi:\omega) = \frac{a v_o e^{j\omega t}}{R} \int_{R_{min}}^{R_{max}} e^{-j\omega r / c_o}\, dr = \frac{a v_o e^{j\omega t}}{jkR}\left[e^{-jkR_{min}} - e^{-jkR_{max}} \right],
$$

where $k = \omega/c_o$ and R_{max} and R_{min} for a concave transducer are given by putting either $\theta = 0$ in Fig. 3.23a, or $\theta = \pi$ in Fig. 3.23c, and for a convex geometry, by putting $\theta = 0$ in Fig. 3.23d. Thus, the pressure phasor is given by

(3.45)
$$\underline{p}(R,0:\omega) = \frac{\rho_o a c_o v_o}{R} \left[e^{-jkR_{min}} - e^{-jkR_{max}} \right],$$
(a)

or

(3.45)
$$\underline{p}(R,0:\omega) = \frac{2j\rho_o a c_o v_o}{R} \sin\{k(R_{max} - R_{min})/2\} e^{-jk(R_{max} + R_{min})/2}.$$
(b)

Alternatively, this result can be obtained by substituting (3.42a) into (2.37b) and then taking the Fourier transform, yielding for the phasor pressure

$$\underline{p}(R,0:\omega_o) = j2\pi\omega_o \rho_o v_o c_o (a/R) \Im\{\mathrm{rect}[(t - \tau_1)/\tau_2]\}|_{\omega=\omega_o},$$

where $\tau_1 = (t_{max} + t_{min})/2$, and $\tau_2 = t_{max} - t_{min}$. After some algebra and on dropping the subscript on ω, this reduces to (3.45).

As an example, the pressure magnitude axial distribution is shown in Fig. 3.24a for a concave transducer with a 4.0 cm radius of curvature and a half-angle of 30 degrees, uniformly excited with a velocity of 1.0 mm/s and radiating into water. In addition, a contour map for the same transducer is shown in Fig. 3.25.

On examining (3.45b) it will be noted that the magnitude of the pressure response at the *geometric* focus ($R = 0$) can be obtained by making use of R_{max} and R_{min} as given in Fig. 3.23a and then taking the limit of (3.45b) as $R \to 0$.

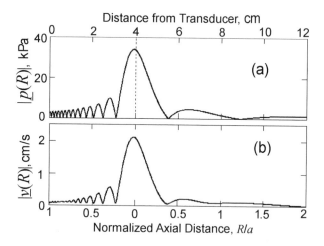

Figure 3.24 Axial CW pressure and velocity profiles for a 1-MHz concave transducer with a 4.0 cm radius of curvature and a half-angle of 30 degrees, uniformly excited with a velocity of 1.0 mm/s radiating into water. (a) Pressure magnitude, calculated from (3.45). (b) Velocity magnitude, calculated from (3.49).

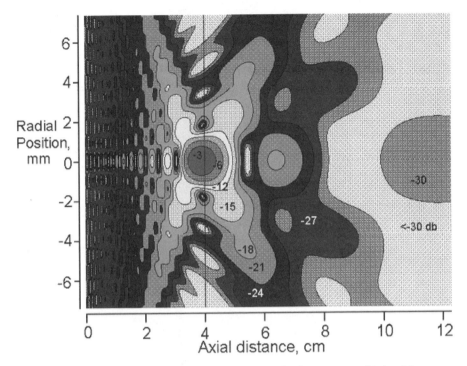

Figure 3.25 Gray-scale-encoded CW pressure magnitude contours obtained from (3.43) for a 1 MHz concave transducer with a 4.0 cm radius of curvature and a half-angle of 30 degrees, uniformly excited with a velocity of 1.0 mm/s radiating into water. Contours are given in -3 dB steps relative to that at the focal point, which is 0.92 mm closer to the transducer than the geometric focus. Note the different scales for the radial and axial directions. The region examined has a radius of 7 mm and a length of 125 mm. (See also color insert.)

If the *gain G* of a transducer is defined as the ratio of the pressure at the focus to that on the transducer surface,[8] and assuming that the geometric focus *a* and the actual focal point are nearly coincident, the transducer gain can be expressed as

(3.46)
$$G = \frac{|p(0,0)|}{\rho_o c_o v_o} = ka(1 - \cos\theta_T),$$
$$= k\hbar = 2\pi\hbar/\lambda$$

where $\hbar = a(1 - \cos\theta_T)$ is the height of the rim. From this, it can be seen that the pressure can be increased by using a higher frequency and/or for a fixed *a*, by making $\theta_T = 90$ degrees (i.e., by using a hemispherical shell). Typically, the maximum pressure does not occur at the geometric focus: it is somewhat

---

8. It should be noted that for a plane piston source, if the focal point is taken to be the last pressure maximum, then from (2.45), $G = 2$.

closer to the transducer. Although an exact implicit expression can be found by differentiating (3.45b) and equating to zero, O'Neil [33] has obtained the following approximate expressions for the normalized maximum pressure and its axial location are

$$
(3.47) \qquad \frac{\left|p(R_m, \pi)\right|}{\rho_o c_o v_o} \approx k\hat{h} + \frac{12}{k\hat{h}}, \quad R_m \approx \frac{12a}{12 + k^2\hat{h}^2},
$$

for $k\hat{h} > 4$.

Taking the example shown in Fig. 3.24a, for which, if $\hat{h} = 3.573\lambda$, the gain is 22.45, and the maximum is located about 2.3% closer to the transducer and the pressure is 1.5% greater than that at the geometric focus. In the limit as $k\hat{h} \rightarrow 0$, corresponding to a flat piston source that has a geometric focus at infinity, the maximum pressure is equal to $2\rho_o c_o v_o$.

Further examination of (3.45b) in comparison to the pressure response of a piston transducer, as given by (2.45b), shows that the ratio of the maximum pressure amplitudes for the same excitation velocity are given by

$$
(3.48) \qquad \frac{\left|p(0, 0:\omega)\right|_{\text{Concave}}}{\left|p(a^2/\lambda:\omega)\right|_{\text{Piston}}} \approx \frac{\pi\hat{h}}{\lambda}
$$

for $k\hat{h} > 4$, which, for the case shown in Fig. 3.24a, is a factor of 11.2.

3.5.4 Velocity and Intensity

At any point (R,θ) the velocity vector is given by $\mathbf{v} = -\text{grad}(\Phi_N) = -\tilde{\mathbf{R}}\dfrac{\partial \Phi_N}{\partial R} - \dfrac{\tilde{\theta}}{R}\dfrac{\partial \Phi_N}{\partial \theta}$, where $\tilde{\mathbf{R}}$ and $\tilde{\theta}$ are unit vectors. Thus, the velocity can be obtained by numerically evaluating the derivatives of (3.43a). For the on-axis observation points, symmetry requires that $\partial \Phi_N/\partial \theta = 0$, and consequently, by evaluating the derivative of (3.44), we find that the velocity phasor is given by

$$
(3.49) \qquad
\begin{aligned}
\underline{v}(R, 0:\omega) = \frac{jav_o}{kR}\Bigg[jk\bigg\{ &\frac{(R - a\cos\theta_T)e^{-jkR_{max}}}{\sqrt{R^2 + a^2 - 2aR\cos\theta_T}} + e^{-jkR_{min}} \bigg\} \\
&- \frac{1}{R}\Big(e^{-jkR_{min}} - e^{-jkR_{max}} \Big) \Bigg],
\end{aligned}
$$

which is plotted in Fig. 3.24b. It can be shown that in the limit as $R \rightarrow a$ the velocity phasor differs from that assumed value of v_o. This was noted by O'Neil [33], who pointed out that this arose from violating the flat surface assumption of the Rayleigh integral, which formed the starting point of the above analysis.

To calculate the intensity distribution, it is necessary to recall that (2.48) gives the time average of the instantaneous intensity vector, $\mathbf{I}(\mathbf{r}:t)$ for a sinusoidal field, i.e., $\bar{\mathbf{I}}(\mathbf{r}) = \frac{1}{2}\text{Re}\{\underline{p}\underline{v}^*\}$. Since an expression for $p(R,0:\omega)$ has already been derived as (3.45), it is simpler to obtain the intensity from the pressure and its phase angle φ by noting that the intensity can be written as:

(3.50)
$$\mathbf{\bar{I}}(R, 0 \text{ or } \pi) = \frac{-|p|^2}{2\rho_o c_o} \frac{\partial(\varphi/k)}{\partial R} \mathbf{\tilde{R}}.$$

Now the pressure phase angle can be obtained from (3.45b) as $\varphi = \frac{\pi}{2} - \frac{k}{2}(R_{max} + R_{min})$. By substituting its derivative into (3.50), the magnitude of the intensity is

(3.51)
$$\bar{I}(R, 0 \text{ or } \pi) = \frac{|p|^2}{2\rho_o c_o}\left(\frac{1}{2} + \frac{a\cos\theta_T - R}{2R_{max}}\right),$$

where R_{max} is given in Fig. 3.23a and the pressure magnitude can be obtained from (3.45). This is plotted in Fig. 3.26 for the same transducer that was considered in Fig. 3.24. At the geometric focus ($R = 0$), (3.51) reduces to

(3.52)
$$\bar{I}(0, 0) = \rho_o c_o (kv_o)^2 h^2 (1 + \cos\theta_T)/4.$$

Thus, the ratio of the peak intensity produced by the concave transducer to that produced by a disk transducer is given by

(3.53)
$$\frac{\bar{I}(0, 0:\omega)|_{\text{Concave}}}{\bar{I}_p(0, a^2/\lambda:\omega)|_{\text{Piston}}} \approx \left(\frac{\pi h}{\lambda}\right)^2 (1 + \cos\theta_T)/2.$$

For the same transducer considered in Fig. 3.24 and Fig. 3.26, this ratio is 118.

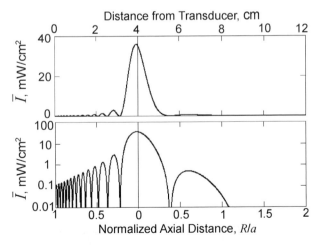

Figure 3.26 Axial CW intensity profile as calculated from (3.51) for a 1 MHz concave transducer with a 4.0 cm radius of curvature, a half-angle of 30 degrees, uniformly excited with a velocity of 1.0 mm/s, and radiating into water. Note the log scale in the lower graph.

3.5.5 Approximate Axial and Lateral Fields Near the Focus

Of particular interest is the pressure field distribution on the focal plane (a plane normal to the axis at the focal point). Using the Fresnel approximation, an approximate expression valid for points close to the axis can be obtained [40, pp. 183–185]. This expression, which was originally derived by O'Neil [33] using a different approach, is given by

$$(3.54) \qquad \left| \underline{p}\left(R, \frac{\pi}{2} : \omega \right) \right| \approx 2\rho_o c_o v_o k \hbar \left[\frac{J_1(kR\mathcal{D}/2a)}{kR\mathcal{D}/2a} \right],$$

where $\mathcal{D} = \sqrt{4\hbar(2a - \hbar)}$ is the aperture diameter. Equation (3.54) is plotted in Fig. 3.27 for the same transducer assumed in Fig. 3.26. For this transducer, the difference between the approximate values predicted by (3.54) and those obtained numerically at the geometric focus were negligible. However, it is to be expected that when the true focal point deviates significantly from the geometric focus, (3.54) will no longer provide a good estimate of the focal plane distribution. Convenient approximate expressions for the intensity distribution in both the axial and lateral planes are those obtained by Cline et al. [41] using the Fresnel approximation. When normalized to the intensity at the geometric focus, these are given by

$$(3.55) \qquad \frac{\bar{I}(R)_{Axial}}{\bar{I}(0)} \approx \left[\frac{\sin[k\hbar R/2(a+R)]}{k\hbar R/2a} \right]^2$$

$$\frac{\bar{I}(R)_{Lateral}}{\bar{I}(0)} \approx \left[2 \frac{J_1(kR\mathcal{D}/2a)}{kR\mathcal{D}/2a} \right]^2.$$

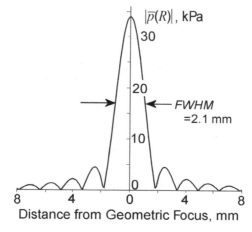

Figure 3.27 Approximate magnitude of the pressure distribution on the geometric focal plane as calculated from (3.54) for a concave transducer with a 4.0 cm radius of curvature, a half-angle of 30 degrees, uniformly excited with a velocity of 1.0 mm/s, and radiating into water.

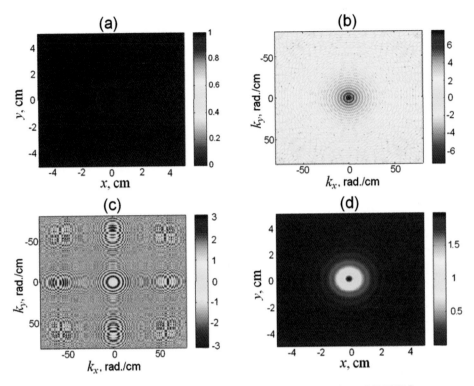

Figure 3.5 Field computation with the angular spectrum method using a 2-D FFT for a piston transducer with a radius $a = 1$ cm, excited at 5 MHz with a normal velocity $v_o = 1$ cm/s. The axial component of the particle velocity was computed on a plane at $z = a^2/\lambda$ ($= 33.3$ cm). (a) Normal particle velocity profile on the transducer plane at $z = 0$. Sampling out to ± 5 cm using 256×256 samples over the entire plane, i.e., $\Delta x = \Delta y = 0.39$ mm per sample. Red corresponds to $v_o = 1$ cm/s, blue to $v_o = 0$. (b) Angular spectrum of the source obtained by taking the 2-D Fourier transform of the source. The source plane was zero padded to ± 10 cm and the color scale is the logarithmic magnitude of the 2-D FFT. The maximum spatial frequencies represent $\pi/\Delta x$ and $\pi/\Delta y$ and have 512×512 samples across the domain. (c) Complex argument of the transfer function $H(k_x, k_y; a^2/\lambda)$, plotted in the spatial frequency domain using 512×512 points. The color map range is from $-\pi$ to π. (d) Normal component of the particle velocity (cm/s) field on the plane $z = a^2/\lambda$. This was obtained by taking the 2-D inverse discrete Fourier transform of the product of the transfer function H and the source angular spectrum. Results are shown out to ± 5 cm using 256×256 points. Note that the distribution peaks at 2.0 cm/s (twice the normal particle velocity), as expected. (See text, p. 144.)

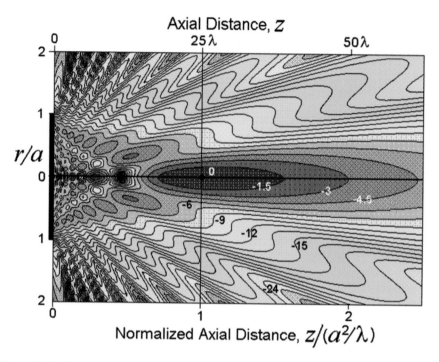

Figure 3.10 Contour map for a disk transducer ($a = 5\lambda$) showing the CW spatial pressure distribution for Rayleigh (i) boundary conditions. Both the axial and radial distances are normalized to the disk radius. The contour lines are expressed in dB's relative to the value at $(0, 5a)$. (See text, p. 149.)

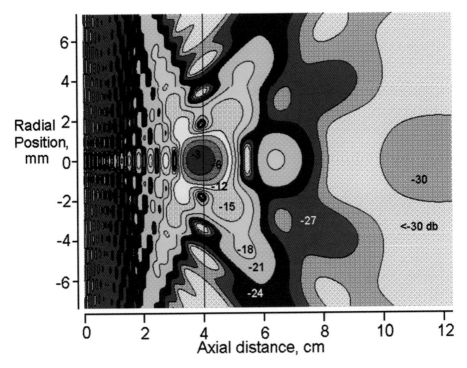

Figure 3.25 Color-encoded CW pressure magnitude contours obtained from (3.43) for a 1 MHz concave transducer with a 4.0 cm radius of curvature and a half-angle of 30 degrees, uniformly excited with a velocity of 1.0 mm/s radiating into water. Contours are given in -3 dB steps relative to that at the focal point, which is 0.92 mm closer to the transducer than the geometric focus. Note the different scales for the radial and axial directions. The region examined has a radius of 7 mm and a length of 125 mm. (See text, p. 169.)

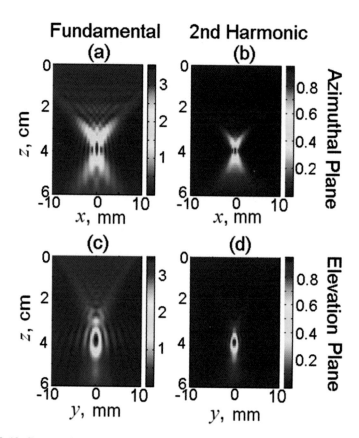

Figure 8.41 Computed transmit profiles for nonlinear propagation in a liver-like medium from a linear phased array excited with a 2-MHz CW signal. Fundamental and second harmonic profiles in: (a), (b) azimuthal plane and (c), (d) elevation plane. The array had 64 elements, each with a height of 20 mm, width of $\lambda/2$, and spacing of $\lambda/4$, giving a total length ≈ 3.7cm. Focusing in both the azimuthal and elevation directions was at a depth of 4 cm. The properties of the medium are the same as those listed Fig. 8.40. The color scale gives the pressure in MPa. The source velocity amplitude was 0.23 m/s (source pressure amplitude ≈ 347 kPa). (Reproduced, with permission, from Zemp et al. [142], *J. Acoust. Soc. Am.*, 113, 139-152, © 2003, Acoustical Society of America.) (See text, p. 552.)

Figure 10.24 Two examples of color flow imaging. For both, the color flow image is added to the gray-scale B-mode image and the color bar scale gives the flow velocity component in the beam direction in cm/s. Vertical tick marks are 1 cm apart. (a) Common carotid artery (red scale) and the jugular vein (blue scale): 15 frames/s, 5.0-MHz center frequency; the focal point is marked by a < close to the RHS. (b) Sector scan showing the umbilical cord (two arteries and one vein) at 29 weeks: 4 frames/s, 2.5-MHz center frequency. (Courtesy Philips Ultrasound.) (See text, p. 695.)

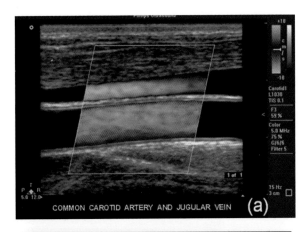

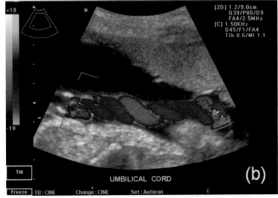

Figure 10.25 Example of a spectral flow display from a sample volume located near the center of the common carotid artery. Two small white lines mark the range-gate boundaries and the white dots show the spectral beam direction. The beam/flow angle was estimated to be 59 degrees, resulting in a peak flow velocity of 43 cm/s. The envelope of the spectral display, indicated by the gray line, gives the variation from within the sample volume of the peak flow velocity over each cycle. (Courtesy Siemens Ultrasound.) (See text, p. 696.)

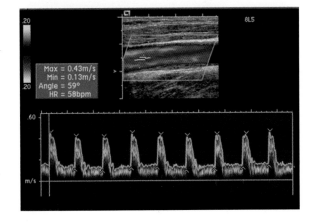

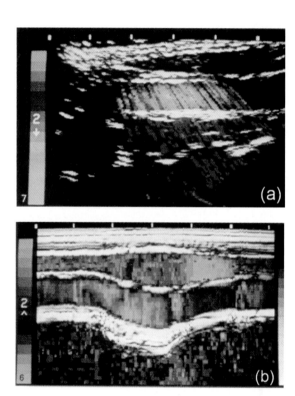

Figure 10.27 Early color-encoded flow images. (a) Common carotid artery flow image superimposed on a gray-scale B-mode image. (b) Three-second M-mode recording showing the movement of tissue and vessel walls in gray scale and blood flow in color. The beam passes through the jugular vein (blue) and then through the common carotid artery. (Reprinted by permission of Elsevier, from Eyer et al. [92], *Ultrasound Med. Biol.*, 7, 21-31, ©1981 World Federation of Ultrasound in Medicine and Biology.) (See text, p. 698.)

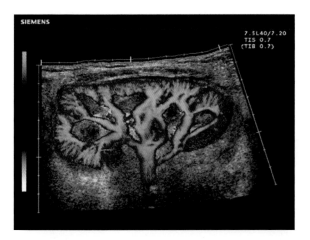

Figure 10.39 Nondirectional power flow image of a kidney. The hue and brightness of the colors indicate the relative power. Note that close to the vessel walls, where the segment volume is only partially in the vessel, the power falls and, in this region, the power scale merges from orange to purple through to black. (Courtesy Siemens Ultrasound.) (See text, p. 722.)

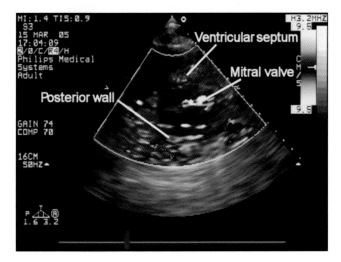

Figure 10.41 Color-encoded tissue velocity image of the heart. The time in the cardiac cycle at which the image was obtained is indicated by the green line. A low-pass filter has been used to suppress the blood flow information. (Courtesy Professor McDicken.) (See text, p. 724.)

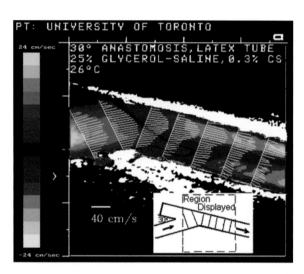

Figure 10.51 Color flow image of a bypass graft model with superimposed vectors showing the 2-D velocity distribution for steady flow (1.4 l/min, Reynolds number = 1600). The B-mode image (7 MHz) and the flow image (5 MHz) are those obtained with a linear-array transducer with the beam in the vertical direction. The color flow image scale gives the flow velocity component in the horizontal direction. The 2-D vectors were calculated from information obtained from color flow images obtained at -20, 0, and +20 degrees. (Reprinted by permission of Elsevier from Maniatis et al. [182], *Ultrasound Med. Biol.*, 20, 559-569, ©1994 World Federation of Ultrasound in Medicine and Biology.) (See text, p. 741.)

3.5.6 Lateral Resolution and Depth of Field

The lateral resolution can be characterized by the full width at half maximum (*FWHM*). From (3.54) it can be readily shown that for a concave transducer the pressure is reduced by 50% when $kR\mathcal{D}/(2a) = 2.215$. Consequently, at the focus $F \approx a$

$$(3.56) \qquad FWHM = 1.4\lambda \frac{\text{Focal Length}}{\text{Aperture}} = 1.4\lambda \frac{F}{\mathcal{D}} \approx 1.4\lambda a/\mathcal{D},$$

which is equal to 2.1 mm for the assumed transducer geometry. The ratio of the focal length to the aperture diameter is generally referred to as the *f-number* of the transducer. Along with the wavelength, it determines the lateral resolution, and as a result it is a very important parameter in specifying the performance of an imaging system. By comparing the *FWHM* for a concave transducer to that of an unfocused disk transducer with the same aperture ($2a = \mathcal{D}$), it can be seen that at the same axial location, the lateral resolutions are identical, i.e., for $z_{disk} = F$, then (3.56) and (3.35) are identical. Thus, *in the Fraunhofer zone*, a focused concave transducer does not result in any improvement in the lateral resolution over that of a simple disk with the same aperture.

The Rayleigh resolution criterion for distinguishing the images of two incoherent point sources created by circular aperture can also be used [40, pp. 185–189]. Specifically, this requires that the maximum of one image lies on the first zero of the other. Since the first zero of the Bessel function in (3.54) occurs when its argument is 3.83, this yields

$$(3.57) \qquad R_L = 1.22\lambda \frac{\text{Focal Length}}{\text{Aperture}} \approx 1.22\lambda a/\mathcal{D} = 1.22\lambda \times \textit{f-number}$$

for the lateral resolution. In the case of the 4 cm geometric focal length transducer considered above, $R_L = 1.83$ mm.

Like the lateral resolution, the depth of field is of major importance in ultrasound imaging system design. It provides a measure of the range of depths over which the transducer maintains reasonably good focusing properties. In the case of a concave transducer Kino [40, p. 191] has shown that a good approximation for the depth of field corresponding to the 3-dB points on the axial pressure response profile is:

$$(3.58) \qquad Z_F(3\,\text{dB}) \approx \frac{1.8\lambda}{\sin^2 \theta_T} = 7.2\lambda \times (\textit{f-number})^2,$$

where the second form makes use of the fact that $\sin \theta_T = \mathcal{D}/(2a)$.

For the 1-MHz transducer with a half-angle of 30 degrees, $Z_F \approx 11$ mm, which is in approximate agreement with that measured from the pressure response curve in Fig. 3.24a.

3.5.7 Comparison with Experimental Results

A number of comparisons of the experimentally measured characteristics of concave transducers with the theoretical predictions have been made for both CW and pulsed conditions [42–44]. In general, the experimental measurements show good quantitative agreement in the focal plane, but significant discrepancies have been found on-axis close to the transducer surface. For example, the on-axis minima of the measured CW response were not found to be zero (see Fig. 3.24). Several possible reasons for these discrepancies have been carefully examined by Cathignol et al. [44], and these include using the Rayleigh integral, which ignores secondary diffraction. They reported carefully conducted experimental measurements on the field and surface displacements produced by a thin piezoceramic bowl using both CW and pulsed excitation. Measurements of the displacement amplitude over the transducer surface were performed with a laser beam and optical interferometer. By means of these measurements, together with theoretical predictions, they showed that a major source of the discrepancy is the generation of Lamb waves.[9] These guided waves appear to originate at the rim of the ceramic where the electric field is non-uniform, resulting in a non-uniform stress. They travel toward the center of the bowl with negligible attenuation, and the resulting focusing effect produces a displacement maximum that can be comparable to the thickness-mode displacement. Since the Lamb waves travel much faster in the ceramic than in the fluid propagation medium, a pressure signal results whose arrival time can precede the edge wave.

Fig. 3.28 illustrates these findings by showing the surface displacement waveform measured at the center of a concave piezoelectric created by a 5-

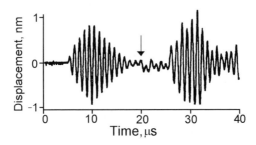

Figure 3.28 Displacement waveform at the center of a concave ceramic piezoelectric transducer with an aperture diameter of 10 cm and a focal length of 10 cm. Measurements were performed using an optical interferometer for an excitation consisting of a 5-cycle 1.0 MHz burst. The first burst, which starts at 5 μs, is due to the thickness mode vibration. Lamb waves from the periphery reach the center at the time marked by the arrow. (Reproduced, with permission, from Cathignol et al. [44], *J. Acoust. Soc. Am.*, 101, 1286–1297, © 1997 Acoustical Society of America.)

---

9. See also the discussion in subsection 3.3.2, which describes evidence for Lamb wave effects in thin disk transducers.

cycle 1 MHz excitation signal. The start of the displacement due to arrival of the Lamb waves from the periphery begins at about 15 µs after the start of the excitation, corresponding to a speed of ~0.35 cm/µs in the ceramic. Fig. 3.29 shows the results of pressure measurements made using a hydrophone placed on-axis close to the transducer using a very short excitation pulse. Comparison of (b) and (c) shows that the head wave, which arrives prior to the edge wave, consists of a component with a lower characteristic frequency (which arrives first) followed by higher-frequency components. Cathignol et al. [44] proposed that the first-arriving component corresponds to the lowest-order symmetrical Lamb waves, whose low-frequency group velocity is ~0.37 cm/µs. All of these measurements provide convincing evidence that Lamb waves play a dominant role in accounting for the discrepancy between the theoretical predictions (based on simple thickness-mode oscillations) and experimental observations.

In a subsequent paper, Cathignol et al. [45] compared the radiated field under pulsed and CW conditions for three spherical transducers of the same geometry: (i) a piezoceramic with air backing, (ii) a piezoceramic with an absorbing backing, and (iii) a piezocomposite material. The piezocomposite material consisted of piezoceramic and a polymer in the form of a matrix. They found that the addition of an absorbing backing layer for the piezoceramic transducer reduced the peak value of the head wave. For the piezocomposite material, the head wave was completely eliminated. When account was taken of the non-sphericity of the piezocomposite transducer, they found that the Rayleigh integral model accurately predicted the on-axis pressure field. In fact,

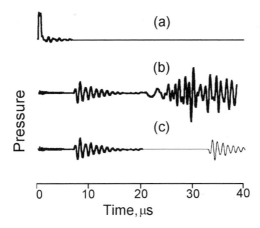

Figure 3.29 Measurement of the on-axis pressure at a distance of 1.0 cm from the center of the concave transducer described in Fig. 3.28. (a) Excitation waveform. (b) Hydrophone signal showing the direct wave, the head wave (arriving before the edge wave), and the edge wave. (c) Reproduction of the hydrophone direct wave signal combined with an inverted replica (thin line) starting at the expected arrival time of the edge wave. (Modified version reproduced, with permission, from Cathignol et al. [44], *J. Acoust. Soc. Am.*, 101, 1286–1297, © 1997 Acoustical Society of America.)

this is in agreement with the earlier work of Coulouvrat [46], who developed a model that takes proper account of secondary diffraction. Comparison of the numerical results with those obtained using the approximate method that neglects secondary diffraction have shown that even for relatively large half-aperture angles, e.g., $\theta_T < 60°$, and over the range $20 < k\mathcal{D} < 100$, where $\mathcal{D}$ is the aperture, the differences were small, especially in the neighborhood of the focal zone.

3.6 Annular Ring, Annulus, and Conical Transducers

The simplest form of a 2-D transducer array consists of annuli of differing radii and a common axis. Because of its cylindrical symmetry, the lateral resolution at a given z-location is angle independent. The idea of using an annular array for achieving a variable focal length originated with a suggestion by Schuck,[10] and the subsequent expansion of this idea by Reid and Wild [47]. Since the basic element of such an array is an annulus, an understanding of its associated field pattern is a useful starting point in phased array design. But even more fundamental is an annular ring whose thickness is small compared to a wavelength. The idea of using a thin annular ring for radio astronomy imaging was reported in the 1960s by Wild [48]. Of key importance was a method for partial cancellation of the high side lobes associated with the J_0 response (see below) of a simple ring structure. Initial reports [49,50,52] on the practical application of this method for ultrasound imaging indicated that major improvements could be achieved in terms of lateral resolution and depth of field. However, implementing this method required that the ring be divided into a number of segments that could be individually addressed, which would have greatly increased the fabrication complexity. In addition, because of the small area, the sensitivity would be significantly reduced. In this subsection we shall start by considering the properties of a simple ring.

3.6.1 Annular Ring

Impulse Response [51]

For an annular ring (Fig. 3.30a) of radius a whose width Δa is small compared to a wavelength, it can be shown (Problem P3) that the velocity impulse response function at (r,z) is given by:

$$(3.59) \qquad h(r, z) = \frac{c_o \Delta a}{\pi r} \left\{ 1 - \frac{\left[a^2 + r^2 + z^2 - c_o^2 t^2 \right]^2}{4a^2 r^2} \right\}^{-1/2},$$

for

$$\left[(a-r)^2 + z^2 \right]^{1/2} < c_o t < \left[(a+r)^2 + z^2 \right]^{1/2},$$

and $h(r,z) = 0$ elsewhere.

10. It is sometimes suggested that this idea originated with Reid and Wild [47], but, as clearly stated their 1958 paper, the idea originated with Schuck.

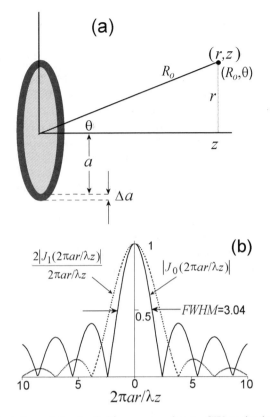

Figure 3.30 Calculation of the far-field response due to CW excitation of a ring of radius a, whose width is Δa and which lies on the plane $z = 0$. (a) Cylindrical geometry used for deriving the response. (b) Bessel function $|J_0(\zeta)|$ lateral pressure response in the Fraunhofer zone. Shown for comparison is the $2|J_1(\zeta)|/\zeta$ lateral response of a circular disk, as given by (3.32), of the same radius.

Fresnel and Fraunhofer Zone Response

One method of obtaining an approximate expression for the harmonic response in the Fraunhofer zone is by taking the Fourier transform of the aperture function and making use of (3.31). Now the aperture function of an infinitesimally narrow ring of radius a is given by the unit-strength impulse of $\Omega(r_1)$ $= \delta([r_1/a] - a)$, and consequently the pressure response can be found by taking the zero-order Hankel transform. From the sifting property of the δ-function and the definition of this transform (Appendix B), at a spatial frequency of k_r $= kr/z$: $\mathcal{H}_0\{\delta([r_1/a] - 1)\} = a^2 J_0(kar/z)$. By substituting this transform into (3.31) and recalling that $\mathfrak{F}[\Omega(r_1)] = 2\pi\mathcal{H}_0[\Omega(r_1)]$, the pressure phasor is given by

(3.60)
$$p(r,z{:}\omega) \approx \frac{j\omega\rho_o v_o a^2}{R_o} e^{-jk\left[z+r^2/(2z)\right]} J_0(kar/z),$$

from which the lateral beam width can be evaluated as $FWHM = 0.48\lambda z/a$.

To compare the lateral beam profiles of the ring with that of a disk of the same diameter, the magnitudes of both $J_0(\zeta)$ and $2J_1(\zeta)/\zeta$ are plotted in Fig. 3.30b. It can be seen that $FWHM$ is about 25% smaller than the disk; however, the first side lobe amplitude is around 3.5 times larger and is only about 8 dB below the central lobe. In medical imaging applications, the use of a transducer that has such large side lobes for both transmission and reception would be unacceptable, since scattering of ultrasound by the annular region surrounding a target could easily create a returned signal that would mask the image information.

The directivity function can be obtained by following the same procedure that led to (3.33) for the disk transducer, though in this case only a single integration is needed. If the ring has an incremental width of Δa, then it can be shown (see Problem P4) that within the Fresnel zone

$$\Delta p(R,\theta{:}\omega) = \frac{j\omega\rho_o v_o}{2\pi R_o} e^{-jk\left(R_o + a^2/2R_o\right)} a\Delta a D(\theta),$$

where the directivity function is given by $D(\theta) = \int_0^{2\pi} e^{jkacos\,\varphi_1 \sin\theta\left[1+\frac{a}{2R_o}cos\,\varphi_1 \sin\theta\right]} d\varphi 1.$

3.6.2 Annulus

Plane

The response of a plane annulus of outer radius a_o and inner radius a_i can be obtained by using the superposition principle illustrated in Fig. 3.31 and one of the previously described equations for the field profile of a disk. Thus, for example, the impulse response of the annulus can be written as $h(\mathbf{r}{:}t) = h_o(\mathbf{r}{:}t) - h_i(\mathbf{r}{:}t)$ where the impulse responses of the two disks can be found from (3.27). Similarly, the CW pressure response can be found from $p(r,z{:}\omega) = p_o(r,z{:}\omega) - p_i(r,z{:}\omega)$ by making use of (3.22). As an example, Fig. 3.32 shows the on-axis CW pressure magnitude response for a annulus with $a_o = 8\lambda$ and $a_i = 5\lambda$ at 5 MHz radiating into water. The axial distance has been normalized to the z-location where the path difference shown in Fig. 3.31 is equal to $\lambda/2$, which is exactly the location of the last maximum.

Concave

A concave annulus forms the basic element of a concave phased-array imaging transducer such as that described by Foster et al. [53]. Arditi et al. [35] have provided a detailed analysis of the annulus and have presented the equations needed to calculate the field profile for both pulsed and CW excitation. The advantage of using such an element as opposed to a plane annulus is that it

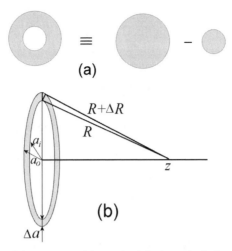

(a)

(b)

Figure 3.31 (a) Use of the superposition principle for calculating the response of a plane annulus. By using the equations for the field profile of a simple disk, the profile for an annulus can be obtained by subtraction. (b) The on-axis z-location corresponding to a path difference between the inner and outer radii of $\lambda/2$ corresponds to the last maximum.

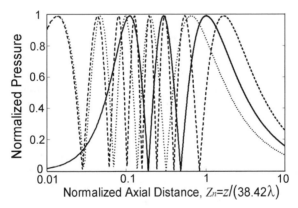

Figure 3.32 Normalized axial pressure magnitude CW response of an annulus with $a_o = 8\lambda$ and $a_i = 5\lambda$ at 5 MHz radiating into water. Solid line shows the annulus; the dashed and dotted curves correspond to disks with radii equal to the outer and inner radii of the annulus, respectively. The logarithmic horizontal axis has been normalized to the z-location where the path length difference between the inner and outer radii is equal to $\lambda/2$.

has a natural (geometric) focal point, and as a result the number of elements needed to achieve a given f-number can be significantly reduced and a smaller time delay is needed to move the focal point over the range of practical interest. Analysis of the field pattern of a concave annulus follows the same approach as used for a plane annulus. Using superposition, the impulse response can be found by using (3.41), while the CW response can be found from (3.43).

3.6.3 Conical (Axicon) Geometry

An important property of the conical transducer geometry shown in Fig. 3.33a is a greatly extended depth of field for the main lobe: approximately the same as the geometric focal range of $z'_1 < z < z'_2$, shown in Fig. 3.33b. If the cone angle is denoted by θ_c and, $\mathcal{D}_1$ and $\mathcal{D}_2$ are the inner and outer diameters, it can be readily shown that the geometric depth of field is given by

$$Z_F \approx \frac{(\mathcal{D}_2 - \mathcal{D}_1)}{2}(\tan\theta_c + \cot\theta_c).$$

The use of a conical ultrasound transducer was first investigated by Burckhardt et al. [54], based on the earlier proposal by McLeod [55] for a new optical element that he called an axicon. Subsequently, Patterson and Foster [56] provided a detailed analysis of the field properties for both pulsed and CW excitation and showed that the predicted patterns were very close to those experimentally measured. Their derivation of expressions for the impulse response assumed was based on the assumption that the integrand in the Rayleigh integral was multiplied by an obliquity factor[11] of $\cos(\tilde{n}, \tilde{R})$. In fact, the inclusion of this factor corresponds to the assumption that the cone behaves like a pressure-release baffle; in other words, they made use of (2.31). Patterson [57] subsequently realized that this factor was not consistent with the rigid baffle assumption and derived the correct equations for the impulse response based on the Rayleigh integral. Moreover, he stated that this factor does not materially affect the results given in [56].

Harmonic Response

Starting from the Rayleigh integral and assuming that the observation point (r,z) radial coordinate r is small compared to the distance from $(0,z)$ to any point on the surface of the cone, Patterson and Foster [56] obtained the following approximate expression for the pressure phasor due to a uniform sinusoidal excitation with a normal velocity amplitude of v_n:

$$(3.61) \quad \underline{p}(r,z{:}\omega) \approx 2\pi\omega\rho_o v_n \cos\theta_c \int_{z_1\cos ec\theta_c}^{z_2\cos ec\theta_c} \frac{\ell}{d} e^{-j2\pi d/\lambda} J_0\left(\frac{2\pi r\ell\cos\theta_c}{\lambda d}\right) d\ell,$$

where $d = \sqrt{\ell^2 + z^2 - 2z\ell\sin\theta_c}$ is the distance from a point on the cone surface to the axis at $(0,z)$, and it has been assumed that $r \ll d$. For on-axis observation points, $J_0(0) = 1$ and the above expression is exact. For the cone dimen-

---

11. See Section 7.2.6 for a discussion of this factor.

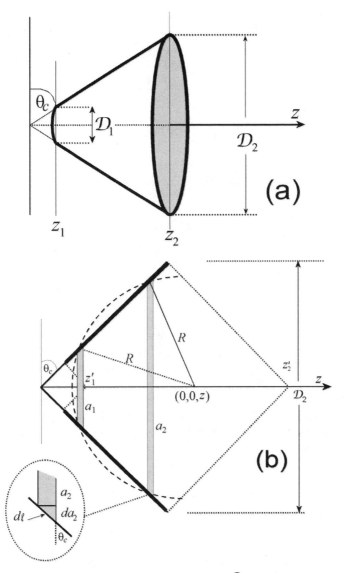

Figure 3.33 Conical transducer (axicon) with aperture $\mathcal{D}_2$ and angle θ_c. (a) General view of structure: the heavy line encloses the transducer element. (b) Cross-sectional view in the plane $x = 0$ for calculating the on-axis impulse response. The portion of a circle (dashed curve) centered at $(0,0,z)$ shows that the two annular rings of radii a_1 and a_2 on the surface of the cone contribute to the impulse response at the on-axis observation point z at the time $t = R/c_o$, provided $z_1' < z < z_2'$.

sions used by Patterson and Foster in their experimental measurements, the normalized on-axis pressure magnitude variation is shown in Fig. 3.34.

When approximations are made to the integral in (3.61), the pressure close to the axis can be expressed as $\underline{p}(r,z{:}\omega) \propto f(\theta_c,\lambda)\sqrt{z}J_0\{2\pi r\sin\theta_c/\lambda\}$, showing

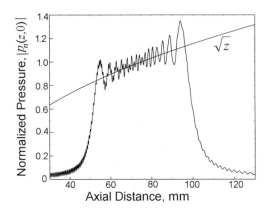

Figure 3.34 Calculated on-axis CW normalized pressure magnitude versus axial distance for a 45-degree cone at 4.0 MHz with $z_1 = 25$, and $z_2 = 50$ mm. The pressure is normalized to that at $z = 75$ mm. The curved line shows that the variation within the geometric focal zone is proportional to $z^{1/2}$.

that the lateral response variation is identical to that of a ring (see (3.60)) whose radius is a is equal to $z \sin \theta_c$. In addition, it will be noted that the axial variation in the geometric focal zone is proportional to $z^{1/2}$, which is plotted in Fig. 3.34. By apodizing the cone, Dietz [58] has shown that this variation can be approximately compensated for, yielding a nearly constant on-axis response over the focal zone. But perhaps of greater significance is that the lateral beam shape is constant over most of the geometric focal zone and the *FWHM* is given by

$$FWHM = 0.48\lambda / \sin \theta_c .$$

For example, if we consider a 45-degree cone at 4 MHz, then *FWHM* = 0.25 mm and the side lobes are >8 dB below the maximum.

3.7 Line, Strip, Triangular, and Rectangular Elements

Our previous discussions of the impulse response have focused on specific geometric shapes. A general method for calculating the impulse response of arbitrary-shaped transducers has been developed by Jensen [16]. It is based on dividing the surface into suitable triangular elements and then calculating the overall impulse response from the impulse response of each. The advantage of this method is that both complex and simple shapes can be readily constructed from a relatively small number of such elements, in much the same manner as that used in many finite-element computational programs; as a result, economies in computational time can be achieved. To obtain an expression for the impulse response of a triangular element, Jensen made use of the

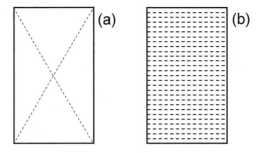

Figure 3.35 Division of a rectangular transducer into (a) four triangular elements, (b) line elements.

acoustic reciprocity theorem.[12] If the field point is considered to act as a point source of a spherical wave, this wave will travel to the transducer element, where the wavefront will form a sequence of arcs. Each point on a given arc corresponds to the same transit time from the point source. From the relative lengths of each arc formed on the transducer surface, Jensen showed how the impulse response could be determined.

From a practical perspective, rectangular transducer shapes are particularly important since medical ultrasound arrays generally use rectangular elements as the basic building blocks. As illustrated in Fig. 3.35a, a rectangular transducer can be synthesized from four triangular elements, and consequently a knowledge of the impulse response of the element enables the overall response to be determined. Alternatively (see Fig. 3.35b), a rectangular transducer can be synthesized from a number of lines [59]. Knowledge of the impulse response of a line element provides an alternative means for calculating the impulse response of transducers, especially those with rectangular and cylindrical geometry.

3.7.1 Line Element

Consider a source of incremental width Δy that is coincident with the x-axis and that extends from x_{min} to x_{max}. For the observation point (x_o, y_o, z) shown in Fig. 3.36, the velocity potential impulse response as given by (2.35) can be written as

$$h(x_1, y_1, z{:}t) = \iint_{S_o} \frac{\xi_o(x)\delta\left(t - \dfrac{R}{c_o}\right)}{2\pi R}\, dS_o,$$

12. In his classical treatise, Lord Rayleigh [3, Vol. 2, p. 145] provided the following statement of the principle of reciprocity attributed to Helmholtz: "If in a space filled with air which is partly bounded by finitely extended fixed bodies and is partially unbounded, sound waves be excited at any point A, the resulting velocity-potential at a second point B is the same both in magnitude and phase, as it would have been at A, had B been the source of sound."

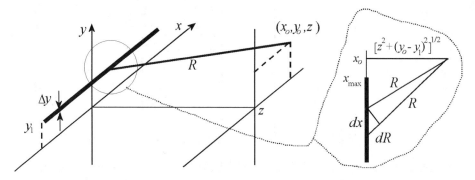

Figure 3.36 Calculating the impulse response at (x_o, y_o, z) of a line element parallel to the x-axis at a height y_1.

where $\xi_o(x)$ is the apodizing function, which we shall take to be unity. But $dS = dx\Delta y$, so that the velocity potential

$$h(x_o, y_o, z:t) = \int_{x_{min}}^{x_{max}} \frac{\Delta y \delta \left(t - \frac{\sqrt{(x_o - x)^2 + (y_o - y_1)^2 + z^2}}{c_o} \right)}{2\pi \sqrt{(x_o - x)^2 + (y_o - y_1)^2 + z^2}} dx$$

By letting $\tau = \dfrac{\sqrt{(x_o - x)^2 + (y_o - y_1)^2 + z^2}}{c_o}$, the impulse response integral can be transformed to

$$h(x_o, y_o, z:t) = \int_{\tau_{min}}^{\tau_{max}} \frac{c_o \Delta y \delta(t - \tau)}{2\pi \sqrt{\left(c_o^2 \tau^2 - (y_o - y_1)^2 - z^2\right)}} d\tau,$$

where $c_o \tau_{max} = \sqrt{(x_{max} - x_o)^2 + (y_o - y_1)^2 + z^2}$,

and $c_o \tau_{min} = \sqrt{(x_{min} - x_o)^2 + (y_o - y_1)^2 + z^2}$

If the δ-function product is evaluated, the response due to an impulse of velocity on the line is given by

(3.62)
$$h(x_o, y_o, z:t) = \frac{c_o \Delta y}{2\pi \sqrt{\left(c_o^2 t^2 - (y_o - y_1)^2 - z^2\right)}}, \quad \text{for } t \in \langle \tau_{max}, \tau_{min} \rangle,$$
$$= 0 \quad \text{elsewhere.}$$

3.7.2 Infinite Strip

If we consider an infinitely long strip of width $2W_{1/2}$ located symmetrically on the plane $z = 0$, the impulse response can be found by integrating (3.62):

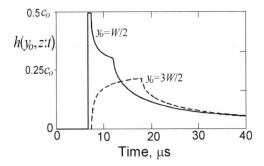

Figure 3.37 Impulse response at $z = 1.0\,\text{cm}$ for a 2.0 cm wide ($W_{1/2} = 1.0\,\text{cm}$), infinitely long baffled strip, as calculated from (3.63). The response is shown for two observation points: one in the geometric shadow, the other outside.

$$h(y_o, z{:}t) = \int_{-W_{1/2}}^{W_{1/2}} \frac{c_o}{2\pi\left(c_o^2 t^2 - (y_o - y)^2 - z^2\right)}\, dy, \quad \text{for } c_o t > c_o t_1$$

where $c_o t_1 = \sqrt{\left(|y_o| - W_{1/2}\right)^2 + z^2}$. This can be evaluated yielding, for the entire range of variables,

$$(3.63) \quad h(y_o, z{:}t) = \frac{c_o}{2}\,\mathcal{H}(t - z/c_o)\mathcal{H}(t_1 - t)\mathcal{H}(W_{1/2} - |y_o|) + \mathcal{H}(t - t_1)h_1(y_o, z{:}t), \quad \text{(a)}$$

where

$$h_1(y_o, z{:}t) = \frac{c_o}{2\pi}\left[\sin^{-1}\left(\frac{(W_{1/2} + y_o)}{\sqrt{c_o^2 t^2 - z^2}}\right) - \sin^{-1}\left(\frac{(y_o - W_{1/2})}{\sqrt{c_o^2 t^2 - z^2}}\right)\right]. \quad \text{(b)}$$

The graph of Fig. 3.37 shows the impulse response for two conditions: one in which the observation point lies in the strip shadow and the second where it lies outside. These conditions and results are the same as those presented by Tupholme [11]. For $y_o = W_{1/2}/2$, it will be noted that there are three times at which there is a change in the shape: the first when the pulse reaches the strip surface, the second when the circle reaches the edge of the strip on the same side as the observation point, and the third when the partial circle reaches the opposite edge.

3.7.3 Rectangular Transducer

In a classic paper published in 1952, Stenzel [60] provided a detailed analysis of the on- and off-axis harmonic response of a rectangular transducer. By using the approach developed by Tupholme [11] and Stepanishen [12], Lockwood and Willette [13] first described a method for calculating the exact impulse response of a rectangular element. Their expressions involved evaluating the integrals of $\cos^{-1}$ functions, and as a result the computation burden was fairly high for ultrasound arrays containing many such elements. A subsequent analysis by San Emeterio and Ullate [61] resulted in analytical expressions, as did the method developed by Jensen [16] using triangular elements. To further reduce the computational burden for 2-D arrays of rectangular elements, methods that approximate the exact impulse function by trapezoidal functions have been described by Turnbull and Foster [62]. All of these techniques are based on evaluation in the time domain.

An alternative approach for obtaining the field response for an arbitrary surface velocity waveform is through a frequency domain approach. This requires that the sinusoidal response of the transducer, i.e., the transfer function, be determined. Since the frequency spectrum of the velocity waveform can be obtained by taking its Fourier transform, the spectrum at the observation point can be obtained. If this is multiplied by the transfer function, then, by an inverse Fourier transform, the temporal signal at the observation point can be recovered. To determine the transfer function in a form that can be readily evaluated, it is usually assumed that the observation point is sufficiently distant so that either the Fresnel or Fraunhofer approximations can be used. It was noted earlier (see Fig. 3.17) that the Fresnel approximation gives good agreement for a piston transducer even when the observation point is quite close to the surface. Consequently, we shall start with this approximation in determining the response of a rectangular transducer.

The Fraunhofer and Fresnel approximation for a rectangular transducer of width W and height H can be obtained from (3.36) as

(3.64)
$$
\underline{p}(x_o,y_o,z{:}\omega) \approx \frac{j\omega\rho_o v_o}{2\pi R} e^{-jk\left[z+\frac{x_o^2+y_o^2}{2z}\right]}
$$
$$
\int_{-\infty}^{\infty}\int_{-\infty}^{\infty} \text{rect}\left(\frac{x_1}{W}\right)\text{rect}\left(\frac{y_1}{H}\right)e^{j\frac{k}{z}(x_ox_1+y_oy_1)}e^{-j\frac{k}{z}(x_1^2+y_1^2)}dx_1dy_1,
$$

where the product of the two rect(.) functions defines the rectangular aperture over the entire plane $z = 0$.

Fraunhofer Approximation

In the Fraunhofer approximation, it is assumed that the exponential term in $(x_1^2 + y_1^2)$ can be ignored, and consequently the integral in (3.64) is simply the 2-D Fourier transform of the aperture function evaluated at the spatial frequencies of $k_x = -kx_o/z$ and $k_y = -ky_o/z$. Consequently, the pressure phasor can be expressed as

(3.65)
$$
\underline{p}(x_o,y_o,z{:}\omega) \approx \frac{j\omega\rho_o v_o}{2\pi R} e^{-jk\left[z+\frac{x_o^2+y_o^2}{2z}\right]}\Im\left\{\text{rect}\left(\frac{x_1}{W}\right)\right\}\Im\left\{\text{rect}\left(\frac{y_1}{H}\right)\right\}.
$$

Now $\Im\{rect(x_1/W)\} = W\dfrac{\sin(Wk_x/2)}{Wk_x/2} = W\dfrac{\sin(\pi Wx_o/\lambda z)}{\pi Wx_o/\lambda z} = W\mathrm{sinc}(Wx_o/\lambda z)$ and

a similar expression for $\Im\{rect(y_1/H)\}$, where $\mathrm{sinc}(\varsigma)$ is defined by:[13] $\mathrm{sinc}(\varsigma) = \sin(\pi\varsigma)/\pi\varsigma$. As a result, (3.65) reduces to

$$(3.66) \quad \underline{p}(x_o,y_o,z{:}\omega) \approx \frac{j\omega\rho_o v_o}{2\pi R}e^{-jk\left[z+\frac{x_o^2+y_o^2}{2z}\right]}WH\mathrm{sinc}\left(\frac{Wx_o}{\lambda z}\right)\mathrm{sinc}\left(\frac{Hy_o}{\lambda z}\right).$$

Now it can be seen that the dependence of the pressure field profile on the x-y location of the observation point is determined by the sinc(.) terms only, and consequently the directivity function (see (3.33)) can be expressed in terms of the lateral and elevation angles shown in Fig. 3.38a:

$$(3.67) \qquad D(\theta,\varphi) \approx \mathrm{sinc}\left(\frac{W\sin\theta}{\lambda}\right)\mathrm{sinc}\left(\frac{H\sin\theta}{\lambda}\right),$$

where $\sin\theta \approx x_o/R$, $\sin\varphi \approx y_o/R$ and it has been assumed that $z \approx R$. Thus, the directivity depends only on the angles subtended by the observation point to the source.

It can be seen from Fig. 3.38b that the angle subtended at the transducer corresponding to the *FWHM* is given by $\theta_{FWHM} \approx 2\sin^{-1}(0.6\lambda/W)$, and therefore a measure of the lateral resolution is

$$(3.68) \qquad FWHM = 2R\sin^{-1}(0.6\lambda/W).$$

It is useful to compare the *FWHM* of two transducers, A and B, at the same far-field radial distance R. If transducer A has a width $W_A = 5\lambda$ and B has a width of $W_B = 1.0\lambda$, then $FWHM_A = 0.187FWHM_B$, i.e., the wider transducer has the smallest beam width. However, since R must be in the far field of both transducers, the minimum distance will be set by the wider transducer (A), and this is 25 times greater $\{(W_B/W_A)^2\}$ than the minimum distance for transducer B.

Fresnel Approximation

An expression for the sinusoidal response in the Fresnel region can be obtained from (3.64) by first noting that it can be written as [29]:

$$(3.69) \quad \underline{p}(x_o,y_o,z{:}\omega) \approx \frac{j\omega\rho_o v_o}{2\pi R}e^{-jk\left[z+\frac{x_o^2+y_o^2}{2z}\right]}\Im\left[rect\left(\frac{x_1}{W}\right)rect\left(\frac{y_1}{H}\right)e^{-j\frac{k}{z}\left(x_1^2+y_1^2\right)}\right], \quad \text{(a)}$$

where the transform is evaluated at the angular spatial frequencies of $k_x = -kx_o/z$ and $k_y = -ky_o/z$. Now with the help of a symbolic math program (MAPLE®) it can be readily shown that

---

13. It should be noted that some authors use the definition $\mathrm{sinc}(\varsigma) = \sin(\varsigma)/\varsigma$.

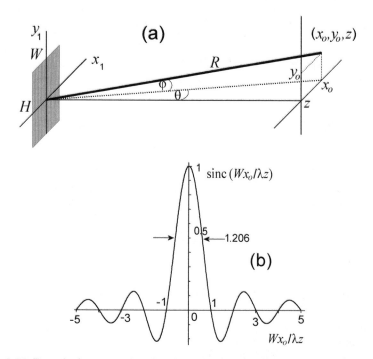

Figure 3.38 Fraunhofer approximation for a rectangular transducer. (a) Geometry defining the spherical coordinate system (R,θ,φ). (b) Response in the lateral direction for $y_o = 0$ as given by the sinc(.) function.

$$
(3.69)\quad p(x_o,y_o,z{:}\omega) \approx \frac{-\omega\rho_o v_o z\lambda}{8\pi R} e^{-jkz}\{\mathrm{erf}[\sigma(W-2x_o)]-\mathrm{erf}[-\sigma(W+2x_o)]\}
$$
$$
\times\{\mathrm{erf}[\sigma(H-2y_o)]-\mathrm{erf}[-\sigma(H+2y_o)]\},\qquad\text{(b)}
$$

where $\sigma=\sqrt{-j\pi/(4\lambda z)}$ and erf(.) is the error function defined by:[14]

$$
\mathrm{erf}(Z)=\frac{2}{\sqrt{\pi}}\int_0^Z e^{-\varsigma^2}d\varsigma\ .
$$

Although this expression for the pressure is in integral form, the error function is very simple to numerically evaluate, and as a result this form is significantly more computationally efficient than direct numerical evaluation of (3.64). To illustrate the accuracy of the Fresnel expression in comparison to the exact (Rayleigh integral) and Fraunhofer approximation, the on-axis harmonic response is shown in Fig. 3.39 for a square transducer of 2×2 cm uniformly excited with a velocity of 1.0 cm/s. It is evident that the Fresnel

---

14. For application in the above equation, it should be noted that Z is complex, leading to a complex value for erf(Z).

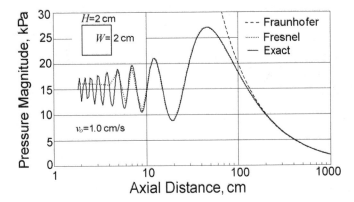

Figure 3.39 Accuracy of the Fresnel approximation in comparison to the Fraunhofer and exact (Rayleigh integral) methods for calculating the on-axis response of a square transducer excited by a 5.0 MHz sinusoid that generates a surface velocity of 1.0 cm/s. The Fresnel approximation was calculated using (3.69) and the Fraunhofer response from (3.66).

approximation gives accurate results well into the near-field region, while the Fraunhofer approximation is accurate only beyond the Rayleigh distance $\{\pi(W/2)^2/\lambda \approx 105\,\text{cm}\}$, similar to the disk transducer results shown in Fig. 3.17.

3.8 Transducer Apodization

3.8.1 Gaussian Apodization

It has long been known that the side lobes that occur with uniform excitation can be greatly reduced by using certain forms of apodization. The primary difficulty with implementing such schemes has been the development of a practical means of achieving such functions without having to use multiple elements. Von Haselberg and Krautkramer [63] appear to have been the first to theoretically analyze the use of a Gaussian excitation function and to have described an approximate means of achieving it in practice. Their analysis was restricted to far-field or on-axis points. Greenspan [67], based on an extension of King's theory [68], developed a more general harmonic analysis of a plane disk radiator having an axisymmetric apodization function. Filipczynski and Etienne [70] demonstrated the use of Gaussian apodization for reducing the side lobes on a concave focusing transducer. They developed approximate equations describing the field characteristics and, with the help of the fabrication technique described by von Haselberg and Krautkramer [63], obtained good qualitative agreement with experimental measurements.

In addition to analyzing the harmonic excitation of a rigid piston with Gaussian apodization, Greenspan [67] also analyzed the transient case by taking the Laplace transform of the harmonic solution, and thereby obtained an expression for the velocity potential impulse response. As noted in section 3.3, the impulse response method was extended by Harris [21] and Tjøtta and Tjøtta [22] to allow for an arbitrary apodization function. For the particular case of a Gaussian apodized axisymmetric transducer with an infinite radius, the velocity impulse response is that given in Problem P1d. In the following, the harmonic solution for a disk of finite size will be considered.

The starting point of King's harmonic analysis[15] was the cylindrical form of the homogeneous Helmholtz free-space wave equation as expressed by (1.63). He pointed out that a solution for the velocity potential could be expressed as[16]

$$(3.70) \qquad \Phi(r, z:\omega) = \int_0^\infty (\sigma^2 - k^2)^{-1/2} e^{-z\sqrt{\sigma^2 - k^2}} J_0(r\sigma)q(\sigma)\sigma d\sigma,$$

where the function $q(\sigma)$ can be established from the boundary conditions specified for the plane $z = 0$. If a disk of radius a exists on the plane $z = 0$ and is excited such that the normal component of the velocity is given by the circularly symmetric distribution $\xi_o(r_1)v_o e^{j\omega t}$, then $q(\sigma)$ can be found by noting that

$v_o\xi_o(r_1) = -\dfrac{\partial \Phi}{\partial z}\Big|_{z=0}$. By differentiating (3.70) with respect to z and putting $z = 0$ we find that[17]

$$v_o\xi_o(r_1) = \int_0^\infty q(\sigma)J_0(r_1\sigma)\sigma d\sigma \equiv \mathcal{H}_0^{-1}\{q(\sigma)\},$$

i.e., it is the inverse Hankel transform of $q(\sigma)$. In view of the self-reciprocal properties of this transform [8], the function $q(\sigma)$ can be expressed as the Hankel transform[18] of $v_o\xi_o(r_1)$:

$$(3.71) \qquad q(\sigma) = v_o \int_0^\infty \xi_o(r_1)J_0(r_1\sigma)r_1 dr_1.$$

15. King's 1934 classical paper made use of the fact that integral solutions in terms of Bessel functions for the cylindrical form of the wave equation were well established in electromagnetic theory. In this regard he gave as a reference a 1915 book by Bateman [71]. Nonetheless, it is clear that King was the first to apply this approach to acoustics, in particular for predicting the radiation from an apodized disk. Using this as a starting point he obtained some of the classical equations for the field of a uniformly excited disk, including the far-field directivity function.

16. This integral is often referred to as King's integral: a helpful derivation is given by Harris [9].

17. It should be noted that $\mathcal{H}_0^{-1}\{\delta(\sigma)/\sigma\} = 1$. Consequently, if $q(\sigma) = v_o\delta(\sigma)/\sigma$, then $\xi_o(r_1) = 1$, which corresponds to a constant velocity over the plane $z = 0$. If this value of $q(\sigma)$ is substituted into (3.70), the velocity potential is given by $\Phi(z:\omega) = -jv_o e^{-jkz}/k$, which describes a plane wave propagating in the $+z$-direction.

18. If $v_o\xi_o(r_1) = K\delta(r_1)/(r_1)$, then $q(\sigma) = K$, where K is a dimensioned constant. If $q(\sigma) = K$ is substituted into (3.70), the resulting inverse Hankel transform is of a standard form (see Appendix B). Consequently, $\Phi(R:\omega) \propto e^{-jkR}/R$, corresponds to spherical wave emanating from a point source at $R = 0$.

Thus, the velocity potential[19] can be determined at any field point (r,z) by substituting (3.71) into (3.70), yielding[20]

$$(3.72) \qquad \Phi(r, z{:}\omega) = \int_0^\infty \frac{v_o J_0(r\sigma)\sigma}{\sqrt{\sigma^2 - k^2}} e^{-z\sqrt{\sigma^2 - k^2}} \int_0^\infty \xi_o(r_1) J_0(r_1\sigma) r_1 dr_1 d\sigma.$$

Let us assume that the apodization is a Gaussian function $\xi_o(r_1) = \mathrm{circ}(r_1/a)e^{-r_1^2/(\varepsilon a)^2}$ where ε describes the degree of truncation ($\varepsilon = \infty$ for uniform excitation) and the circ function sets $\xi_o(r_1)$ to zero outside the transducer area. With this function, the integral expression for $q(\sigma)$ is not in a standard form. However, it should be noted that if $\varepsilon < 0.5$, then $\xi_o(a) \approx 0$, and consequently $\xi_o(r_1) \approx e^{-r_1^2/(\varepsilon a)^2}$. With this approximation (3.71) can be evaluated [72, eqn. 11.4.29], yielding $q(\sigma) = (v_o\varepsilon^2 a^2/2)e^{-(\varepsilon a\sigma/2)^2}$. Consequently, by substituting this into (3.70) the pressure phasor ($p = j\omega\rho_o\Phi$) can be expressed in terms of a single integral:

$$(3.73) \quad p(r, z{:}\omega) = \frac{j\omega\rho_o v_o (\varepsilon a)^2}{2} \int_0^\infty (\sigma^2 - k^2)^{-1/2} e^{-z\sqrt{\sigma^2 - k^2} - (\varepsilon a\sigma/2)^2} J_0(r\sigma)\sigma d\sigma,$$

for $\varepsilon \le 0.5$.

For on-axis observation points ($r = 0$) and any value of ε, it can be easily shown that the following much simpler expression can be obtained directly from the Rayleigh integral (see Problem P2 in Chapter 2):

$$(3.74) \qquad p(0, z{:}\omega) = j\omega\rho_o v_o \int_z^{\sqrt{z^2 + a^2}} e^{-jkR} e^{-(R^2 - z^2)/(\varepsilon a)^2} dR,$$

which can be readily evaluated. From the examples shown in Fig. 3.40 it is evident that if a nearly complete Gaussian apodization function is present on the disk ($\varepsilon < 0.5$), the near-field fluctuations are essentially eliminated. The removal of side lobes can be understood by noting that for a Gaussian apodized transducer, the velocity amplitude undergoes a smooth reduction to near zero at the edge of the disk, whereas for a uniformly excited disk there is an abrupt transition at the edge. Because of the smooth reduction the effects of the edge-wave contribution are reduced. However, it should be pointed out that because the transmitted power for the Gaussian apodized transducer will be less (for the same v_o), the maximum pressure is reduced.

To calculate the off-axis profile, the double integral in (3.72) must be evaluated. As noted earlier, for Gaussian apodization such that $\varepsilon \le 0.5$, a good approximation for the inner integral is available; however, the presence of a pole at $k = \sigma$ complicates the evaluation. Fortunately, the contributions of this

---

19. That the Rayleigh integral expression for an apodized disk can be reduced to King's form of solution was first shown by Bouwkamp [69]; the reverse of this statement was proven by Greenspan [67].

20. For a uniformly apodized disk of radius a, i.e., $\xi_o(r_1) = \mathrm{circ}(r_1/a)$, it can be readily shown that this equation simplifies to an equation for the velocity potential identical to (3.13), which was obtained by the angular spectrum method.

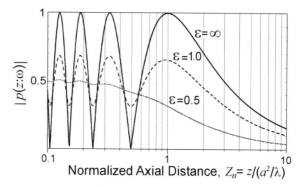

Figure 3.40 The normalized pressure magnitude versus normalized axial distance for various degrees of Gaussian apodization on a disk of radius $a = 10\lambda$. The value $\varepsilon = \infty$ corresponds to no apodization and $\varepsilon = 0.5$ to a nearly complete Gaussian on the disk. Exact pressure magnitudes were calculated from (3.74) and normalized by $2\rho_o c v_o$.

pole and beyond are negligible, and it is sufficient to replace the upper limit by $0.99k$. The graph of Fig. 3.41 clearly shows the greatly reduced side lobes for the Gaussian apodized transducer and the relatively constant pressure distribution profile up to $Z_n = 0.3$. It is also clear that the beam diverges in the far-field region. A uniformly excited disk of the same radius and the same peak excitation velocity gives twice the peak pressure, but side lobes are clearly evident and, as indicated by Fig. 3.40, the profile shows large fluctuations in the near-field region.

A number of methods have been proposed for achieving a Gaussian apodization. In one scheme, Du and Breazeale [64] used a quartz crystal with a back electrode that was much smaller than the front. The resulting electric field distribution approximated a Gaussian function. On the other hand, Hsu et al. [65] used non-uniform poling of a lead zirconate titanate (PZT) piezoelectric rod. Both groups reported good agreement with theoretical predictions.

In the Fraunhofer zone, it can be shown that for a circularly symmetric apodization $\xi_o(r_1)$, the directivity function can be expressed as [2, p. 600; 66, pp. 475–476; also see the derivation leading to (3.33)]

$$(3.75) \qquad D(\theta) \approx \frac{2}{a^2} \int_0^a \xi_o(r_1) J_0(kr_1 \sin\theta) r_1 dr_1,$$

which, as noted earlier, is the zero-order Hankel transform of the apodization function. By letting $w = kr_1$, this can be written in the more convenient form

$$(3.76) \qquad D(\theta) \approx \frac{2}{(ka)^2} \int_0^{ka} \xi_o\left(\frac{w}{k}\right) J_0(w \sin\theta) w \, dw.$$

If the transducer is uniformly excited ($\xi_o(r_1) = 1$), then, in view of the Bessel function identity: $\int_0^y x J_0(x) dx = y J_1(y)$, it can be readily shown that (3.76)

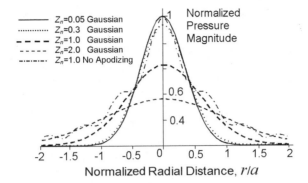

Figure 3.41 The effects of Gaussian apodization on the near- and far-field radial pressure profile for a disk of radius $a = 10\lambda$. The response is shown for four different normalized axial distances, $Z_n = z/(a^2/\lambda)$, as calculated from (3.73) using a normalizing pressure of $\rho_o c v_o$ and $\varepsilon = 0.5$. In addition, the radial profile is shown for a uniformly excited disk with the pressure normalized to $2\rho_o c v_o$.

reduces to the previously derived expression for the directivity function, namely (3.33b). For the Gaussian apodization $\xi_o(r_1) = e^{-r_1^2/(\varepsilon a)^2}$, considered previously, the directivity function is

$$(3.77) \qquad D(\theta) \approx \frac{2}{(ka)^2 D_o} \int_0^{ka} e^{-(w/(k\varepsilon a))^2} J_0(w \sin\theta) w\, dw,$$

where division by $D_o = \varepsilon^2(1 - e^{-1/\varepsilon^2})$ ensures that $D(0) = 1$. This is plotted in Fig. 3.42 for three different values of ε. In (a) the degree of truncation is quite small, and as a result most of the Gaussian function is close to the center of the disk, and thus the beam divergence as measured by the half-angle θ_R is large. For (c) the Gaussian is highly truncated and consequently the directivity function is almost identical to the uniform apodization case shown in Fig. 3.20b.

Depth of Field and Lateral Resolution: Unfocused

The depth of field corresponds roughly to the region over which the lateral beam width remains substantially constant. From Fig. 3.40 it can be seen that this extends from the transducer surface to the location where the pressure magnitude starts to diminish substantially, e.g., the Rayleigh distance. Since the effective aperture radius is approximately εa, the depth of field is roughly given by [39]

$$Z_F \approx \pi(\varepsilon a)^2 / \lambda.$$

The lateral resolution is also governed by the effective aperture radius and is [39] $FWHM \approx 1.67\varepsilon a$. For example, if these results are applied to the transducer considered in Figs. 3.40 and 3.41 ($a = 10\lambda$, $\varepsilon = 0.5$, $f = 5.0$ MHz), we find that $Z_F = 24$ mm and $FWHM = 2.5$ mm.

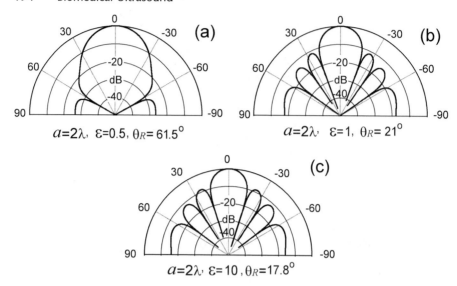

Figure 3.42 Far-field directivity function for Gaussian apodization for disks of the same radius but different degrees of truncation. (a) $\varepsilon = 0.5$, (b) $\varepsilon = 1.0$, (c) $\varepsilon = 10$. The truncation in (c) is very large, so that it corresponds approximately to a uniform distribution.

Depth of Field and Lateral Resolution: Focused

A focused field pattern can be achieved with a piston transducer through the use of a radial dependent phase shift or delay. For example, in the case of CW excitation, the complex apodization function

$$\xi_o(r_1) = \text{circ}\left(\frac{r_1}{a}\right) e^{-jk\left(\sqrt{F^2 + r_1^2} - F\right)},$$

where F is the focal length and a is the piston radius, corresponds to a spherical phase shifter that causes the waves originating from each incremental ring on the piston to arrive with the same phase at F. For such a scheme, the lateral beam profile at the focal point can be shown to be given approximately by $\left[\dfrac{J_1(kr\mathcal{D}/2F)}{kr\mathcal{D}/2F}\right]$, where $\mathcal{D} = 2a$ is the aperture diameter. Since this is the same as for a concave transducer, the FWHM is given by (3.56), i.e.,

$$FWHM = 1.4\lambda \frac{\text{Focal Length}}{\text{Aperture}} \approx 1.4\lambda F/\mathcal{D}.$$

If Gaussian apodization is also included with the focusing phase shift, then the apodization equation is modulated as follows:

$$\xi_o(r_1) = \text{circ}\left(\frac{r_1}{a}\right) e^{-r_1^2/(\varepsilon a)^2} e^{-jk\left(\sqrt{F^2 + r_1^2} - F\right)},$$

where ε is the factor governing the truncation of the Gaussian function on the disk. If $\varepsilon^2 \ll 1$ corresponding to a small degree of truncation, and $F^2 \gg (\varepsilon a)^2$, then Lu and Greenleaf [87] have shown that the lateral resolution on the focal plane is given by $\left[\dfrac{J_1(kr\mathcal{D}/2F)}{kr\mathcal{D}/2F} \right]$, where $\mathcal{D}_e = 2\varepsilon a$ is the effective aperture diameter. In addition, the depth of field is given approximately by [39]

$$Z_F(3\,\mathrm{dB}) \approx 2\frac{\lambda F^2}{\pi(\varepsilon a)^2}\sqrt{1 + 2\left(\frac{\lambda F}{\pi(\varepsilon a)^2}\right)^2},$$

for $(\lambda/\pi\varepsilon a)^2 \ll (\varepsilon a)^2/F^2$.

3.9 Diffractionless and Limited Diffraction Beams

The question as to whether it is possible to generate beams with a small divergence angle, much like a laser beam, is of considerable practical interest. As will be seen, if the transducer is of infinite extent and is appropriately excited throughout its surface area, the resulting beam should show no diffractive spreading. When the same excitation is applied to a transducer of finite extent, diffraction will be present and the resulting beam is generally described as a *limited diffraction* beam. Thus, the search for solutions to the homogeneous wave equation that could enable beams to be achieved that have a very large depth of field has been actively pursued.

In 1987 Durnin [76] proposed solutions to the free-space wave equation that predicted diffractionless optical wave propagation, and he and his colleagues [77] described experiments to verify the beam properties. This work sparked a great deal of interest. In essence, the starting point was the inviscid form of the wave equation, i.e.,

$$\left[\nabla^2 - \frac{1}{c_o^2}\frac{\partial^2}{\partial t^2} \right]\phi(\mathbf{r}{:}t) = 0$$

In Cartesian coordinates they proposed a separable solution (one that had been obtained some 46 years earlier by Stratton [78, p. 365]), which can be written as

(3.78)
$$\phi = 2\pi\phi_o e^{j(\omega_o t)} \int_0^{2\pi} A(\varphi)e^{-j(x\alpha_B\cos\varphi + y\alpha_B\sin\varphi + \beta_B z)}\,d\varphi$$

where $\beta_B = k/a$, $\alpha_B = k\sqrt{1 - a^{-2}}$, $\alpha_B^2 + \beta_B^2 = k^2 = (\omega_o/c_o)^2$, φ is the polar angle, and $A(\varphi)$ is an arbitrary complex function. Stratton pointed out that the integrand represents a plane wave with wave-vector components $(\alpha_B\cos\varphi, \alpha_B\sin\varphi, \beta_B)$, traveling in a direction that makes an angle θ with respect to the z-axis. Thus, the integral represents plane waves whose directions form a cone about the z-axis and that are weighted by $A(\varphi)$. In symmetrical cylindrical coordinates such that $x = r \cos \theta$, $y = r \sin \theta$, and since $A(\varphi)$ is independent of φ, (3.78) transforms to

$$\phi = 2\pi\phi_o e^{j(\omega_o t - \beta_B z)} \int_0^{2\pi} e^{-j\alpha_B r \cos(\theta - \varphi)} d\varphi,$$

which can be evaluated with the help of Appendix C to yield

(3.79)
$$\phi_B(r, z:t) = \phi_o e^{j(\omega_o t - \beta_B z)} J_0(\alpha_B r).$$

From this form, which was derived by Durnin [76], it can be seen that the transverse profile retains the same shape in the radial direction for all $z > 0$ and α_B determines the central beam width. Moreover, it is necessary that $0 \leq \alpha_B < k$ to avoid having an evanescent beam. Durnin noted that if $\alpha_B = 0$, then (3.79) corresponds to a plane wave and that as $\alpha_B \to k$, the central region diameter approaches $3\lambda/4$. The above-noted papers created much interest and were responsible for initiating research projects in several areas, including ultrasound.

The Bessel beam is one of many solutions to the homogeneous wave equation that have been investigated. It is a highly localized solution in space, though not in time. More generally, solutions that are highly localized both in space and time are often referred to as *localized wave* solutions. Much earlier work, which went unnoticed for several years, was the fundamental paper of 1983 by Brittingham [79]. It is generally considered to be the first to describe localized wave nondiffracting solutions and was followed shortly thereafter by the work of Ziolkowski [80].

The first ultrasonic proposals and experimental investigations appear to be those reported in the Russian scientific literature in 1988 by Karpelson [81,82]. In these papers, which were accepted before Durnin's publications appeared, he specified the requirement for a non-divergent beam in the far field and then, though a synthesis approach based on a far-field approximation to the Rayleigh integral, specifically (3.75), he derived the Bessel function apodization equation. Subsequent ultrasound experimental work has been reported by Hsu et al. [83] and Campbell and Soloway [84]: both groups described the fabrication of a Bessel beam transducer and reported good agreement of the experimental results with calculations. Theoretical performance comparisons of the approximate Bessel beam transducer with an axicon have been described by Holm [85].

In what follows, a more general approach is used to construct a variety of diffractionless solutions to (3.78), and some of the solutions previously noted will be obtained. The joint 2-D spatial Fourier transform and Fourier transform with respect to time in a symmetric cylindrical coordinate system (r, z) can be defined. Denoting the spatial-temporal Fourier transform operator by $\Im_{r,z:t}$, the transform of the velocity potential is

$$\Phi(k_r, k_z:\omega) \equiv \Im_{r,z} \Im_t \{\phi(r, z:t)\} \equiv \Im_{r,z:t} \{\phi(r, z:t)\}$$

(3.80)
$$= \int_0^\infty dr \, r J_o(k_r r) \int_{-\infty}^\infty dz \, e^{jk_z z} \int_{-\infty}^\infty dt \, \phi(r, z:t) e^{-j\omega t},$$

where $r^2 = x^2 + y^2$, the spatial frequencies $[L^{-1}]$ are denoted by k_z and k_r, and $k_r^2 = k_x^2 + k_y^2$. In addition, the inverse spatio-temporal Fourier transform is:

(3.81)
$$\phi(r, z{:}t) \equiv \mathfrak{I}_{r,z{:}t}^{-1}\{\Phi(k_r, k_z{:}\omega)\}$$
$$= \frac{1}{(2\pi)^3} \int_0^\infty dk_r \; k_r J_o(k_r r) \int_{-\infty}^\infty dk_z \; e^{-jk_z z} \int_{-\infty}^\infty d\omega \; \Phi(k_r, k_z{:}\omega) e^{j\omega t}.$$

Now the wave equation in symmetrical cylindrical coordinates can be written as

$$\left[\frac{\partial^2}{\partial r^2} + \frac{1}{r}\frac{\partial}{\partial r} + \frac{\partial^2}{\partial z^2} - \frac{1}{c_o^2}\frac{\partial^2}{\partial t^2}\right]\phi(r, z{:}t) = 0,$$

and by taking the spatio-temporal Fourier transform we find that

(3.82)
$$\boxed{\left[k_r^2 + k_z^2 - \frac{\omega^2}{c_o^2}\right]\Phi(k_r, k_z{:}\omega) = 0}.$$

Donnelly and Ziolkowski [73,74] have formulated a systematic method of obtaining solutions to the above "algebraic" equation through the use of generalized functions [8, pp. 92–98], and several examples are given in the following subsections, leading to some of the solutions previously mentioned. Specifically, suitable functions $\Phi(k_r, k_z{:}\omega)$ need to be determined that will constrain the transformation variables so that $k_r^2 + k_z^2 - \omega^2/c_o^2$ in (3.82) will be zero. For example, a solution to (3.82) can be written as

(3.83)
$$\Phi(k_r, k_z{:}\omega) = \sigma(k_r{:}\omega)\delta\{\omega/c_o - g(k_r)\}\delta\{k_z - f(k_r)\},$$

where $g(k_r)$, $f(k_r)$, and $\sigma(k_r{:}\omega)$ are well-behaved functions. In (3.82), if the Φ term is nonzero, the term in square brackets must be zero, which occurs when $\omega/c_o = g(k_r)$ and $k_z = f(k_r)$. By substituting these into the term in square brackets, it can be seen that $g(k_r)$ and $f(k_r)$ are related by

(3.84)
$$k_r^2 + f^2(k_r) - g^2(k_r) = 0.$$

By making appropriate choices for one of these functions as well as for $\sigma(k_r{:}\omega)$ and then taking the inverse spatio-temporal Fourier transform of (3.83), $\phi(r, z{:}t)$ can be determined. Donnelly and Ziolkowski used this approach for constructing a variety of nondiffracting localized wave solutions. Sushilov et al. [86] also used this approach for generating the solutions described in the subsequent subsections, together with new X-wave solutions.

3.9.1 Plane Wave Solution

One of the simplest solutions to (3.82) occurs when the second δ-function in (3.83) is $\delta(R_2 \pm \omega/c_o)$. Because $k_r^2 + k_z^2 - \omega^2/c_o^2 = 0$, it follows that the other δ-function is $\delta(k_r)$. If it is also assumed that $\sigma(k_r{:}\omega) = (2\pi)^3\phi_o\sigma_\omega(\omega)/k_r$, where ϕ_o is the velocity potential amplitude, the solution to (3.82) can be written as

(3.85)
$$\Phi(k_r, k_z : \omega) = \frac{\phi_o (2\pi)^3 \sigma_\omega(\omega)}{k_r} \delta(k_r) \delta(k_z \pm \omega/c_o),$$

By substituting (3.85) into (3.81), the inverse spatio-temporal Fourier transform is given by

$$\phi_B(z:t) = \int_0^\infty dk_r \int_{-\infty}^\infty dk_z \int_{-\infty}^\infty d\omega\, J_o(k_r r) \phi_{o\sigma\omega}(\omega) \delta(k_r) \delta(k_z \pm \omega/c_o) e^{-j(k_z z - \omega t)},$$

which simplifies to the following equation for the weighted sum of plane waves traveling in the positive z-direction:

(3.86)
$$\phi_B(z:t) = \phi_o \int_{-\infty}^\infty \sigma_\omega(\omega) e^{j\omega\left(t - \frac{z}{c_o}\right)} d\omega.$$

If $\sigma_\omega = \delta(\omega - \omega_o)$, then (3.86) reduces to

$$\phi_B(z:t) = \phi_o e^{j\omega_o\left(t - \frac{z}{c_o}\right)},$$

which is a simple plane wave of frequency ω_o propagating in the positive z-direction.

3.9.2 Bessel Function Beam

As a second example we will derive Durnin's Bessel beam equation by following the assumptions proposed by Li and Bharath [75]. Specifically, in (3.83) we assume that $g(k_r) = \pm a k_r / \sqrt{a^2 - 1}$, where a is a constant. By substituting this into (3.84), the other function can be found as $f(k_r) = \pm k_r / \sqrt{a^2 - 1}$, and therefore the solution to (3.82) is

(3.87)
$$\Phi(k_r, k_z : \omega) = \sigma(k_r : \omega) \delta\left\{ \frac{\omega}{c_o} \pm \frac{a k_r}{\sqrt{a^2 - 1}} \right\} \delta\left\{ k_z \pm \frac{k_r}{\sqrt{a^2 - 1}} \right\}.$$

As will be shown, by an appropriate choice of the parameter a, this solution enables several field profiles to be produced.

For monochromatic waves of angular frequency ω_o, it will be assumed that

(3.88)
$$\sigma(k_r : \omega) = \frac{(2\pi)^3}{k_r} e^{-jk_r r} \frac{a}{\sqrt{a^2 - 1}} \phi_o \delta(\omega - \omega_o),$$

where ϕ_o is the velocity potential amplitude, and that $|a| > 1$. From (3.88) and (3.87) the transform domain solution can be obtained by using (3.81) and written as

$$\phi_B(r, z:t) = \int_0^\infty dk_r \int_{-\infty}^\infty dk_z \int_{-\infty}^\infty d\omega\, J_0(k_r r) \phi_o \delta\{\omega - \omega_o\} \delta\left\{ k_z - \frac{k_r}{\sqrt{a^2 - 1}} \right\}$$

$$\times \delta\left\{ \frac{\omega}{c_o} - \frac{a k_r}{\sqrt{a^2 - 1}} \right\} e^{-jk_z z} e^{j\omega t}.$$

Evaluating the integrals results in

(3.89)
$$\phi_B(r, z:t) = \phi_o e^{j\omega_o\left(t - \frac{z}{ac_o}\right)} J_0\left(r\frac{\omega_o}{c_o}\sqrt{1-a^{-2}}\right).$$

By using the notation used earlier, i.e., $\alpha_B = k\sqrt{1-a^{-2}}$ and $\beta_B = k/a$, where $k = \omega_o/c_o$ and noting that $\alpha_B^2 + \beta_B^2 = k^2$, (3.89) transforms to (3.79), i.e.,[21]

(3.79)
$$\phi_B(r, z:t) = \phi_o e^{j(\omega_o t - \beta_B z)} J_0(\alpha_B r).$$

To generate this diffractionless beam on the plane $z = 0$, the transducer must have an infinite radius and the normal component of velocity on that plane must be:

(3.90)
$$v_o\xi(r_0:t) = -\frac{\partial\phi_B}{\partial z}\bigg|_{z=0} = \phi_o\beta_B e^{j\omega_o t} J_0(\alpha_B r_0).$$

From (3.89) it can be seen that the speed with which the wave propagates is given by $c = ac_o$, which, since $a > 1$ for waves in the +z-direction waves, implies a phase speed greater than c_o. However, because a steady-state situation is being considered, the field at any given location on the z-axis consists of all contributions out to infinity from the source plane, and consequently it can be argued that it is really a group speed that is being measured.

Both α_B and β_B in (3.79) are proportional to the frequency, and this has important implications when pulse excitation is considered. The frequency dependence of α_B makes the beam width frequency-dependent. To make it independent over a given range of frequencies such as those associated with a pulse, $(1 - a^{-2})^{1/2} \propto \omega^{-1}$. However, because the phase speed is given by $c = ac_o$, the frequency dependence of a causes dispersion, resulting in distortion as the pulse travels down the z-axis. Campbell and Soloway [84] pointed out that under these conditions the group speed will be less than c_o.

The beam lateral characteristics at any z-location are shown in Fig. 3.43a for a 2.5 MHz transducer of infinite radius apodized by $\xi_o(r_1) = \beta_B J_0(\alpha_B r_1)$, as given by (3.90). To show how the frequency affects the apodization, the required apodization for 2.0 MHz is also shown. From this it is clear that there will be some deterioration of the beam characteristics under pulsed conditions. In practice, the transducer diameter is limited and the influence of truncating the Bessel function must be considered. For example, if we consider a transducer of radius $a = 25$ mm, and assume that $\alpha_B = 1224$ m^{-1}, then the truncated Bessel function will contain the 10 annular regions shown in Fig. 3.43c. The exact on-axis pressure response for this function was calculated from (see Problem P2 in Chapter 2)

$$p(0, z:\omega) = j\omega\rho v_o \int_z^{\sqrt{z^2+a^2}} J_0\left(\alpha_B\sqrt{R^2-z^2}\right)e^{-jkR}dR,$$

21. Lu and Greenleaf [89] have given a more general form as $\phi_B(r,\theta,z:t) = \phi_o e^{j(\omega_o t - \beta_B z + n\theta)} J_n(\alpha_B r)$, where $n = 0, 1, 2, \ldots$ The axisymmetric form, given in (3.79), corresponds to $n = 0$.

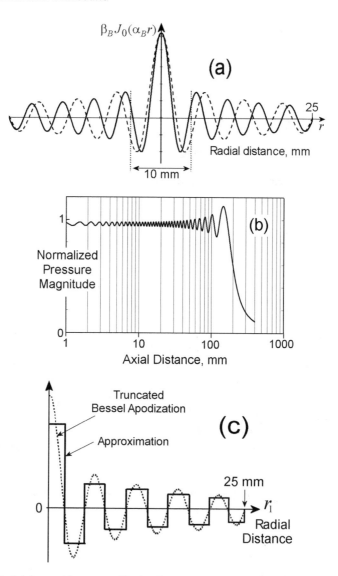

Figure 3.43 (a) Lateral beam profile for Bessel apodization (solid line) for 2.5 MHz excitation and $\alpha_B = 1224\,\text{m}^{-1}$. Dashed curve is for 2.0 MHz. (b) On-axis normalized pressure response for a 50 mm diameter disk excited at 2.5 MHz with $\alpha_B = 1224\,\text{m}^{-1}$ using the truncated apodization function given in (c). A practical approximation to the truncated function is shown.

and this is illustrated in Fig. 3.43b. It is apparent that the beam retains its original narrow divergence up to about 200 mm (i.e., the depth of field is about 200 mm). As reported by Lu and Greenleaf [87,88] in their experiments and simulations with a 10-element 50-mm-diameter annular array used under both CW and pulsed conditions, it is necessary to use a constant excitation amplitude in each of the 10 zones (see Fig. 3.43c). The depth of field and lateral beam width are given by [87] $Z_F \approx a\sqrt{(k/\alpha_B)^2 - 1}$, and $FWHM = 3/\alpha_B$. For example, for the 50 mmdiameter disk and apodization considered in Fig. 3.43, $Z_F = 212\,mm$ and $FWHM = 2.5\,mm$.

3.9.3 Superluminal Pulse

Up to this point we have considered only monochromatic localized waves. Of great importance in ultrasound is the use of pulses to generate minimally diffracting beams. As will be seen, the solutions are nonseparable and the resulting waves are localized both in time and space. In this and the next subsection, two types of waves will be considered [74,90].

If we let $\gamma = 1/a$, where $0 < \gamma < 1$, and assume that $\sigma(k_r, \omega)$

$$\sigma(k_r) = \frac{(2\pi)^3 \gamma^2}{1 - \gamma^2} e^{-z_o \gamma k_r / \sqrt{1 - \gamma^2}},$$

where $z_o > 0$ is arbitrary, then (3.87) can be written as

(3.91) $$\Phi(k_r, k_z : \omega) = \frac{(2\pi)^3 \gamma^2}{1 - \gamma^2} e^{-z_o \gamma k_r / \sqrt{1 - \gamma^2}} \delta\left\{ k_z - \frac{\gamma k_r}{\sqrt{1 - \gamma^2}} \right\} \delta\left\{ \frac{\omega}{c_o} - \frac{k_r}{\sqrt{1 - \gamma^2}} \right\}.$$

By substituting (3.91) into (3.81) and evaluating the integrals over k_z and ω, it can be shown that the velocity potential can be expressed as

$$\phi(r, z : t) = \frac{\gamma^2}{1 - \gamma^2} \int_0^\infty k_r J_0(k_r r) \phi_o e^{-k_r (jz + z_o - jc_o t / \gamma) \gamma / \sqrt{1 - \gamma^2}} \, dk_r.$$

With the help of $\int_0^\infty k_r J_0(m k_r) e^{-nk_r} dk_r = n(n^2 + m^2)^{-3/2}$ [91, eq. 6.623.2], this can be evaluated as

(3.92) $$\phi(r, z : t) = \frac{z_o + j(z - c_o t / \gamma)}{\left[\{z_o + j(z - c_o t / \gamma)\}^2 + r^2 (1 - \gamma^2) / \gamma^2 \right]^{3/2}},$$

which, on the z-axis, reduces to

$$\phi(0, z : t) = [z_o + j(z - c_o t / \gamma)]^{-2}.$$

To interpret the properties of the pulse represented by this velocity potential, it is helpful to consider what an observer would see when moving with the pulse center, i.e., with a speed of c_o/γ. By setting $z = c_o t / \gamma$, it can be seen that the observer in this moving coordinate system will see a pulse whose shape is independent of time. At any on-axis observation point, the imaginary term is zero, so that $|\phi(0, z : z\gamma/c_o)| = 1/z_o^2$. Because $0 < \gamma < 1$, the group speed along the z-axis (c_o/γ) is greater than the speed of sound, and by analogy with the optical case, the pulse is said to be *superluminal*. The incremental components produced on the source plane all move with the speed of sound, but the axially directed pulse produced as a result of constructive or destructive interference of these components can move at a speed that is substantially greater.

In Fig. 3.44a, the real part of the velocity potential is shown for four different z-locations and $\gamma = 0.2$, as calculated from (3.92). All four waveforms are identical but occur at different times corresponding to a propagation speed of $5c_o = 7500$ m/s. Figure 3.44b shows the normalized surface velocity waveforms in the z-direction at $z = 0$ for three different radial locations. These were calculated from (3.90) using $v_{no} = \mathrm{Re}\{-\mathrm{grad}(\phi)\}_{z=0}$. Because these waveforms differ both in their time and radial dependence, significant difficulties exist in realizing such a source. Moreover, a finite aperture transducer can be expected to result in some performance deterioration. In Fig. 3.44c are shown the normalized pressure waveforms at $z = 50$ mm for three different radial locations. It will be noted that the amplitude decays rapidly in the radial direction, approximately as $1/r^3$.

3.9.4 X-Waves

These were first described by Lu and Greenleaf [89] and experimentally verified by them [92]. Additional forms of X-waves propagating in inviscid media and media with classical loss originating from both infinite- and finite-size apertures have been described by Sushilov et al. [86,93]. Let us assume that $\gamma = \cos\zeta$, $k = k_r/\sin\zeta$, where $0 < \cos\zeta < 1$, and $k = \omega/c_o$, and that $\sigma(k_r,\omega)$ is given by

$$(3.93) \qquad \sigma(k_r) = \frac{(2\pi)^3}{k_r \sin\zeta} B(k_r/\sin\zeta) e^{-b_o k_r/\sin\zeta},$$

where b_o is a constant with dimensions of length and $B(.)$ is any function of k. Substitution into (3.91) yields an expression for the transformed velocity potential, which can be inverse-transformed to yield an expression identical to the zero-order equation originally obtained by Lu and Greenleaf [89]

$$\phi(r,z{:}t) = \int_0^\infty B(k)J_0(kr\sin\zeta)e^{k[b_o - j(z\cos\zeta - c_o t)]}dk.$$

If $B(k) = \phi_o$ (a constant) and noting that $\int_0^\infty J_0(mk)e^{-nk}dk = (n^2 + m^2)^{-1/2}$ [91, eq. 6.611.1], this evaluates to

$$(3.94) \qquad \phi(r,z{:}t) = \frac{\phi_o}{\sqrt{[b_o - j(z\cos\zeta - c_o t)]^2 + (r\sin\zeta)^2}}.$$

If we set $z = c_o t/\cos\zeta$ in (3.94), corresponding the center of the pulse, it will be noted that the amplitude is independent of the z-location. In addition, it can be seen that the speed of propagation is $c_o/\cos\zeta$, which is greater than c_o, corresponding to a superluminal pulse.

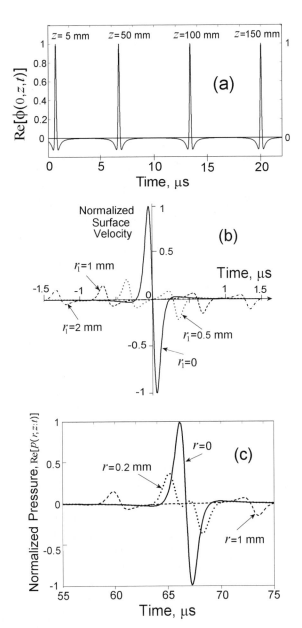

Figure 3.44 Superluminal pulse waveforms for $\gamma = 0.2$, $z_o = 1.0$ mm, $c_o = 1500$ m/s, originating from a disk of infinite radius. (a) The normalized real part of the velocity potential waveform is shown at four z-axis locations. (b) Normal component of the surface velocity waveform for three radial locations. Note the presence of waveforms at negative times. (c) Normalized pressure waveforms at three radial locations for $z = 50$ mm.

203

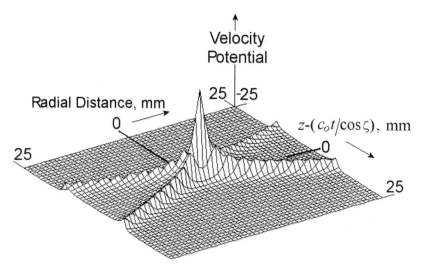

Figure 3.45 X-wave velocity potential for $\zeta = 22.5$ degrees, $b_o = 0.05$ mm. The values of z and c_o are in mm and mm/s, respectively.

In Fig. 3.45 the velocity potential pulse for $\zeta = 22.5$ degrees, $b_o = 0.05$ mm is shown as a function of the radial distance and $(z\text{-}c_o t/\cos\zeta)$ and clearly demonstrates the X-shape of the waveform. Because the shape is independent of z, the graph shows both the time variation of velocity potential at a fixed z-location and the velocity potential z-variation at a specified time, i.e., a snapshot.

Shown in Fig. 3.46a are the velocity potentials at various radial locations on the plane $z = 0$. These were calculated from the real part of (3.94) using the values of ζ and b_o assumed by Lu and Greenleaf [92] in their simulation and experimental studies of X-waves. The value of ζ corresponds to a pulse speed of $1.00244c_o$, which is just superluminal. For an infinite radius transducer, the lateral beam characteristics are independent of the z-location and decay inversely with the radial distance (see Fig. 3.46b). The latter should be contrasted with the superluminal pulse described in the previous subsection, whose lateral profile decays as $1/r^3$.

Experimental verification of the predicted behavior of X-waves using a 5 cm diameter, 10-element annular array has been described by Lu and Greenleaf [92]. Because of the non-zero element size and the limited number of annular rings, the on-axis waveform was found to suffer appreciable decay. At approximately 35 cm from the source plane, the signal was reduced by 6 dB, which was in agreement with the predicted depth of field ($Z_F = a \cot \zeta$) [89] of a finite-aperture source of radius a. In addition, measurement of the lateral and axial beam -6 dB widths showed good agreement with those predicted [89], specifically with the values: $R_L = 2b_0\sqrt{3}/\sin\zeta = 2.5$ mm, and $R_A = 2b_0\sqrt{3}/\cos\zeta = 0.17$ mm , respectively.

For a finite-aperture realization, generating the required pulse waveforms on the source plane presents a number of practical difficulties. Specifically,

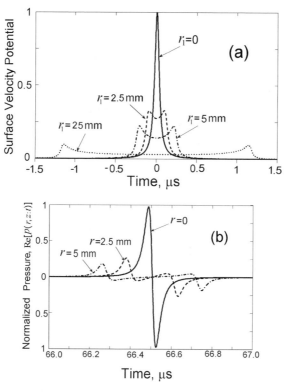

Figure 3.46 X-wave simulations for $\zeta = 4.0$ degrees, $b_o = 0.05$ mm, an infinite-radius disk at $z = 0$, and $c_o = 1500$ m/s. (a) Normalized velocity potential on the surface $z = 0$ at four different radii. (b) Normalized pressure waveforms at 100 mm from the disk showing the amplitude decay.

because the transducer bandwidth will be limited, special attention must be paid to the spectral characteristics of the velocity waveforms needed to generate a limited diffraction beam and to the manner in which the driving waveforms are modified by the transducer transfer function.

3.10 Effects of Attenuation

Absorption is the process of conversion of the ultrasound energy into heat or other energy forms. During its passage through a medium, an ideal plane wave will be subject to energy loss through absorption and a redirection of some of its energy by scattering due to non-uniformities in compressibility and density. The effects of both absorption and scattering are incorporated into the attenuation coefficient. Methods for measuring absorption and attenuation in biological tissue, together with experimental results, have been reviewed by Bamber [94] and earlier by Wells [95].

So far in this chapter, the field response from transducers of various geometric shapes has been described by assuming that adsorption and the related phenomenon of dispersion can be ignored. Since the attenuation of soft tissue can be large, especially at higher frequencies, it is particularly important that its effects be properly accounted for. Complications arise in seeking to derive a wave equation whose solution can represent the frequency dependence of both absorption and dispersion corresponding to the characteristics of a variety of tissues and fluids. Part of the difficulty is due to an incomplete understanding of the physical processes involved. As will be seen, the classical viscous loss equation gives rise to an absorption coefficient that has very nearly a square-law frequency dependence. While water and other fluids exhibit this dependence, this is not the case for most biological soft tissues. A number of approximate methods for dealing with the effects of attenuation have been described, and these will be reviewed following a brief discussion of the relation between dispersion and absorption.

3.10.1 Kramers-Kronig Relationships

The change in the phase velocity of a propagated wave with frequency is known as *dispersion*. In an unbounded medium, dispersion is caused by absorption. In fact, absorption is a necessary and sufficient condition for dispersion to exist, and as a result it is not surprising to find that there exists a direct relation between the two quantities. Kronig and Kramers independently obtained the relations for electromagnetic waves, and these are generally known as the Kramers-Kronig (K-K) relationships. Since they are a direct result of linearity and causality (an effect cannot precede its cause), they are independent of the detailed mechanisms and are applicable to other types of waves, including acoustic waves. It appears that Ginzberg [96] in 1955 was the first to formulate a form of the K-K equations applicable to acoustic waves. Since then, a number of derivations have been given, among which are those of Futerman [97], O'Donnell et al. [98], and Weaver and Pao [99]. Generally, a frequency-domain approach is used to arrive at the integral form of the K-K relations. However, a time-domain analysis can also be used to arrive at dispersion relations for media whose attenuation obeys a power law frequency dependence [101–103].

For acoustic waves, the K-K equations can be expressed in terms of the components of a complex propagation constant that can be defined by

$$(3.95) \qquad \underline{k}(\omega) = \beta(\omega) - j\alpha(\omega) = \frac{\omega}{c_o(\omega)} - j\alpha(\omega),$$

in which $c_o(\omega)$ denotes the phase speed and $\alpha(\omega)$ is the attenuation coefficient. The pair of equations relating these two quantities can be expressed in the following form:

$$\alpha(\omega) = \frac{-2\omega^2}{\pi} \int_0^\infty \left[\frac{1}{c_o(\omega')} - \frac{1}{c_o(\omega)} \right] \frac{d\omega'}{\omega'^2 - \omega^2} \qquad (a)$$

(3.96)
$$\frac{1}{c_o(\omega)} = \frac{2}{\pi}\int_0^\infty [\alpha(\omega') - \alpha(\omega)]\frac{d\omega'}{\omega'^2 - \omega^2}$$
(b)

From these it is evident that given the functional form of the attenuation coefficient, the form of the dispersion can be determined, and vice versa.

As noted in 1.8.1 (see footnote 35), longitudinal wave propagation in most soft tissue is found to have a frequency-dependent attenuation that is generally well approximated by

(3.97)
$$\alpha = \alpha'_o |\omega|^n,$$

where α'_o is the angular frequency attenuation factor and n is a real positive number that typically lies in the range $1 \le n \le 2$. By making use of generalized functions, Szabo [102] obtained equations that relate $\alpha(\omega)$ and $c_o(\omega)$ for values of n in the range from 0 to 3. Similar relations, valid for positive frequencies but based on the differential K-K relations, were subsequently obtained by Waters et al. [100,101]. For both positive and negative frequencies, these relations can be written as

(3.98)
$$\frac{1}{c_\omega} \equiv \frac{1}{c_o(\omega)} = \frac{1}{c_o} + \alpha'_o \tan\left(\frac{\pi n}{2}\right)\left(|\omega|^{n-1} - |\omega_o|^{n-1}\right), \quad \text{for} \quad 0 < n < 1$$
(a)

and $1 < n < 3$,

(3.98)
$$\frac{1}{c_{0\omega}} \equiv \frac{1}{c_o(\omega)} = \frac{1}{c_o} - \frac{2}{\pi}a'_o \ln\left|\frac{\omega}{\omega_o}\right|, \quad \text{for} \quad n = 1,$$
(b)

where c_o is the phase velocity at the reference frequency ω_o. In fact, in the limit as $n \to 1$, (3.98a) reduces to (b).

The case $n = 2$ corresponds closely to that of water and certain other fluids. Since $\tan(\pi) = 0$, it follows from (3.98a) that dispersion should be absent. On the other hand, for $n = 1$, corresponding to that frequently observed in soft tissue, dispersion is present. Fig. 3.47 shows the fractional change in speed, as predicted by (3.98), for various values of n. It should be noted that at the reference frequency of 1.0 MHz, the attenuation for all values of n is assumed to have the same value of $\alpha = 5.756$ Np/m, corresponding to that typically seen in soft tissue. It will be noted that for $n > 2$ the speed decreases with increasing frequency and normal dispersion is said to be present. For $n < 2$ the opposite is true, and the dispersion is said to be anomalous. The presence of dispersion increases the difficulty of obtaining an exact account of its effects, and consequently it is sometimes ignored. For narrow-band signals the effect of this simplification on the resulting transient wave is likely to be small.

3.10.2 Transfer Function and Impulse Response

To determine the transient response due to plane wave propagating in tissue, one can simply convolve the tissue impulse response with the incident wave-

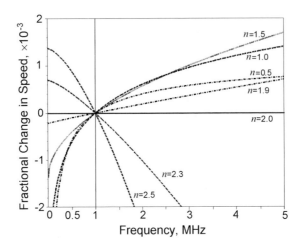

Figure 3.47 Fractional change in phase propagation speed versus frequency for different values of the exponent n. At the assumed reference frequency of 1.0 MHz, $c_o = 1500$ m/s. An attenuation coefficient of 0.5 dB/[cm.(MHz)^n] was assumed. This corresponds to an angular frequency coefficient of $\alpha'_0 = 5.76/(2\pi \times 10^6)^n$, m^{-1}(rad/s)^n. (Reproduced, with permission, from Cobbold et al. [111], *J. Acoust. Soc. Am.*, 116, 3294–3303, © 2004 Acoustical Society of America.)

form. The impulse response can be determined by taking the inverse Fourier transform of the transfer function. However, this may not be a straightforward process. For example, if we assume that the attenuation varies linearly with frequency, then the transfer function for transmission of a harmonic wave through a thickness z of tissue might be written as

$$(3.99) \qquad H_\alpha(f) \approx K e^{-\alpha_0 |f| z} e^{-j2\pi f z/c_o},$$

where the approximation sign serves to emphasize the fact that the phase term has been assumed to be a linear function of distance. The difficulty arises from the fact that this expression does not account for the effects of dispersion, which, in view of the K-K relations, will be present if attenuation is non-zero. Even though the effects of dispersion may be small, especially for narrow-band waveforms, failure to account for it in the above expression will generally result in a noncausal impulse response. For example, the inverse Fourier transform of (3.99) can be obtained using a symbolic math program (e.g., MAPLE®), yielding

$$h_\alpha(t) = \frac{2K\alpha z}{(\alpha z)^2 + 4\pi^2 \left(t - \dfrac{z}{c_o}\right)^2}.$$

For $t < z/c_o$, it can be seen that $h_\alpha(t)$ is non-zero, and consequently this expression for the impulse response is noncausal and may not properly represent the actual response.

To obtain a causal expression for the impulse response, Gurumurthy and Arthur [112] and Kuc [113] assumed that the tissue phase response is that of a causal minimum phase filter. Because the log-magnitude and the phase characteristics of such a filter form a Hilbert transform pair, the phase response of the transfer function can be calculated from the magnitude response. By taking the inverse Fourier transform of this self-consistent transfer function, the impulse response $h_\alpha(t)$ can be computed. The transfer function obtained by Gurumurthy and Arthur [112] is

$$(3.100) \qquad H_\alpha(f) = K e^{-\alpha_o |f| z} e^{-j2\pi f z \eta} e^{j \frac{2}{\pi} f \alpha_o z \ln(2\pi f)},$$

where $\eta = 1/c_o + 20\alpha_o/\pi^2$.

The results illustrated in Fig. 3.48 were obtained by taking the inverse Fourier transform of (3.100) and assuming an attenuation of 0.87 dB/(cm.MHz). For both graphs the actual start of each waveform is

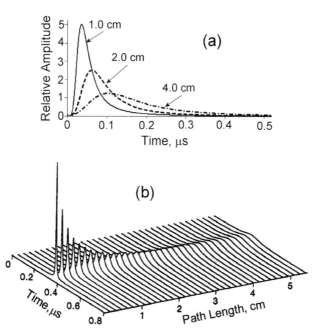

Figure 3.48 Impulse response of a medium with a propagation speed of 1500 m/s (6.67 μs/cm) and with an attenuation that varies linearly with frequency and is given by $\alpha = 0.1$ Np/(cm.MHz) or $\alpha = 0.87$ dB/(cm.MHz). The calculations used the Hilbert dispersive model of the transfer function as given by (3.100). (a) Response at 1, 2, and 4 cm. The pulses have been displaced so as to align their starting times, e.g., for the 1 cm depth the delay is 6.67 μs. (b) The impulse response over a range of depths (steps of 1.5 mm): each response has been displaced so that the peaks are aligned. (Reproduced, with permission, from Gurumurthy and Arthur [112], *Ultrasonic Imaging*, 4, 355–377, © 1982 Dynamedia Inc.)

delayed in time by nearly z/c_o, but for convenience in presentation the waveforms have been aligned. It can be seen from that with increasing depth, the higher frequencies are more heavily attenuated, thereby causing the pulse duration to increase with increasing depth.

3.10.3 Some Simplified Models

If the fractional bandwidth of the time-domain signal is small, then it is probably sufficient to assume that the attenuation is constant and equal to that at the center frequency. This suggests that the impulse response function (see (2.35)) can be written as

$$(3.101) \qquad h(\mathbf{r}{:}t) = \iint_{S_o} \frac{\xi_o(x,y)e^{-\alpha_c R}\delta\left(t - \dfrac{R}{c_o}\right)}{2\pi R}\,dS_o,$$

where α_c is the attenuation constant at the center frequency, ξ_o is the apodization function, and dispersion effects are assumed negligible. In the case of a simple disk transducer of radius a, for on-axis locations this simplifies to

$$(3.102) \qquad h(0,z{:}t) = c_o \mathcal{H}\left(t - \frac{z}{c_o}\right)\mathcal{H}\left(\frac{\sqrt{a^2 + z^2}}{c_o} - t\right)\xi_o\left(\sqrt{(c_o t)^2 - z^2}\right)e^{-\alpha_c c_o t}.$$

For a uniformly apodized disk, an analytic expression for the on-axis harmonic response can be obtained (see problem P7b). The response for a disk of radius $a = 5\lambda$ at 5.0 MHz is shown in Fig. 3.49a for: $\alpha_c = 0$, $\alpha_c = 0.288\,\text{cm}^{-1}$ (2.5 dB.cm^{-1}), and $\alpha_c = 0.576\,\text{cm}^{-1}$ (5.0 dB.cm^{-1}). It will be noted that while the general characteristics of the zero attenuation response are maintained, the positions of the maxima shift toward the transducer with increasing attenuation.

A more accurate model to account for frequency-dependent attenuation is based on linear systems theory (assuming linear propagation) [106]. This suggests that (3.101) can be rewritten as

$$(3.103) \qquad h(\mathbf{r}{:}t) = \int_T \iint_{S_o} h_\alpha(R{:}t - \tau)\frac{\xi_o(x,y)\delta\left(\tau - \dfrac{R}{c_o}\right)}{2\pi R}\,dS_o\,d\tau,$$

where $h_\alpha(.)$ is the attenuation impulse response that can be calculated from the attenuation transfer function, as described in the previous subsection.

If the field point is sufficiently far from the transducer surface so that all the wavelets arriving there have approximately the same attenuation, the task is considerably simplified. Specifically, (3.103) can be replaced by the convolution

$$(3.104) \qquad h(\mathbf{r}{:}t) = h_{\alpha m}(\mathbf{r}{:}t) * h_S(\mathbf{r}{:}t),$$

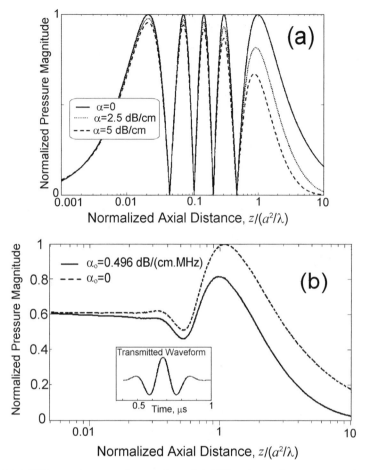

Figure 3.49 Effects of attenuation on the axial CW and transient response for a uniformly excited disk transducer with a radius of 5λ ($a = 1.5$ mm) at 5.0 MHz, propagating into media with different attenuation. (a) Response for CW excitation at 5.0 MHz. (b) Pressure response for a wideband ($\sigma = 1 \times 10^7 \text{s}^{-1} \equiv 75\%$ bandwidth) Gaussian transmitted pulse with a center frequency of 5.0 MHz, propagating into media whose attenuation is proportional to the frequency.

where h_s is the spatial velocity impulse response in the absence of attenuation and $h_{\alpha m}$ is the attenuation impulse response corresponding to the mean distance of the observation point from the transducer surface. However, since $h_{\alpha m}$ is a function of time, (3.104) is a non-stationary convolution. As described by Jensen et al. [106], the computational task can be simplified if it is also assumed that $h_{\alpha m}$ remains constant for non-zero values h_s, and its value is taken to be equal to that corresponding to the mid-point of h_s.

3.10.4 Accounting for Attenuation and Dispersion

One method of obtaining the response due to a wideband transient is to make use of the Rayleigh-Sommerfeld diffraction equations appropriate to the case where the normal component of the velocity is specified on the boundary [105]. If the normal inward component of the velocity spectrum on the boundary is denoted by $v_n(\omega)$, then, from (2.29), the velocity potential at **r** is given by the modified Rayleigh-Sommerfeld diffraction equation

$$(3.105) \qquad \Phi(\mathbf{r}{:}\omega) = \frac{1}{2\pi} \iint_{S_o} \frac{e^{-jkR}}{R} v_n(\omega) dS_o,$$

where $\underline{k}$ is now the complex wave number, as defined in (3.95). Justification for replacing the real wave number in the original Rayleigh-Sommerfeld diffraction equation has been given in [104].

As an example, we consider a piston source of radius a, excited by a Gaussian waveform. The particle velocity at $z = 0$ can be written as

$$v_n(0{:}t) = v_{no} e^{j\omega_o t} e^{-\sigma^2 t^2/2}$$

so that the spectrum is given by

$$(3.106) \qquad v_n(0{:}\omega) = v_{no} \Im\{e^{j\omega_o t} e^{-\sigma^2 t^2/2}\} = v_{no} \frac{\sqrt{2\pi}}{\sigma} e^{-(\omega-\omega_o)^2/2\sigma^2}.$$

If the propagation medium has an attenuation that is proportional to the frequency ($n = 1$), then from (3.95) and (3.98b)

$$(3.107) \qquad \underline{k} = \frac{\omega}{c_o(\omega_o)} - \frac{2}{\pi}\alpha_o'\omega \ln\left|\frac{\omega}{\omega_o}\right| - j\alpha_o'|\omega|.$$

The pressure waveform can be obtained from (3.105) by recalling that $p = \rho_o \partial \phi(\mathbf{r}{:}t)/\partial t$ and by an inverse Fourier transform, yielding

$$\underline{p}(\mathbf{r}{:}t) = \frac{\rho_o}{2\pi} \frac{\partial}{\partial t}\left\{\Im^{-1}\left[\iint_{S_o} \frac{e^{-jkR}}{R} v_n(\omega) dS_o\right]\right\}.$$

If the observation point is on the z-axis, this reduces to

$$\underline{p}(z{:}t) = \rho_o \frac{\partial}{\partial t}\left\{\Im^{-1}\left[\int_0^a \frac{e^{-jkr}}{r} v_n(\omega) dr\right]\right\} = j\rho_o \Im^{-1}\left[\int_z^{\sqrt{z^2+a^2}} \omega e^{-jkR} v_n(\omega) dR\right].$$

Substituting (3.106), this simplifies to

$$(3.108) \qquad \underline{p}(z{:}t) = \rho_o v_{no} \frac{\sqrt{2\pi}}{\sigma} \Im^{-1}\left[\frac{\omega}{\underline{k}} e^{-(\omega-\omega_o)^2/(2\sigma^2)}\left(e^{-jkz} - e^{-jk\sqrt{z^2+a^2}}\right)\right],$$

which accounts for both attenuation and dispersion. The CW response of a disk transducer is illustrated in Fig. 3.49a. For this narrow-band case, there is no dispersion, and an analytical expression can be obtained either by evaluating the transform or more directly as described in [105]. For a wide-band Gaussian pulse, the peak pressure response as calculated from (3.108) is shown in Fig. 3.49b. While the waveforms are affected by dispersion at the greater depths, over the range of axial distances shown, the peak pressure remains virtually independent. To illustrate the effects of dispersion on the waveforms, Fig. 3.50 shows the influence of including and excluding the dispersion term. Significant changes in the wave shape are present, and in addition the waveform is slightly expanded in duration as compared to that close to the transducer.

3.10.5 Classical Viscous Loss

In a seminal paper published in 1845 [107], Stokes derived an equation for wave propagation in a classical viscous medium in the absence of thermal conduction. For a plane wave propagating in the x-direction, his equation can be written as (see Chapter 1 (1.38)):

$$(3.109) \qquad \frac{1}{c_o^2} \frac{\partial^2 \phi}{\partial t^2} - \frac{\partial^2 \phi}{\partial x^2} = \kappa \left(\mu_B + \frac{4}{3}\mu \right) \frac{\partial}{\partial t} \left(\frac{\partial^2 \phi}{\partial x^2} \right).$$

Although the steady-state solution of this equation is well known, having been studied in the mid-1800s, transient problems have proven rather more difficult to address. It is well established that approximate solutions to such problems do not satisfy causality in the strict sense, i.e., a propagated pulse does not have a sharp front but extends asymptotically to plus and minus infinity, similar to solutions of the second-order diffusion equation. Exact transient solutions

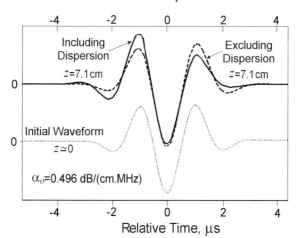

Figure 3.50 Effects of dispersion on the on-axis waveform for the same conditions illustrated in Fig. 3.49. The initial Gaussian wideband waveform is shown together with the waveforms at a normalized distance of 10 with and without the dispersion term (the second term in (3.107)).

have been obtained using the Laplace transform. Of particular importance is the work of Hanin [108] in 1957, who obtained a solution for a δ-function source in terms of power series expansions. More recently, Ludwig and Levin [109] also obtained a δ-function solution, which they expressed in terms of two real integrals suitable for numerical evaluations for a wide range of conditions. Approximation methods have also been used to obtain solutions valid for small absorption coefficients and observation points that are not very close to the source. In an important contribution, Blackstock [110] considered the 1-D problem in which a sinusoidal source was abruptly switched on. By assuming the absorption to be small, specifically that $\alpha\omega \ll c_0$, where α is the absorption coefficient, he showed that (3.109) could be reduced to a second-order parabolic diffusion or heat conduction equation. If $\alpha = \alpha_o'\omega^2$, the above approximation can be written as $\alpha_o\omega^3 \ll c_0$, from which it can be seen that for a transient source the observation point must not be too close.

The much simpler steady-state solution for a sinusoidal source on the plane $x = 0$ can be found by letting $\Phi = \phi e^{j\omega t}$, enabling (3.109) to be reduced to

$$(3.110) \qquad \underline{k}^2\Phi + \frac{\partial^2\Phi}{\partial x^2} = 0,$$

where $\underline{k}$ is the complex propagation constant as defined in (3.95). Thus

$$(3.111) \qquad \underline{k}^2 = \frac{\omega^2/c_o^2}{1 + j\omega\kappa\left(\mu_B + \dfrac{4}{3}\mu\right)} = \frac{k_o^2}{1 + j\omega\kappa\left(\mu_B + \dfrac{4}{3}\mu\right)},$$

in which $k_o = \omega/c_o$, $c_o(= 1/\sqrt{\kappa\rho_o})$ is the propagation speed in the absence of dispersion, and the compressibility κ is taken to be real. If the imaginary term in the denominator is much less than unity, then (3.111) can be expanded as:

$$(3.112) \qquad \underline{k} = \pm k_o\left[1 - \frac{j\omega\kappa}{2}\left(\mu_B + \frac{4}{3}\mu\right) - \frac{3\omega^2\kappa^2}{8}\left(\mu_B + \frac{4}{3}\mu\right)^2 - \cdots\right]$$

$$= \pm(\beta - j\alpha),$$

where α is given by

$$(3.113) \qquad \alpha \approx \frac{\omega^2\kappa}{2c_o}\left(\mu_B + \frac{4}{3}\mu\right) = \frac{\omega^2}{2\rho_o c_o^3}\left(\mu_B + \frac{4}{3}\mu\right),$$

so that the absorption coefficient increases as the square of the frequency provided $1 \gg j\omega\kappa\left(\mu_B + \dfrac{4}{3}\mu\right)$, and the attenuation factor is given by

$$\alpha_o' = \frac{\left(\mu_B + \dfrac{4}{3}\mu\right)}{2\rho_o c_o^3}.$$

The real part of the propagation constant is

$$\text{(3.114)} \qquad \beta \approx k_o \left(1 - \frac{3\omega^2\kappa^2}{8} \left(\mu_B + \frac{4}{3}\mu \right)^2 \right).$$

For a plane wave propagating in the $+x$-direction, the velocity potential is

$$\Phi(x{:}t) = \Phi_o e^{j(\omega t - kx)}$$
$$= \Phi_o e^{j(\omega t - \beta x)} e^{-\alpha x}.$$

But the phase speed is given by $c_\omega = \omega/\beta$, which from (3.114) can be expressed as

$$\text{(3.115)} \qquad c_\omega(\omega) = c_o \left(1 - \frac{3\omega^2\kappa^2}{8} \left(\mu_B + \frac{4}{3}\mu \right)^2 \right)^{-1} \approx c_o \left(1 + \frac{3\omega^2\kappa^2}{8} \left(\mu_B + \frac{4}{3}\mu \right)^2 \right);$$

consequently, if the same approximation holds true, the dispersion, which can be expressed by the excess speed $\Delta c(\omega) = c_\omega - c_o$, also increases as the square of the frequency. If the absorption varied *exactly* as the square of the frequency, then, according to the K-K equations (see subsection 3.10.1), there should be no dispersion. However, because the dependence is not exactly parabolic, dispersion is predicted, though it can be very small.

Thus, the differential equation expressed by (3.109) has a plane wave solution characterized by absorption coefficient and excess speed, both of which increase approximately as the square of the frequency. As noted earlier, pure water has been found to have an absorption coefficient that accurately obeys the square-law frequency dependence over a very wide frequency range extending from the sub-MHz range to above 1 GHz [114]. This is used as the basis for determining the μ_B for water as well as for other fluids whose absorption coefficients have quadratic frequency dependence. A quick calculation of the excess speed at 10 MHz for water at 15°C using $\kappa = 4.7 \times 10^{-10}\,\text{Pa}^{-1}$ and $\mu_B = 2.81\,\mu = 0.0031\,\text{kg/m.s}$ yields $1.0 \times 10^{-5}\,\text{m/s}$, which is well beyond the range of current measurement techniques. Such a small value is in agreement with (3.98a), which predicts that for $n = 2$ there should be no dispersion.

3.10.6 Formulations for an Attenuation Power Law

As noted earlier, many of the experimental measurements for soft biological media indicate that the frequency dependence of the attenuation can be approximately represented by $\alpha = \alpha_o' \omega^n$, where n lies in the range from 1 to 2. Consequently, the simple viscous loss mechanism assumed in the classical dissipative wave equation of (3.109) cannot properly account for propagation in such media unless $n = 2$.

A number of efforts have been made to develop a wave equation that properly accounts for the attenuation characteristics of tissue. Some initial work is that published in the early 1980s by Leeman and his colleagues [115,116]. Based on the assumption that the attenuation arises from a multiplicity of relaxation processes, Nachman et al. [117] derived a causal linearized wave equation for fluids from first principles. By a suitable choice of the relaxation processes, it is possible to obtain a good fit to a variety of the experimentally observed frequency-dependent attenuation characteristics. However, for N relaxation mechanisms, the equation is of the order $N + 2$, making analytical solutions difficult to obtain.

Berkhoff et al. [118] used this multiple relaxation model in simulating ultrasound B-mode image formation with a 132-element linear array. To represent the complex wave number of homogenized beef liver, they used a two-parameter model and obtained the parameter values by a best fit to the experimentally measured [119] attenuation versus frequency characteristics. From this model they calculated the dispersion and found that the speed of sound increased by approximately 2.2 m/s (a fractional change of 0.14%) over the frequency range 1 to 10 MHz. Although this is small, it can significantly affect a wideband signal (see Fig. 3.50) such as that used in a B-mode imaging system. By including dispersion, Berkhoff et al. found that the computed pulse waveforms were affected, although the B-mode image quality was unaffected.

In 1994 Szabo [103] proposed the causal linear convolutional wave equation to describe the ultrasound radiation propagation in media whose attenuation obeys a frequency power law. In 1-D, his equation for the pressure can be written as

$$(3.116) \qquad \frac{\partial^2}{\partial z^2} p(\mathbf{r};t) - \frac{1}{c_o^2} \frac{\partial^2}{\partial t^2} p(\mathbf{r};t) + \mathcal{L}(t) * p(\mathbf{r};t) = 0,$$

where c_o is the phase velocity at a reference frequency of ω_o and $\mathcal{L}(t)$ is the loss operator that guarantees causality and that accounts for the effects of dispersion and attenuation. More recently, an integral solution to this equation has been obtained [105], which can be expressed as

$$(3.117) \qquad p(z;t) = \frac{1}{2\pi} \int_{-\infty}^{\infty} p(0;\omega) e^{-j[\omega/c_\omega - j\alpha(\omega)]z + j\omega t} d\omega.$$

By substituting this into (3.116), the loss operator can be obtained as

$$\mathcal{L}(t) = \frac{1}{2\pi} \int_{-\infty}^{\infty} \left\{ \left[\frac{\omega}{c_\omega} - j\alpha(\omega) \right]^2 - \frac{\omega^2}{c_o^2} \right\} e^{j\omega t} d\omega$$

When the attenuation is governed by the power law given by (3.97) and n is in the range $0 < n < 3$, the equations for $\alpha(\omega)$ and c_ω are given by (3.98).

If n in the range for $0 < n < 3$, it has been shown that the particle velocity can be expressed as [111]

$$(3.118) \qquad \frac{v(x,t)}{v_{no}} = \Im^{-1}\left\{ \Im[v(0,t)] \exp\left(-\alpha_o' x |\omega|^n - j\omega x \left\{ \frac{1}{c_o} + \alpha_o' \tan\left(n\frac{\pi}{2} \right) \right. \right.$$
$$\left. \left. \times \left[|\omega|^{n-1} - |\omega_o|^{n-1} \right] \right\} \right) \right\}. \qquad \text{(a)}$$

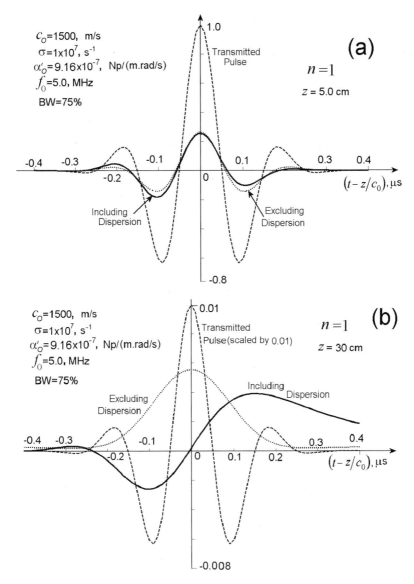

Figure 3.51 Effects of dispersion on the propagation of a Gaussian pulse with a 75% bandwidth in a tissue-like medium ($n = 1.0$). The results were calculated from (3.118). The transmitted pulse and the received pulse when dispersion is ignored and included are shown for depths of (a) 5.0 cm and (b) 30 cm. (Reproduced, with permission, from Cobbold et al. [111], *J. Acoust. Soc. Am.*, 116, 3294–3303, © 2004 Acoustical Society of America.)

When $n = 1$, a more convenient computational form is

(3.118) $$\frac{v(x,t)}{v_{no}} = \Im^{-1}\left\{\Im[v(0,t)]\exp\left(-\alpha'_o x|\omega| - j\omega x\left[\frac{1}{c_o} - \frac{2}{\pi}\alpha'_o \ln\left|\frac{\omega}{\omega_o}\right|\right]\right)\right\}.$$ (b)

The effect of dispersion on the transmission of a Gaussian pulse with a band-width of 50% in a tissue-like medium is illustrated in Fig. 3.51. It can be seen that the particle velocity waveform suffers significant changes due to the effects of attenuation, even when the effects of dispersion are ignored and the two-way path is 5 cm. However, when the two-way path is 30 cm, the effects of dispersion produce major changes in the shape and its spectrum.

Problems

P1. This problem concerns a generalization of the impulse response method to take account of the case where an arbitrary planar source is apodized [22].

a. Using the figure shown below, show that (3.24) can be transformed

$$\text{to } h(r, z{:}t) = \int_0^\infty \frac{\delta\left(t - \frac{\sqrt{b^2 + z^2}}{c_o}\right)}{2\pi\sqrt{b^2 + z^2}} b\Xi(b)db \text{ where}$$

$$\Xi(b) = \int_0^{2\pi} \xi_o(x + b\cos\alpha, y + b\sin\alpha)d\alpha$$

in which $\xi_o(x_1,y_1)$ is the apodization function, where the subscript has been used to avoid confusion with the coordinates of the observation point.

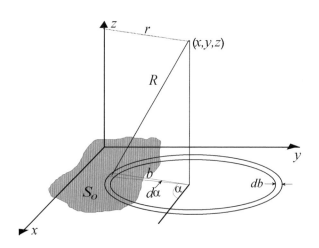

b. If $\xi_o(x_1, y_1)$ contains no discontinuities, show that the above expression for the velocity impulse response reduces to

$$h(r, z{:}t) = \frac{c_o}{2\pi} \Xi\left(\sqrt{c_o^2 t^2 - z^2}\right) \quad \text{for} \quad c_o t \geq z$$

$$= 0 \qquad\qquad\qquad \text{for} \quad c_o t < z.$$

c. If the source is axisymmetric, show that the on-axis impulse response is given by

$$h(0, z{:}t) = c_o \xi_o\left(\sqrt{c_o^2 t^2 - z^2}\right) \quad \text{for} \quad c_o t \geq z$$

$$= 0 \qquad\qquad\qquad \text{for} \quad c_o t < z.$$

d. If it is assumed that the apodization function is given by $\xi_o(r_1) = \operatorname{circ}\left(\dfrac{r_1}{a}\right) e^{-r_1^2/(\varepsilon a)^2}$, where ε describes the degree of truncation ($\varepsilon = \infty$ for uniform excitation), a is the transducer radius, and the circ function sets $\xi_o(r_1)$ to zero for $r_1 > a$, then the apodization function is discontinuous. However, the analysis is much simpler if the transducer is assumed to have an infinite radius, and the apodization is taken to be the continuous Gaussian function $\xi_o(r_1) = e^{-r_1^2/\sigma^2}$, where σ is a constant. With this assumption show that:

$$h(r, z{:}t) = c_o J_0\left(\frac{2r}{\sigma^2}\sqrt{c_o^2 t^2 - z^2}\right) e^{-(r^2 + c_o^2 t^2 - z^2)/\sigma^2} \mathcal{H}(c_o t - z),$$

where $J_0(.)$ is a cylindrical Bessel function of the first kind and zero order and $\mathcal{H}(.)$ is the Heaviside step function. Appendix C may be helpful.

P2. Consider an infinite narrow strip of width Δy whose center of symmetry coincides with the x-axis and whose surface is on the plane $z = 0$. Assuming CW excitation of angular frequency ω with a surface velocity amplitude of v_o, a medium of density of ρ_o, and propagation speed c_o, derive an expression for the z-axis pressure assuming that $z \gg \Delta y$. If $\rho_o = 1000\,\text{kg/m}^3$, $c_o = 1500\,\text{m/s}$, $v_o = 0.1\,\text{m/s}$, $\Delta y = 1\,\text{mm}$, and a $f = 5\,\text{MHz}$, plot a graph of the pressure amplitude along the z-axis from 1 to 100 cm and show that the far-field pressure falls off as $1/\sqrt{z}$.

P3. Show that the velocity impulse response at the cylindrical coordinate (r, z) due to a thin annulus of radius a and width Δa that lies on the plane $z = 0$ is given by:

$$h(r, z) = \frac{c_o \Delta a}{\pi r}\left\{1 - \frac{\left[a^2 + r^2 + z^2 - c_o^2 t^2\right]^2}{4a^2 r^2}\right\}^{-1/2}$$

for $[(a - r)^2 + z^2]^{1/2} < c_o t < [(a + r)^2 + z^2]^{1/2}$, and $h(r, z) = 0$ elsewhere. See [51] for further details.

P4. a. By making use of the fact that the aperture weighting function for a ring of radius r_{11} is given by $\delta(r_{11} - r_1)$, and that the Fraunhofer far-field response is proportional to the Fourier transform of the aperture function, show that for a disk of radius a whose aperture weighting is the circularly symmetric function $\xi_o(r_1)$, the directivity function is given by (3.75).

b. For a uniformly excited transducer $[\xi_o(r_1) = 1]$, show that (3.75) reduces to (3.33b).

c. Show that the pressure response in the Fresnel zone due to CW excitation of a narrow ring of radius a and incremental width Δa is given by

$$\underline{\Delta p}(R, \theta{:}\omega) = \frac{j\omega\rho_o v_o}{2\pi R_o} e^{-jk\left(R_o + a^2/2R_o\right)} a\Delta a D(\theta),$$

where the directivity function is given by

$$D(\theta) = \int_0^{2\pi} e^{jkacos\,\varphi_1\,\sin\theta\left[1 + \frac{a}{2R_o}\cos\varphi_1\,\sin\theta\right]} d\varphi1.$$

P5. Starting from (3.22), which gives the pressure phasor for a piston transducer of radius a at any cylindrical coordinate location (r,z), and assuming the hard baffle boundary condition, derive (3.32) giving the far-field (Fraunhofer) approximation for the pressure phasor, i.e.,

$$\underline{p}(r, z{:}\omega) \approx \frac{j\omega\rho_o v_o a^2}{2R}\left[\frac{2J_1(kar/z)}{kar/z}\right]e^{-jk\left[z + r^2/(2z)\right]}, \text{ where } k = \omega/c_o, J_1 \text{ is}$$

a cylindrical Bessel function of the first kind, and (r,z) are the cylindrical coordinates of the field point. You will find it helpful to make use of a "standard" result that expresses the Bessel function as an integral.

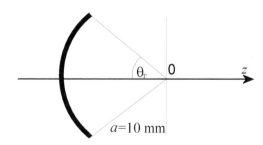

P6. The concave transducer shown above has a radius of curvature of 10 mm and a half-angle of $\theta_T = 20$ degrees.

a. Starting from the Rayleigh integral, derive an expression for the *on-axis* velocity potential response for a δ-function of velocity at the surface, and state any approximations used.

    b. The transducer is excited such that the normal component of the surface velocity is a single cycle of a 10 MHz sinusoidal waveform. From the result of part (a), determine the on-axis pressure waveform, at $z = -5.0, 0$ and 100 mm.

P7. Using the simplified model for the frequency-independent attenuation given by (3.101) and assuming a simple disk of radius a with an apodization function ξ_o:

    a. Obtain the equation for the axial velocity impulse response as given by (3.102).

    b. Show that the axial harmonic pressure response for a uniformly excited disk is given by

$$p(0, z : \omega) = \frac{\rho_o V_o c_o}{1 - j c_o \alpha_c / \omega} \left[e^{-[\alpha_c + j\omega/c_o]z} - e^{-[\alpha_c + j\omega/c_o]\sqrt{z^2 + a^2}} \right].$$

References

1. Zemanek, J., Beam behavior within the nearfield of a vibrating piston, *J. Acoust. Soc. Am.*, 49, 181–191, 1970.
2. Skudrzyk, E., *The Foundations of Acoustics; Basic Mathematics and Basic Acoustics*, Springer-Verlag, New York, 1971.
3. Rayleigh, J.W.S, *The Theory of Sound* (in two vols., 2nd edn., 1894), republished, Dover Publications, New York, 1945.
4. Archer-Hall, J.A., and Gee, D., A single integral computer method for axisymmetric transducers with various boundary conditions, *NDT International*, 13, 95–101, 1980.
5. Markiewicz, A., and Chivers, R.C., Effects of baffle conditions on the near-field of piston disk radiators, *Acustica*, 60, 289–294, 1986.
6. Fung, C.C.W., Cobbold. R.S.C., and Bascom, P.A.J., Radiation coupling of a transducer-target system using the angular spectrum method, *J. Acoust. Soc. Am.*, 92, 2239–2247, 1992.
7. Steel, R., and Fish, P.J., A simulation study of sample volume sensitivity for oblique pulsed finite beam insonation of Doppler ultrasound flow phantom cylindrical vessels, *IEEE Trans. Ultrason. Ferroelect. Freq. Contr.*, 50, 58–67, 2000.
8. Bracewell, R.N., *The Fourier Transform and its Applications*, 3rd edn., McGraw-Hill, New York, 2000.
9. Harris, G.R., Review of transient field theory for a baffled planar piston, *J. Acoust. Soc. Am.*, 70, 10–20, 1981.
10. Hutchins, D.A., and Hayward, G., Radiated Fields of Ultrasonic Transducers, Ch. 1, pp. 1–80 in: *Physical Acoustics: Ultrasonic Measurement Methods*, Vol. 19, Thurston, R.N., and Pierce, A.D. (Eds.), Academic Press, New York, 1990.
11. Tupholme, G.E., Generation of acoustic pulses by baffled plane pistons, *Mathematika*, 16, 209–224, 1969.
12. Stepanishen, P.R., Transient radiation from pistons in an infinite baffle, *J. Acoust. Soc. Am.*, 49, 1629–1638, 1971.
13. Lockwood, J.C., and Willette, J.G., High speed method for computing the exact solution for the pressure variations in the nearfield of a bafflled piston, *J. Acoust. Soc. Am.*, 53, 735–741, 1973.

14. Ohtsuki, S., Ring function method for calculating nearfield of sound source, *Bull. Tokyo Inst. Tech.*, No. 123, 23–27, 1974. Also published in Japanese as: Calculation method for the nearfield of a sound source with ring function, *J. Acoust. Soc. Japan*, 30, 76–81, 1974.

15. Penttinen, A., and Luukkala, M., The impulse response and pressure nearfield of a curved ultrasonic radiator, *J. Phys. D*, 9, 1547–1557, 1976.

16. Jensen, J.A., Ultrasound fields from triangular apertures, *J. Acoust. Soc. Am.*, 100, 2049–2056, 1996.

17. Kozina, O.G., and Makarov, G.I., Transient processes in the acoustic fields generated by a piston membrane of arbitrary shape, *Soviet Physics Acoustics*, 7, 39–43, 1961.

18. Tupholme, G.E., Generation of an axisymmetrical acoustic pulse by a deformable sphere, *Proc. Cambridge Phil. Soc*, 63, 1285–1308, 1967.

19. Schoch, A., Betrachtungen uber das schallfeld einer kolbenmembran, *Akust. Zeitschr.*, 6, 318–326, 1941.

20. Cathignol, D., Faure, P., and Chavrier, F., Acoustic field of plane or spherical transducers, *Acustica*, 83, 410–418, 1997.

21. Harris, G.R., Transient field of a baffled planar piston having an arbitrary vibration amplitude distribution, *J. Acoust. Soc. Am.*, 70, 186–204, 1981.

22. Tjøtta, J.N., and Tjøtta, S., Nearfield and farfield of pulsed acoustic radiators, *J. Acoust. Soc. Am.*, 71, 824–834, 1982.

23. Delannoy, B., Bruneel, C., Haine, F., and Torguet, R., Anomolous behavior in the radiation pattern of piezoelectric transducers induced by parasitic Lamb waves, *J. Appl. Phys.*, 51, 3942–3948, 1980.

24. Weight, J.P., Ultrasonic beam structures in fluid media, *J. Acoust. Soc. Am.*, 76, 1184–1191, 1984.

25. Hayman, A.J., and Weight, J.P., Transmission and reception of short ultrasonic pulses by circular and square transducers, *J. Acoust. Soc. Am.*, 66, 945–951, 1979.

26. Baboux, J.C., Lakestani, F., and Perdix, M., Theoretical and experimental study of the contribution of radial modes to the pulsed ultrasonic field radiated by a thick piezoelectric disk, *J. Acoust. Soc. Am.*, 75, 1722–1731, 1984.

27. Jia, X., Berger, J., and Quentin, G., Experimental investigations of Lamb waves on pulsed piezoelectric transducers and their ultrasonic radiation into liquids, *J. Acoust. Soc. Am.*, 90, 1181–1183, 1991.

28. Wright, F.J., and Berry, M.V., Wave-front dislocations in the soundfield of a pulsed circular piston radiator, *J. Acoust. Soc. Am.*, 75, 733–748, 1984.

29. Crombie, P., Bascom, P.A.J., and Cobbold, R.S.C., Calculating the pulsed response of linear arrays: accuracy versus computational efficiency, *IEEE Trans. Ultrason. Ferroelect. Freq. Contr.*, 44, 997–1009, 1997.

30. Harris, G.R., Hydrophone measurements in diagnostic ultrasound fields, *IEEE Trans. Ultrason. Ferroelect. Freq. Contr.*, 35, 87–101, 1988.

31. Shombert, D.G., Smith, S.W., and Harris, G.R., Angular response of miniature ultrasonic hydrophones, *Med. Phys.*, 9, 484–492, 1982.

32. Williams, A.O., Acoustic intensity distribution from a "piston" source. II. The concave piston, *J. Acoust. Soc. Am.*, 17, 219–227, 1946.

33. O'Neil, H.T., Theory of focusing radiators, *J. Acoust. Soc. Am.*, 21, 516–526, 1949.

34. Kikuchi, Y., Transducers for ultrasonic systems, Ch. 4, pp. 289–342, in: *Ultrasound: its Applications in Medicine and Biology*, F.F. Fry (Ed.), Elsevier, Amsterdam, 1978.

35. Arditi, M., Foster, F.S., and Hunt, J.W., Transient fields of concave annular arrays, *Ultrasonic Imaging*, 3, 37–61, 1981.

36. Gibson, W.G.R., Cobbold, R.S.C., and Foster, F.S., Ultrasonic fields of a convex semi-spherical transducer, *J. Acoust. Soc. Am.*, 94, 1923–1929, 1993.

37. de Hoop, A.T., Zeroug, S., and Kostek, S., Transient analysis of the transmitting properties of a focused acoustic transducer with an arbitrary rim, *J. Acoust. Soc. Am.*, 98, 1767–1777, 1995.

38. Schmerr, L.W., Sedov, A., and Lerch, T.P., A boundary diffraction wave model for a spherically focused ultrasonic transducer, *J. Acoust. Soc. Am.*, 101, 1269–1277, 1997.

39. Lu, J-y, Zou, H., and Greenleaf, J.F., Biomedical ultrasound beam forming, *Ultrasound in Med. Biol.*, 20, 403–428, 1994.

40. Kino, S., *Acoustic Waves: Devices, Imaging and Analog Signal Processing*, Prentice-Hall, Englewood Cliffs, NJ, 1986.

41. Cline, H.E., Hynynen, K., Hardy, C.J., Watkins, R.D., Schenck, J.F., and Jolesz, F.A., MR temperature mapping of focused ultrasound surgery, *Magn. Reson. Med.*, 31, 628–636, 1994.

42. Madsen, E.L., Goodsitt, M.M., and Zagzebski, J.A., Continuous waves generated by focused radiators, *J. Acoust. Soc. Am.*, 70, 1508–1517, 1981.

43. Mair, H.D., and Hutchins, D.A., Axial focusing by phased concentric annuli, pp. 619–626 in: *Progress in Underwater Acoustics*, H.M. Merklinger (Ed.), Plenum Press, New York, 1986.

44. Cathignol, D., Sapozhnikov, O.A., and Zhang, J., Lamb waves in piezoelectric focused radiator as a reason for discrepancy between O'Neil's formula and experiment, *J. Acoust. Soc. Am.*, 101, 1286–1297, 1997.

45. Cathignol, D., Sapozhnikov, O.A., and Theillere, Y., Comparison of acoustic fields radiated from piezoceramic and piezocomposite focused transducers, *J. Acoust. Soc. Am.*, 105, 2612–2617, 1999.

46. Coulouvrat, F., Continuous field radiated by a geometrically focused transducer: numerical investigation and comparison with an approximated model, *J. Acoust. Soc. Am.*, 94, 1663–1675, 1993.

47. Reid, J.M., and Wild, J.J., Current developments in ultrasonic equipment for medical diagnosis, *Proc. Nat. Electronics Conf.*, 12, 1002–1015, 1956.

48. Wild, J.P., A new method for image formation with annular apertures and an application in radio astronomy, *Proc. Roy. Soc. A*, 286, 499–509, 1965.

49. Burckardt, C.B., Grandchamp, P.A., and Hoffmann, H., Methods for increasing the lateral resolution of B-scan, in *Acoustical Holography and Imaging*, Vol. 5, pp. 391–413, P.S. Green (Ed.), Plenum Press, New York, 1973.

50. Vilkomerson, D., Acoustic imaging with thin annular apertures, in *Acoustical Holography and Imaging*, Vol. 5, pp. 283–316, P.S. Green (Ed.), Plenum Press, New York, 1973.

51. Foster, S.F., Patterson, M.S., Arditi, M., and Hunt, J.W., The conical scanner: a two transducer ultrasound scatter imaging technique, *Ultrasonic Imaging*, 3, 62–82, 1981.

52. Burckardt, C.B., Grandchamp, P.A., and Hoffmann, H., Focussing ultrasound over a large depth with an annular aperture: an alternative method, *IEEE Trans. Sonics Ultrasonics*, SU-22, 11–15, 1975.

53. Foster, S.F., Larson, J.D., Mason, M.K., Shoup, T.S., Nelson, G., and Yoshida, H., Development of a 12-element annular array transducer for realtime ultrasound imaging, *Ultrasound Med. Biol.*, 15, 649–659, 1989.

54. Burckardt, C.B., Hoffmann, H., and Grandchamp, P.A., Ultrasound axicon: a device for focusing over a large depth, *J. Acoust. Soc. Am.*, 54, 1628–1630, 1973.

55. McLeod, J.H., The axicon: a new type of optical element, *J. Opt. Soc. Am.*, 44, 592–597, 1954.

56. Patterson, M.S., and Foster, F.S., Acoustic fields of conical radiators, *IEEE Trans. Sonics Ultrasonics*, SU-29, 83–92, 1982.

57. Patterson, M.S., *The Application of Axicon Transducers to Medical Ultrasound Imaging*, PhD thesis, University of Toronto, 1984.

58. Dietz, D.R., Apodixed conical focusing for ultrasound imaging, *IEEE Trans. Sonics Ultrasonics*, SU-29, 128–138, 1982.

59. Lasota, H., Salamon, R., and Delannoy, B., Acoustic diffraction analysis by the impulse response method: a line impulse response approach, *J. Acoust. Soc. Am.*, 76, 280–290, 1984.

60. von Stenzel, H., Die akustische strahlung der rechteckigen kolbenmembran, *Acustica*, 2, 263–281, 1952.

61. San Emeterio, J.L., and Ullate, L.G., Diffraction impulse response of rectangular transducers, *J. Acoust. Soc. Am.*, 92, 651–662, 1992.

62. Turnbull, D.H., and Foster, F.S., Beam steering with pulsed two-dimensional transducer arrays, *IEEE Trans. Ultrason. Ferroelect. Freq. Contr.*, 38, 320–333, 1991.

63. von Haselberg, K., and Krautkramer, J., Ein ultraschall-strahler fur die werkstoffprufung mit verbessertem nahfeld, *Acustica*, 9, 359–364, 1959.

64. Du, G., and Breazeale, M.A., The ultrasonic field of a Gaussian transducer, *J. Acoust. Soc. Am.*, 76, 2083–2088, 1985.

65. Hsu, D.K., Margeten, F.J., Hasselbusch, M.D., Wormley, S.J., Hughes, M.S., and Thompson, D.O., Technique for nonuniform poling of piezoelectric element and fabrication of Gaussian transducers, *IEEE Trans. Ultrason. Ferroelect. Freq. Contr.*, 37, 404–410, 1990.

66. Ziomek, L.J., *Fundamentals of Acoustic Field Theory and Space-Time Signal Processing*, CRC Press, Boca Raton, FL, 1995.

67. Greenspan, M., Piston radiator: some extensions of the theory, *J. Acoust. Soc. Am.*, 65, 608–621, 1979.

68. King, L.V., On the acoustic radiation field of the piezo-electric oscillator and the effect of viscosity on transmission, *Can. J. Res.*, 11, 135–155, 1934.

69. Bouwkamp, C.J., A contribution to the theory of acoustic radiation, *Philips Res. Reports*, 1, 251–277, 1945/46.

70. Filipczynski, L., and Etienne, J., Theoretical study and experiments on spherical focusing transducers with Gaussian surface velocity distribution, *Acustica*, 28, 121–128, 1973.

71. Bateman, H., *The Mathematical Analysis of Electrical and Optical Wave-Motion on the Basis of Maxwell's Equations*, Cambridge University Press, Cambridge, 1915.

72. Abramowitz, M, and Stegun, I.A. (Eds.), *Handbook of Mathematical Functions*, Dover, New York, 1965.

73. Donnelly, R., and Ziolkowski, R.W., A method for constructing solutions of homogeneous partial differential equations: localized waves, *Proc. Roy. Soc. Lond. A*, 437, 673–692, 1992.

74. Donnelly, R., Ziolkowski, R.W., Designing localized waves, *Proc. Roy. Soc. Lond. A*, 440, 541–563, 1993.

75. Li, G., and Bharath, A.A., Numeric study of limited diffraction, bandlimited, acoustic waves: a novel solution family of the homogeneous scalar wave equation, *Wave Motion*, 28, 203–213, 1998.

76. Durnin, J., Exact solutions for nondiffracting beams. I. The scalar theory, *J. Opt. Soc. Am. A*, 4, 651–654, 1987.

77. Durnin, J., Miceli, J.J., and Eberly, J.H., Diffraction-free beams, *Phys. Rev. Lett.* 58, 1499–1501, 1987.

78. Stratton, J.A., *Electromagnetic Theory*, McGraw-Hill, New York, 1941.

79. Brittingham, J.N., Focus wave modes in Maxwell's equations: transverse electric mode, *J. Appl. Phys.*, 54, 1179–1189, 1983.

80. Ziolkowski, R.W., Exact solutions of the wave equation with complex source locations, *J. Math. Phys.*, 26, 861–863, 1985.

81. Karpelson, A., Possibilities of forming narrow weakly divergent ultrasonic beams, *Sov. J. NDT*, No. 5, 10–18, 1988 [in Russian].

82. Karpelson, A., Ultrasonic piezotransducer that forms a specified directivity pattern, *Sov. J. NDT*, No. 7, 496–502, 1988 [in Russian].

83. Hsu, D.K., Margeten, F.J., and Thompson, D.O., Bessel beam ultrasonic transducer: fabrication method and experimental results, *Appl. Phys. Lett.*, 55, 2066–2068, 1989.

84. Campbell, J.A., and Soloway, S., Generation of a nondiffracting beam with frequency-independent beamwidth, *J. Acoust. Soc. Am.*, 88, 2467–2477, 1990.

85. Holm, S., Bessel and conical beams and approximations with annular arrays, *IEEE Trans. Ultrason. Ferroelect. Freq. Contr.*, 45, 712–718, 1998.

86. Sushilov, N.V., Tavakkoli, J., and Cobbold, R.S.C., New X-wave solutions of free-space scalar wave equation and their finite size realization, *IEEE Trans. Ultrason. Ferroelect. Freq. Contr.*, 48, 274–284, 2001.

87. Lu, J-Y., and Greenleaf, J.F., Ultrasonic nondiffracting transducer for medical imaging, *IEEE Trans. Ultrason. Ferroelect. Freq. Contr.*, 37, 438–447, 1990.

88. Lu, J-Y., and Greenleaf, J.F., Producing deep depth of field and depth-independent resolution in NDE with limited diffraction beams, *Ultrasonic Imaging*, 15, 134–149, 1993.

89. Lu, J-Y., and Greenleaf, J.F., Nondiffracting X waves: exact solutions to free-space scalar wave equation and their finite aperture realizations, *IEEE Trans. Ultrason. Ferroelect. Freq. Contr.*, 39, 19–31, 1992.

90. Donnelly, R., Power, D., Templeman, G., and Whalen, A., Graphical simulation of superluminal acoustic localized wave pulses, *IEEE Trans. Ultrason. Ferroelect. Freq. Contr.*, 41, 7–12, 1994.

91. Gradshteyn, I.M., and Ryzhik, I.M., *Table of Integrals, Series, and Products*, 4th edn., Academic Press, New York, 1980.

92. Lu, J-Y., and Greenleaf, J.F., Experimental verification of nondiffracting X-waves, *IEEE Trans. Ultrason. Ferroelect. Freq. Contr.*, 39, 441–446, 1992.

93. Sushilov, N.V., Tavakkoli, J., and Cobbold, R.S.C., Propagation of limited-diffraction X-waves in dissipative media, *IEEE Trans. Ultrason. Ferroelect. Freq. Contr.*, 49, 75–82, 2002.

94. Bamber, J.C., Attenuation and absorption, Ch. 4 in: *Physical Principles of Medical Diagnosis*, 2nd edn., C.R. Hill, J.C. Bamber, and G.R. ter Haar (Eds.), Wiley, Chichester, UK, 2004.

95. Wells, P.N.T., *Biomedical Ultrasonics,* Academic Press, New York, 1977.

96. Ginzberg, V.L., Concerning the general relationship between absorption and dispersion of sound waves, *Soviet Physics Acoustics*, 1, 32–41, 1955.

97. Futerman, W.I., Dispersive body waves, *J. Geophysical Res.*, 67, 5279–5291, 1962.

98. O'Donnell, M., Jaynes, E.T., and Miller, J.G., Kramers-Kronig relationship between ultrasonic attenuation and phase velocity, *J. Acoust. Soc. Am.*, 69, 696–701, 1981.

99. Weaver, R.L., and Pao, Y-H, Dispersion relations for linear wave propagation in homogeneous and inhomogeneous media, *J. Math. Phys.*, 22, 1909–1918, 1981.

100. Waters, K.R., Hughes, M.S., Mobley, J., Brandenburger, G.H., and Miller, J.G., On the applicability of Kramers-Kronig relations for ultrasonic attenuation obeying a frequency power law, *J. Acoust. Soc. Am.*, 108, 556–563, 2000.

101. Waters, K.R., Hughes, M.S., Brandenburger, G.H., and Miller, J.G., On a time-domain representation of the Kramers-Kronig dispersion relations, *J. Acoust. Soc. Am.*, 108, 2114–2119, 2000.

102. Szabo, T.L., Causal theories and data for acoustic attenuation obeying a frequency power law, *J. Acoust. Soc. Am.*, 97, 14–24, 1995.

103. Szabo, T.L., Time domain wave equations for lossy media obeying a frequency power law, *J. Acoust. Soc. Am.*, 96, 491–500, 1994.

104. Sushilov, N.V., Tavakkoli, J., and Cobbold, R.S.C., Propagation of limited-diffraction X-waves in dissipative media, *IEEE Trans. Ultrason. Ferroelect. Freq. Contr.*, 49, 675–682, 2002.

105. Sushilov, N.V., and Cobbold, R.S.C., Frequency-domain wave equation and its time-domain solutions in attenuating media, *J. Acoust. Soc. Am.*, 115, 1431–1436, 2004.

106. Jensen, J.A., Gandhi, D., and O'Brien, W.D., Ultrasound fields in an attenuating medium, pp. 943–946 in: *1993 IEEE Ultrasonics Symp. Proc.*, 1994.

107. Stokes, G.G., On the theories of the internal friction of fluids in motion, and of the equilibrium and motion of elastic solids, *Trans. Cambridge Phil. Soc.*, 8, 287–319, 1845.

108. Hanin, M., Propagation of an aperiodic wave in a compressible viscous medium, *J. Math. Phys.*, 37, 234–249, 1957.

109. Ludwig, R., and Levin, P.L., Analytical and numerical treatment of pulsed wave propagation into a viscous fluid, *IEEE Trans. Ultrasonics, Ferroelect. Freq. Contr.*, 42, 789–792, 1995.

110. Blackstock, D.T., Transient solution for sound radiated into a viscous fluid, *J. Acoust. Soc. Am.*, 41, 1312–1319, 1967.

111. Cobbold, R.S.C., Sushilov, N.V., and Weathermon, A.C., Transient propagation in media with classical or power-law loss, *J. Acoust. Soc. Am.*, 116, 3294–3303, 2004.

112. Gurumurthy, K.V., and Arthur, R.M., A dispersive model for the propagation of ultrasound in soft tissue, *Ultrasonic Imaging*, 4, 355–377, 1982.

113. Kuc, R., Modeling acoustic attenuation of soft tissue with a minimum-phase filter, *Ultrasonic Imaging*, 6, 24–36, 1984.

114. Davidovich, L.A., Makhkamov, S., Pulatova, L., Khabibullaev, P.K., and Khaliulin, M.G., Acoustic properties of certain organic liquids at frequencies 0.3 to 3 GHz, *Soviet Physics Acoustics*, 18, 264–266, 1972.

115. Leeman, S., Ultrasound pulse propagation in dispersive media, *Phys. Med. Biol.*, 25, 481–488, 1980.

116. Leeman, S., Hutchins, L., and Jones, J.P., Pulse scattering in dispersive media, pp. 139–147 in: *Acoustical Imaging*, Vol. 11, J. P. Powers (Ed.), Plenum Press, New York, 1982.

117. Nachman, A.I., Smith, J.F., and Waag, R.C., An equation for acoustic propagation in inhomogeneous media with relaxation losses, *J. Acoust. Soc. Am.*, 88, 1584–1595, 1990.

118. Berkhoff, A.P., Thijssen, J.M., and Homan, R.J.F., Simulation of ultrasonic imaging with linear arrays in causal absorptive media, *Ultrasound Med. Biol.*, 22, 245–259, 1996.

119. Jongen, H.A.H., Thijssen, J.M., van den Aarssen, M., and Verhoef, W.A., A general model for the absorption of ultrasound by biological tissues and experimental verification, *J. Acoust. Soc. Am.*, 79, 535–540, 1986.

4

Nonlinear Ultrasonics

Up to this point, it has generally been assumed that the excitation is sufficiently small so that linearity can be assumed. In practice, for both ultrasound diagnostic and therapeutic applications, this condition is frequently exceeded. For diagnostic applications where a short, high-amplitude transmit pulse is used to obtain good resolution and sensitivity, the amplitude is often sufficiently large that nonlinear effects become apparent [7–9]. As will be discussed in Chapter 8 (section 8.6), the presence of nonlinearity in B-mode imaging enables harmonic imaging to be achieved with the potential advantage of improved spatial resolution [10]. In therapeutic use, such as in lithotripsy, where a shock wave is generated near the focal zone for the purpose of kidney stone fragmentation, a high degree of nonlinearity occurs in the propagation process, especially as the wavefront approaches the focal zone. Similarly, when high-intensity focused ultrasound is used to raise the temperature of a localized zone, nonlinear effects often become important. Further details of the biomedical aspects of nonlinear ultrasound are contained in the reviews by Carstensen and Bacon [11] and Duck [12]. A number of excellent books and chapters devoted to nonlinear acoustics provide a much more detailed account at both the advanced and introductory levels [1–6].

4.1 Introduction

In his classic chapter on the propagation of finite amplitude acoustic waves in viscous media, Lighthill [13] points out that there are two influences at work that tend to change the shape of a waveform as it propagates. The first concerns the effect of a frequency-dependent attenuation. This was discussed in Chapter 1 (subsection 1.8.1) in the context of linear propagation theory and typically causes a down-shift in the transmitted center frequency. The second arises from a combination of the effects of changes in the speed of propagation and the effects of convection (see section 4.4). Because the speed with which a wave propagates varies with the density of the medium, it propagates faster during the compression phase and diminishes during rarefaction. This causes portions of the waveform to become steeper as the wave progress, resulting in the generation of higher harmonics. Because the medium moves in the direction of wave propagation during compression and in the opposite direction during expansion, the propagating wave is also convected. This causes waveform distortion similar to that created by the speed variation. Both of these nonlinear effects can lead to the formation of a shock wave, depending on the attenuation characteristics of the medium.

Incorporating the effects of nonlinearity into the propagation process makes the theoretical analysis[1] a good deal more complex, and as a result it is usually necessary to make certain simplifying approximations to arrive at algorithms that enable computational evaluation to be carried out in a reasonable time. When the pressure is sufficiently high that the effects of nonlinearity dominate, a shock wave can form. For example, such a wave is characterized by an abrupt change in the pressure and density. Shock waves can form, for example, in the focal zone region of a lithotripsy system, and they provide the means for disintegrating the kidney stone. An exact analysis is made particularly difficult when the effects of attenuation and diffraction are incorporated. In this chapter we shall begin by examining the propagation of finite-amplitude plane waves in an ideal nonlinear fluid, and we will study the changes that occur in the particle velocity, density, and pressure during this process.

4.2 Lagrangian and Eulerian Coordinate Systems

In previous chapters it was generally assumed that the amplitudes of the variables were sufficiently small compared to their undisturbed values that nonlinear propagation effects could be ignored. When this approximation is no longer valid, it is helpful to express the equations in terms of a coordinate system that tracks the behavior of a particular acoustic particle rather than by using a fixed coordinate that describes what happens at a specific location. As first explained in Chapter 1, an equation is said to have the *Lagrangian* form when it describes what happens to a particular acoustic particle. For example, the Lagrangian form of the expression for acoustic velocity describes how the velocity of a particle varies with time. This should be contrasted with the fixed (*Eulerian* or laboratory) coordinate system, in which the velocity at a specific location is described. To avoid possible confusion, we shall begin by discussing

---

1. A valuable historical account that also serves as a useful introduction to the field has been written by Blackstock [14].

the relation between these two systems, and this will be based on the very clear presentation given in the paper by Lee and Wang [15].

For an incident plane wave, the displacements can be examined by using a 1-D sequence of acoustic particles to represent the elements of volume. In Fig. 4.1a, the equilibrium positions of particles A and B are denoted by a_A and a_B. The presence of an acoustic wave will cause the positions of A and B to change and, as shown in Fig. 4.1b, at a particular instant of time t their positions are $X_A(t) = a_A + \xi_A(t)$ and $X_B(t) = a_B + \xi_B(t)$, where ξ is the displacement. In general, the position of any particle can be written as $X(a\!:\!t) = a + \xi(a\!:\!t)$, in which the independent variables a and t are called the *Lagrangian coordinates*. If field quantities such as the particle velocity or pressure are expressed in terms of these variables, then the resulting expressions correspond to the Lagrangian form. Field quantities, when expressed in Lagrangian coordinates, will be distinguished from the Eulerian form through the use of a subscript L. For example, the particle velocity is given by $v_L(a,t) = \partial X(a\!:\!t)/\partial t = \partial \xi(a\!:\!t)/\partial t$. The Eulerian velocity will be simply denoted by $v(x\!:\!t)$, without the use of a subscript.

It is useful to relate the field quantities expressed in one coordinate system to those of the other. If the field quantity is denoted by q, then $q_L(a\!:\!t)$ can be related to the Eulerian form $q(x\!:\!t)$ by using a Taylor series expansion and retaining just the lowest-order term in ξ, i.e.,

$$q_L(a\!:\!t) = q(x\!:\!t)\big|_{x = a + \xi(a\!:\!t)} \approx q(a\!:\!t) + \frac{\partial q}{\partial x}\bigg|_{x=a} \xi(a\!:\!t).$$

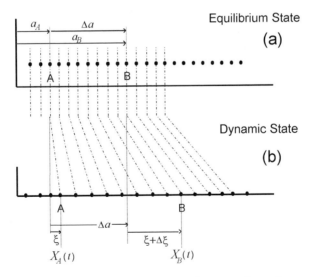

Figure 4.1 Illustrating how the acoustic particles (representing volume elements) move for an incident plane wave. (a) Under equilibrium (unperturbed) conditions, particles A and B are separated by Δa. (b) In the presence of a plane wave and at a particular instant of time, particle A has been displaced from its equilibrium by ξ and particle B by $\xi + \Delta\xi$. The volume between A and B is shown as having increased (corresponding to a reduction in pressure), so that the density would be decreased.

Similarly, the Eulerian form can be written as

$$q(x{:}t) = q_L(a{:}t)\big|_{a=x-\xi(a{:}t)} \approx q_L(x{:}t) - \frac{\partial q_L}{\partial a}\bigg|_{a=x} \xi(x{:}t).$$

For example, with the help of the above equations, the particle velocity relations can be written as:

$$v_L(a{:}t) = v(a{:}t) + \frac{\partial v}{\partial x}\bigg|_{x=a} \xi(a{:}t) \quad \text{and} \quad v(x{:}t) = v_L(x{:}t) - \frac{\partial v_L}{\partial a}\bigg|_{a=x} \xi(x{:}t).$$

4.2.1 Density in Terms of Displacement

To obtain a wave equation in Lagrangian coordinates, we shall need to express the Lagrangian density in terms of the particle displacement. In Fig. 4.1a, the volume associated with each particle is the volume between successive parallel planes normal to the x-axis. If the y-z area is $dydz$, then the *equilibrium* volume associated with the particles that lie between A and B is $\Delta V_o = \Delta a dydz$, which in the limit as $\Delta a \to 0$ can be written as $dV_o = da dydz$. At a time t in the presence of a plane wave (see Fig. 4.1b), the volume changes to $\Delta V(t) = (\Delta \xi + \Delta a)dydz$, which in the limit as $\Delta a \to 0$ can be expressed as $dV(t) = da\left(1 + \frac{\partial \xi}{\partial a}\right)dydz$. But, since the mass between two planes remains constant and the y- and z-dimensions are unchanged, $\rho_o dV_o = \rho_L dV(t)$ and hence

$$\rho_o dadydz = \rho_L da\left(1 + \frac{\partial \xi}{\partial a}\right)dydz,$$

yielding

(4.1)
$$\rho_L = \rho_o\left(1 + \frac{\partial \xi}{\partial a}\right)^{-1}$$

Alternatively, noting that $dX = da + \frac{\partial \xi}{\partial a}da$, this can also be written as

(4.2)
$$\rho_L = \rho_o\left(\frac{dX}{da}\right)^{-1}.$$

4.3 Exact 1-D Wave Equation for an Inviscid Medium

The Lagrangian form of the 1-D momentum equation can be readily derived[2] by noting that the force per unit area acting on a plane at X is equal to the

2. The 3-D form of the momentum equation was previously derived in Chapter 1 as (1.19), from which the 1-D form could have been written down. However, because the 1-D form can be so readily derived, we have chosen to do this.

Lagrangian pressure p_L, while that acting on a plane at $X + \delta X$ is $p_L + \delta X(\partial p_L/\partial X)$. Consequently, the net force acting in the positive x-direction on this unit area incremental volume is equal to $-\delta X(\partial p_L/\partial X)$. Because the element has a mass of $\rho_L \delta X$ and its Lagrangian acceleration is $\partial^2 \xi/\partial t^2$, it follows from Newton's law that

(4.3)
$$\boxed{\rho_L \frac{\partial^2 \xi}{\partial t^2} = -\frac{\partial p_L}{\partial X}}.$$

In view of (4.2), this can be written as:

$$\rho_o \frac{\partial^2 \xi}{\partial t^2} = -\frac{\partial p_L}{\partial a}.$$

Because it can be assumed that p_L is a function only of ρ_L, it follows that

(4.4)
$$\rho_o \frac{\partial^2 \xi}{\partial t^2} = -\frac{\partial p_L}{\partial \rho_L} \frac{\partial \rho_L}{\partial a}.$$

Taking the partial derivative of (4.2) yields $\dfrac{\partial \rho_L}{\partial a} = -\rho_o \left(1 + \dfrac{\partial \xi}{\partial a}\right)^{-2} \dfrac{\partial^2 \xi}{\partial a^2}$, which can then be substituted into (4.4) to give

(4.5)
$$\boxed{\frac{\partial^2 \xi}{\partial t^2} = \frac{\partial p_L}{\partial \rho_L} \left(1 + \frac{\partial \xi}{\partial a}\right)^{-2} \frac{\partial^2 \xi}{\partial a^2}}.$$

This is an "exact" wave equation for an inviscid uniform medium for finite-amplitude disturbances due to a plane wave. It describes the time behavior of a particle whose equilibrium position is a in terms of its displacement, density, and pressure.

It should be noted that for small-displacement amplitudes, such that $1 \gg \partial \xi/\partial a$, it is unnecessary to distinguish between a and x; consequently, (4.5) reduces to the 1-D wave equation for an inviscid medium under small-signal conditions:

(4.6)
$$\frac{\partial^2 \xi}{\partial t^2} = c_o^2 \frac{\partial^2 \xi}{\partial x^2},$$

where $c_o^2 = \dfrac{\partial p}{\partial \rho}\bigg|_S$ is defined to be the small-signal speed of sound under isentropic conditions.

4.3.1 Exact Equation for an Adiabatic Gas

We shall assume that the propagation medium is an ideal gas whose equation of state under adiabatic conditions is

(4.7)
$$\frac{p}{p_o} = \left(\frac{\rho}{\rho_o}\right)^\gamma,$$

where γ is the ratio of the specific heats. This relation applies in both Eulerian and Lagrangian coordinate systems. Thus, under adiabatic conditions, the partial derivatives give

$$(4.8) \qquad \left.\frac{\partial p}{\partial \rho}\right|_s = \left.\frac{\partial p_L}{\partial \rho_L}\right|_s = \frac{\gamma p_o}{\rho_o}\left(\frac{\rho}{\rho_o}\right)^{\gamma-1} = c_o^2\left(1+\frac{\partial \xi}{\partial a}\right)^{1-\gamma},$$

in which $c_o = \sqrt{\gamma p_o/\rho_o}$ is the small-signal adiabatic speed and the right-hand side results from using (4.2). By substituting (4.8) into the wave equation as given by (4.5) yields

$$(4.9) \qquad \boxed{\frac{\partial^2 \xi}{\partial t^2} = c_o^2\left(1+\frac{\partial \xi}{\partial a}\right)^{-(\gamma+1)}\frac{\partial^2 \xi}{\partial a^2}.}$$

This is an "exact" form of the wave equation for a perfect gas.

4.3.2 First Integral of Exact Wave Equation

To obtain the first partial integral of (4.9), we shall follow the procedure used by Earnshaw [24] in his classic paper of 1859. Specifically, we shall tentatively assume that the Lagrangian particle velocity v_L ($= \partial X/\partial t = \partial \xi/\partial t$) can be expressed as a function of $\partial \xi/\partial a$, i.e.,

$$(4.10) \qquad \boxed{\partial \xi/\partial t = F\left(\frac{\partial \xi}{\partial a}\right).}$$

Differentiating this first with respect to t and then with respect to a yields the following two equations:

$$(4.11) \qquad \frac{\partial^2 \xi}{\partial t^2} = \frac{\partial^2 \xi}{\partial a \partial t}F'\left(\frac{\partial \xi}{\partial a}\right), \quad \frac{\partial^2 \xi}{\partial a \partial t} = \frac{\partial^2 \xi}{\partial a^2}F'\left(\frac{\partial \xi}{\partial a}\right),$$

resulting in

$$\frac{\partial^2 \xi}{\partial t^2} = \left[F'\left(\frac{\partial \xi}{\partial a}\right)\right]^2\frac{\partial^2 \xi}{\partial a^2}.$$

If this is compared to (4.9), it can be seen that the assumed form of (4.10) is valid provided

$$(4.12) \qquad F'\left(\frac{\partial \xi}{\partial a}\right) = \pm c_o\left(1+\frac{\partial \xi}{\partial a}\right)^{\frac{-(\gamma+1)}{2}},$$

and consequently (4.10) is a partial first integral of (4.9).

By integrating (4.12) and noting (4.10), the particle velocity can then be obtained as

$$v_L = F\left(\frac{\partial \xi}{\partial a}\right) = C_1 \mp \frac{2c_o}{\gamma - 1}\left(1 + \frac{\partial \xi}{\partial a}\right)^{\frac{1-\gamma}{2}}.$$

The integration constant C_1 can be found by first observing that if $v_L = 0$, then the Lagrangian particle density $\rho_L = \rho_o$, and thus by using (4.2), we find that $C_1 = \pm 2c_o/(\gamma - 1)$, yielding

(4.13)
$$v_L = F\left(\frac{\partial \xi}{\partial a}\right) = \pm \frac{2c_o}{\gamma - 1}\left[1 - \left(1 + \frac{\partial \xi}{\partial a}\right)^{\frac{1-\gamma}{2}}\right].$$

Alternatively, this can be written in terms of the pressure, by making use of (4.1) and substituting into the adiabatic gas law (4.7), yielding

(4.14)
$$\frac{p_L}{p_o} = \left[1 \mp \frac{(\gamma - 1)v_L}{2c_o}\right]^{\frac{2\gamma}{\gamma - 1}}.$$

4.4 Wave Propagation Speed in a Gas

The propagation speed of a wave can be defined as the rate at which any given phase point on the wave propagates. For example, the speed can be found by determining the rate at which a specific value of the particle velocity, pressure, or density is propagated. We shall do this for a gas under adiabatic conditions by first determining the Lagrangian wave propagation speed and, from this, the Eulerian speed [17, pp. 177–186].

Consider two acoustic particles separated by a known distance. The Lagrangian speed can be found by determining the time taken for a specific value of the Lagrangian particle velocity v_L to occur on the second particle after it occurred on the first. Since v_L is a function of a and t, we can write the total differential relation as

$$dv_L = (\partial v_L / \partial t)dt + (\partial v_L / \partial a)da.$$

The condition $dv_L = 0$ corresponds to the same acoustic particle velocity v_L being transmitted from the particle at a to that at $a + da$ in a time interval of dt. Consequently, Lagrangian wave propagation speed is given by

(4.15)
$$\left.\frac{da}{dt}\right|_{v_L = \text{const.}} = -\left(\frac{\partial v_L}{\partial t} \bigg/ \frac{\partial v_L}{\partial a}\right).$$

But (4.11) and (4.12) state $\dfrac{\partial v_L}{\partial t} = \dfrac{\partial v_L}{\partial a} F'\left(\dfrac{\partial \xi}{\partial a}\right)$, and $F'\left(\dfrac{\partial \xi}{\partial a}\right) = \pm c_o\left(1 + \dfrac{\partial \xi}{\partial a}\right)^{-(\gamma+1)/2}$,

so that (4.15) reduces to

(4.16)
$$\left.\frac{da}{dt}\right|_{v_L=\text{const.}} = \mp c_o\left(1+\frac{\partial\xi}{\partial a}\right)^{-(\gamma+1)/2},$$

Making use of (4.1) to express this equation in terms of the Lagrangian density and denoting the Lagrangian wave propagation speed by C_L, we obtain

(4.17)
$$C_L = \pm c_o\left(1+\frac{\partial\xi}{\partial a}\right)^{-(\gamma+1)/2} = \pm c_o\left(\frac{\rho_L}{\rho_o}\right)^{(\gamma+1)/2}.$$

It should be noted that C_L^2 is exactly equal to the coefficient of $(\partial^2\xi/\partial a^2)$ in (4.9), so that the exact wave equation is identical in form to the small-signal equation, except that C_L is no longer a constant. The Lagrangian speed can also be expressed in terms of the Lagrangian particle velocity by substituting (4.13) into (4.17), yielding

(4.18)
$$C_L = \mp c_o\left(1\mp\frac{\gamma-1}{2c_o}v_L\right)^{\frac{\gamma+1}{\gamma-1}}.$$

To obtain the Eulerian speed [17, pp. 177–186], the total change in $x\ (= a+\xi)$ can be expressed as

$$dx = \frac{\partial(a+\xi)}{\partial a}da + \frac{\partial(a+\xi)}{\partial t}dt = \left(1+\frac{\partial\xi}{\partial a}\right)da + \frac{\partial\xi}{\partial t}dt,$$

or

(4.19)
$$\left.\frac{dx}{dt}\right|_{v=\text{const.}} = \left(1+\frac{\partial\xi}{\partial a}\right)\left.\frac{da}{dt}\right|_{v_L=\text{const.}} + \frac{\partial\xi}{\partial t}.$$

By substituting (4.16) and (4.8) into (4.19), noting that $v_L = \partial\xi/\partial t$, and observing that the difference between v_L and v is small, the Eulerian wave speed can be expressed as

$$C_E(t) = \left.\frac{dx}{dt}\right|_{v=\text{const.}} = \mp\left(\frac{\partial p}{\partial\rho}\right)^{1/2} + v(t) = \mp c_o\left(\frac{\rho}{\rho_o}\right)^{\frac{\gamma-1}{2}} + v(t).$$

Alternatively, by making use of (4.13) and (4.16), (4.19) can also be expressed as

(4.20)
$$C_E = \mp c_o + \frac{\gamma+1}{2}v(t).$$

It therefore follows that for an observer at a fixed location, the speed with which the wave propagates fluctuates about c_o and will vary spatially, as illustrated in Fig. 4.2. Moreover, an observer moving with a speed of c_o, instead of seeing a constant density, will see changes in the density that vary in time and that depend on the excitation amplitude.

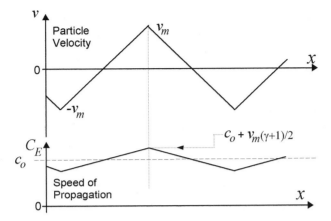

Figure 4.2 Variation in the speed of propagation versus distance for an triangular particle velocity waveform.

4.4.1 Why Does the Speed Vary?

If isothermal conditions exist and the medium obeys Boyle's law, the pressure/density relation will be linear. The Lagrangian and Eulerian speed equations can then be obtained by putting $\gamma = 1$ in (4.18) and (4.20), and these are listed in Table 4.1 for outgoing waves (positive x-direction). Evidently, since different parts of a given waveform move at different speeds, waveform distortion occurs. In the case of propagation under isothermal conditions, the speed is modulated by the particle velocity in a simple additive manner. At a fixed point in space, during times when there are positive particle velocities the speed is increased, while during the times of negative velocities the speed is diminished. This suggests that the wave is transported by the particle motion, i.e., it is convected, and is generally referred to as the *convection* contribution to the nonlinear propagation. The expression for the speed in Lagrangian coordinates under isothermal propagation conditions depends on the particle density: the denser the region, the greater the speed, and vice

Table 4.1. Wave Propagation Speeds in Ideal Gases for Isothermal and Adiabatic Conditions

	Isothermal	Adiabatic
Coordinate System	$\dfrac{p}{p_o} = \dfrac{\rho}{\rho_o}$	$\dfrac{p}{p_o} = \left(\dfrac{\rho}{\rho_o}\right)^{\gamma}$
Lagrangian	$C_L = c_o \dfrac{\rho_L}{\rho_o}$	$C_L = c_o \left(\dfrac{\rho_L}{\rho_o}\right)^{\frac{\gamma+1}{2}} = c_o \left(1 + \dfrac{\gamma-1}{2c_o} v_L\right)^{\frac{\gamma+1}{\gamma-1}}$
Eulerian	$C_E = c_o + v$	$C_E = c_o + \dfrac{\gamma+1}{2} v = c_o + v + \dfrac{\gamma-1}{2} v$

versa. Thus, for example, a specific value of pressure takes less time to move through a crowded portion of the medium than through a portion that is less crowded.

Under adiabatic conditions the Eulerian speed has been written in two forms, the second of which indicates that the propagation speed is modulated by the effects of both *convection* and the *nonlinearity of the medium*. The non-linearity of the medium refers to the nonlinear pressure/density relation, which is present for an adiabatic gas as well as for most fluids. In the case of a gas such as air, $\gamma = 1.4$, and consequently the ratio of the nonlinearity of the medium to that of convection is $(\gamma - 1)/2 = 0.2$, i.e., the convective effect dominates. However, for liquids, as will be seen, the reverse is generally true, so that the nonlinearity of the medium dominates the change in propagation speed with the particle velocity.

4.4.2 Coefficient of Nonlinearity and Parameter of Nonlinearity for Liquids and Gases

In the above analysis, the pressure/density relation has been assumed to be that of an ideal gas, under either isothermal or adiabatic conditions. For liquids, the pressure/density relation can be written as $p = p(\rho,s)$, where $p = p_o + p_1$ and $\rho = \rho_o + \rho_1$. The subscripts refer to the equilibrium and excess values, respectively, and s is the entropy. A Taylor series expansion leads to

$$(4.21) \quad p_1 = \left.\frac{\partial p}{\partial \rho}\right|_0 \rho_1 + \frac{1}{2!}\left.\frac{\partial^2 p}{\partial \rho^2}\right|_0 \rho_1^2 + \ldots = A\frac{\rho_1}{\rho_o} + \frac{B}{2!}\left(\frac{\rho_1}{\rho_o}\right)^2 + \frac{C}{3!}\left(\frac{\rho_1}{\rho_o}\right)^3 + \ldots$$

where $\quad A = \rho_o\left.\frac{\partial p}{\partial \rho}\right|_0, B = \rho_o^2\left.\frac{\partial^2 p}{\partial \rho^2}\right|_0, C = \rho_o^3\left.\frac{\partial^3 p}{\partial \rho^3}\right|_0 + \ldots$

and the subscript 0 indicates that the partial derivatives are evaluated at the equilibrium density, pressure, and entropy. In the above it should be noted that $A = \rho_o(\partial p/\partial \rho)|_0 = \rho_o c_o^2$, where c_o is the small-signal adiabatic speed of sound.

Now, (4.7) for an adiabatic gas can be written as: $1 + p_1/p_o = (1 + \rho_1/\rho_o)^\gamma$, which can be expanded as

$$(4.22) \quad p_1 = p_o\left[\gamma\frac{\rho_1}{\rho_o} + \frac{\gamma(\gamma - 1)}{2!}\left(\frac{\rho_1}{\rho_o}\right)^2 + \frac{\gamma(\gamma - 1)(\gamma - 2)}{3!}\left(\frac{\rho_1}{\rho_o}\right)^3 + \cdots\right].$$

By comparing (4.22) term by term with (4.21), it can be seen that: $c_o = \sqrt{\gamma p_o/\rho_o}$, $B/A = \gamma - 1$, and $C/A = (\gamma - 1)(\gamma - 2)$. The first-order measure of nonlinearity, B/A, is the *parameter of nonlinearity*, though it is often simply referred to as the B/A ratio. Using this parameter, the "exact" wave equation as given by (4.9) can now be expressed in a form that is approximate for liquids and is "exact" for gases by substituting $\gamma = B/A + 1$, yielding

(4.23)
$$\frac{\partial^2 \xi}{\partial t^2} = c_o^2 \left(1 + \frac{\partial \xi}{\partial a}\right)^{-(B/A+2)} \frac{\partial^2 \xi}{\partial a^2}.$$

Subsequent equations can similarly be re-expressed in terms of B/A. Specifically, from Table 4.1, the Eulerian propagation speed under adiabatic conditions can now be written as

(4.24)
$$C_E = c_o + v + \frac{B}{2A}v,$$

from which it can be seen that the ratio of the nonlinearity of the medium to the convective nonlinearity is simply $B/2A$. Generally, a *coefficient of nonlinearity* is introduced, defined by

(4.25)
$$\beta = 1 + \frac{B}{2A}$$

so that (4.24) can be written as

(4.26)
$$C_E = c_o + \beta v.$$

Note that for a linear medium, $\beta = 1$, which from (4.25) corresponds to $B/A = 0$.

The two most widely used methods for measuring the B/A ratio are the finite-amplitude and the thermodynamic methods. In the finite-amplitude method, the relative amplitude of the second harmonic is measured, and this can be shown to be related to B/A. On the other hand, the thermodynamic method makes use of an expansion of the B/A ratio in terms of both the change in speed of sound with hydrostatic pressure $(\partial c_o/\partial p)_T$ and with temperature $(\partial c_o/\partial T)_p$, both of which can be measured. Details for both measurement techniques have been described by Law et al. [20] for biological media. Listed in Table 4.2 are some representative values, but a much more complete tabulation is given in [21] and in Table 1.8 for biological media.

Table 4.2. Representative Values of the Nonlinearity Parameter, B/A

Substance	T, °C	c_o, m/s	B/A	Ref.
Distilled water	20	1482	5.0	[21]
Distilled water	30	1509	5.3	[20]
Glycerol	20	1923	8.8	[22]
Glycerol	30	1901	9.1	[22]
Whole beef liver	30	1573	6.5	[22]
Human breast fat	37	1436	9.6	[22]
Pig fatty tissue	30	1447	11.1	[20]
Pig whole blood	30	—	6.3	[23]

4.5 Reduced Equations

4.5.1 Exact Form

In considering 1-D small-signal waves, it was noted in section 1.4.2 that the general solution consisted of the superposition of outgoing and incoming waves, each of which are solutions to two reduced first-order equations for the velocity potential. For large-displacement amplitudes, the reduced wave equation in Eulerian coordinates for outgoing plane waves in a non-dissipative medium is [19, p. 67]

$$(4.27) \qquad \frac{\partial v}{\partial t} + (c_o + \beta v)\frac{\partial v}{\partial x} = 0.$$

This can be regarded as an extension of the linear reduced equation by making the propagation speed linearly dependent on the particle velocity, i.e., by replacing c_o by $(c_o + \beta v)$ as given by (4.26), thereby resulting in a nonlinear equation. Equation 4.27 is exact for an ideal gas and a very good approximation for most liquids [19, p. 67]. To determine the speed with which a given phase point propagates, this equation can be combined with the differential relation $dv = (\partial v/\partial t)dt + (\partial v/\partial x)dx$. Noting that for a given phase point, $dv = 0$, yields

$$\frac{dx}{dt}\bigg|_{v=\text{const}} = c_o + \beta v,$$

which shows that the propagation speed varies from point to point on the waveform.

Three different implicit forms of the solution to (4.27) will be considered. The first two can be expressed in the functional forms

$$(4.28) \qquad v = G\{x - (\beta v + c_o)t\}$$

and

$$(4.29) \qquad v = F\left\{t - \frac{x}{\beta v + c_o}\right\}.$$

That these are solutions can be verified by substitution into (4.27). The first form is the solution for an initial value problem in which the velocity is specified for all values of $x > 0$ at time $t = 0$, i.e., the boundary value $v(x,0) = G(x)$ is given. Even though Poisson obtained it for isothermal conditions, it is generally referred to as the Poisson solution. The second form, which is a modified form of the Poisson solution, is a boundary value solution since the velocity v is specified at a specific plane $(x = 0)$, i.e., $v(0; t) = F(t)$ is given. The third form of solution, as first described by Earnshaw [24] in 1860, is the solution to the classic piston problem in which a source consisting of a planar piston starts moving at $t = 0$. If the location of the piston face at any time t is given by $X(t)$, then Earnshaw's solution of (4.27) for outgoing waves is

(4.30)
$$v = \frac{\partial X(\varphi)}{\partial t} \mathcal{H}(c_o t - x),$$
(a)

where

$$\varphi = t - \frac{x - X(\varphi)}{\beta \partial X(\varphi)/\partial t + c_o}$$
(b)

and $\mathcal{H}(.)$ is the unit step function.

In the expression for φ, the term $X(\varphi)$ accounts for the fact that the piston face is a moving source whose location at a given time t generally differs from $x = 0$. In addition, it should be noted that φ is the time at which a specific value of the velocity left the piston face. For example, the leading edge of the velocity wave corresponds to $\varphi = 0$. If the piston displacement is small compared to x, then (4.30) reduces to (4.29), i.e., $\partial X(\varphi)/\partial t = F$.

4.5.2 Approximate Form: Quadratic Nonlinearity

An approximate reduced equation [27, pp. 46–47] can be obtained from the "exact" form by rearranging (4.27) as

(4.31)
$$\frac{\partial v}{\partial x} = \frac{-1}{c_o(1 + \beta v/c_o)} \frac{\partial v}{\partial t},$$

and then by assuming that $\beta v/c_o \ll 1$, yielding

(4.32)
$$\frac{\partial v}{\partial x} \approx \frac{-1(1 - \beta v/c_o)}{c_o} \frac{\partial v}{\partial t}.$$

An alternative and simpler form can be obtained by transforming to a retarded time coordinate system, (x', τ) in which $x' = x$ and $\tau = t - x/c_o$. Since the partial derivatives in (4.32) can be written as

$$\frac{\partial v}{\partial x} = \frac{\partial v}{\partial x'}\frac{\partial x'}{\partial x} + \frac{\partial v}{\partial \tau}\frac{\partial \tau}{\partial x} = \frac{\partial v}{\partial x'} - \frac{\partial v}{\partial \tau}\frac{1}{c_o}, \quad \text{and} \quad \frac{\partial v}{\partial t} = \frac{\partial v}{\partial x'}\frac{\partial x'}{\partial t} + \frac{\partial v}{\partial \tau}\frac{\partial \tau}{\partial t} = \frac{\partial v}{\partial \tau}$$

we find that the approximate equation describing the particle velocity in the new coordinate system $v(x', \tau) = v(x, \tau)$ is given by

(4.33)
$$\frac{\partial v}{\partial x} = \frac{\beta v}{c_o^2} \frac{\partial v}{\partial \tau}.$$

A solution to this is given by Blackstock [16] as

(4.34)
$$v(x, \tau) = G\{\tau + \beta vx/c_o^2\}.$$

4.6 Sinusoidal Excitation

4.6.1 Particle Velocity

Consider a 1-D piston whose displacement is given by $X(t) = X_o(1 - \cos \omega t)\mathcal{H}(t)$, i.e., the position of the piston face is at $x = 0$ at time $t = 0$ and has a total displacement of X_o. Consequently, for $t > 0$ the piston velocity is $\partial X(t)/\partial t = \omega X_o \sin(\omega t)\mathcal{H}(t)$, and from (4.30), the implicit solution is

$$(4.35) \quad v = \omega X_o \sin(\omega\varphi)\mathcal{H}(c_o t - x), \quad \text{where} \quad \varphi = t - \frac{x - X_o(1 - \cos \omega\varphi)}{\beta \omega X_o \sin \omega\varphi + c_o}.$$

From (4.27), it is evident that this solution is valid only up to times or distances where $\partial v/\partial x$ or $\partial v/\partial t$ remain finite.

As an example we consider the piston velocity and displacement waveforms shown in Fig. 4.3 for a lossless water-like medium. The spatial distribution of v, as calculated from (4.35), is plotted in Fig. 4.4a for the parameters given in the caption. Also shown is the small-signal spatial distribution of v, i.e., the peak velocity is many times less than c_o. The graph is a snapshot of the velocity distribution from the source location at $x \approx 0$ to the position where the slope becomes infinite. Since the piston movement is very small (~4 µm), the fact that the source location is moving could have been ignored in the calculation without incurring a significant error. It is clearly seen that those portions of the waveform that correspond to the higher particle velocities travel faster than the small-signal wave, while those with negative velocities travel slower. At the location where the slope becomes infinite, a shock wave forms

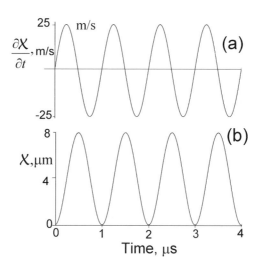

Figure 4.3 Velocity and displacement profile for an infinite plane piston source. (a) Sinusoidal velocity waveform that is initiated at $t = 0$, with an amplitude of 25 m/s. (b) Source displacement waveform.

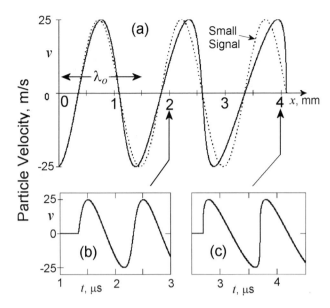

Figure 4.4 Particle velocity waveforms. (a) Snapshot view of sinusoidal wave propagation into a lossless water medium showing the nonlinear distortion of the particle velocity waveform as a function of distance from the source as calculated from (4.35) for the excitation waveform shown in Fig. 4.3. It was assumed that β = 3.5, c_o = 1500 m/s, and the following conditions at the piston: v_o = 25 m/s (X_o = 3.98 μm), f_o = 1.0 MHz (λ_o = 1.5 mm). The snapshot is at t = 2.73 μs, corresponding to the time at which the leading edge reaches 4.09 mm. Note that at $x \sim 4.09$ mm, $\partial v/\partial x \rightarrow -\infty$, corresponding to the development of a shock wave at the leading edge. The small-signal velocity is shown as the dashed curve. The graphs in (b) and (c) show the time waveforms at the spatial positions indicated in (a). In (c) the slope is nearly infinite at the leading edge.

consisting of a discontinuity in the pressure, density, and velocity. At the two indicated x-locations, the velocity waveforms are plotted as a function of time in Fig. 4.4b and c. These also clearly demonstrate the increasing harmonic distortion with distance from the source.

4.6.2 Pressure Distribution

To determine the pressure distribution, we can make use of the perfect gas relation between v and p, as given by (4.14). A binomial expansion of (4.14) yields to a second order in v

$$\frac{p + p_o}{p_o} \approx 1 \mp \frac{\gamma}{c_o} v + \frac{\gamma(\gamma + 1)}{4c_o^2} v^2,$$

where $p + p_o$ is the total instantaneous pressure. Since $p_o = \rho_o c_o^2/\gamma$, the pressure signal can be expressed as

$$p \approx \rho_o c_o^2 \left[\frac{v}{c_o} + \frac{(\gamma+1)}{4} \left(\frac{v}{c_o} \right)^2 \right]$$

It was previously noted that approximate expressions for a liquid can be obtained from those for an ideal gas by substituting $\beta = (\gamma + 1)/2$. Hence the pressure signal is

(4.36)
$$p \approx \rho_o c_o^2 \left[\frac{v}{c_o} + \frac{\beta}{2} \left(\frac{v}{c_o} \right)^2 \right],$$

which reduces to the usual small-signal impedance relation $p/v = \rho_o c_o$ if $v \ll 2c_o/\beta$. It can be seen from (4.36) that the pressure waveform deviates from the velocity waveform only if v becomes comparable to c_o. For the case considered in Fig. 4.4, the shape of the spatial pressure distribution is very similar to the velocity distribution, except that the pressure varies from +38.6 MPa to −36.4 MPa, i.e., the mean pressure is somewhat higher than p_o, and the small-signal peak pressures ($\rho_o c_o v_o$) of ±37.5 MPa lies between the two.

4.7 Harmonic Content

4.7.1 Inviscid Medium

For ultrasound transducers that make use of the piezoelectric effect, the source displacement is generally very small compared to a wavelength. With this assumption Fubini [25] obtained an explicit form for the steady-state Earnshaw solution [24]. Taking the sinusoidal piston excitation assumed earlier, namely $X(t) = X_o(1 - \cos \omega t)$, and assuming small piston displacements, the steady-state form of (4.35) is

(4.37)
$$v = v_o \sin(\omega\varphi),$$

where
$$\omega\varphi \approx \omega t - \frac{\omega x}{\beta v_o \sin \omega \varphi + c_o}$$

and in which $v_o = \omega X_o$ is the piston velocity amplitude. By assuming that $\beta v_o/c_o \ll 1$, the second term in the expression for $\omega\varphi$ can be expanded and higher-order terms can be neglected. This yields

$$\omega\varphi \approx \omega t - \frac{\omega x}{c_o} \left(1 - \frac{\beta v_o \sin \omega \varphi}{c_o} \right),$$

and consequently

(4.38)
$$v = v_o \sin \left[\omega t - \frac{\omega x}{c_o} (1 - \beta v/c_o) \right].$$

By expressing this in terms of the wave number $k = \omega/c_o$ and the shock formation distance $\bar{x} = c_o^2/(\beta \omega v_o)$ as derived in the next section, it is found that

(4.39)
$$\frac{v}{v_o} = \sin\left[\omega t - kx + \frac{xv}{\bar{x}v_o}\right].$$

Since this is an odd function of $(\omega t - kx)$, a solution to this transcendental equation can be obtained by expressing v/v_o as the Fourier series: $\dfrac{v}{v_o} = \sum\limits_{m=1}^{\infty} A_m$ sin $m(\omega t - kx)$. If the standard integral expression for the coefficients A_m is evaluated by making use of the properties of Bessel functions, it can be readily shown that

(4.40)
$$v = 2v_o \sum_{n=1}^{\infty} \frac{J_m(mx/\bar{x})\sin m(\omega t - kx)}{mx/\bar{x}},$$

for $x/\bar{x} \le 1$, $\beta v_o/c_o \ll 1$, and where $J_m(.)$ is an m'th-order cylindrical Bessel function. Consequently, the velocity amplitude of the m'th harmonic is given by $v_m = 2v_o J_m(mx/\bar{x})/(mx/\bar{x})$.

Changes in the fundamental and four harmonics of the particle velocity are shown in Fig. 4.5a. It will be noted that the fundamental amplitude decreases by only 12% at the shock formation distance. From the linear plot of Fig. 4.5b it is clear that the amplitude ratio of the second harmonic to the first is nearly a linear function of the normalized distance. Using an approximate analysis of nonlinear plane wave propagation in a non-attenuating medium, Thuras et al. [26] showed that the ratio of the second harmonic to the first was proportional to the distance from the source. Their expression for the pressure amplitude is valid provided that x is much less than the shock formation distance so that harmonics higher than the second could be neglected. Moreover, in their 1935 publication they experimentally confirmed this behavior. Their expression can be written as

(4.41)
$$p_2 \approx p_1 \frac{(1+B/2A)p_0\omega}{2\rho_o c_o^3}x \approx p_1 \frac{\beta v_o\omega}{2c_o^2}x$$
$$\frac{p_2}{p_1} \approx \frac{x/\bar{x}}{2}$$

where ω is the fundamental frequency, p_1 and p_2 are the fundamental and second harmonic pressure amplitudes, and p_0 and v_0 are the pressure and velocity amplitudes at the source.

4.7.2 Effect of Attenuation

To account for the effects of attenuation, Thuras et al. [26] assumed that the fundamental and the second harmonic were attenuated as though each was the only wave present. They obtained

(4.42)
$$\frac{p_2}{p_1} \approx p_0 \frac{\beta\omega}{2\rho_o c_o^3}\left[\frac{e^{-\alpha_2 x} - e^{-2\alpha_1 x}}{2\alpha_1 - \alpha_2}\right],$$

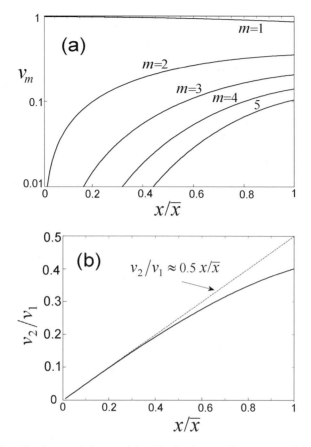

Figure 4.5 Amplitudes v_n of the particle velocity harmonics generated by an initially sinusoidal plane wave as the shock formation distance is approached. (a) First five harmonics assuming that the fundamental component, $m = 1$, had a unit velocity amplitude at $x = 0$. (b) The ratio of the second to the first harmonic is close to linear for $x/\bar{x} < 0.4$.

in which α_1 and α_2 are the attenuation coefficients at the fundamental and second harmonic frequencies. Subsequently other derivations of the same equation have been described [19]. Fig. 4.6 shows an example of a medium whose acoustical properties are not too far different from tissue. The shock formation distances for the three source pressure amplitudes assumed in the figure are $\bar{x}(0.04\,\text{MPa}) = 230\,\text{cm}$, $\bar{x}(0.4\,\text{MPa}) = 23\,\text{cm}$, $\bar{x}(0.8\,\text{MPa}) = 11.5\,\text{cm}$.

4.8 Shock Wave Formation [16]

A shock wave consists of a very abrupt change in the pressure and particle velocity that propagates spatially in such a manner as to cause large and highly

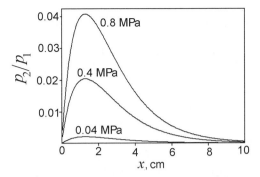

Figure 4.6 Ratio of the second harmonic pressure amplitude to the fundamental versus distance from the source for a plane CW 2.0 MHz wave as calculated from (4.42). Curves are shown for three different values of the source pressure amplitude. The medium was assumed to be castor oil at 20°C. For castor oil: $B/A = 8.96$, $\alpha = 0.096 f^{5/3}$ Np/(cm.MHz$^{5/3}$), $c_o = 1492$ m/s, and $\rho_o = 953$ kg/m^3. Thus, $\alpha_1 = 0.305$ Np/cm and $\alpha_2 = 0.968$ Np/cm for 2 and 4 MHz, respectively.

localized stresses in the propagating medium. In the application of shock-wave therapy to kidney stone destruction (lithotripsy), it is currently believed that the stresses created by the passage and reflection of the shock wave, together with the secondary shock waves due to cavitation, are primarily responsible for stone disintegration.

4.8.1 Plane Shock Waves

For plane waves traveling in a non-attenuating medium, a shock wave forms when $\partial v/\partial t \to \infty$, and this first occurs at the shock formation distance $\bar{x}$ corresponding to a time $\bar{t}$. Expressions for both these quantities can be obtained for a piston source by making use of Earnshaw's equation (4.30). In the discussion that followed the earlier presentation of this equation, it was noted that the value of φ is the time at which a particular incremental portion of the signal left the piston face. Evidently, at the shock formation distance there will be no change of x with an incremental change in φ, i.e., $(\partial x/\partial \varphi)_{\bar{x}} = 0$ and at the corresponding time $\bar{t}$, $(\partial t/\partial \varphi)_{\bar{t}} = 0$. These conditions, when applied to (4.30), enable both $\bar{x}$ and $\bar{t}$ to be found for any given excitation. This will be illustrated for the particular case of the sinusoidal excitation shown in Fig. 4.3. By finding $\partial x/\partial \varphi$ and $\partial t/\partial \varphi$ from (4.35) and equating each to zero, it can be readily shown that

(4.43a)
$$\hat{t} = \varphi - \frac{c_o + (\beta - 1)X_o \omega \sin(\omega\varphi)}{\beta\omega^2 X_o \cos(\omega\varphi)}$$

and

(4.43b) $\hat{x} = X_o(1 - \cos \omega\varphi) + \dfrac{[c_o + (\beta - 1)X_o\omega \sin \omega\varphi][c_o + \beta X_o\omega \sin \omega\varphi]}{\beta\omega^2 X_o \cos(\omega\varphi)}.$

From (4.43) it can be seen that the minimum value of $\bar{t} = c_o/(\beta\omega^2 X_o)$ occurs when $\varphi = 0$, which corresponds to the leading edge of the excitation wave. Consequently, $\bar{t} = c_o/(\beta\omega^2 X_o)$ and $\bar{x} = c_o^2/(\beta\omega^2 X_o)$. For the conditions listed in the caption of Fig. 4.4, we find that $\bar{x} = 4.09\,\text{mm}$ and $\bar{t} = 2.73\,\mu s$, in agreement with the curves shown in Fig. 4.4a and c. Since the assumed excitation wave-form is periodic, subsequent shocks will also be present, but these will occur at distances that are closer to the source, depending on the amplitude of the source movement (~0.5% reduction for the case considered above). This is because the initial shock front forms in an undisturbed medium, while subsequent shocks form in a medium that has already been disturbed.

4.8.2 Shock Parameter

The shock formation distance for a sinusoidal plane wave can be expressed in terms of the ratio of the source velocity amplitude to the small-signal speed of sound, i.e., $v_o/c_o = \varepsilon_M$, which is called the acoustic *Mach* number. Since the source velocity for the sinusoidal excitation being considered is given by $v_o = \omega X_o$ and $k = \omega/c_o$, the shock formation distance for a plane sinusoidal wave traveling in a non-attenuating medium can be written as

(4.44) $\bar{x} = 1/(\beta k \varepsilon_M).$

It is helpful to define a plane wave normalized shock parameter by

(4.45) $\sigma_s = \dfrac{x}{\bar{x}} = \beta k \varepsilon_M x,$

so that at the shock formation distance $\bar{x}$, $\sigma_s = 1$, while $\sigma_s < 1$ corresponds to the pre-shock regime. For regions beyond $\bar{x}$ the originally sinusoidal wave-form becomes more distorted and energy is lost, especially in the shock transition region (shock front). Thus, σ_s provides a convenient means for characterizing the various stages of shock formation. In the case of a spherically converging wave, it can be shown [19] that when the effects of absorption are not significant, the radial distance (from the center of curvature) where the shock first occurs is given by

(4.46) $\bar{r} = a e^{-1/(\beta k a \varepsilon_M)},$

where a is the radius of curvature of the wave. The shock parameter for this case is given by

(4.47) $\sigma_s = 1 + \beta k a \varepsilon_M \ln(\bar{r}/r) = -\beta k a \varepsilon_M \ln(r/a),$

where r is measured from the center of curvature. Note that for this case $\sigma_s = 1$ at $r = \bar{r}$ and $\sigma_s = 0$ at $r = a$.

As noted earlier, the shock region is a transition region where the pressure and velocity change very rapidly. For real fluids, in locations where $\partial v/\partial t$

becomes large, energy is more rapidly dissipated, and as a result $\partial v/\partial t$ is large but not infinite. Analyses of what happens to the wave beyond $\bar{x}$ have to take into account the absorption, and this has been addressed though several approximate approaches [19]. One of the simplest is the weak shock theory [18], which among other things assumes that dissipation of energy is associated only with the shock region. Since this assumption implies that the energy loss due to ordinary absorption is much smaller, it is evident that this theory does not apply to very weak shocks, as its name would seem to imply. It requires that the nonlinearity must be sufficiently strong that shocks of significant strength can be formed. Based on the Fubini solution given by (4.40), which is valid for $\sigma_S \leq 1$, and other approximate analyses that are valid for $\sigma_S > 1$, the waveforms over a full range of distances from the source can be estimated. Sketches [19] for a strong wave are shown in Fig. 4.7. It should be noted that at $\sigma_S = 3$ a sawtooth wave forms that has a rich harmonic content. Beyond $\sigma_S = 3$ the higher harmonics of the sawtooth wave are rapidly dissipated and the shock front disappears. It can be shown that the amplitude of the wave at $\sigma_S \gg 1$ becomes independent of the source amplitude, a phenomenon called *acoustical saturation*. The explanation for this is that any further increase in the source energy is exactly balanced by the increased energy lost in the shock front over the preceding region.

4.9 Effects of Nonlinearity, Diffraction, and Attenuation

In the last chapter we examined the influence of diffraction and attenuation on the radiation field characteristics of different transducer geometries under small-signal conditions. It therefore remains to extend this discussion to the nonlinear propagation regime.

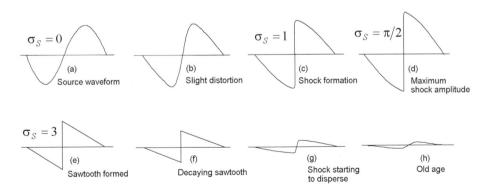

Figure 4.7 Sketches of the time-domain velocity waveform at increasing distances from a sinusoidal source when the amplitude is sufficient to create a strong wave (based on Blackstock et al. [4.19]). The shock parameter σ_S is unity at the shock formation distance $\bar{x}$ and is directly proportional to the distance from the source.

Because nonlinear effects are involved in diagnostic ultrasound and are an inherent part of many therapeutic ultrasound methods, considerable efforts have been made to develop theoretical models that provide reasonably accurate predictions of the field profiles. The approximations used to arrive at methods that can be transformed into computationally efficient algorithms often limit the range of spatial locations where good accuracy can be expected.

4.9.1 Burgers' Equations

An *evolution equation*, as the name implies, describes the manner in which a process develops temporally, spatially, or both. A nonlinear evolution equation, such as the reduced wave equation of (4.27), describes how the particle velocity changes both in time and space. In the framework of quadratic nonlinearity, the reduced wave equation in retarded time[3] $(\tau = t - z/c_o)$, as given by (4.33), can be rewritten as

$$(4.48) \qquad \frac{\partial v(z, \tau)}{\partial z} = \frac{\beta v}{c_o^2} \frac{\partial v}{\partial \tau},$$

where the right-hand side of the equation describes the nonlinearity. In the case $\beta = 0$, the solution is simply a plane progressive wave traveling in the z-direction. An exact solution of (4.48) can be written as

$$v(z, \tau) = f(\tau + \beta z v/c_o^2).$$

For a sinusoidal excitation of $v(0,t) = v_o \sin(\omega t)$, the solution is

$$(4.39) \qquad v(z, t) = v_o \sin[\omega(t - z/c_o) + \omega \beta z v/c_o^2],$$

which is identical to the approximate form of Earnshaw's solution derived earlier.

To account for the effects of weak absorption due to viscous loss, it can be shown [28] that an additional term should be added to the right-hand side of (4.48), resulting in

$$(4.49) \qquad \frac{\partial v(z, \tau)}{\partial z} = \frac{\beta v}{c_o^2} \frac{\partial v}{\partial \tau} + \frac{1}{2 c_o^3 \rho_o} \frac{\partial^2 v}{\partial \tau^2} \left(\mu_B + \frac{4}{3} \mu \right), \qquad \text{(a)}$$

where μ and μ_B are the shear and bulk viscosity coefficients. This equation, often referred to as *Burgers' equation*,[4] is one of the simplest models used to describe the propagation of a finite-amplitude plane progressive wave in a

---

3. Since 3-D propagation is considered in this section and most authors take the z-direction as the beam axis, we have switched to this system.

4. The full form includes a term that accounts for thermal conduction loss, but in the case of water-like fluids, this term is much smaller than the viscous loss term and consequently is ignored in this and subsequent equations.

classic viscous loss medium [27]. An interesting historical account of its development has been given by Blackstock et al. [19]. Derivations from first principles are given in [32, Chapter 2] as well as in [13].

By using the classic linear relation $p = \rho_o c_o v$, this equation can also be written in terms of the pressure

(4.49)
$$\frac{\partial p}{\partial z} = \frac{\beta}{\rho_o c_o^3} p \frac{\partial p}{\partial \tau} + \frac{\delta}{2c_o^3} \frac{\partial^2 p}{\partial \tau^2},$$
(b)

where $\delta = \left(\mu_B + \frac{4}{3}\mu \right) \Big/ \rho_o$.

A further form can be obtained that expresses the excess wave speed ($u = \beta v$) in terms of a frame of reference that moves with the speed c_o. Using slightly different approximations from those used to obtain (a) and (b), Lighthill [13] has shown that

(4.49)
$$\frac{\partial u}{\partial t} + u \frac{\partial u}{\partial Z} = \frac{\delta}{2} \frac{\partial^2 u}{\partial Z^2},$$
(c)

where $Z = z - c_o t$. It should be noted that although (c) does not directly transform into (a), they were both derived using the same order of approximation.

A useful method of obtaining a frequency domain solution to (4.49a) is to assume a complex Fourier series solution of the form [33, 34, 37, p. 313]

$$v(z, \tau) = \frac{1}{2} \sum_{m=-\infty}^{\infty} v_m(z) e^{j2\pi m f_1 \tau},$$

where $v_m(z)$ is the amplitude of the particle velocity of the m'th harmonic of the fundamental f_1. Substituting this into (4.49) and from (3.113), noting that

the attenuation coefficient is given by $\alpha \approx \frac{2\pi^2 f^2}{\rho_o c_o^3} \left(\mu_B + \frac{4}{3}\mu \right) = \alpha_o f^2$, it can be shown that [33]

$$\frac{\partial v_m(z)}{\partial z} = j \frac{\beta 2\pi f_1}{2c_o^2} \sum_{i=-\infty}^{\infty} (m-i) v_i v_{m-i} - \alpha_o (m f_1)^2 v_m.$$

Now, to a first order,

$$v_m(z + \Delta z) = v_m(z) + \frac{\partial v_m(z)}{\partial z} \Delta z.$$

which enables the iterative description of the propagating wave to be written as

$$v_m(z + \Delta z) = v_m(z) + \left[j \frac{\beta 2\pi f_1}{2c_o^2} \sum_{i=-\infty}^{\infty} (m-i) v_i v_{m-i} - \alpha_o (m f_1)^2 v_m \right] \Delta z.$$

The summation term can be rewritten in a form that is more convenient for computation, yielding

$$(4.50) \quad v_m(z + \Delta z) = v_m(z) + \left[j \frac{\beta 2\pi f_1}{2c_o^2} \left(\sum_{i=1}^{m-1} i v_i v_{m-i} + \sum_{i=m+1}^{N} m v_i v_{m-1}^* \right) - \alpha_o (m f_1)^n v_m \right] \Delta z,$$

where the star indicates the complex conjugate, N is the number of harmonics to be retained in the computation process, and we have assumed $v_{m=0} = 0$ [37]. In addition, it has been assumed that the frequency dependence of the attenuation coefficient can be more generally written as $\alpha(f) = \alpha_o f^n$.

As an example, we consider an initial 1 MHz sinusoidal plane wave with a velocity amplitude of 0.4 m/s propagating in a medium whose attenuation increases linearly ($n = 1$) with frequency with values of 0.3 and 1.0 dB/(cm.MHz). The magnitude of the harmonic amplitudes were calculated using (4.50) and are plotted as a function of the normalized distance from the source in Fig. 4.8 for two attenuation values. It will be noted that the harmonics reach a maximum at a distance from the source that increases with harmonic number. Moreover, it can be shown that for zero attenuation the results are the same as those obtained with the Fubini method, i.e., $v_m = 2v_o J_m (mx/\bar{x})/(mx/\bar{x})$, as discussed earlier (see subsection 4.7.1).

The 1-D Burgers' equation can be extended to apply for convergent (+) or divergent (−), spherical ($n' = 1$) or cylindrical waves ($n' = 2$) and takes the form [29]

$$(4.51) \quad \frac{\partial v(r, \tau)}{\partial r} + \frac{v(r, \tau)}{n'r} = \pm \left[\frac{\beta v}{c_o^2} \frac{\partial v}{\partial \tau} + \frac{1}{2c_o^3 \rho_o} \frac{\partial^2 v}{\partial \tau^2} \left(\mu_B + \frac{4}{3} \mu \right) \right],$$

for $kr \gg 1$, which is known as the *generalized Burgers' equation* [27]. In addition, it should be noted that an augmented form that accounts for nonlinearity, thermoviscous absorption, and multiple relaxation phenomena has been derived by Pierce [35]. Cleveland et al. [36] have used this formulation and have obtained time-domain numerical solutions that are in excellent agreement with a previously derived analytic solution for the special case of a thermoviscous mono-relaxing fluid.

4.9.2 Khokhlov-Zabolotskaya-Kuznetsov (KZK) Equation

To account for the combined effects of diffraction, absorption, and nonlinearity, Kuznetsov [30] extended the work of Zabolotskaya and Khokhlov [31] through the inclusion of the viscous loss term and arrived at the following approximate 3-D equation for the velocity potential expressed in real time:

$$(4.52) \quad \frac{\partial^2 \phi}{\partial t^2} - c_o^2 \nabla^2 \phi = \frac{\partial}{\partial t} \left[\frac{1}{\rho_o} \left(\mu_B + \frac{4}{3} \mu \right) \nabla^2 \phi + (\nabla \phi)^2 + \frac{(\beta - 1)}{c_o^2} \left(\frac{\partial \phi}{\partial t} \right)^2 \right],$$

where the right-hand side accounts for absorption and nonlinearity. In seeking a quasi-planar solution for a wave propagating in the z-direction of a Carte-

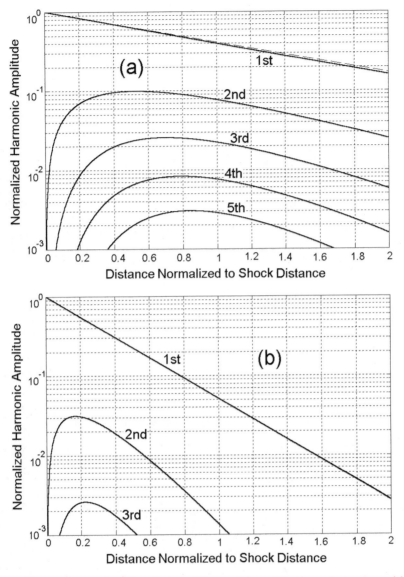

Figure 4.8 Frequency-domain solution of Burgers' equation for a plane wave with a fundamental frequency of 1 MHz propagating in a medium with $\beta = 3.5$, $\rho_o = 1000\,\text{kg/m}^3$, $c_o = 1500\,\text{m/s}$, and an initial particle velocity amplitude of 0.4 m/s corresponding to a peak pressure of 0.6 MPa. The distance is with respect to the source and is normalized to the shock distance of 25.6 cm. The particle velocity, normalized to 0.4 m/s, is shown for the fundamental and each harmonic. Calculations were performed using (4.50). (a) Attenuation of 0.3 dB/(cm.MHz). The dashed line corresponds to $\exp[-\alpha_o f_0 z]$. (b) Attenuation of 1.0 dB/(cm.MHz).

sian coordinate system, Kuznetsov showed that when expressed in retarded
time ($\tau = t - z/c_o$) this could be expressed as[5]

$$
(4.53) \qquad \frac{\partial^2 \phi}{\partial \tau \partial z} - \frac{c_o}{2} \nabla_\perp^2 \phi = \frac{\partial}{\partial \tau} \left[\frac{1}{2 c_o^3 \rho_o} \left(\mu_B + \frac{4}{3} \mu \right) \frac{\partial^2 \phi}{\partial \tau^2} + \frac{\beta}{2 c_o^3} \left(\frac{\partial \phi}{\partial \tau} \right)^2 \right],
$$

in which $\nabla_\perp^2 = \dfrac{\partial^2}{\partial x^2} + \dfrac{\partial^2}{\partial y^2}$ is a transverse Laplacian that operates in a plane

normal to the direction of propagation. In regard to the viscosity term ($\mu_B +$
$4\mu/3$), it should be recalled (from Chapter 1) that the presence of the same
term for a 1-D linear wave gives rise to an attenuation proportional to ω^2. Consequently, the presence of this term in (4.53) can be expected to result in
approximately the same frequency dependence. To express this parabolic wave
equation in terms of the pressure distribution, we can assume that $p \approx$
$\rho_o(\partial\phi/\partial t) = \rho_o(\partial\phi/\partial\tau)$, which is consistent with the order of the approximations
used in (4.53). Taking the partial derivative of (4.53) with respect to time and
substituting in this the relation between p and $\partial\phi/\partial\tau$ yields

$$
(4.54) \qquad \frac{\partial^2 p}{\partial \tau \partial z} - \frac{c_o}{2} \nabla_\perp^2 p = \frac{1}{2 c_o^3 \rho_o} \frac{\partial}{\partial \tau} \left[\left(\mu_B + \frac{4}{3} \mu \right) \frac{\partial^2 p}{\partial \tau^2} + \beta \frac{\partial p^2}{\partial \tau} \right],
$$

which is widely known as the KZK [30,31] equation.

As stated by Hamilton and Morfey [27], the KZK equation is an augmen-
tation of Burgers' equation that accounts for the combined effects of diffraction, absorption, and nonlinearity in directional beams. It is frequently used
for calculating the radiated field when nonlinear effects must be accounted
for. Moreover, it provides a reasonably good approximation to the field distribution for sources whose apertures are large compared to a wavelength (ka
$\gg 1$) so that they produce fairly directional waves (quasi-plane), for observation points that are not too close to the source $\{z > a(ka)^{1/3}\}$, and for points
that lie within a reasonably narrow cone so that their off-axis locations are not
too large [38]. It should also be noted that to express the KZK equation in
terms of the z-component of the particle velocity, we can substitute $v_z \approx$
$p/(\rho_o c_o)$, which is an approximation that is also consistent with the approximations used in obtaining (4.54). For sources with cylindrical symmetry, cylindrical coordinates (r,z) can be used, in which case (4.54) is still applicable, but
now the transverse Laplacian is given by $\nabla_\perp^2 = \dfrac{\partial^2}{\partial r^2} + \dfrac{1}{r} \dfrac{\partial}{\partial r}$.

4.9.3 Attenuation

The assumption of a simple viscous loss model (which as noted earlier implies
an ω^2 frequency dependence) for the attenuation presents problems if absorp-

---

5. In obtaining this equation the parabolic approximation has been made, which implies that
the angular spectrum is narrow so that the wave will be close to planar.

tion is to be incorporated in a more general manner. For most biological tissues the attenuation can be characterized by an attenuation constant $\alpha(\omega) = \alpha_0 f^n$, where n is generally around 1 but may lie in the range $1 \leq n < 2$. As noted in the last subsection, incorporating such a dependence into a frequency-domain method of solution is straightforward, but for a time-domain method it is more complex. When a finite difference method is used, the effects of some general frequency-dependent absorption processes can be represented by first determining the transfer function between two incrementally separated planes [39] and then obtaining the impulse response. Finally, by convolving this with the waveform at a point on the plane at z, the waveform at the corresponding point on the plane $z + dz$ can be calculated. The computational burden of this approach can be reduced through the use of a wavelet (time-frequency) method described by He [40], which uses a bank of digitally implemented Gaussian filters to decompose the original signal into a number of narrow-band components. Each narrow-band component propagates at a speed determined by the dispersion relation associated with the attenuation characteristics and is subject to attenuation governed by the frequency dependence of the attenuation coefficient. An alternative approach is to Fourier transform the waveform, multiply by the transfer function, and then perform an inverse Fourier transform to obtain the attenuated waveform.

An augmented version of the KZK equation in cylindrical coordinates that includes the effects of absorption and dispersion by a medium with multiple independent relaxation processes has been presented by Cleveland et al. [36].

4.10 Numerical Methods and Results

4.10.1 Using the KZK Equation

A number of techniques have been developed to enable reasonably efficient numerical prediction of the field profiles under conditions that result in significant nonlinear behavior. Moreover, comparisons of experimental and numerical predictions indicate that within the domain of validity, methods based on the KZK equation enable good agreement to be achieved for both pulsed and CW excited ultrasound transducers. The original work of Bakhvalov et al. in the application of numerical methods for solving the KZK equation has been summarized in their book [5]. More recently, Ginsberg and Hamilton [37] have reviewed many of the computational methods and have pointed out that in general the techniques can be divided into three categories: frequency-domain, time-domain, and combined time- and frequency-domain methods.

Frequency-domain methods are appropriate when the source waveform is either periodic or quasi-periodic. Since the waveform maintains its periodicity as it progresses from the source, a Fourier series can be used to represent the waveform, and consequently the explicit time dependence can be eliminated. Basically, this technique leads to a system of coupled differential equations that can be solved by marching forward in incremental steps. The solution enables the Fourier coefficient to be determined, and from this the time-domain waveform can be calculated.

For solving the KZK equation in the time domain, the starting point is the integral of (4.54), i.e.,

$$(4.55) \qquad \frac{\partial p}{\partial z} = \frac{c_o}{2} \int_{-\infty}^{\tau} \nabla_{\perp}^2 p \, d\tau + \frac{1}{2 c_o^3 \rho_o} \left[\left(\mu_B + \frac{4}{3} \mu \right) \frac{\partial^2 p}{\partial \tau^2} + \beta \frac{\partial p^2}{\partial \tau} \right],$$

where the first term on the right-hand side represents the effects of diffraction. Time-domain methods enable pulsed or short-burst source waveforms to be treated and generally employ a finite difference computational approach. If the operator-splitting technique is used (also called the method of fractional steps: see, for example [47, pp. 847–848]), then (4.55) is split into the following three equations:

$$\frac{\partial p}{\partial z} = \frac{\beta p}{c_o^3 \rho_o} \frac{\partial p}{\partial \tau} \equiv \mathcal{L}_1 \cdot p \qquad \text{(a)}$$

$$(4.56) \qquad \frac{\partial p}{\partial z} = \frac{\left(\mu_B + \frac{4}{3} \mu \right)}{2 c_o^3 \rho_o} \frac{\partial^2 p}{\partial \tau^2} \equiv \mathcal{L}_2 \cdot p \qquad \text{(b)}$$

$$\frac{\partial p}{\partial z} = \frac{-c_o}{2} \int_{-\infty}^{\tau} \nabla_{\perp}^2 p \, d\tau \equiv \mathcal{L}_3 \cdot p, \qquad \text{(c)}$$

and the total change in pressure is assumed to be given by

$$(4.57) \qquad \frac{\partial p}{\partial z} = \mathcal{L}_1 \cdot p + \mathcal{L}_2 \cdot p + \mathcal{L}_3 \cdot p,$$

in which $\mathcal{L}_n$ denotes an operator that can be nonlinear. Thus, this method assumes that over an incremental distance Δz, all three effects are independent of each other, and the total change in pressure can be approximated by their sum. Partial justification for its use is based on the fact that by integrating the KZK equation with respect to retarded time, a form equivalent to (4.57) is obtained. A second-order operator-splitting approach is illustrated in Fig. 4.9 [41]. Over each incremental distance Δz, three calculations are performed. Two of these account for the effects of attenuation and diffraction over two half-steps and can be in the frequency domain using the angular spectrum approach for diffraction and the frequency-dependent power-law for attenuation. The third calculation accounts for nonlinear propagation over a full step, and this can be performed in either the time or frequency domain using an appropriate form of Burgers' equation.

It should be noted that the first of the three equations is identical in form to the reduced wave equation of (4.33), so that its analytical solution, as given

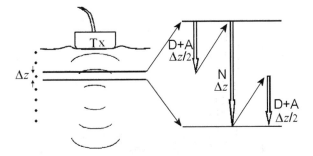

Figure 4.9 Fractional step marching scheme and the second-order operator-splitting approach described by (4.57). The acoustic field from the transducer (*Tx*) is propagated plane by plane in incremental steps. Each step involves the propagation of diffraction (*D*), attenuation (*A*), and nonlinearity (*N*). (Reproduced, with permission, from Zemp et al. [41], *J. Acoust. Soc. Am.*, 113, 139–152, © 2003 Acoustical Society of America.)

by (4.34), can be used in an incremental form. For a transient waveform, the waveform is generally uniformly sampled, but following evaluation of (4.56a) these uniform samples become non-uniformly spaced at $z + \Delta z$ because their local speed of propagation will differ from c_o, and therefore the waveform at $z + \Delta z$ must be resampled before continuing with subsequent steps in the procedure.

Measurements of the harmonic field patterns generated by piston transducers using large-signal CW excitation were reported by Gould et al. [42] in 1966. They stated, "The higher harmonics in a definitely nonlinear case have as their source the whole three-dimensional fundamental beam, not the piston, and so it is not evident that these harmonic components should either closely resemble or greatly differ from a linear fundamental beam." Comparisons of experimental results with those predicted by numerical solution of the KZK equation have been presented by a number of authors. Some of the on-axis measurements of the various harmonic components of the pressure, as reported by Nachef et al. [43], are shown in Fig. 4.10. It is evident that one of the effects of high excitation levels is to shift the near-field structures closer to the transducer. For example, the last maximum under small-signal conditions occurs approximately at 36 cm (a^2/λ), whereas the measured value for the fundamental shown in Fig. 4.10a is close to 26 cm. This shift can be readily understood from the observation that the nonlinearity causes energy to be depleted from the fundamental to feed the harmonics. From the graphs shown in Fig. 4.10b it can be seen that, except in the near-field region, the KZK theoretical predictions are in good qualitative agreement with the measured values.

The off-axis measurements for CW excited piston transducers compared with numerical predictions have been reported by TenCate [44]. Shown in Fig. 4.11a is the transverse field under small-signal conditions. For high excitation

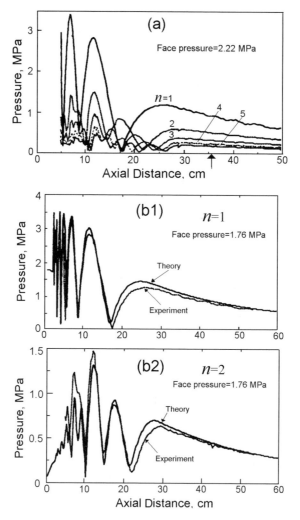

Figure 4.10 Measured on-axis pressure distributions in degassed, deionized water for the fundamental, second, third, fourth, and fifth harmonics from a CW excited (1.0 MHz) plane piston transducer with an effective radius of 23.2 mm. The theoretical results were obtained from numerical solutions to the KZK equation using the following: coefficient of nonlinearity, $\beta = 3.5$; Rayleigh distance, $z_R = \pi a^2/\lambda$ = 112.6 cm; absorption coefficient at 1 MHz, $\alpha = 6.04 \times 10^{-4}$ Np/cm. (a) Comparison of measured results for five harmonics. The arrow marks the location of the last maximum for small-signal excitation conditions. (b) Comparison of measured and computed results for the first four harmonics. (Reproduced, with permission, from Nachef et al. [43], *J. Acoust. Soc. Am.*, 98, 2303–2323, © 1995 Acoustical Society of America.)

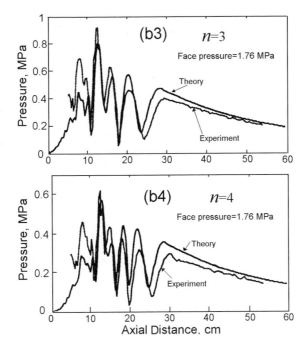

Figure 4.10 *Continued*

levels it can be seen from Fig. 4.11b that harmonics are generated that have transverse profiles with unexpected extra side lobes, which have been termed "fingers." As explained by Berntsen et al. [45], these arise from the scattering of sound by sound. In the absence of absorption and far from the source, it has been predicted that they should decay with the axial distance as $1/z$, which has been experimentally confirmed [44]. It should also be observed that the harmonic side lobes fall off more quickly than the fundamental. It is likely that this is due to the harmonic generation being amplitude-dependent: in locations where the fundamental amplitude is reduced, the harmonic amplitude will be much smaller.

4.10.2 Other Frequency- and Time-Domain Methods

Methods that avoid the use of the KZK equation, with the limitations that are imposed by the parabolic approximation, have been described by several groups [37], and two of these will now be described.

Frequency Domain

In the method proposed and studied by Christopher and Parker [46], a phenomenological approach was taken in which over incremental distances the individual processes involved (diffraction, absorption, nonlinear propagation)

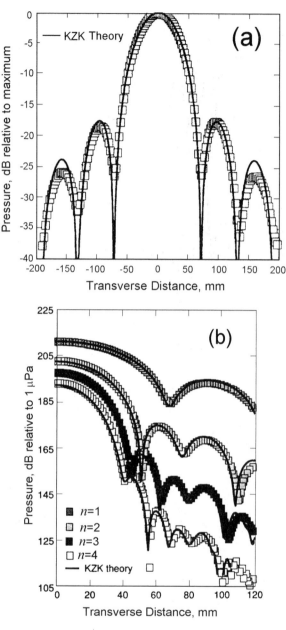

Figure 4.11 Measured off-axis pressure distributions for a CW excited (1.0 MHz) plane piston transducer with a radius of 12.1 mm in water compared to theory. (a) At a range $z = 1000$ mm for small-signal radiation conditions. (b) The fundamental and three harmonics for a source level of 223 dB relative to 1 μPa at a range $z = 894$ mm. The theoretical results were obtained from numerical solutions to the KZK equation. (Reproduced, with permission, from TenCate [45], *J. Acoust. Soc. Am.*, 94, 1084–1089, © 1993 Acoustical Society of America.)

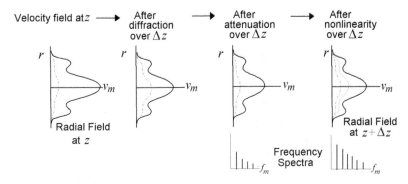

Figure 4.12 Computation process developed by Christopher and Parker [47] for a step size of Δz. The solid curves show the fundamental normal component of the particle velocity as a function of the radial position for a cylindrically symmetrical transducer. The dashed and dotted curves are the harmonics. (Based on similar drawings in Christopher and Parker [47].)

are assumed to be independent and can be superimposed, i.e., the operator-splitting technique just described. In calculating the effects of diffraction they made use of the equation for the point-spread function derived on the basis of the free space wave equation in Chapter 2 as (2.74). This can be written as

$$h_p(x, y, z|z + \Delta z) = \frac{\Delta z e^{-jk_m R}}{2\pi R^2} \left[\frac{1}{R} + jk_m \right],$$

where $R = \sqrt{x^2 + y^2 + (\Delta z)^2}$, and the index corresponds to the m'th harmonic of the fundamental. According to (2.67), by convolving this with the velocity potential on the plane z, the velocity potential on the plane at $z + \Delta z$ can be obtained, i.e.,

$$\Phi(x, y, z + \Delta z) = \Phi(x, y, z) * h_p(x, y, z|z + \Delta z).$$

This can be evaluated[6] by taking the spatial Fourier transforms of both quantities, and then taking the inverse transform of the product of the two transformed quantities. The result of this step is illustrated by the left-hand side of Fig. 4.12. Also illustrated are the attenuation and nonlinearity calculations, details of which are given in [46].

The results obtained with this technique are illustrated in Fig. 4.13 for a simple uniformly apodized piston transducer radiating into water. It was assumed that the CW source intensity was $3.3\,\text{W/cm}^2$, corresponding to a source pressure of $100\,\text{kPa}$. With increasing distance from the transducer the

---

6. To improve the computational efficiency for their assumed axisymmetric geometry, Christopher and Parker used the discrete Hankel transform as described in [48].

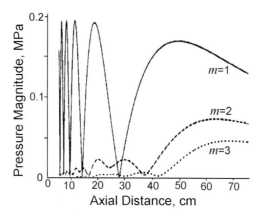

Figure 4.13 On-axis CW computed pressure profile for a 2.25 MHz piston transducer with a radius of 1.9 cm and an initial pressure amplitude of 100 kPa, and radiating into water ($c_o = 1500$ m/s, $\alpha = 0.00025$ Np/cm). The fundamental and two harmonics are shown. (Reproduced, with permission, from Christopher and Parker [7], *J. Acoust. Soc. Am.*, 90, 488–499, © 1991 Acoustical Society of America.)

waveform can be expected to become increasingly distorted, and this is reflected in the increasing amplitudes of the harmonics. The fundamental reaches its last maximum somewhat prior to a^2/λ, while for the harmonics they lie beyond it. Good agreement was demonstrated with experimental measurements, and these results suggest that the field can be more accurately computed close to the source, where the parabolic approximation used for the KZK equation breaks down.

Computed results for the normal component of the acoustic particle velocity in both the axial and radial directions are shown in Fig. 4.14 for a focused transducer, details of which are given in the caption. It should be noted from Fig. 4.14b that for the higher harmonics the lateral beam width is reduced, a result that might have been expected from considering the reduction in wavelength. In addition, the figure clearly shows the presence of the fingers discussed earlier.

Time Domain

Tavakkoli et al. [49] have described a time-domain technique that is well suited for calculating the field for transient transmitted waveforms from both focused and plane transducers. They also used the operator-splitting technique but employed a second-order method using a gridding scheme with planes normal to the z-direction and a step size that depended on the operator being used. All calculations were performed in the time domain. The attenuation term was evaluated by calculating the convolution of the acoustic velocity and the impulse response of a causal minimum-phase filter that characterized the dis-

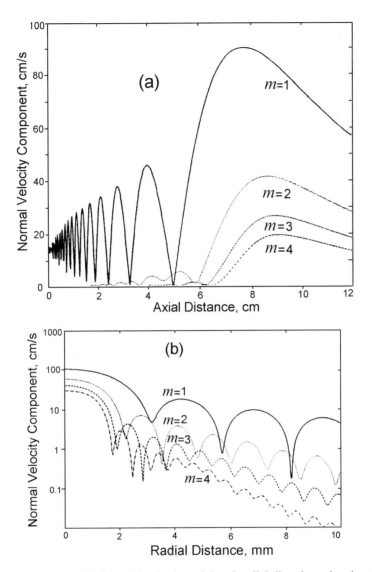

Figure 4.14 Computed field profiles in the axial and radial directions showing the normal component of the acoustic particle velocity for a 3.0 MHz focused transducer using uniform CW excitation. The transducer was assumed to have an aperture diameter of 2.0 cm and a geometric focal length of 10 cm and to be radiating into water (c_o = 1500 m/s, α = 0.00025 Np/cm, β = 3.5). In addition, a spherically symmetrical focusing phase factor was used. The profiles for the fundamental and three harmonics are shown for (a) the axial direction at a source intensity of 3 W/cm^2 and (b) the radial direction at the focal plane (z ~ 7.7 cm) for 10 W/cm^2. (Reproduced, with permission, from Christopher and Parker [47], *J. Acoust. Soc. Am.*, 90, 488–499, © 1991 Acoustical Society of America.)

sipative and dispersive characteristics of soft tissue, as described in section 4.9.3. By numerical evaluation of the Rayleigh integral they calculated the change in pressure and normal component of the velocity between the gridding planes. The nonlinear term was evaluated from the approximate form of the Earnshaw equation as given by (4.34). The technique has been validated by comparison with the nonlinear results obtained for a piston transducer using the KZK equation and with experimental measurements [52].

Experimental and computational field profiles have been compared for a large-aperture multi-element concave transducer that was used for high-energy shock-wave therapy [50]. The dimensions of this transducer are given in Fig. 4.15. Also shown in this figure are the fluid media and their characteristics. For the water, the attenuation coefficient is proportional to ω^2, while for the tissue-mimicking fluid (1,3-Butandiol) it is approximately proportional to ω. For the measurements shown in Fig. 4.16, all the elements were excited with an impulse, giving rise to the pressure waveform shown in Fig. 4.16a close to the surface. Measurements of the pressure waveform at the focal point were performed using a 1-mm^2 PVDF hydrophone specifically developed for recording shock wave pressures [51], and these are shown in Fig. 4.16b and c

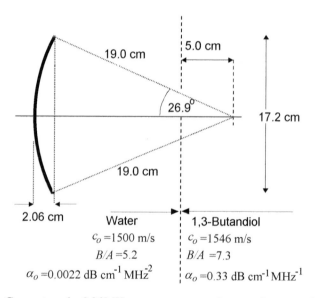

Figure 4.15 Geometry of a 0.36 MHz concave composite transducer used to generate shock waves in the volume around the focal point [50]. The transducer small-signal gain was ~30. The transducer field was measured and simulated in the focal zone. The medium was degassed, deionized water up to 5 cm from the focal point. Beyond this, a tissue-mimicking fluid (1,3-Butandiol) was used. Simulations were performed using the time-domain scheme developed by Tavakkoli et al. [4.50]; measurements were performed using a PVDF hydrophone specifically developed for recording shock wave pressures [51].

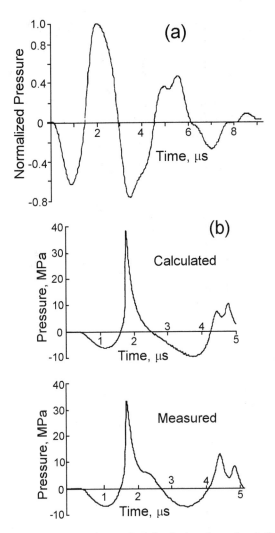

Figure 4.16 Comparison of experimental and calculated results at the focal point of the concave transducer shown in Fig. 4.15. (a) Measured pressure waveform at the surface of the source. This waveform was used as the input for the computations. Measured and computed results for a peak input pressure of (b) 0.476 MPa and (c) 0.85 MPa. (Reproduced, with permission, from Tavakkoli et al. [4.50], *J. Acoust. Soc. Am.*, 104, 2061–2072, © 1998 Acoustical Society of America.)

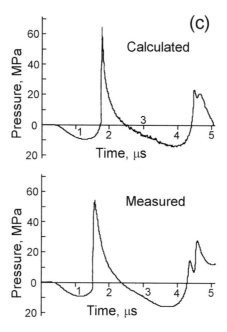

Figure 4.16 *Continued*

for two different input pressures. For both inputs the field becomes highly non-linear in the volume surrounding the focal point and a very rapid increase in pressure occurs, which is characteristic of a shock wave.

References

1. Naugolnykh, K., and Ostrovsky, L., *Nonlinear Wave Processes in Acoustics*, Cambridge Univ. Press, Cambridge, UK, 1998.
2. Beyer, R.T., and Letcher, S.V., *Physical Ultrasonics* (Ch. 7, Nonlinear Acoustics), Academic Press, New York, 1969.
3. Blackstock, D.T., Nonlinear acoustics (theoretical), Chapter 3, pp. 3–185 to 3–205 in: *American Institute of Physics Handbook*, D.E. Grey (Ed.), 3rd Edn., McGraw-Hill, New York, 1972.
4. Beyer, R.T., *Nonlinear Acoustics*, Navy Sea Systems Command, Washington, DC, 1974 (reprinted, with a new appendix containing more recent references and published by: Acoustical Society of America, Woodbury, NY, 1997).
5. Bakhvalov, N.S., Zhileikin, Y.M., and Zabolotskaya, E.A., *Nonlinear Theory of Sound*, American Institute of Physics, New York, 1987.
6. Hamilton, M.F., and Blackstock, D.T. (eds.), *Nonlinear Acoustics*, Academic Press, New York, 1998.
7. Bacon, D.R., Finite amplitude distortion of the pulsed fields used in diagnostic ultrasound, *Ultrasound Med. Biol.*, 10, 189–195, 1984.
8. Parker, K.J., Observation of nonlinear acoustic effects in a B-scan imaging instrument, *IEEE Trans. Sonics Ultrasonics*, 32, 4–8, 1985.

9. Li, S., McDicken, W.N., and Hoskins, P.R., Nonlinear propagation in Doppler Ultrasound, *Ultrasound Med. Biol.*, 19, 359–364, 1993.

10. Ward, B., Baker, A.C., and Humphrey, V.F., Nonlinear propagation applied to the improvement of resolution in diagnostic medical imaging, *J. Acoust. Soc. Am.*, 101, 143–154, 1997.

11. Carstensen, E.L., and Bacon, D.R., Biomedical applications, Chapter 15 in: *Nonlinear Acoustics*, M.F. Hamilton and D.T. Blackstock (Eds.), Academic Press, New York, 1998.

12. Duck, F.A., Nonlinear acoustics in diagnostic ultrasound, *Ultrasound Med. Biol.*, 28, 1–18, 2002.

13. Lighthill, M.J., Viscosity effects in sound waves of finite amplitude, pp. 250–351 in: *Surveys in Mechanics*, G.K. Batchelor and R.M. Davis (Eds.), University Press, Cambridge, 1956.

14. Blackstock, D.T., History of Nonlinear Acoustics: 1750s-1930s, Chapter 1 in: *Nonlinear Acoustics*, M.F. Hamilton and D.T. Blackstock (Eds.), Academic Press, New York, 1998.

15. Lee, C.P., and Wang, T.G., Acoustic radiation pressure, *J. Acoust. Soc. Am.*, 94, 1099–1109, 1993.

16. Blackstock, D.T., Propagation of plane sound waves of finite amplitude in nondissipative fluids, *J. Acoust. Soc. Am.*, 34, 9–30, 1962.

17. Lamb, H., *The Dynamical Theory of Sound*, 2nd edn., Edward Arnold & Co., London, 1925.

18. Blackstock, D.T., Connection between the Fay and Fubini solutions for plane sound waves of finite amplitude, *J. Acoust. Soc. Am.*, 39, 1019–1026, 1966.

19. Blackstock, D.T., Hamilton, M.F., and Pierce, A.D., Progressive waves in lossless and lossy fluids, Chapter 4 in: *Nonlinear Acoustics*, M.F. Hamilton and D.T. Blackstock (Eds.), Academic Press, New York, 1998.

20. Law, W.K., Frizzell, L.A, and Dunn, F., Determination of the nonlinearity parameter B/A of biological media, *Ultrasound Med. Biol.*, 11, 307–318, 1985.

21. Beyer, R.T., The parameter B/A, Chapter 2 in: *Nonlinear Acoustics*, M.F. Hamilton and D.T. Blackstock (Eds.), Academic Press, New York, 1998.

22. Sehgal, C.M., Bahn, R.C., and Greenleaf, J.F., Measurement of the acoustic nonlinearity parameter B/A in human tissues by a thermodynamic method, *J. Acoust. Soc. Am.*, 76, 1023–1029, 1984.

23. Law, W.K., Frizzell, L.A, and Dunn, F., Ultrasonic determination of the nonlinearity parameter *B/A* for biological media, *J. Acoust. Soc. Am.*, 69, 1210–1212, 1981.

24. Earnshaw, S., On the mathematical theory of sound, *Trans. Royal Soc.*, 150, 133–148, 1860.

25. Fubini, E., Anomalie nella propagazione di ande acustiche de grande ampiezza. *Alta Frequenza*, 4, 530–581, 1935.

26. Thuras, A.L., Jenkins, R.T., and O'Neil, H.T., Extraneous frequencies generated in air carrying intense sound waves, *J. Acoust. Soc. Am.*, 6, 173–180, 1935.

27. Hamilton, M.F., and Morfey, C.L., Model Equations, Chapter 3 in: *Nonlinear Acoustics*, M.F. Hamilton and D.T. Blackstock (Eds.), Academic Press, New York, 1998.

28. Khokhlov, R.V., and Soluyan, S.I., Propagation of acoustic waves of moderate amplitude through dissipative and relaxing media, *Acustica*, 14, 241–247, 1964.

29. Naugol'nykh, K.A., Soluyan, S.I., and Khokhlov, R.V., Spherical waves of finite amplitude in a viscous thermally conducting medium, *Sov. Phys. Acoust.*, 9, 42–46, 1963.

30. Kuznetsov, V.P., Equations of nonlinear acoustics, *Sov. Phys. Acoust.*, 16, 467–470, 1971.
31. Zabolotskaya, E.A., and Khokhlov, R.V., Quasi-plane waves in the non-linear acoustics of confined beams, *Sov. Phys. Acoust.*, 15, 35–40, 1969.
32. Rudenko, O.V., and Soluyan, S.I., *Theoretical Foundations of Nonlinear Acoustics*, Consultants Bureau, New York, 1977.
33. Haran, M.E., and Cook, B.D., Distortion of finite amplitude ultrasound in lossy media, *J. Acoust. Soc. Am.*, 73, 774–779, 1983.
34. Trivett, D.H., and Van Buren, A.L., Comments on "Distortion of finite amplitude ultrasound in lossy media" by M.E. Haran and B.D. Cook [*J. Acoust. Soc. Am.*, 73, 774–779, 1983]. *J. Acoust. Soc. Am.*, 76, 1257–1258, 1984.
35. Pierce, A.D., *Acoustics: An Introduction to Its Physical Principles and Applications*, Acoustical Society of America Publications, New York, 1989.
36. Cleveland, R.O., Hamilton, M.F., and Blackstock, D.T., Time-domain modeling of finite-amplitude sound in relaxing fluids, *J. Acoust. Soc. Am.*, 99, 3312–3318, 1996.
37. Ginsberg, J.H., and Hamilton, M.F., Computational methods, Chapter 11 in: *Nonlinear Acoustics*, M.F. Hamilton and D.T. Blackstock (Eds.), Academic Press, New York, 1998.
38. Tjottta, J.N., and Tjotta, S., An analytical model for the nearfield of a baffled piston transducer, *J. Acoust. Soc. Am.*, 68, 334–339, 1980.
39. Kuc, R., Modeling acoustic attenuation of soft tissue with a minimum-phase filter, *Ultrasonic Imag.*, 6, 24–36, 1984.
40. He, P., Simulation of ultrasound pulse propagation in loss media obeying a frequency power law, *IEEE Trans. Ultrason. Ferroelect. Freq. Contr.*, 45, 114–125, 1998.
41. Zemp, R.J., Tavakkoli, J., and Cobbold, R.S.C., Modeling of nonlinear ultrasound propagation in tissue from array transducers, *J. Acoust. Soc. Am.*, 113, 139–152, 2003.
42. Gould, R.K., Smith, C.W., Williams, Jr., A.O., and Ryan, R.P., Measured structure of harmonics self-generated in an acoustic beam, *J. Acoust. Soc. Am.*, 40, 2539–2548, 1997.
43. Nachef, S., Cathignol, D., Tjotta, J.N., Berg, A.M., and Tjotta, S., Investigation of a high-intensity sound beam from a plane transducer. Experimental and theoretical results, *J. Acoust. Soc. Am.*, 98, 2303–2323, 1995.
44. TenCate, J.A., An experimental investigation of the nonlinear pressure field produced by a plane circular piston, *J. Acoust. Soc. Am.*, 94, 1084–1089, 1993.
45. Berntsen, J., Tjottta, J.N., and Tjotta, S., Interaction of sound waves. Part IV: Scattering of sound by sound, *J. Acoust. Soc. Am.*, 86, 1968–1983, 1989.
46. Christopher, P.T., and Parker, K.J., New approaches to nonlinear diffractive field propagation, *J. Acoust. Soc. Am.*, 90, 488–499, 1991.
47. Press, W.H., Teukolsky, S.A., Vetterling, W.T., and Flannery, B.P., *Numerical Recipes in FORTRAN: The Art of Scientific Computing*, 2nd edn., Cambridge University Press, UK, 1992.
48. Christopher, P.T., and Parker, K.J., New approaches to linear propagation of acoustic fields, *J. Acoust. Soc. Am.*, 90, 507–521, 1991.
49. Tavakkoli, J., Cathignol, D., Souchon, R., and Sapozhnikov, O.A., Modeling of pulsed finite-amplitude focused sound beams in time domain, *J. Acoust. Soc. Am.*, 104, 2061–2072, 1998.
50. Tavakkoli, J., Birer, J., Arefiev, A., Prat, F., Chapelon, J-Y., and Cathignol, D., A piezocomposite shock wave generator with electronic focusing capability: applica-

tion for producing cavitation-induced lesions in rabbit liver, *Ultrasound Med. Biol.*, 23, 107–115, 1997.

51. Tavakkoli, J., Birer, and Cathignol, D., Development of a PVDF low-cost shock-wave hydrophone, *Shock Waves*, 5, 369–374, 1996.

52. Khokhlova, V.A., Souchon, R., Tavakkoli, J., Sapozhnikov, O.A., and Cathignol, D., Numerical modeling of finite-amplitude sound beams: shock formation in the near field of a cw plane piston source, *J. Acoust. Soc. Am.*, 110, 95–108, 2001.

5

Scattering of Ultrasound

Because of the complex structure of most biological media, the scattered signal arising from an incident pulsed ultrasound beam is generally difficult to fully interpret, even when details of the structure are available. To address this problem, it is helpful to start by assuming a plane harmonic wave incident on a simple symmetrical scattering structure. Now any incident harmonic wave can be treated as a superposition of plane harmonic waves, and any pulse can be transformed into a spectrum of frequencies, so that a solution to the plane harmonic wave scattering problem enables a more general problem to be solved. Many methods of solution have been used, all of which are based on either exact or approximate solution of the wave equation. The boundary value method, initially used by Rayleigh [1,2] to obtain approximate solutions for spherical and cylindrical scatterers by acoustic waves, will first be studied. Small spherical scatterers are frequently used to model the structure of soft biological media [3], and in addition a simple spherical scatterer or a small-diameter wire is sometimes used to measure the pulse-echo response of an ultrasound transducer. Moreover, an array of such objects can be used to determine the performance of an imaging system. A Green's function approach can be used to arrive at an integral solution for the scattered wave, and this is especially helpful when the density and compressibility of the scattering region vary in a continuous manner. Since the integrand involves the sum of the incident and scattered fields, it is generally appropriate to make the Born approximation in which the scattered field is assumed to be small compared to that incident. Other approximations, such as the assumption of an observation point in the far field and scatterer dimensions that are small compared to a wavelength, enable explicit equations to be written for the scattered field. These methods, along with the boundary value approach, are reviewed in standard texts [4–6]. For CW scattering by structures with relatively simple shapes such as spheres and cylinders, the volume edited by Bowman et al. [7] and the chapter by Varadan et al. [8] are particularly helpful. Matrix methods can also be used and can be applied to structures of complex shape. One such method will be described and illustrated for calculating the scattering by a red blood cell (RBC).

Based on the assumptions of linear systems theory, a general model for the pulse-echo response can be obtained by combining the impulse response for the transmission, scattering, and reception processes. Both 1-D and 3-D approaches will be discussed. In the final part of this chapter, some approaches are described for determining the backscattered signal from a volume that contains a distribution of scatterers whose maximum dimensions are small compared to a wavelength. The particular case of backscattering by blood is examined in some detail.

5.1 Spherical and Cylindrical Representations of a Plane Wave

One method for obtaining exact solutions for scattering of a plane wave incident on spheres and cylinders is to express the incident wave as the sum of either spherical or cylindrical components. Alternatively, in the case of spherical scatterers, a point source can be assumed and the scattered field calculated. If the source is moved very far away from the scatterer, the incident field will be nearly plane, enabling the plane wave scattered field to be obtained. For the first method, the wave expansion expressions are given below.

For a harmonic plane incident wave propagating in the z-direction with an amplitude p_{im}, the pressure can be written as $p(z{:}t) = p_{im}e^{j\omega(t - z/c_o)}$. If the polar coordinates r and θ are used to specify the plane z, then $z = r\cos\theta$, so that $p(r,\theta{:}t) = p_{im}e^{j(\omega t - kr\cos\theta)}$. It can be shown that this can be expressed as the sum of a series of spherical waves given by [2, pp. 272–273]

$$(5.1) \quad p(r,\theta{:}t) = p_{im}e^{j(\omega t - kr\cos\theta)} = p_{im}e^{j\omega t}\sqrt{\frac{\pi}{2kr}}\sum_{n=0}^{\infty}(-j)^n(2n+1)\mathcal{P}_n(\cos\theta)J_{n+\frac{1}{2}}(kr),$$

in which $\mathcal{P}_n(.)$ is a Legendre polynomial of the first kind of order n and $J_{n+1/2}(.)$ is a cylindrical Bessel function of non-integer order. The latter can be expressed in terms of an nth-order spherical Bessel function through the relation $J_n(kr) = \sqrt{\frac{\pi}{2kr}}J_{n+1/2}(kr)$. We shall also need an expression for the radial component of the particle velocity, which can be obtained from (1.37) and (1.39) as $\underline{v}_r = (j/\omega\rho_o)\partial p/\partial r$, and the derivative of Bessel functions as given in Appendix C. Applying these to (5.1) enables the radial velocity phasor component to be expressed as

$$(5.2) \quad \underline{v}_r(r,\theta) = -\frac{p_{im}k}{\omega\rho_o}\sqrt{\frac{\pi}{2kr}}\sum_{n=0}^{\infty}(-j)^{n+1}(2n+1)\left[J_{n+\frac{3}{2}}(kr)-\frac{n}{kr}J_{n+\frac{1}{2}}(kr)\right]P_n(\cos\theta).$$

Similarly, a plane wave traveling in the z-direction when expressed in cylindrical coordinates (r,φ) can be expanded in terms of cylindrical waves [2, p. 309]:

$$(5.3) \quad p(r,\varphi{:}t) = p_{im}e^{j(\omega t - kr\cos\varphi)} = p_{im}e^{j\omega t}\left[J_0(kr)+2\sum_{n=1}^{\infty}(-j)^n J_n(kr)\cos(n\varphi)\right],$$

and the radial component of the particle velocity phasor is

$$(5.4) \quad \underline{v}_r(r,\varphi) = -\frac{p_{im}k}{\omega\rho_o}\left[jJ_1(kr)+\sum_{n=1}^{\infty}(-j)^{n+1}[J_{n-1}(kr)-J_{n+1}(kr)]\cos(n\varphi)\right].$$

In both the spherical and cylindrical expansions, it should be noted that a given component, e.g., $n = 1$, has an amplitude that depends on the radial distance through a Bessel function, but which also is angle-dependent through either the Legendre polynomial or the cosine function.

5.2 Scattering Cross-Sections

In discussing the scattered field characteristics, it is helpful to define the following quantities for an incident plane wave: (i) *total cross-section*, (ii) *scattering cross-section*, and (iii) *differential scattering cross-section*.

For an incident plane wave, the total cross-section is defined as

$$(5.5) \quad \sigma_t = \frac{\text{Time Averaged Total (Scattered + Absorbed) Power}}{\text{Time Averaged Incident Intensity}} = \frac{\overline{W_t}}{\overline{I}}. \quad (a)$$

Because the intensity can be expressed in Watts/m² and the power in Watts, the units of σ_t are square meters, as implied by the use of the term "cross-section." Physically, σ_t is that area of the incident wavefront that contains an amount of incident power equal to the total scattered power plus the power absorbed by the scatterer. Thus, the ratio of the total scattering cross-section to the physical cross-sectional area of the scatterer provides a useful measure of the scattering strength.

In a similar manner, the scattering cross-section is defined by

$$(5.5) \quad \sigma_s = \frac{\text{Time Averaged Total Scattered Power}}{\text{Time Averaged Incident Intensity}} = \frac{\overline{W_s}}{\overline{I}}. \quad (b)$$

If the absorption cross-section (σ_a) is defined as the ratio of the time-averaged total absorbed power to the average incident intensity, then it follows from (a) and (b) that

$$\sigma_t = \sigma_s + \sigma_a.$$

The differential scattering cross-section describes the variation of the scattered power with angular direction. It can be defined by

$$\sigma_d(\theta,\varphi) = \frac{\text{Time Averaged Scattered Power in the Direction } (\theta,\varphi) \text{ per Unit Solid Angle}}{\text{Time Averaged Incident Intensity}}.$$

It should be noted that a sphere has a solid angle of 4π steradians (sr), while an elementary solid angle is given by $d\Omega = \sin\theta d\theta d\varphi$. If $\overline{dW}(\theta,\varphi)$ is the power scattered in the direction (θ,φ) into a solid angle of $d\Omega$, then the above definition is equivalent to

(5.5)
$$\sigma_d(\theta,\varphi) = \frac{\overline{dW}}{d\Omega}\frac{1}{\overline{I}} = \frac{d\sigma_s}{d\Omega}.$$
(c)

Of major importance is the differential scattering in the opposite direction to the incident beam: this is called the (differential) *backscattering* cross-section and is given by

$$\sigma_b = \sigma_d(\pi,0).$$

The differential and backscattering cross-sections are often expressed in cm^2/sr.

5.3 Exact Analysis: Boundary Value Method

A well-established method for obtaining an exact solution for the scattered field due to a plane, cylindrical, or spherical wave incident on a scatterer of relatively simple geometry consists of expressing the Helmholtz equation solution in terms of an infinite series of orthogonal polynomials. Appropriate boundary conditions can then be imposed on the scatterer surface to determine the expansion coefficients. This method will be first illustrated for a plane wave incident on a rigid sphere. Two situations will be discussed, both of which were originally examined by Rayleigh [1] in his classic paper of 1872. In the first, the sphere is assumed to be infinitely dense so that the force created by the incident wave will cause no movement, while in the second the density condition is relaxed. The same approach will then be used to obtain a solution for scattering of a plane wave by an infinitely long compressible cylinder. Similar methods can be used for the prolate spheroid [9], of which the sphere and cylindrical rod are special cases.

5.3.1 Rigid Spherical Scatterer

Immobile Sphere

It should be recalled from Chapter 1 that the pressure at a given location $\mathbf{r}$ is the sum of the incident pressure p_i (when the scatterer is absent) and the scattered pressure p_s, i.e.,

$$(5.6) \qquad p(\mathbf{r}{:}t) = p_i(\mathbf{r}{:}t) + p_s(\mathbf{r}{:}t).$$

As illustrated in Fig. 5.1, we shall assume an incident plane harmonic wave, a spherical scatterer of radius a, zero compressibility ($\kappa_v = 0$), and infinite density ($\rho_v = \infty$). The last condition ensures that the sphere will remain stationary.

To obtain an expression for the scattered pressure p_s, we shall take the center of the sphere as the origin of a spherical coordinate system (r,θ,φ) and note that due to symmetry, the field at any location $\mathbf{r}$ is independent of φ. For a harmonic wave $p(r,\theta)$ must satisfy the spherical form of the Helmholtz equation given by (1.61). Because $p(r,\theta)$ is independent of φ, this simplifies to

$$(5.7) \qquad \frac{1}{r^2}\frac{\partial}{\partial r}\left(r^2\frac{\partial p}{\partial r}\right) + \frac{1}{r^2 \sin\theta}\frac{\partial}{\partial\theta}\left(\sin\theta\frac{\partial p}{\partial\theta}\right) + k^2 p(r,\theta) = 0.$$

If the variables in the solution are assumed to be separable, we can write

$$(5.8) \qquad p(\mathbf{r}) = R(r)P(\theta).$$

Substituting this into (5.7), it can be shown that two independent differential equations result, the first of which is the Legendre equation given by

$$(5.9) \qquad \left(1-\eta^2\right)\frac{d^2 P}{d\eta^2} - 2\eta\frac{dP}{d\eta} + n(n+1)P(\eta) = 0,$$

where $n = 0, 1, 2, 3 \ldots$ and $\eta = \cos\theta$. Solutions to this are the Legendre polynomials of the first kind, $P_n(\cos\theta)$. The second is Bessel's equation, which can be expressed as

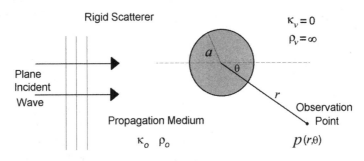

Figure 5.1 Geometry for calculating the pressure field that results from the scattering of an incident plane wave by a rigid sphere.

(5.10) $$\frac{d^2R}{d(kr)^2} + \frac{2}{kr}\frac{dR}{d(kr)} + \left(1 + \frac{n(n+1)}{(kr)^2}\right)R(kr) = 0:$$

a solution to which can be expressed in terms of *spherical* Bessel and Neumann functions. If the wave is traveling away from the source, then a solution is

(5.11) $$R_n = A_n[J_n(kr) - jn_n(kr)],$$ (a)

where the A_n is a constant, and the spherical Bessel and Neumann functions $J_n(.)$ and $n_n(.)$ can be expressed in terms of the cylindrical Bessel and Neumann functions by

(5.11) $$J_n(kr) = \sqrt{\frac{\pi}{2kr}} J_{n+\frac{1}{2}}(kr) \quad \text{and} \quad n_n(kr) = \sqrt{\frac{\pi}{2kr}} \mathcal{N}_{n+\frac{1}{2}}(kr).$$ (b)

A complete solution to (5.7) is therefore given by substituting into (5.8) the sum of all elementary solutions to Legendre's and Bessel's equations. Making use of the above relations, the scattered pressure at **r** can be expressed as

(5.12) $$\underline{p}_s(\mathbf{r}) = \sum_{n=0}^{\infty} A_n \sqrt{\frac{\pi}{2kr}} \left[J_{n+\frac{1}{2}}(kr) - j\mathcal{N}_{n+\frac{1}{2}}(kr) \right] P_n(\cos\theta).$$

The values of expansion coefficients A_n can be determined by making use of the boundary conditions on the surface of the sphere. Since the sphere has been assumed to have zero compressibility and to be infinitely dense, the radial component of the velocity will be zero. Now the radial velocity component is given by $\underline{v}_r = (j/\omega\rho_o)\partial p/\partial r$, so that by differentiating (5.6) and equating to zero the required boundary condition can be written as

$$\underline{v}_{ri}(a) + (\partial\underline{p}_s/\partial r)_{r=a} = 0.$$

By evaluating the partial derivative of (5.12) at $r = a$ and substituting (5.2) for the previously derived expression for radial velocity of an incident plane wave, an equation is obtained that contains all the terms of the summation. Because the wave functions are orthogonal, the boundary condition applies to each harmonic component, enabling the expansion coefficients to be expressed by

$$A_n = p_o \frac{(-j)^{n+2}(2n+1)}{1 + jK_n(ka)},$$

where
$$K_n(ka) = \frac{\frac{n}{ka}\mathcal{N}_{n+\frac{1}{2}}(ka) - \mathcal{N}_{n+\frac{3}{2}}(ka)}{J_{n+\frac{3}{2}}(ka) - \frac{n}{ka}J_{n+\frac{1}{2}}(ka)}.$$

By substituting this into (5.12), the scattered pressure phasor is given by

(5.13) $\underline{p}_s(\mathbf{r}) = p_{im} \sqrt{\dfrac{\pi}{2kr}} \displaystyle\sum_{n=0}^{\infty} \dfrac{(-j)^{n+2}(2n+1)}{1+jK_n(ka)} \left[J_{n+\frac{1}{2}}(kr) - j\mathcal{N}_{n+\frac{1}{2}}(kr) \right] P_n(\cos\theta).$

For observation points sufficiently distant such that $kr \gg 1$, this can be simplified by making use of the fact that the Bessel and Neumann functions can be replaced by their limiting forms. Moreover, for scatterers that are much smaller than a wavelength ($ka \ll 1$), it can be shown that in the far field (5.13) simplifies to

(5.14) $$\underline{p}_s(r,\theta) \approx -p_{im} \dfrac{k^2 a^3}{3r} e^{-jkr} \left(1 - \dfrac{3}{2}\cos\theta \right),$$ (a)

so that the scattered time-averaged intensity, $\bar{I} = p_s p_s^* / (2\rho_o c_o)$, is given by

(5.14) $$\bar{I}_s(r,\theta) \approx p_{im}^2 \dfrac{k^4 a^6}{18\rho_o c_o r^2} \left(1 - \dfrac{3}{2}\cos\theta \right)^2.$$ (b)

This shows that *the intensity falls off as the square of the distance, increases as the sixth power of the radius (or as the square of the volume) and varies inversely as the fourth power of the wavelength[1] (or is proportional to the fourth power of the frequency).*

The scattering and differential scattering cross-sections can be found from the definitions given by (5.5). The total scattered power can be found by evaluating $\overline{W}_s = \int_0^{\pi} \bar{I}_s(r,\theta) 2\pi r^2 \sin\theta d\theta$ and this, with the help of (5.14b) and (5.5b), enables the scattering cross-section to be expressed as

(5.15) $$\sigma_s = \dfrac{7\pi k^4 a^6}{9}.$$ (a)

The average power scattered at an angle θ into an elementary area $r^2 \sin\theta d\theta d\varphi$ on the surface of a sphere of radius r can be written as $d\overline{W} = \bar{I}_s r^2 \sin\theta d\theta d\varphi$. Now, the definition of a solid angle enables an incremental solid angle to be expressed as $d\Omega = \sin\theta d\theta d\varphi$. Consequently, $d\overline{W}/d\Omega = \bar{I}_s r^2$ and from (5.5c) and (5.14) the differential scattering cross-section is given by

(5.15) $$\sigma_d(\theta) = \dfrac{k^4 a^6}{9} \left(1 - \dfrac{3}{2}\cos\theta \right)^2, \quad \text{for} \quad ka \ll 1, \quad r \gg 1.$$ (b)

To illustrate the angle dependence of the scattered pressure, we show in Fig. 5.2 polar graphs for $kr = 50$ and six different values of ka, all results being computed directly from (5.13). For $ka = 0.1$, the results are virtually identical

---

1. For incident light, the inverse fourth-power intensity dependence on wavelength for small scatterers formed the basis of Rayleigh's celebrated explanation as to why the sky is blue [10].

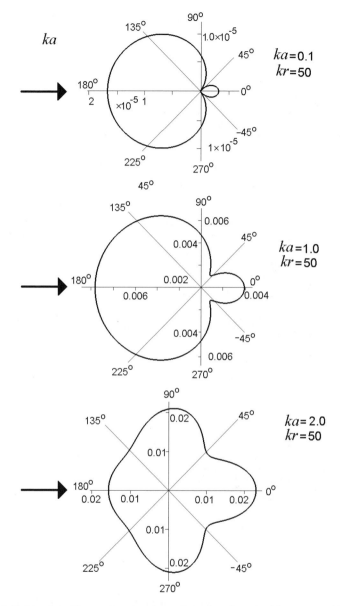

Figure 5.2 Polar plots illustrating the scattering of a plane incident wave (direction given by arrow) by a small rigid sphere that is fixed in space. The magnitudes of the ratios of the scattered to the incident pressures for six different values of ka are shown: the numerical values of the ratios are given on the horizontal and vertical axes.

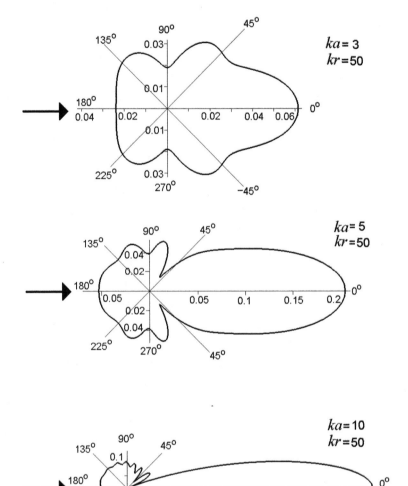

Figure 5.2 *Continued*

to that given by (5.14a). With increasing *ka* it can be seen that the scattered wave contains an increasing component in the forward scattering direction, which as expected corresponds to the field that destructively interferes with the incident field in the shadow region.

Free Rigid Sphere

In the last subsection it was assumed that the sphere was infinitely dense, thereby enabling the effect of the incident pressure on its vibration to be neglected. Rayleigh [1] relaxed this assumption but did not account for the influence of viscous damping on the movement, which was subsequently included by Sewell [11] in a paper published in 1910. It can be shown that for a small sphere and in the far field, this results in [12]

$$(5.16) \qquad \underline{p}_s(r,\theta) \approx p_{im} \frac{k^2 a^3}{3r} e^{-jkr} \left\{ 1 - \frac{3}{2} \left[\frac{(\rho_v - \rho_o) K_\mu}{\rho_v - \rho_o + \frac{3}{2} \rho_o K_\mu} \right] \cos\theta \right\},$$

for $ka \ll 1$, $kr \gg 1$, in which $K_\mu = 1 - \frac{3}{a} \sqrt{\frac{\mu}{j\omega\rho_o}} \left[1 - \frac{1}{a} \sqrt{\frac{\mu}{j\omega\rho_o}} \right]$ and where μ is

the shear viscosity. For an infinitely dense sphere the term in brackets reduces to unity, making the equation identical in magnitude to (5.14a), while for an inviscid fluid it reduces to

$$(5.17) \qquad \underline{p}_s(r,\theta) \approx p_{im} \frac{k^2 a^3}{3r} e^{-jkr} \left\{ 1 - \frac{3}{2} \left[\frac{\rho_v - \rho_o}{\rho_v + \rho_o/2} \right] \cos\theta \right\},$$

for $ka \ll 1$, $kr \gg 1$, and $\mu = 0$. This shows that if the scatterer and fluid densities are the same, the scattering will be isotropic.

5.3.2 Compressible Spherical Scatterer

A similar approach used for the rigid sphere can also be used to determine the scattered field caused by a sphere of finite density and non-zero compressibility freely suspended in a fluid medium. As mentioned earlier, movement of the center of the sphere is caused by the net effect of the incident and scattered waves and will be in the direction of the incident wave. In addition, movement of the sphere causes a movement of the surrounding fluid, and this depends on the fluid viscosity. In the case of a solid sphere, wave-mode conversion can occur at the boundary, making it necessary to account for the presence of both longitudinal and transverse waves in the sphere. As first discussed by Faran [14], the presence of these waves becomes particularly significant when the incident frequency approaches that associated with certain normal modes of free vibration. In fact, for a transient incident wave, the received waveform appears to bear little relationship to that transmitted. Hickling [15] corrected an error in Faran's original paper and reported a comparison of predictions with experimental measurements for both CW and transient conditions. Similar comparisons have been reported by Neubauer et al. [16] and Dragonette et al. [17]. Subsequently, Lin and Raptis [18] accounted for the effects of the fluid viscosity. More recently, Numrich and Uberall [19] and Hackman [20] have provided extensive reviews of scattering by elastic solids that also include an analysis of the effects of Rayleigh surface waves and other modes of vibration in spheres and cylinders.

To simplify the analysis, we shall ignore the above effects and will begin the analysis by using (5.12) to write the scattered pressure outside the sphere as

$$\underline{p}_s(\mathbf{r}) = \sum_{n=0}^{\infty} A_n \sqrt{\frac{\pi}{2k_o r}} \left[J_{n+\frac{1}{2}}(k_o r) - j\mathcal{N}_{n+\frac{1}{2}}(k_o r) \right] P_n(\cos\theta),$$

for $r \geq a^+$, in which the subscript o on the wave number k denotes its value outside the sphere and a^+ denotes the outer surface of the scatterer. Due to the differing speed of propagation, this wave number will generally differ from that inside, for which we will use the subscript v.

Inside the sphere there are no sources and the solution must be continuous at $r = 0$. Because the spherical Neumann function is discontinuous when the argument is zero $\{n_n(0) = -\infty\}$, it would be inappropriate to use this function in constructing an expansion for the field in the sphere. Consequently, we write the pressure as

$$\underline{p}_v(\mathbf{r}) = \sum_{n=0}^{\infty} B_n \sqrt{\frac{\pi}{2k_v r}} J_{n+\frac{1}{2}}(k_v r) P_n(\cos\theta), \quad \text{for } r \leq a^-.$$

To determine the constants A_n and B_n in the above equations, it is necessary to make use of the surface boundary conditions. These express the equalities of the pressures and the normal velocity components on the two sides of the surface and can be expressed as

$$\underline{p}_i(k_o a^+) + \underline{p}_s(k_o a^+) = \underline{p}_v(k_o a^-)$$
$$\underline{v}_{ri}(k_o a^+) + \underline{v}_{rs}(k_o a^+) = \underline{v}_{rv}(k_v a^-).$$

Implicit in these equations is the assumption that the displacement of the spherical surface is very small in comparison to the equilibrium radius a. Because $\underline{v}_r = (j/\omega\rho_o)\partial p/\partial r$, the latter can be written as

$$\rho_o \left[\frac{\partial \underline{p}_i}{\partial r} + \frac{\partial \underline{p}_s}{\partial r} \right]_{k_o r = k_o a^+} = \rho_v \left[\frac{\partial \underline{p}_v}{\partial r} \right]_{k_v r = k_v a^-}.$$

By applying these to the n'th harmonic component, the values of A_n and B_n can be obtained. After considerable algebra, it can be shown that the scattered pressure field is given by

(5.18)
$$\underline{p}_s(\mathbf{r}) = p_{im} \sum_{n=0}^{\infty} C_n (-j)^n (2n+1) h_n^o(k_o r) P_n(\cos\theta),$$
(a)

where

(5.18)
$$h_n^o(k_o r) = \sqrt{\frac{\pi}{2k_o r}} \left[J_{n+\frac{1}{2}}(k_o r) - j\mathcal{N}_{n+\frac{1}{2}}(k_o r) \right]$$
(b)

is a spherical Hankel function of the second kind of order n, and

(5.18)
$$C_n = \frac{\rho_v c_v j_n^v j_n^{\prime o} - \rho_o c_o j_n^o j_n^{\prime v}}{\rho_o c_o h_n^o j_n^{\prime v} - \rho_v c_v j_n^v h_n^{\prime o}},$$
(c)

in which the prime indicates the partial derivative with respect to r evaluated either just inside (superscript v) or just outside (superscript o) the spherical boundary.[2] In the far field ($k_o r \gg 1$) and for small scatterers ($k_v a \ll 1$), it can be shown that (5.18) reduces to

(5.19)
$$\underline{p}_s(r,\theta) \approx p_{im} e^{-jkr} \frac{k^2 a^3}{3r} \left\{ \frac{\kappa_v - \kappa_o}{\kappa_o} + \frac{3(\rho_v - \rho_o)}{2\rho_v + \rho_o} \cos\theta \right\},$$

which was originally derived by Rayleigh [1, 2, pp. 282–284].

The above equation will appear again in a slightly different form in describing the Green's function approach to solving the inhomogeneous wave equation and will prove to be valuable in discussing the scattering from blood.[3] Consequently, it is profitable to consider its interpretation and physical meaning at this point. First, it can be seen that (5.19) comprises two terms representing the fractional changes in compressibility and density. The compressibility term is independent of the angle θ and is referred to as a *monopole* term since it corresponds to a pulsating point source. On the other hand, the density term is angle-dependent and is known as the *dipole* term because it arises from oscillatory motion like a dipole source. Thus, one can see that mismatches in the mechanical properties will cause the obstacle to undergo different modes of vibrations. A mismatch in density causes the obstacle to oscillate back and forth about the undisturbed position, whereas a mismatch in compressibility causes the obstacle to pulsate (expand and contract). For most soft biological media, the dipole term contributes less than the monopole. For example, Fig. 5.3 shows the scattering of a plane wave by a single RBC in plasma when the wavelength is much greater than the maximum dimensions ($ka = 0.1$). It is evident that the dipole contribution is relatively small compared to the monopole contribution.

For an infinitely dense and incompressible scatterer, it can be seen that (5.19) reduces to (5.14a), as expected. The opposite extreme is that of small spherical gaseous bubble in a fluid. For example, using the values given in Table 1.1 for air bubble in water, the monopole term is $(\kappa_v - \kappa_o)/\kappa_o \approx (7047 - 0.46)/0.46 \approx 15000$, while the dipole term is $3(\rho_v - \rho_o)/(2\rho_v + \rho_o) \approx 3(1.2 - 1000)(2.4 + 1000) \approx 3$. Hence the dipole term can be neglected and because $\kappa_v \gg \kappa_o$, (5.19) simplifies to

$$\underline{p}_s(r,\theta) \approx p_{im} e^{-jkr} \frac{k^2 a^3}{3r} \frac{\kappa_v}{\kappa_o}.$$

2. By using (5.11b), the spherical Bessel functions in the expression for C_n can be expressed in terms of cylindrical Bessel functions of non-integer order, which are more commonly available in packages for numerical computation.

3. A major portion of this paragraph has been extracted from [21].

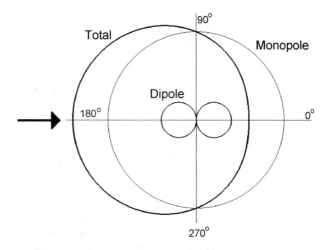

Figure 5.3 Monopole and dipole contributions to scattering by a single RBC in blood plasma when insonated by a plane wave. The RBC was modeled as a sphere and the graph shows the pressure distribution ($|p| \propto \sqrt{\sigma_d}$) as a function of the scattering angle. The dipole and monopole contributions to the total pressure were calculated from (5.19) using the following values for horse blood RBCs in plasma as measured by Urick [13]: $\rho_o = 1021\,\text{kg/m}^3$, $\rho_v = 1091\,\text{kg/m}^3$, $\kappa_o = 0.409\,\text{GPa}^{-1}$, $\kappa_v = 0.341\,\text{GPa}^{-1}$, together with $ka = 0.1$, $kr = 50$. If the RBC equivalent radius is taken to be 2.7 μm (volume = 82 μm³), then $ka = 0.1$ corresponds to a frequency of ~8.8 MHz.

Comparison of the ratio of the scattered intensity for an air bubble to that of a rigid sphere of the same radius in water shows that the air bubble has a scattering strength that is ~10^8 greater.

In a similar manner to that for a rigid sphere, the scattering cross-section and the differential scattering cross-section for the compressible sphere can be obtained from (5.19) and the definitions of (5.5), yielding

(5.20)
$$\sigma_s = \frac{4\pi k^4 a^6}{9}\left[\left|\frac{\kappa_v - \kappa_o}{\kappa_o}\right|^2 + 3\left|\frac{\rho_v - \rho_o}{2\rho_v + \rho_o}\right|^2\right],$$
(a)

(5.20)
$$\sigma_d(\theta) = \frac{k^4 a^6}{9}\left[\frac{\kappa_v - \kappa_o}{\kappa_o} + \frac{3(\rho_v - \rho_o)}{2\rho_v + \rho_o}\cos\theta\right]^2.$$
(b)

As a further example, Fig. 5.4 shows the backscattering cross-section variation as a function of ka for sphere with a radius of 2.7 μm, making its volume the same as that of 82 μm³ RBC. The calculations were made with the series expansion equation of (5.18) using the parameters given in the figure caption. It can be seen that the backscattering cross-section obeys the approximate equation of (5.20b) even for values of ka considerably beyond 0.1. For $ka > 1$, e.g., $f > 90\,\text{MHz}$, the behavior is dominated by resonance effects.

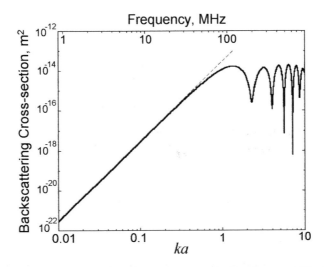

Figure 5.4 Backscattering cross-section for a 2.7 μm radius compressible "RBC" sphere in saline over a wide range of *ka* values using (5.18) with 20 terms in the expansion (no change occurred with further terms). The dashed line shows the results given by the approximate (small *ka*) equation, which corresponds to an f^4 frequency dependence. The following parameters were used: $\rho_v = 1078\,\text{kg/m}^3$, $\kappa_v = 0.39115\,\text{GPa}^{-1}$, $\rho_o = 1004\,\text{kg/m}^3$, $\kappa_o = 0.44206\,\text{GPa}^{-1}$, $kr = 50$, $a = 2.7\,\mu\text{m}$.

5.3.3 Compressible Cylindrical Scatterer

With reference to Fig. 5.5, the general problem consists of a plane wave incident at an arbitrary angle α on an infinitely long cylinder of radius *a*, whose axis coincides with the *z*-axis. In general, both longitudinal and transverse waves will be excited in the cylinder; and, depending on the fluid viscosity, a transverse wave can also be propagated in the surrounding fluid. For normal incidence (α = 0), the problem becomes much simpler if the fluid is assumed to be inviscid and wave-mode conversion effects are neglected. Indeed, Rayleigh [2, pp. 309–311] was the first to analyze the scattering for this case, though with the added assumptions that the observation point was in the far field and the radius was small compared to the wavelength. The effects of fluid viscosity [18,22], wave-mode conversion for both normally [14] and obliquely incident [23,24] waves, and anisotropy of the cylindrical scatterer [25] have also been described.

The analysis of this problem follows the same scheme used for the sphere. Expressions are written for the incident wave in terms of cylindrical harmonics, the scattered wave, and the wave inside the cylinder. The incident wave is given by modifying (5.3) to include the incident angle:

$$\underline{p}_i(r,z,\varphi) = p_{im}e^{-jkz\sin\alpha}\left[J_0(kr)+2\sum_{n=1}^{\infty}(-j)^n J_n(kr\cos\alpha)\cos(n\varphi)\right]$$

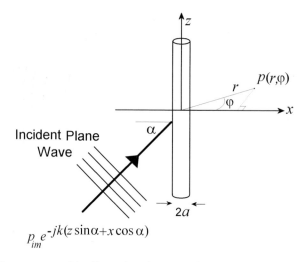

$$p_{im}e^{-jk(z\sin\alpha + x\cos\alpha)}$$

Figure 5.5 Geometry used in discussing the scattering of a plane wave incident at an angle α on an infinitely long cylinder.

The scattered wave can be expressed in terms of cylindrical Bessel and Neumann functions as

$$\underline{p}_s(r,z,\varphi) = p_{im}e^{-jkz\sin\alpha}\sum_{n=0}^{\infty} A_n[J_n(kr\cos\alpha) - j\mathcal{N}_n(kr\cos\alpha)]\cos(n\varphi),$$

and, if wave mode conversion can be ignored, then the wave inside the cylinder is represented by

$$\underline{p}_v(r,z,\varphi) = p_{im}e^{-jkz\sin\alpha}\sum_{n=0}^{\infty} B_n J_n(kr\cos\alpha)\cos(n\varphi).$$

By applying the boundary conditions, the constants A_n and B_n can be determined and it can be shown that the scattered wave pressure in the far field $(kr \gg 1)$ and for a small-radius cylinder $(ka \ll 1)$ reduces to [4, p. 464]

(5.21)

$$\underline{p}_s(r,z,\varphi) \approx p_{im}\frac{k^2a^2}{2}\sqrt{\frac{\pi\cos^3\alpha}{2kr}}\left\{\frac{\kappa_v - \kappa_o}{\kappa_o} + \frac{2(\rho_v - \rho_o)}{\rho_v + \rho_o}\cos\varphi\right\}e^{-j\left[\frac{\pi}{4} + k(r\cos\alpha + z\sin\alpha)\right]}.$$

It should be noted that this expression contains a compressibility term giving isotropic scattering and a density term that is angle-dependent, similar to that of a small sphere. But in contrast to a sphere, the scattering varies inversely as $\sqrt{r}$ and as $\omega^{3/2}$. For a rigid immobile cylinder $(\kappa_v = 0, \rho_v = \infty)$ and normal incidence $(\alpha = 0)$, (5.21) reduces to an equation originally obtained by Rayleigh [2, p. 311]:

$$\underline{p}_s(r,z,\varphi) \approx -p_{im}\frac{k^2a^2}{2}\sqrt{\frac{\pi}{2kr}}\{1-2\cos\varphi\}e^{-j\left[\frac{\pi}{4}+kr\right]}.$$

It is of interest to note that cylindrical scatterers are sometimes used to model the scattering from tissue. For example, ultrasound scattering by trabecular bone has been modeled in this way. Trabecular bone consists of a 3-D lattice in which the spaces are filled with bone marrow media. In the approach used by Wear [26], ultrasound scattering was modeled by cylinders whose diameters were small compared to a wavelength, and whose lengths were greater than the beam cross-section.

5.4 Integral Equation Methods

Most media possess some degree of inhomogeneity. For example, in the ocean there are slight variations in salinity and temperature from region to region: these will cause slight changes in the path of an acoustic wave and cause scattering. In tissue, the cellular nature of the media causes local variations of compressibility and density: these are responsible for the speckle background patterns seen in ultrasound B-mode images. To characterize the effects of such variations, it is first necessary to obtain a wave equation that describes propagation in an inhomogeneous medium.

5.4.1 Wave Equation for an Inhomogeneous Region

In this task we follow the derivation given by Morse and Ingard [4, pp. 407–410], though derivations have been given by others [5, p. 282; 27–29]. It should be noted that the foundations of this approach and some of the results were originally developed and derived by Rayleigh [1; see also 2, pp. 149–152] in 1872.

We assume that the density and compressibility at any location $\mathbf{r}$ can be represented by values of $\Delta\rho(\mathbf{r})$ and $\Delta\kappa(\mathbf{r})$ superimposed on uniform background values of ρ_o and κ_o, and that $\Delta\rho(\mathbf{r})$ and $\Delta\kappa(\mathbf{r})$ are not restricted in their magnitudes. Thus, in the presence of an acoustic field the total density and compressibility can be expressed as

(5.22)
$$\begin{cases}\rho(\mathbf{r}{:}t) = \rho_o + \Delta\rho(\mathbf{r}) + \rho_1(\mathbf{r}{:}t) = \rho_v(\mathbf{r}) + \rho_1(\mathbf{r}{:}t) \\ \kappa(\mathbf{r}) = \kappa_o + \Delta\kappa(\mathbf{r}) = \kappa_v(\mathbf{r})\end{cases}$$

where $\rho_1(\mathbf{r}{:}t)$ is the small-signal acoustic density component, $\rho_v(\mathbf{r})$ is the equilibrium density, and $\kappa_v(\mathbf{r})$ is the equilibrium compressibility.

Now the Eulerian form of the equation of state, as given by (1.25), can be expressed as

$$\frac{\partial\rho_1}{\partial t} + \mathbf{v}\cdot\nabla\rho = \kappa_v\rho_v\left[\frac{\partial p}{\partial t} + \mathbf{v}\cdot\nabla p\right]$$

in which p is the acoustic pressure and $\mathbf{v}$ is the particle velocity. For small signals such that $c_o \gg |\mathbf{v}|$, $\partial p/\partial t \gg \mathbf{v} \cdot \nabla p$, so that this equation reduces to

(5.23)
$$\frac{\partial \rho_1}{\partial t} + \mathbf{v} \cdot \nabla \rho \approx \kappa_v \rho_v \frac{\partial p}{\partial t}$$

In addition, the Eulerian form of the continuity equation, as given by (1.22), is

$$\frac{\partial \rho_1}{\partial t} + \nabla \cdot (\rho \mathbf{v}) = 0,$$

which can then be expanded to[4]

(5.24)
$$\frac{\partial \rho_1}{\partial t} + \mathbf{v} \cdot \nabla \rho + \rho \nabla \cdot \mathbf{v} = 0.$$

Subtracting (5.23) and (5.24) and noting that for small signal conditions $\rho_1 \ll \rho_v$, so that from (5.22) $\rho \approx \rho_v$, we obtain

$$\kappa_v \rho_v \frac{\partial p}{\partial t} = -\rho \nabla \cdot \mathbf{v} \approx -\rho_v \nabla \cdot \mathbf{v},$$

or

(5.25)
$$\kappa_v \frac{\partial \rho}{\partial t} + \nabla \cdot \mathbf{v} = 0.$$

Now for an inviscid fluid, Euler's equation, as given by (1.21) for small-signal conditions, can be written as

(5.26)
$$\rho_v \frac{\partial \mathbf{v}}{\partial t} + \nabla p = 0.$$

By taking the partial derivative with respect to time of (5.25) and using (5.26) to substitute for $\partial \mathbf{v}/\partial t$, we obtain

(5.27)
$$\kappa_v \frac{\partial^2 p}{\partial t^2} = \nabla \cdot [(1/\rho_v)\nabla p].$$

The final form of the wave equation can be obtained by adding $\frac{1}{\rho_o}\left(\nabla^2 p - \frac{1}{c_o^2}\frac{\partial^2 p}{\partial t^2}\right)$ to both sides of (5.27) and noting that the wave speed in the background region (where $\Delta\rho(\mathbf{r}) = \Delta\kappa(\mathbf{r}) = 0$) is denoted by $c_o = 1/\sqrt{\rho_o\kappa_o}$.

4. By using the vector relation $\nabla \cdot (w\mathbf{u}) = \mathbf{u} \cdot \nabla w + w\nabla \cdot \mathbf{u}$.

These steps enable the following form of the inhomogeneous wave equation to be obtained:

(5.28)
$$\boxed{\nabla^2 p - \frac{1}{c_o^2}\frac{\partial^2 p}{\partial t^2} = \frac{1}{c_o^2}\frac{\partial^2 p}{\partial t^2}\left[\frac{\kappa_v - \kappa_o}{\kappa_o}\right] + \nabla\cdot\left[\frac{\rho_v - \rho_o}{\rho_v}\nabla p\right].}$$
    (a)

On examining this equation, it will be noted that the left-hand side consists of the wave equation terms for a uniform medium, while the right-hand side corresponds to a radiation source that represents the scattering of energy due to the non-uniform nature of the medium.

An alternative form of (5.28a) can be obtained [27] by first noting that the wave speed in the scattering medium is given by $c(\mathbf{r}) = 1/\sqrt{\rho_v \kappa_v}$. By substituting into (5.27) and transforming[4] the right-hand side, it can be readily shown that the wave equation reduces to $\nabla^2 p - \dfrac{1}{c^2}\dfrac{\partial^2 p}{\partial t^2} = \nabla(\ln\rho_v)\cdot\nabla p$. If $c = c_o + \Delta c$, $\Delta c/c_o \ll 1$, and $\Delta\rho/\rho_o \ll 1$, this can be expressed as

(5.28)
$$\boxed{\nabla^2 p - \frac{1}{c_o^2}\frac{\partial^2 p}{\partial t^2} \approx -\frac{2\Delta c}{c_o^3}\frac{\partial^2 p}{\partial t^2} + \nabla(\ln\rho_v)\cdot\nabla p,}$$
    (b)

whose right-hand side is the "source" scattering term.

5.4.2 Integral Scattering Equation

Consider the arbitrary-shaped scattering volume shown in Fig. 5.6 with acoustic properties of κ_v and ρ_v that can vary throughout V_s. The scattering volume is assumed to be imbedded in an infinite background medium whose acoustic properties are constant (κ_o, ρ_o). To obtain an integral equation that

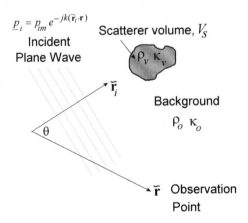

$\underline{p}_i = p_{im}e^{-jk(\tilde{\mathbf{r}}_i\cdot\mathbf{r})}$
Incident
Plane Wave

Scatterer volume, V_S

$\rho_v \kappa_v$

$\tilde{\mathbf{r}}_i$

Background
$\rho_o \kappa_o$

θ

$\tilde{\mathbf{r}}$ Observation
Point

Figure 5.6 Scattering volume within which the density and compressibility vary, imbedded in a uniform region. The unit vectors $\tilde{\mathbf{r}}_i$ and $\tilde{\mathbf{r}}$ are in the directions of the incident wave and observation point, respectively.

expresses the total acoustic pressure field (incident + scattered) due to an incident wave, we make use of (5.28a), which applies to points both within and outside the scatterer (outside the scatterer $(\kappa_v - \kappa_o) = (\rho_v - \rho_o) = 0$). For the problem at hand it is convenient to write the wave equation as

$$\nabla^2 p - \frac{1}{c_o^2}\frac{\partial^2 p}{\partial t^2} = -f(\mathbf{r}:t),$$

where the "source" term $f(\mathbf{r}:t)$ is given by (see (5.28a))

(5.29) $$f(\mathbf{r}:t) = \frac{-1}{c_o^2}\frac{\partial^2 p}{\partial t^2}\left[\frac{\kappa_v - \kappa_o}{\kappa_o}\right] - \nabla \cdot \left[\frac{\rho_v - \rho_o}{\rho_v}\nabla p\right],$$

whose Fourier transform is

(5.30) $$F(\mathbf{r}:\omega) = k^2\left[\frac{\kappa_v - \kappa_o}{\kappa_o}\right]\underline{p} - \nabla \cdot \left[\frac{\rho_v - \rho_o}{\rho_v}\nabla\underline{p}\right].$$

In using the Green's function approach for obtaining an integral equation for the scattered pressure field, we write the Fourier transformed version of the wave equation and the equation governing the Green's function as

$$(\nabla^2 + k^2)\underline{p} = -F(\mathbf{r}:\omega)$$
$$(\nabla^2 + k^2)G(\mathbf{r}|\mathbf{r}_o) = -\delta(\mathbf{r} - \mathbf{r}_o)$$

in which G is the Green's function and $k = \omega/c_o$ is the wave number for the background medium. We then proceed in the manner previously described in Chapter 2 (see (2.8)), i.e., multiplying the above two equations by G and F respectively, subtracting, integrating over a volume V that *includes* the scatterer volume V_s, and then making use of Green's theorem. These steps enable the acoustic pressure to be expressed as

(5.31) $$\underline{p}(\mathbf{r}:\omega) = \iint_S\left[G\frac{\partial\underline{p}}{\partial n} - \underline{p}\frac{\partial G}{\partial n}\right]dS_o + \iiint_{V_s}G(\mathbf{r}|\mathbf{r}_o)F(\mathbf{r}_o:\omega)dV_o,$$

where the partial derivatives are in the outward direction normal to the surface, and the subscript o serves to remind us that the integrations are with respect to $\mathbf{r}_o$. Moreover, as noted earlier, outside V_s but within the enclosing surface S, $\rho_v - \rho_o = 0$ and $\kappa_v - \kappa_o = 0$, so that in this region it follows from (5.30) that $F(\mathbf{r}_o:\omega) = 0$. Consequently, as indicated, the volume integral can be written as being over the scatterer volume V_s.

Because the background medium has been assumed to be unbounded, the appropriate Green's function is $G(\mathbf{r}|\mathbf{r}_o) \equiv G(|\mathbf{r} - \mathbf{r}_o|) = e^{-j\omega R/c_o}/4\pi R$, in which $R = |\mathbf{r} - \mathbf{r}_o|$ is the distance to the observation point $\mathbf{r}$. It can be shown that if the surface is a sphere of very large radius so that the incident pressure wave enters from infinity, then the surface integral in (5.31) is exactly equal to the incident pressure wave p_i. Thus, using (5.30) and (5.31) and noting that $\underline{p}_s = \underline{p} - \underline{p}_i$, the scattered field pressure can be expressed as

(5.32)

$$\underline{p}_s(\mathbf{r}{:}\omega) = \iiint_{V_s} \left\{ k^2 \underline{p}(\mathbf{r}_o) \left[\frac{\kappa_v - \kappa_o}{\kappa_o} \right] G(\mathbf{r}|\mathbf{r}_o) - \nabla \cdot \left[\frac{\rho_v - \rho_o}{\rho_v} \nabla \underline{p}(\mathbf{r}_o) \right] G(\mathbf{r}|\mathbf{r}_o) \right\} dV_o,$$

in which the operator ∇ is with respect to the coordinates of $\mathbf{r}_o$. The second term can be transformed by means of a vector relation[4] to $\nabla \cdot \left[\frac{\rho_v - \rho_o}{\rho_v} G \nabla \underline{p}(\mathbf{r}_o) \right] - \frac{\rho_v - \rho_o}{\rho_v} [\nabla G \cdot \nabla \underline{p}(\mathbf{r}_o)]$. Moreover, by using Gauss' theorem,[5] the volume integral of the divergence term can then be converted to an integral over the surface enclosing the scatterer. Because this surface integral vanishes, (5.32) reduces to

(5.33)

$$\underline{p}_s(\mathbf{r}{:}\omega) = \iiint_{V_s} \left\{ k^2 \underline{p}(\mathbf{r}_o) \left[\frac{\kappa_v - \kappa_o}{\kappa_o} \right] G(\mathbf{r}|\mathbf{r}_o) + \left[\frac{\rho_v - \rho_o}{\rho_v} \right] [\nabla G(\mathbf{r}|\mathbf{r}_o) \cdot \nabla \underline{p}(\mathbf{r}_o)] \right\} dV_o,$$

which is often referred to as the *scattering equation*. It should be noted that (5.33) is valid for a scattering region in which both the compressibility and density can be spatially varying throughout the volume V_s, in which case both terms enclosed by square brackets would be functions of $\mathbf{r}_o$. In addition, it is valid when the scattering region has constant acoustic properties. The first monopolar term is the contribution arising from the difference in compressibility and the second (dipolar) term arises from the density difference. It will be noted that both terms depend on the total pressure $\overline{p} = \overline{p}_s + \overline{p}_i$ and, because this is not known, an approximation method must be used to evaluate the scattered pressure.

5.4.3 Scattering Approximations

If the scattering is sufficiently weak so that the scattered pressure is much less than the incident pressure, the incident wave will remain virtually unchanged as it progresses through the scattering volume, i.e., $p(\mathbf{r}_o) \approx p_i(\mathbf{r}_o)$. This is known as the *Born approximation* and it enables the scattered pressure to be evaluated without having to use, for example, the method of successive approximations. The assumption of weak scattering also implies that multiple scattering (scattering of the scattered wave) can be ignored.

In addition to the Born approximation, it can often be assumed that the observation point is sufficiently far from the scattering region so that an approximate expression can be used for the point source Green's function and its gradient. With the help of Fig. 5.7, in which it is assumed that $r \gg r_o$, the Green's function is approximately given by

5. Gauss' divergence theorem: $\iiint_V \text{div}\,\mathbf{u}\,dV = \iint_S \mathbf{u} \cdot \tilde{\mathbf{n}}\,dS.$

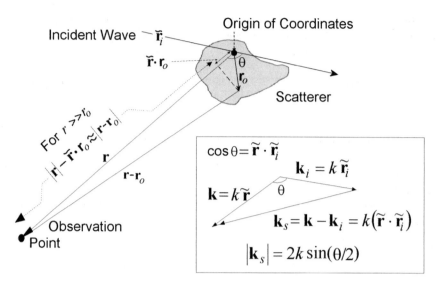

Figure 5.7 Obtaining an approximate expression for the point source Green's function in the far field. The insert shows how the scattering vector k_s is defined and related to θ. The expression for $|k_s|$ was obtained by noting that

$$|\mathbf{k}_s| = k[\tilde{\mathbf{r}}^2 + \tilde{\mathbf{r}}_i^2 - 2(\tilde{\mathbf{r}} \cdot \tilde{\mathbf{r}}_i)]^{1/2} = 2k\left[\frac{1 - \cos\theta}{2}\right]^{1/2}.$$

$$G(\mathbf{r}|\mathbf{r}_o) = e^{-jk|\mathbf{r}-\mathbf{r}_o|}/4\pi|\mathbf{r}-\mathbf{r}_o| \approx e^{-jk(r-\tilde{\mathbf{r}}\cdot\mathbf{r}_o)}/(4\pi r),$$

in which $\tilde{\mathbf{r}}$ is a unit vector in the direction of the observation point $\mathbf{r}$. In addition, the gradient is approximated by

$$\nabla G(\mathbf{r}|\mathbf{r}_o) \approx jk\tilde{\mathbf{r}}G(\mathbf{r}|\mathbf{r}_o).$$

For an incident plane wave in the direction of the unit vector $\tilde{\mathbf{r}}_i$, the incident pressure and its gradient at a position $\mathbf{r}$ are given by

$$\underline{p}_i = p_{im}e^{-jk(\tilde{\mathbf{r}}_i \cdot \mathbf{r})}, \quad \nabla\underline{p}_i = -jk\tilde{\mathbf{r}}_i\underline{p}_i,$$

where p_{im} is the pressure amplitude. Using the Born approximation, substituting the above four relations into (5.33), and denoting the angle between the incident direction and the observation direction by θ, i.e., $\cos\theta = \tilde{\mathbf{r}}_i \cdot \tilde{\mathbf{r}}$, the scattered pressure can be written as

$$(5.34) \quad \underline{p}_s(\mathbf{r}, \tilde{\mathbf{r}}_i) = p_{im}\frac{e^{-jkr}k^2}{4\pi r}\iiint_{V_s}\left\{\left[\frac{\kappa_v - \kappa_o}{\kappa_o}\right] + \left[\frac{\rho_v - \rho_o}{\rho_v}\right]\cos\theta\right\}e^{jkr_o \cdot (\tilde{\mathbf{r}} - \tilde{\mathbf{r}}_i)}dV_o.$$

It is convenient to define a scattering vector $\mathbf{k}_s$ by: $\mathbf{k}_s = k(\tilde{\mathbf{r}} - \tilde{\mathbf{r}}_i)$. With the help of the insert in Fig. 5.7, the magnitude of this vector is related to the scattering angle by $|\mathbf{k}_s| = 2k\sin(\theta/2)$. Thus, (5.34) can be expressed as:

$$(5.35) \qquad \boxed{\underline{p}_s(r, \mathbf{k}_s) = p_{im} \frac{e^{-jkr}}{r} \Theta(\mathbf{k}_s),} \qquad \text{(a)}$$

where

$$(5.35) \qquad \Theta(\mathbf{k}_s) = \frac{k^2}{4\pi} \iiint_{V_s} [\gamma_\kappa(\mathbf{r}_o) + \gamma_\rho(\mathbf{r}_o) \cos\theta] e^{j(\mathbf{r}_o \cdot \mathbf{k}_s)} dV_o, \qquad \text{(b)}$$

describes the angular distribution of the scattered pressure, and the γ functions are given by $\gamma_\kappa(\mathbf{r}_o) = (\kappa_v - \kappa_o)/\kappa_o$ and $\gamma_\rho(\mathbf{r}_o) = (\rho_v - \rho_o)/\rho_v$. Equation (5.35) shows that the scattered pressure at an observation point consists of a spherical wave originating from the center of the scattering volume V_s with an amplitude that depends on the scattering angle. The derivation assumed an incident plane, weak scattering ($\gamma_\kappa \ll 1$, $\kappa_\rho \ll 1$), and that the observation point was in the far field.

Now the 3-D spatial Fourier transforms of the compressibility and density functions can be defined by:

$$\Gamma_\kappa(\mathbf{k}_s) = \iiint \gamma_\kappa(\mathbf{r}_o) e^{j\mathbf{r}_o \cdot \mathbf{k}_s} dV_o,$$

and

$$\Gamma_\rho(\mathbf{k}_s) = \iiint \gamma_\rho(\mathbf{r}_o) e^{j\mathbf{r}_o \cdot \mathbf{k}_s} dV_o.$$

By using these in (5.35), the scattered pressure can be re-expressed in terms of the 3-D spatial Fourier transforms of the compressibility and density functions [4, pp. 411–414], i.e.,

$$(5.36) \qquad p(\mathbf{k}_s : t) = p_{im} \frac{e^{j(\omega t - kr)}}{4\pi r} k^2 \{\Gamma_\kappa(\mathbf{k}_s) + \Gamma_\rho(\mathbf{k}_s) \cos\theta\}.$$

The differential scattering cross-section of V_s can be readily obtained from (5.35) and the definition given by (5.5c) as

$$(5.37) \qquad \sigma_d = |\Theta(\mathbf{k}_s)|^2.$$

Further simplification of (5.34) is possible if the maximum dimension of the scattering region is small compared to a wavelength (the long wavelength limit). Specifically, for $ka \ll 1$, where a is the maximum dimension of the volume V_s, the exponential term under the integral sign is approximately unity and the integral reduces to the product of the scatterer volume and the spatially averaged compressibility and density terms. Consequently, the scattered pressure can be written as

$$(5.38) \qquad \underline{p}_s(\mathbf{r} : \omega) = p_{im} \frac{k^2 V_s}{4\pi r} \left[\frac{\kappa_v - \kappa_o}{\kappa_o} + \frac{\rho_v - \rho_o}{\rho_v} \cos\theta \right] e^{-jkr}, \qquad \text{(a)}$$

which is independent of the scatterer shape, is proportional to the scatterer volume [2, p. 152], and depends on the mean values of the κ's and ρ's over V_s. This enables the differential scattering cross-section to be obtained as

$$(5.39) \qquad \sigma_d(\theta) = \frac{k^4 V_s^2}{16\pi^2} \left[\frac{\kappa_v - \kappa_o}{\kappa_o} + \frac{\rho_v - \rho_o}{\rho_v} \cos\theta \right]^2 .$$

For the particular case of a spherical scatterer of radius a ($V_s = 4\pi a^3/3$) whose compressibility and density are constant over the scatterer volume, (5.38a) enables the scattered pressure to be expressed as

$$(5.38) \qquad \underline{p}_s(\mathbf{r}{:}\omega) = p_{im} \frac{k^2 a^3}{3r} \left(\frac{\kappa_v - \kappa_o}{\kappa_o} + \frac{\rho_v - \rho_o}{\rho_v} \cos\theta \right) e^{-jkr} . \qquad (b)$$

Comparison of (5.38b) with (5.19), derived from the boundary value approach, reveals that the two expressions differ in the dipole term. This appears to be the result of making the Born approximation, which assumed that the perturbation of the incident wave by the scattering medium was small, i.e., $\Delta\rho(\mathbf{r})/\rho$ and $\Delta\kappa(\mathbf{r})/\kappa \ll 1$. By making the additional assumption that the density change is small ($|\rho_v - \rho_o| \ll \rho_o$), the two equations become identical.

5.5 Matrix Methods

For more complex scatterer geometries, a variety of methods are available for calculating the scattering. One of these, proposed and developed by Waterman [30], is particularly well suited for scatterers that have some degree of symmetry. Subsequent to the initial description for acoustic waves, Waterman [31] and Varatharajulu and Pao [32] extended the method to take account of wave-mode conversion and the presence of transverse waves. Moreover, the method has been applied for calculating the scattering from an arbitrary number of scatterers [33,34]. An outline of Waterman's technique will be given and illustrated for a scatterer with rotational symmetry.

5.5.1 The T-Matrix of Waterman

In the method devised by Waterman [30], the field components and the Green's function are expanded as an orthonormal set of wave functions. By applying the Helmholtz theorem (see Chapter 2) to regions that are interior and exterior to the surface encompassing the scatterer, two relations are obtained. These, together with the boundary conditions, are of key importance in obtaining the *transition* T-matrix that relates the expansion coefficients of the scattered and incident fields. In his review of scattering by elastic solids, Hackman [20] gives a useful summary of the technique and its application.

The velocity potential at the observation point $\mathbf{r}$ can be written as the sum of the incident and scattered fields, i.e., $\Phi(\mathbf{r},\omega) = \Phi_i(\mathbf{r},\omega) + \Phi_s(\mathbf{r},\omega)$. A scatterer

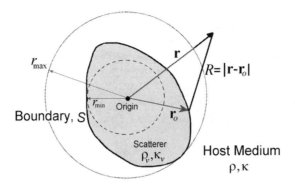

Figure 5.8 Geometry of an arbitrary scatterer with a bounding surface denoted by S. The field point at r is shown as being exterior to S.

is shown in Fig. 5.8 bounded by a surface S, which is assumed to be piecewise smooth. For field points exterior to the scatterer surface, the Helmholtz theorem enables the velocity potential of the scattered field to be expressed as

$$\Phi_i(\mathbf{r}:\omega) = -\iint_S (G\nabla_+\Phi - \Phi_+\nabla G)\cdot \tilde{\mathbf{n}}dS_o, \quad \text{for } \mathbf{r} \text{ outside } S \tag{a}$$

(5.40)

where $G = G(k|\mathbf{r} - \mathbf{r}_o|)$ is taken to be the free space Green's function, $\tilde{\mathbf{n}}$ is a unit vector normal to the surface pointing in an outward direction, Φ_+ is the total field on the outside surface, and $\nabla_+\Phi$ is the gradient of the total field on the surface approached from the outside. In addition, it should be noted that the subscript o is a reminder that the integration is with respect to the source point $\mathbf{r}_o$. For field points inside the scatterer, the Helmholtz theorem provides a relation between the incident field and that on the surface S.

$$\Phi_i(\mathbf{r}:\omega) = \iint_S (G\nabla_+\Phi - \Phi_+\nabla G)\cdot \tilde{\mathbf{n}}dS_o, \quad \text{for } \mathbf{r} \text{ inside } S. \tag{b}$$

(5.40)

Now the free space Green's function can be expressed as a zero-order spherical Hankel function of kR, i.e.,

$$G(k|\mathbf{r} - \mathbf{r}_o|) = e^{-jkR}\bigg/ 4\pi R = -\frac{jk}{4\pi}h_0(kR),$$

In spherical coordinates (r,θ,φ) the Green's function can be expanded in terms of outgoing partial wave solutions to the Helmholtz equation. If $\{\psi_n(k\mathbf{r})\}$ is a set of outgoing spherical wave solutions, then, using a simplified notation,[6] the Green's function can be written as [30]

---

6. Here, a single index n has been used to represent the indices m, n, and σ in the full expansion form given below.

(5.41)
$$G(k|\mathbf{r} - \mathbf{r}_o|) = -\frac{jk}{4\pi} \sum_n \psi_n(k\mathbf{r}_>) \mathrm{Re}\{\psi_n(k\mathbf{r}_<)\}, \tag{a}$$

where Re denotes the real part, $r_>$ is the greater of (r, r_o), and $r_<$ is the lesser of (r, r_o). In spherical coordinates these wave functions can be expressed in terms of associated Legendre[7] polynomials P_n^m of the first kind, spherical Hankel functions h_n, and spherical Bessel functions J_n as:

(5.41)
$$\begin{cases} \psi_{m,n,\sigma}(k\mathbf{r}) \\ \mathrm{Re}\{\psi_{m,n,\sigma}(k\mathbf{r})\} \end{cases} = \gamma_{m,n}^{1/2} \begin{cases} h_n(kr) \\ J_n(kr) \end{cases} P_n^m(\cos\theta) \begin{cases} \cos(m\varphi); \sigma = 1 \\ \sin(m\varphi); \sigma = 2 \end{cases}, \tag{b}$$

where $n = 1, 2, 3, \ldots \infty, m = 0, 1, 2, \ldots n, \sigma = 1, 2, \gamma_{m,n} = \varepsilon_m(2n+1)\dfrac{(n-m)!}{(n+m)!}$ and $\varepsilon_0 = 1$ and $\varepsilon_m = 2$ for $m > 0$.

Both forms of the Helmholtz equation given by (5.40) are used in obtaining the final results. For the first equation, in which the observation point lies outside S, $(r > r_o)$, if (5.41a) is substituted into (5.40a), then, for $r > r_{max}$,

(5.42)
$$\Phi_s(k\mathbf{r}) = \sum_n B_n \psi_n(k\mathbf{r}), \tag{a}$$

where the expansion coefficients for the scattered wave are given by

(5.42)
$$B_n = \frac{jk}{4\pi} \iint_S \{\mathrm{Re}\{\psi_n(k\mathbf{r}_o)\}\nabla_+\Phi - \Phi_+\nabla[\mathrm{Re}\{\psi_n(k\mathbf{r}_o)\}]\} \cdot \tilde{\mathbf{n}} dS. \tag{b}$$

For the incident wave we can make use of an expansion similar to that used for a plane wave in (5.1). If the observation point lies inside S, we substitute this expansion together with (5.41a) into (5.40b), so that for $r < r_{min}$

$$\Phi_i = \sum_n A_n \mathrm{Re}\{\psi_n(k\mathbf{r})\}$$
$$= \frac{-jk}{4\pi} \sum_n \mathrm{Re}\{\psi_n(k\mathbf{r})\} \iint_S \{\psi_n(k\mathbf{r}_o)\nabla_+\Phi - \Phi_+\nabla[\psi_n(k\mathbf{r})]\} \cdot \tilde{\mathbf{n}} dS_o,$$

where the coefficients A_n are all known. Because the set of wave functions ψ_n are orthogonal, these coefficients are given by

(5.43)
$$A_n = -\frac{jk}{4\pi} \iint_S \{\psi_n(k\mathbf{r}_o)\nabla_+\Phi - \Phi_+\nabla[\psi_n(k\mathbf{r}_o)]\} \cdot \tilde{\mathbf{n}} dS_o.$$

To determine the unknown values of $\nabla_+\Phi$ and Φ_+, boundary conditions must be imposed on the surface S. For example, they could consist of the Neumann's condition ($\tilde{\mathbf{n}} \cdot \nabla_+\Phi = 0$) or Dirichlet's condition ($\Phi_+ = 0$). For the more general

---

7. The associated Legendre polynomials of the first kind can be defined by:
$$P_n^m(r) = (-1)^m(1 - r^2)^{m/2}[d^n P_n(r)/dr^m].$$

case considered in Fig. 5.8 in which the fields penetrate the scatterer, the conditions are that the pressure and the normal component of the particle velocity are continuous across the interface, i.e., $\rho\Phi_+ = \rho_v\Phi_-$ and $\tilde{\mathbf{n}}\cdot\nabla_+\Phi = \tilde{\mathbf{n}}\cdot\nabla_-\Phi$. Now the field inside S can be expanded in terms of the set of wave functions $\Phi = \Sigma C_n \mathrm{Re}\{\psi_n(k_v\mathbf{r})\}$ with expansion coefficients C_n, i.e., $\Phi = \Sigma C_n \mathrm{Re}\{\psi_n(k_v\mathbf{r})\}$, where k_v is the propagation constant inside S. Consequently, Φ_- and, $\tilde{\mathbf{n}}\cdot\nabla_-\Phi$ and therefore Φ_+ and $\tilde{\mathbf{n}}\cdot\nabla\Phi_+$, can be expressed in terms of C_n. By means of (5.43), the coefficients C_n can be expressed in terms of the known incident wave expansion coefficients A_n. Consequently, with the help of (5.42b), the scattered wave expansion coefficients B_n can be determined. Specifically, Waterman [30] showed that the scattered wave expansion coefficients are related to the incident wave coefficients by

$$(5.44) \qquad\qquad B_n = \sum_{m=0} T_{m,n} A_n$$

where $T_{m,n}$ are the elements of the transition matrix $\mathbf{T}$ given by

$$(5.45) \qquad\qquad \mathbf{T} = -\frac{\mathrm{Re}\{\mathbf{Q}\}}{\mathbf{Q}} \qquad\qquad (a)$$

in which

$$(5.45)$$
$$Q_{mn} = \frac{k}{4\pi} \iint_S \left[\frac{\rho_v}{\rho}\mathrm{Re}\{\psi_m(k_v\mathbf{r})\}\nabla\psi_n(k\mathbf{r}) - \psi_n(k\mathbf{r})\nabla[\mathrm{Re}\{\psi_m(k_v\mathbf{r})\}]\right]\cdot\tilde{\mathbf{n}}dS_o. \qquad (b)$$

Evaluation of this surface integral using spherical coordinates requires that the coordinates of the scatterer surface be expressed in the form $r = r(\theta,\varphi)$.

It can be seen that (5.44) enables the scattered wave expansion coefficients to be determined, and hence the attributes of the scattered wave are fully described by (5.42a). Because the transition matrix depends only on the shape and properties of the scatterer, it is independent of the form of the incident wave. Consequently, provided the incident wave can be expanded in the assumed form, the same matrix can be used to analyze scattering for different incident waves. For observation points that are in the far field, the expansion coefficients can be simplified and the number of matrix elements required to achieve reasonable accuracy can be greatly reduced.

5.5.2 Scattering by a Red Blood Cell

To illustrate the method devised by Waterman, we consider scattering of a plane incident wave by an RBC. At lower ultrasonic frequencies, where the maximum dimensions are much less than a waveleigh, it is a good approximation to assume that an RBC behaves as a Rayleigh scatterer ($ka \ll 1$) for which the radius a is taken to be that of a sphere whose volume is equal to that of an RBC. Under these circumstances the differential scattering cross-section is given by (5.20b). For example, if the maximum dimension of an RBC

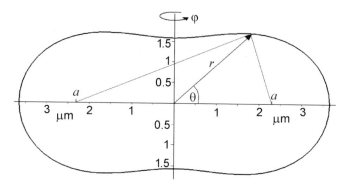

Figure 5.9 Biconcave disk model of an RBC in which the surface is given by $r^4 + a^4 - 2a^2r^2\cos(2\theta) = b^4$, where $b > a > 0$ and the major axis is $\sqrt{a^2+b^2}$. The graph is plotted for $a = 2.337\,\mu m$, $b = a/0.83$. (Based on Kuo and Shung [35].)

is taken to be $8\,\mu m$, and it is assumed that the condition $ka \ll 1$ can be written as $10ka \le 1$, then 6 MHz is an estimate of the maximum frequency for which an RBC behaves as a Rayleigh scatterer. In practice, much higher frequencies are sometimes used for imaging and Doppler ultrasound measurements, and consequently it is important to know the frequency at which the scattering can no longer be assumed to be Rayleigh and to know how the scattering cross-section depends on the RBC shape and orientation.

Kuo and Shung [35] used the T-matrix method of Waterman to investigate some of these questions. They calculated the backscattering from an RBC assuming that the shape can be approximated either by a sphere, a flat disk, or a biconcave disk. The biconcave disk is the best approximation: its geometric form, together with the equation for its surface,[8] is given in Fig. 5.9. Because of the rotational symmetry, the form of the wave function given by (5.41) simplifies to one that is independent of φ. Moreover, if the observation point is in the far field, the large argument Hankel function approximation[9] can be used.

The RBC and the suspending fluid (saline) were assumed to have the following properties: $\rho_v = 1078\,kg/m^3$, $\kappa_v = 0.3911\,GPa^{-1}$, $\rho_o = 1004.6\,kg/m^3$, $\kappa_o = 0.4421\,GPa^{-1}$, from which the speed of sound was calculated. In calculating the backscattering cross-section, Kuo and Shung [35] assumed that the off-diagonal terms of the transition matrix could be neglected. They stated that these terms represent mode coupling between different orders of the spherical harmonics and consequently, in the absence of wave-mode conversion at the scatterer boundary, it is reasonable to assume a diagonal transition matrix.

---

8. The curve is called the Cassini (17th century) oval, which is defined as the set of points such that the product of the distances from each point on the surface to the two "foci" is equal to b^2.

9. The large argument approximation for a spherical Hankel function of the second kind is $h_m(kr) \approx (j)^{m+1}e^{-jkr}/kr$, for $kr \gg (m + 0.5)^2/2$ with $m = 1, 2, 3, \ldots$, representing an outgoing spherical wave.

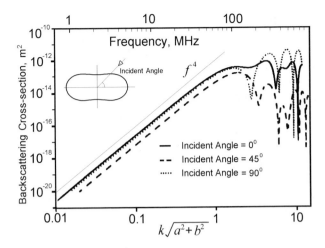

Figure 5.10 Backscattering cross-section as a function of frequency for a biconcave "RBC" calculated using the T-matrix method for different plane wave incident angles. The dimensions of a and b are those given in Fig. 5.9 and correspond to a volume of 110.5 μm^3. (Reproduced, with permission, from Kuo and Shung [5.35], *IEEE Trans. Biomed. Eng.*, 41, 29–33, © 1994 IEEE.)

Based on the above assumptions they calculated the backscattering cross-section over a range of $k\sqrt{a^2 + b^2}$ values for a volume[10] of 110.5 μm^3. The results shown in Fig. 5.10 indicate that the cross-section obeys a f^4 frequency dependence well beyond $k\sqrt{a^2 + b^2} = 0.1$, and that resonance effects become important only at much higher frequencies. Moreover, the results are in qualitative agreement with those of Fig. 5.4, which shows the backscattering cross-section for a spherical scatterer[11] as calculated using the exact boundary value approach.

5.6 Time-Domain Scattering Equations

The complex structure of most biological media requires that substantial approximations must be made to arrive at tractable scattering models. For soft biological media, one such model is based on the assumption that the medium consists of a distribution of discrete scatterers imbedded in a background whose acoustic properties are constant. An alternative model is based on the assumption that the acoustic properties of the medium vary in a continuous manner and that scattering is caused by the changes encountered by the incident wave. As discussed in the next section, both models can be used to determine the pulse-echo response.

---

10. This corresponds to the dimensions given in [35, Fig. 4] but differs from the value of 80 μm^3 given in the paper (private communication from Dr. Kuo).

11. The rather smaller assumed volume (82 μm^3 vs. 110.5 μm^3) should be noted.

In the particle approach, the scatterers are assumed to be discrete entities, perhaps with varying geometry and differing acoustic properties, and to have a certain spatial distribution. At a given observation point the scattering contributions can constructively or destructively interfere. If the scatterers are small compared to a wavelength, they will behave like Rayleigh scatterers, and the contribution to the total scattered signal can be determined in a fairly straightforward manner provided the scattering is sufficiently weak so that multiple scattering can be neglected. For an incident plane wave and an isotropic scatterer, the scattered field can be determined from the pressure impulse response, $h_s(|r_o - r|:t)$, where r_o is the location of the scatterer and r is the field position.

In the continuum model the variations in the acoustic properties are assumed to create scattering of the incident wave and give rise to the received signal. We shall first obtain a time-domain integral expression for the scattered pressure created by variations in compressibility and density in the volume V_s and this will be used in the next section to determine the pulse-echo response.

In Chapter 2 expression (2.17) was obtained for the velocity potential in an unbounded medium exterior to a source contained within a volume V_s. This can be converted to the following equation for the total pressure[12]

$$(5.46) \qquad p(r{:}t) = p_i(r{:}t) + \iiint_{V_s} \int_{-\infty}^{\infty} g(r|r_o{:}t|t_0) f(r|r_o{:}t|t_0) dt_0 dV_o,$$

in which the unbounded Green's function is given by

$$(5.47) \qquad g(r|r_o{:}t|t_0) = \frac{1}{4\pi|r - r_o|} \delta\left[t - \left(t_0 + \frac{|r - r_o|}{c_o}\right)\right],$$

also $-f(r{:}t)$ is the source term in the wave equation and $\rho_v(r)$ and $\kappa_v(r)$ describe the spatial dependence of the equilibrium density and compressibility. Now the source term, expressed in terms of the κ's and ρ's, is given by the right-hand side of (5.28a), and if we assume that $p_s(r{:}t) \ll p_i(r{:}t)$, then the scattered pressure is given by

(5.48)

$$p_s(r{:}t) = -\iiint_{V_s} \int_{-\infty}^{\infty} \left\{ \frac{1}{c_o^2} \frac{\partial^2 p_i}{\partial t^2} \left[\frac{\kappa_v - \kappa_o}{\kappa_o} \right] + \nabla \cdot \left[\frac{\rho_v - \rho_o}{\rho_v} \nabla p_i \right] \right\} g(r|r_o{:}t|t_0) dt_0 dV_o. \qquad \text{(a)}$$

From (5.28b), the following alternative form can also be obtained using the Born approximation:

---

12. While the equations given in Chapter 2 are for the velocity potential, it should be noted that the wave equation for the pressure is identical, and consequently the equations referred to are applicable by a simply replacing $\Phi(r{:}t)$ by $p(r{:}t)$, though the source term $f(r{:}t)$ now has different dimensions.

$$(5.48) \qquad p_s(\mathbf{r}:t) = -\iiint_{V_s} \int_{-\infty}^{\infty} \left\{ \frac{2\Delta c}{c_o^3} \frac{\partial^2 p_i}{\partial t^2} - \nabla(\ln \rho_v) \cdot \nabla p_i \right\} g(\mathbf{r}|\mathbf{r}_o:t|t_0) dt_0 dV_o . \qquad \text{(b)}$$

For subsequent derivations, it is helpful to simplify the notation by denoting volume and surface integrals with a single integral sign and letting $dV_o \equiv d^3 r_o$ and $dS_o \equiv d^2 r_o$. Thus, (5.48) can be written as

$$(5.49) \qquad p_s(\mathbf{r}:t) = \int_{V_s} \int_{-\infty}^{\infty} g(\mathbf{r}|\mathbf{r}_o:t|t_0) f_{op}[p_i] dt_0 d^3 r_o , \qquad \text{(a)}$$

where, for $\rho_o \gg \Delta \rho(\mathbf{r}_o)$, the operator f_{op} is given by

$$(5.49) \qquad f_{op} = \frac{1}{\rho_o} \nabla(\Delta \rho) \cdot \nabla - \frac{2\Delta c}{c_o^3} \frac{\partial^2}{\partial t^2} . \qquad \text{(b)}$$

In evaluating this operator it should be remembered that the differential operator ∇ is with respect to $\mathbf{r}_o$ and that in general both $\Delta \rho$ and Δc are functions of $\mathbf{r}_o$. Equation (5.49a) will be used in the next section in order to obtain a relation for the pulse-echo response of a transmitter–receiver system.

5.7 Pulse-Echo Response

In a simple ultrasound pulse-echo system, such as that used in early diagnostic systems, ultrasonic pulses are transmitted from a fixed location and cause scattered signals to be produced, some of which are back-scattered. These can be detected by the receiving transducer that typically will be the same as the transmit transducer. If the speed of propagation is nearly constant, then these signals will be detected at times that are approximately equal to the depth at which the scattering occurs. Consequently, the variation of the received signal over time provides a mapping of the acoustic properties through which the transmitted pulse propagates. However, as will be seen, the acoustic properties become partially obscured by a number of effects, such as the frequency-dependent attenuation, the spatial distribution of the transmitted pulse, the acoustic properties of the surrounding tissue, and the transducer geometry.

A simplified representation of the pulse-echo response is shown in Fig. 5.11. The *sample volume* can be defined as a region within which the received signal will be no less than −6 dB of the peak value for a point scatterer placed anywhere within it. The transmitted pulse convolved with the transmit–receive impulse response, in combination with the receiver gating pulse, governs its shape.

In 1977 Gore and Leeman [36] reported an analytical approach to the problem of calculating the pulse-echo response using the continuum model for scattering. They obtained a frequency-domain expression for the scattered pressure but without accounting for the receiving transducer geometry. A similar approach was subsequently used by Fatemi and Kak [37], who may not

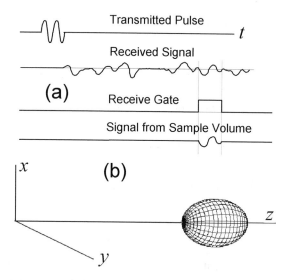

Figure 5.11 Simplified representation of the pulse-echo response. (a) Transmitted and gated received waveform. (b) Sample volume resulting from a pulse propagated in the z-direction in combination with the receive gating waveform. In practice, the shape may differ substantially from that indicated.

have been aware of Gore and Leeman's earlier work. Subsequently, Stepanishen [38] used the particle approach to obtain an expression for the received signal voltage waveform for a specified excitation voltage waveform using a linear system approach. Assuming that the scatterer was a simple point source monopole scatterer and that the electromechanical response of the transmission and reception transducers could be represented by their transfer function, he obtained frequency- and time-domain expressions for the reception transducer output signal. The continuum model has also been used by Dickinson and Nassiri [39] and by Jensen [40] for calculating the pulse-echo response; the latter derivation forms the basis of the next subsection.

5.7.1 Continuum Model

In describing a simple pulse-echo system, we shall assume that the effects of attenuation can be ignored and will make use of the geometry shown in Fig. 5.12 to determine the output voltage from a receiving transducer by scattering of a wave produced by a transmitting transducer. It will also be assumed that within the volume V_s the variations in the compressibility and density are small compared to the constant values in the background medium. If the transmitting transducer is excited so as to produce a velocity waveform $v_n(t)$ on its surface, the inhomogeneities within V_s will scatter the incident wave and the scattered field will propagate to the receiving transducer surface. We shall assume that the receiving transducer is phase-sensitive so that the output

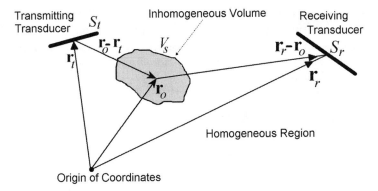

Figure 5.12 Coordinate system for calculating the pulse-echo response due to a scattering volume V_s, within which both the density and compressibility can change. For generality, separate plane transmitting and receiving transducers are shown.

signal depends on both the amplitude and phase of the signals arriving at each element of its area. The net force acting on its surface arises from the pressure created at $\mathbf{r_r}$ on each elementary area dS_r of the receiving transducer by the scattered pressure field. Thus, the total force $f(t)$ is given by

$$f(t) = K \int_{S_r} p_r(\mathbf{r_r}{:}t) d^2\mathbf{r_r}$$

where S_r is the receiver transducer area, $p_r(\mathbf{r_r}{:}t)$ is the pressure distribution on its surface, and the constant K will be assumed to be 2, corresponding to an ideal reflecting plane. If the transducer conversion process is assumed to be linear, it can be characterized by the transducer electromechanical impulse response $w_r^\delta(t)$, so that

(5.50)
$$e_o(t) = w_r^\delta(t) * \int_{S_r} 2p_r(\mathbf{r_r}{:}t) d^2\mathbf{r_r}.$$

Now (5.49a) can be used to express the pressure distribution on the receiving transducer surface at $\mathbf{r_r}$, and therefore is written as

(5.51)
$$p_r(\mathbf{r_r}{:}t) = \int_{V_s} \int_{-\infty}^{\infty} \frac{\delta[t - t_0 + |\mathbf{r_r} - \mathbf{r_o}|/c_o]}{4\pi|\mathbf{r_r} - \mathbf{r_o}|} f_{op}[p_i(\mathbf{r_o}{:}t)] dt_0 \, d^3r_o,$$

in which $\dfrac{\delta[t - t_0 + |\mathbf{r_r} - \mathbf{r_o}|/c_o]}{4\pi|\mathbf{r_r} - \mathbf{r_o}|}$ is the free space Green's function as given by (5.47) and the operator f_{op} was defined in (5.49b) by $f_{op} = \dfrac{1}{\rho_o}\nabla(\Delta\rho)\cdot\nabla - \dfrac{2\Delta c}{c_o^3}\dfrac{\partial^2}{\partial t^2}$. In addition, it should again be noted that both $\Delta\rho$ and Δc are functions of $\mathbf{r_o}$ and that the ∇ operator is with respect to $\mathbf{r_o}$.

To obtain the pulse-echo response it is necessary to relate the pressure incident on the scattering region $p_i(\mathbf{r}_o:t)$ to the normal component of the velocity waveform $v_n(t)$ on the transmitting transducer surface. Such a relation was derived from the Rayleigh integral in Chapter 2 and was written in (2.37b) as the time convolution:

(5.52)
$$p_i(\mathbf{r}_o:t) = \rho_o \frac{\partial v_n(t)}{\partial t} * h_t(\mathbf{r}_o:t),$$

where $h_t(\mathbf{r}_o:t)$ is the velocity potential impulse response given by

(5.53)
$$h_t(\mathbf{r}_o:t) = \int_{S_t} \frac{\delta[t - |\mathbf{r}_o - \mathbf{r}_t|/c_o]}{2\pi|\mathbf{r}_o - \mathbf{r}_t|} d^2\mathbf{r}_t,$$

and the normal component of the velocity on the transducer surface is related to the input voltage waveform $e_i(t)$ by the transmitter electromechanical impulse response $w_t^\delta(t)$ through

$$v_n(t) = w_t^\delta(t) * e_i(t).$$

By substituting (5.52) into (5.51) and the resulting expression into (5.50) and then rearranging the integration order, the output voltage waveform can be written as

$$e_o(t) = w_r^\delta(t) * \rho_o \int_{V_s} \int_{-\infty}^{\infty} f_{op} \left[\frac{\partial v_n(t)}{\partial t} * h_t(\mathbf{r}_o:t) \right] \int_{S_r} \frac{\delta[t - t_0 + |\mathbf{r}_r - \mathbf{r}_o|/c_o]}{2\pi|\mathbf{r}_r - \mathbf{r}_o|} d^2\mathbf{r}_r \, dt_0 d^3\mathbf{r}_o.$$

This can be re-expressed as

$$e_o(t) = w_r^\delta(t) * \rho_o \int_{V_s} f_{op} \left[\frac{\partial v_n(t)}{\partial t} * h_t(\mathbf{r}_o:t) \right] * h_r(\mathbf{r}_o:t) d^3\mathbf{r}_o$$

where $h_r(\mathbf{r}_o:t) = \int_{S_r} \frac{\delta[t - |\mathbf{r}_o - \mathbf{r}_r|/c_o]}{2\pi|\mathbf{r}_o - \mathbf{r}_r|} d^2\mathbf{r}_r$ is the impulse response of the receiving transducer. If the two transducers are identical and are at the same location, then the above expression for the output voltage reduces to

$$e_o(t) = \rho_o w_r^\delta(t) * \frac{\partial v_n(t)}{\partial t} * \int_{V_s} f_{op}[h_{tr}(\mathbf{r}_o:t)] d^3\mathbf{r}_o,$$

where $h_{tr}(\mathbf{r}_o:t) = h_t(\mathbf{r}_o:t) * h_r(\mathbf{r}_o:t)$ characterizes the pulse-echo response due to a point scatterer at $\mathbf{r}_o$ and that depends on the distance of the transducer from the scatterer. Jensen [40] then makes the assumption that the scattering volume is in the far field so that $h_{tr}(\mathbf{r}_o:t)$ varies gradually over V_s, enabling the integral in the above convolution to be written as

$$\int_{V_s} f_{op}[h_{tr}]d^3\mathbf{r}_o = \int_{V_s}\left\{\frac{1}{\rho_o}[\Delta\rho(\mathbf{r}_o)]\cdot\nabla h_{tr} - \frac{2\Delta c(\mathbf{r}_o)}{c_o^3}\frac{\partial^2 h_{tr}}{\partial t^2}\right\}d^3\mathbf{r}_o.$$

$$\approx \int_{V_s}\left\{\frac{\Delta\rho}{\rho_o}\nabla^2 h_{tr} - \frac{2\Delta c}{c_o^3}\frac{\partial^2 h_{tr}}{\partial t^2}\right\}d^3 r_o$$

As noted above, $h_{tr}(\mathbf{r}_o{:}t)$ is a function of the distance of the transducer from the scatterer, and consequently it can be expressed in terms of the time taken for a pulse to travel this distance. If the variations in the propagation speed are assumed to be small, this time can be written as $t = |r_t - r_o|/c_o$, so that $\nabla^2 h_{tr} = (1/c_o^2)\partial^2 h_{tr}/\partial t^2$. With the above approximations, the output voltage can be expressed as

$$(5.54)\quad e_o(t) = \rho_o w_r^\delta(t)*\frac{\partial v_n(t)}{\partial t}*\int_{V_s}\left\{\frac{\Delta\rho(\mathbf{r}_o)}{\rho_o} - \frac{2\Delta c(\mathbf{r}_o)}{c_o}\right\}\left\{\frac{1}{c_o^2}\frac{\partial^2 h_{tr}(\mathbf{r}_o{:}t)}{\partial t^2}\right\}d^3\mathbf{r}_o.\quad(a)$$

An alternative form can be obtained by noting that $c^2\kappa\rho = 1$, which approximates to

$$2\kappa_o\rho_o c_o\Delta c + c_o^2\rho_o\Delta\kappa + c_o^2\kappa_o\Delta\rho = 0,$$

i.e., $-2\Delta c/c_o = \Delta\kappa/\kappa_o + \Delta\rho/\rho_o$. By substitution, (5.54a) becomes

$$(5.54)\quad e_o(t) = \rho_o w_r^\delta(t)*\frac{\partial v_n(t)}{\partial t}*\int_{V_s}\left\{\frac{2\Delta\rho(\mathbf{r}_o)}{\rho_o} + \frac{\Delta\kappa(\mathbf{r}_o)}{\kappa_o}\right\}\left\{\frac{1}{c_o^2}\frac{\partial^2 h_{tr}(\mathbf{r}_o{:}t)}{\partial t^2}\right\}d^3\mathbf{r}_o.\quad(b)$$

It will be noted that the integrand contains two terms. As discussed by Jensen [40], the first term corresponds to the acoustic properties of the medium. From a measurement perspective, this term is unfortunately obscured by the effects of spatial and time convolutions. The time convolution is with the excitation velocity waveform and the spatial convolution is with a spatially dependent pulse-echo response.

5.7.2 Single Particle Model [38]

For the geometry of Fig. 5.13, in which a single point scatterer exists at $\mathbf{r}_o$, and the discussion given in the last subsection, it is straightforward matter to obtain the output voltage in terms of the input voltage waveform. With the help of the linear system representation of Fig. 5.14, the following three equations can be written down:

$$p_r(\mathbf{r}_r{:}t) = e_i(t)*w_t^\delta(t)*\rho_o\frac{\partial h_t(\mathbf{r}_o{:}t)}{\partial t}*h_s(\mathbf{r}_r{:}t)\tag{a}$$

$$(5.55)\qquad f(t) = 2\int_{S_r} p_r(\mathbf{r}_r{:}t)d^2\mathbf{r}_r\tag{b}$$

$$e_o(t) = f(t)*w_r^\delta(t)\tag{c}$$

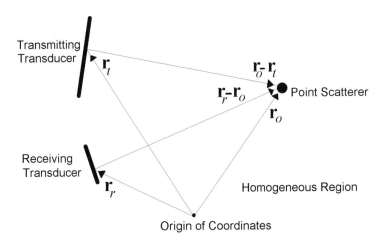

Figure 5.13 Geometry for determining the transmit–receive response due to a point scatterer located at r_o.

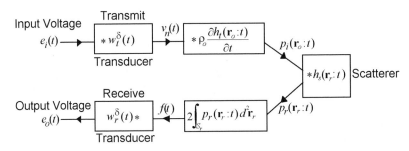

Figure 5.14 Time-domain representation of the transmit–receive response for a point scatterer in a non-attenuating medium. The pressure impulse response of the isotropic scatterer (i.e., the scattered pressure at an observation point due to an incident plane wave impulse) is denoted by $h_s(r_r:t)$, where r_r is a point on the surface of the receiving transducer.

where $w_t^\delta(t)$ and $w_r^\delta(t)$ are the electromechanical responses of the transmitter and receiver transducers and $h_s(r_r:t)$ is the pressure impulse response of the scatterer. By substituting (5.55a) and (b) into (c), the output voltage is given by

$$(5.56) \qquad e_o(t) = \rho_o e_i(t) * w_t^\delta(t) * \frac{\partial h_t(r_o:t)}{\partial t} * \left[2 \int_{S_r} h_s(r_r:t) d^2r_r \right] * w_r^\delta(t). \qquad (a)$$

Now a point scatterer in the absence of dipole and higher-order terms has an impulse response given by[13]

---

13. This can be more readily seen by first expressing the transfer function of a point scatterer as $H(r_r|r_o:\omega) = S(\omega)e^{-\omega|r_r-r_o|/c_o}/4\pi|r_r - r_o|$. The inverse Fourier transform is given by $h(r_r|r_o:t) = \mathcal{F}^{-1}\{S(\omega)\} * \mathcal{F}^{-1}\{G(r_r|r_o:\omega)\} = s(t) * \delta(t - |r_r - r_o|/c_o)/4\pi|r_r - r_o|$.

$$h_s(\mathbf{r}_r : t) = s(t) * \frac{\delta(t - |\mathbf{r}_r - \mathbf{r}_o|/c_o)}{4\pi |\mathbf{r}_r - \mathbf{r}_o|},$$

where $s(t)$ describes the scattering strength. Consequently, if the transmission and receiver transducers are the same, the integral term in (5.56) can be written as

$$2 \int_{S_r} h_s(\mathbf{r}_r : t) d^2\mathbf{r}_r = s(t) * \int_{S_r} \frac{\delta(t - |\mathbf{r}_r - \mathbf{r}_o|/c_o)}{2\pi |\mathbf{r}_r - \mathbf{r}_o|} d^2\mathbf{r}_r = s(t) * h_t(\mathbf{r}_o : t),$$

so that (5.56) becomes

(5.56) $$e_o(t) = \rho_o \frac{\partial e_i(t)}{\partial t} * w_t^\delta(t) * h_t(\mathbf{r}_o : t) * h_t(\mathbf{r}_o : t) * s(t) * w_r^\delta(t).$$ (b)

This was given by Stepanishen [38] together with its equivalent form in the frequency domain.

As an example, we consider a circular transducer of radius a used both as a transmitter and receiver. For simplicity, it will be assumed that the scatterer is on-axis and that $s(t) = s_o\delta(t)$, $w_t^\delta(t) = \delta(t)$, $w_r^\delta(t) = \partial\delta(t)/\partial t$. Furthermore, the input voltage will be taken to be a Heaviside step function $\mathcal{H}(t)$, which results in the normal surface velocity component being a δ-function. From (2.38), the velocity potential impulse response is given by

$$h_t(z : t) = \mathcal{H}\left(t - \frac{z}{c_o}\right) - \mathcal{H}\left(t - \frac{\sqrt{z^2 + a^2}}{c_o}\right).$$ These values, in combination with either (5.56b) or Fig. 5.14, can be used to evaluate the velocity potential and pressure at the scatterer location and the resulting force on the transducer and output voltage, all of which are sketched in Fig. 5.15.

5.8 One-Dimensional Scattering

In the 3-D analysis presented in section 5.4, scattering of an incident wave was assumed to be caused by variations in the density and compressibility throughout a specified volume. As illustrated in Fig. 5.16, a much simpler situation arises for an incident plane wave if the scattering arises from density and compressibility variations in the direction of propagation. This problem was first addressed by Wright [43] and Jones [44] by representing the acoustic properties of the scattering medium by its distance-dependent characteristic impedance and making use of the equations derived in Chapter 1 for the reflection and transmission coefficients at normal incidence. They obtained approximate expressions for the pressure impulse response of the medium, i.e., the reflected pressure wave for a plane incident pressure impulse. An alternative approach described by Bamber and Dickinson [42] started with the time-domain form of the 1-D scattering equation for small changes in compressibility ($\Delta\kappa = \kappa_v - \kappa_o$)

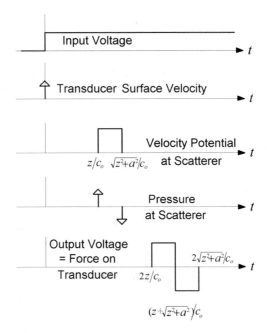

Figure 5.15 Sketch showing the transmit–receive response for a piston transducer of radius a and a point scatterer at a near-field on-axis location of z.

and density ($\Delta\rho = \rho_v - \rho_o$). This equation can be obtained from the 3-D form given by (5.48a) and is:

$$(5.57) \quad p_s(z{:}t) \approx -\int dz_o \int \left\{ \frac{1}{c_o^2} \frac{\partial^2 p_i}{\partial t_0^2} \left[\frac{\Delta\kappa}{\kappa_o} \right] + \frac{\partial}{\partial z_o} \left[\frac{\Delta\rho}{\rho_o} \frac{\partial p_i}{\partial z_o} \right] \right\} g(z|z_o{:}t|t_0) dt_0,$$

where $g(z|z_o{:}t|t_0)$ is now the 1-D Green's function. Expanding the differential coefficient of the product and noting that an incident plane wave traveling

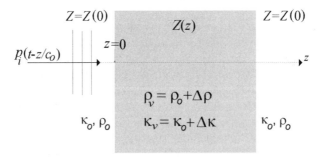

Figure 5.16 A 1-D scattering problem in which a plane wave is incident on a region whose density and compressibility vary in the direction of propagation. The scattering region can be treated as having a characteristic impedance that is a function z.

in the positive z-direction is given by $p_i = p_o(t_o - z_o/c_o)$, which satisfies $\dfrac{1}{c_o^2}\dfrac{\partial^2 p_i}{\partial t_0^2} = \dfrac{\partial^2 p_i}{\partial z_0^2}$ as well as the reduced wave equation, $\dfrac{\partial p_i}{\partial z_o} = -\dfrac{1}{c_o}\dfrac{\partial p_i}{\partial t_o}$, (5.57) can be written as

$$p_s(z\!:\!t) = \int dz_o \int \frac{1}{c_o}\left\{ -\frac{1}{c_o}\frac{\partial^2 p_i}{\partial t_0^2}\left[\frac{\Delta\kappa}{\kappa_o} + \frac{\Delta\rho}{\rho_o}\right] + \frac{\partial}{\partial z_o}\left[\frac{\Delta\rho}{\rho_o}\right]\frac{\partial p_i}{\partial t_o}\right\} g(z|z_o\!:\!t|t_0)\,dt_0.$$

Now Morse and Feshbach [41] have shown that the Green's function for the 1-D wave equation can be written in terms of the Heaviside step function as

$$g(z|z_o\!:\!t|t_0) = \frac{c_o}{2}\,\mathcal{H}[(t - t_0) - |z - z_o|/c_o].$$

By substituting this into the above expression for the scattered pressure, then performing the integration with respect to t_o, Bamber and Dickinson [42] obtained

$$p_s(z\!:\!t) = \int \left\{ \frac{1}{4c_o}\frac{\partial p_i\left(t + \dfrac{z}{c_o} - \dfrac{2z_o}{c_o}\right)}{\partial t}\left[\frac{\Delta\kappa(z_o)}{\kappa_o} + \frac{\Delta\rho(z_o)}{\rho_o}\right] \right.$$
$$\left. + \frac{1}{2}p_i\left(t + \frac{z}{c_o} - \frac{2z_o}{c_o}\right)\frac{\partial}{\partial z_o}\left[\frac{\Delta\rho(z_o)}{\rho_o}\right] \right\} dz_o.$$

Finally, by integrating the first term by parts and combining with the second, they obtained the following convolution integral:

$$(5.58)\qquad p_s(z\!:\!t) = \frac{1}{4}\int p_i\left(t + \frac{z}{c_o} - \frac{2z_o}{c_o}\right)\frac{\partial}{\partial z_o}\left[\frac{\Delta\rho(z_o)}{\rho_o} - \frac{\Delta\kappa(z_o)}{\kappa_o}\right]dz_o.$$

To interpret this expression it is helpful to consider the special case in which the scattering region consists of a step change in the acoustic properties at $z = z_1$ with uniform properties elsewhere. For the incident wave $p_i = p_i(t - z/c_o)$ traveling in the positive z-direction, this step change in impedance will cause a reflected wave to be generated that moves in the negative z-direction. Because the derivative of a step is a δ-function, it follows from (5.58) that the reflected wave will be given by $p_r(z\!:\!t) \propto p_i\{t + (z - 2z_1)/c_o\}$, which describes a wave moving in the negative z-direction but delayed in time by $2z_1/c_o$. For example, if the incident wave is a δ-function $p_i = A\delta(t - z/c_o)$, then the reflected wave will be given by $p_r \propto \delta\{t + (z - 2z_1)/c_o\}$ for $z < z_1$.

In the general case for a plane wave incident on a region whose characteristic impedance varies in the z-direction, reflections will arise from different depths and, depending on the magnitude of the impedance variations, multiple reflections may be present. In fact, the reflection properties of the medium can be characterized by its pressure impulse response $h(z)$, which is the reflected pressure wave for an incident δ-function. Thus, for the incident wave $p_i = p_i(t - z/c_o)$, the reflected wave is given by the convolution $p_r(z:t) = p_i(t + z/c) * h(z)$. When the impedance changes are small so that multiple reflections can be ignored and the effects of attenuation are negligible, it is evident that the impulse response can be identified with the differential term in (5.58), i.e.,

$$h(z) = \frac{1}{4} \frac{\partial}{\partial z_o} \left[\frac{\Delta\rho}{\rho_o} - \frac{\Delta\kappa}{\kappa_o} \right],$$

which, as described below, is related to the variation of the characteristic impedance with distance.

With reference to Fig. 5.16, let $Z(z)$ denote characteristic impedance of the medium at a given location z. Since $Z(z) = \rho c = \sqrt{\rho(z)/\kappa(z)}$ then by differentiation $2ZdZ\kappa + Z^2 d\kappa = d\rho$ or $2dZ/Z = d\rho/\rho - d\kappa/\kappa$. Thus, for small density and compressibility changes

$$\frac{1}{4} \frac{\partial}{\partial z} \left[\frac{\Delta\rho}{\rho_o} - \frac{\Delta\kappa}{\kappa_o} \right] \approx \frac{1}{2Z(z)} \frac{dZ(z)}{dz},$$

so that the pressure impulse can also be expressed as

$$h(z) = \frac{1}{2Z(z)} \frac{dZ(z)}{dz} = \frac{1}{2} \frac{d[\ln Z(z)]}{dz}.$$

An identical expression for the impulse response was published first by Wright [43], and subsequently by Jones [44] and Kak et al. [45]. They represented the scattering region as a sequence of small impedance steps and found the impulse response by taking limit as the number of steps became large and the step size became small. They also obtained expressions for the impulse response when multiple reflections were present. Subsequently, using a rather simpler derivation, Leeman [46] obtained the same equations.

5.9 Scattering by Distributions

Much attention has been paid to the problem of determining the scattered signal when a distribution of particles is insonated by a plane wave. Simplifying approximations are generally needed to make the analysis tractable, and these typically include neglecting the effects of multiple scattering. If the scatterers are randomly distributed, the position of a given scatterer would be uncorrelated with any other, and the scattered power should increase with the scatterer number density. On the other hand, correlation between the scatterer positions (implying organization) results in interference effects, and these play an important role in governing how the scattered power varies with the scatterer number density. Added complications result if the scatterers have differing size, shape, or acoustic properties, as may occur in real tissue. Moreover, if the scatterers are moving, as occurs with blood flowing in a vessel, the scattered signal will be non-stationary and will exhibit a Doppler frequency shift.

An important example is that of RBCs suspended in a medium known to inhibit the formation of aggregates, such as physiological saline. If the concentration of RBCs in the suspending fluid is small (e.g., the Hct is <2%), the scattered power is found to be directly proportional to the number density. As the Hct is increased, the average distance between RBCs decreases and their positions become partially correlated, which, as will be seen, has a profound effect on the scattered power. These and other issues related to scattering by RBCs will be discussed.

5.9.1 Random Distributions of Point Scatterers

One of the earliest papers (1945) to address the problem of determining the scattering due to a random distribution of isotropic *point* scatterers, including the effects of multiple scattering, was that by Foldy [47]. He used a consistent wave-equation approach to obtain expected values of the wave function (e.g., the velocity potential or pressure), the flux, and the intensity. For N point scatterers randomly distributed throughout a specified volume, there can be an infinite number of possible arrangements, all of which differ from one another in terms of the scatterer locations. A specific distribution will be called a *realization*, and the *expected* (statistical average) quantity such as the pressure or intensity will be denoted by $E[.]$.

For a given realization, the scattered pressure at a given observation point $\mathbf{r}$ can be obtained, and if this process is repeated for many different realizations, then the expected pressure $E[p(\mathbf{r})]$ and the expected value of the square of the pressure $E[p^2(\mathbf{r})]$ can be determined. Foldy showed that the expected pressure within a volume V_s that contains a random distribution of point scatterers satisfies the Helmholtz equation for a uniform medium in which there are no scatterers present, though with a speed of propagation that depends on the average number density of scatterers and their scattering properties. Consequently, no contribution to the *expected pressure* can arise from within V_s, though a contribution may arise from the effects of the impedance change that an incident wave encounters at the bounding surface to V_s.

Foldy also showed that the *expected square* of the pressure, $E[p^2(\mathbf{r})]$, is governed by an integral equation that is of fundamental significance to the problem of multiple scattering. This equation states that for many realizations of a random distribution of point scatterers, $E[p^2(\mathbf{r})]$ is the sum of two terms. The first is equal to the square of the expected pressure at the observation point. The second term consists of an integral over the volume occupied by the scatterers, and this accounts for the contributions from all scatterers within the insonated volume. If the effects of multiple scattering are small, then the integrand is proportional to the product of the square of the expected pressure at a particular scatterer and a scattering cross-section per unit volume at the same point. This second term is an *incoherent* contribution in the sense that the scatterer positions for a given realization are uncorrelated with those for any other realization, and therefore the scattered signal from different real-izations will be uncorrelated.[14] In contrast, the first term represents a *coherent* scattered wave that can arise from the incident wave encountering a scattering region that has different average acoustic properties from that outside.

In view of the above, the expected value of the square of the pressure can be written as

$$E\left[|p(\mathbf{r})|^2\right] = E^2\left[|p_c(\mathbf{r})|\right] + E\left[|p_{inc}(\mathbf{r})|^2\right],$$

in which the subscripts c and inc stand for the coherent and incoherent parts, respectively, $E^2[.] \equiv \{E[.]\}^2$, and $E[|p_{inc}(\mathbf{r})|] = 0$. In practice, it is often assumed that measurements are made from a sample volume that lies within a region whose *average* acoustic properties are the same as the sample volume. In this case, the coherent term is zero and only the incoherent intensity need be considered.

5.9.2 Backscattering Coefficient

The differential scattering cross-section σ_d and its backscattering cross-section σ_b were defined in section 5.2 with a discrete scatterer in mind. If the scattering volume consists either of a collection of discrete scatterers or a region in which the acoustic properties fluctuate spatially, then the *incoherent* portion of the scattered power can be expected to vary in proportion to the scattering volume and incident intensity. A useful measure of the scattering strength of a distribution of scatterers when insonated by a plane harmonic wave is the *differential scattering coefficient*, defined by

$$(5.59) \qquad \sigma_{dsc}(\theta,\varphi) = \frac{\text{Time Average Scattered Intensity in the Direction } (\theta,\varphi) \text{ per United Solid Angle}}{\text{Time Average Incident Intensity} \times \text{Elementary Volume of Scatterers}}, \qquad (a)$$

in which the elementary volume is assumed to be large enough so that it would contain a representative distribution of scatterers. In the case of a statistically varying distribution, then the scattered intensity would be the ensemble-averaged value. The MKS units are $(\text{m.sr})^{-1}$, though $(\text{cm.sr})^{-1}$ are frequently used. It is important to note that we have used the same symbol (but a different subscript) as the scattering cross-section to denote the differential scattering *coefficient*, even though the units differ. Since the same transducer is often used both for transmission and reception, the (differential) *backscattering coefficient* (BSC)

$$\sigma_{BSC} = \sigma_{dsc}(\pi,0),$$

---

14. In this context the term "incoherent" does not refer to the temporal signal observed for a given realization: such a signal will be highly correlated with the incident waveform. It refers to the relation between signals obtained from different realizations.

is particularly important. If p_1 is the backscattered pressure for a unit volume of scatterers at a unit distance away and the incident pressure wave is given by $p_{im}\cos(\omega t)$, then, because the time-averaged intensity of the incident wave is equal to $p_{im}^2/(2\rho_o c_o)$, the backscattering coefficient is given by

$$(5.59) \qquad\qquad \sigma_{BSC} = 2E\left[\overline{p_1^2}\right]/p_{im}^2 , \qquad\qquad (b)$$

in which the bar denotes the time average.

5.9.3 A Random Distribution of Scatterers (Hct << 1)

It is the aim here to obtain an expression for the backscattering coefficient due to a large number N of scatterers that are randomly distributed within a sample volume V and that have a random distribution of volumes. Any particular realization can be described by the set $\{(\mathbf{r}_1,V_1^s), (\mathbf{r}_2,V_2^s). \ldots (\mathbf{r}_N,V_N^s)\}$, in which $\mathbf{r}$ denotes the position vector and V^s denotes the scatterer volume. Four different realizations for 2-D distribution of 50 scatterers are illustrated in Fig. 5.17, together with the backscattered signal for a sinusoidal incident plane wave. For the present, it will be assumed that each scatterer is small compared to a wavelength and that the number density is small enough so that the effects of position correlation due to the finite size of the scatterers can be neglected. It will also be assumed that the distance of the observation point from the sample volume V is much greater than its maximum dimension and that scattering is sufficiently weak so that multiple scattering can be neglected. This model will serve as an introduction to the more difficult task of calculating the BSC from blood. The statistical distribution of volumes corresponds to the

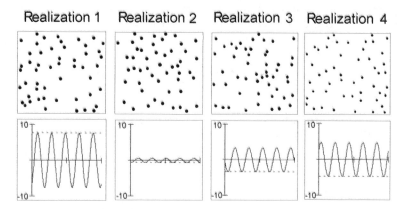

Figure 5.17 Four 2-D scatterer realizations for $N = 50$ and the corresponding backscattered signal. The scatterers are randomly distributed with a uniform distribution and have a volume that is a random variable. The amplitudes (dashed line) are Gaussian distributed and the phases (relative to the incident waveform) are uniformly distributed over 2π.

known RBC size distribution and the assumption of a very small number density corresponds to a low Hct, i.e., less than 2%.

Suppose that a uniform field is seen by all N scatterers and that each has the same acoustic properties but can differ in volume. By applying the principle of superposition, the total backscattered pressure phasor for a particular realization can be found from (5.35) by putting $\theta = \pi$, noting that $\mathbf{k}_s = 2k\tilde{\mathbf{r}}_i$, and then summing the contributions from all N scatterers yielding,

$$\underline{p}_s(r{:}\omega) = p_{im} \frac{k^2 e^{-jkr}}{4\pi r} \left\{ \left[\frac{\kappa_v - \kappa_o}{\kappa_o} \right] - \left[\frac{\rho_v - \rho_o}{\rho_v} \right] \right\} \sum_{n=1}^{N} \iiint_{V_n^s} e^{j2k(\mathbf{r}_o \cdot \tilde{\mathbf{r}}_i)} dV_o,$$

where V_n^s denotes the volume of the n'th scatterer. Because each particle is assumed to be small compared to a wavelength, the exponential term under the integral sign remains nearly constant, enabling the integral to be reduced to the volume of the n'th particle multiplied by the exponential term. By multiplying the pressure phasor by an exponential time factor and then taking the real part, the scattered pressure becomes

(5.60)
$$p_s(r{:}t) = \frac{p_{im}}{r} \frac{\sqrt{\sigma_b}}{E[V_s]} \sum_{n=1}^{N} V_n^s \cos[\omega t + \phi_n],$$

where σ_b is the backscattering cross-section for a particle whose volume is equal to the expected volume $E[V_s]$, which is, from (5.39), given by

$$\sigma_b = \left(\frac{k^2 E[V_s]}{4\pi} \right)^2 \left[\frac{\kappa_v - \kappa_o}{\kappa_o} - \frac{\rho_v - \rho_o}{\rho_v} \right]^2.$$

In addition, the phase angle $\phi_n = 2k(\mathbf{r}_n \cdot \tilde{\mathbf{r}}_i) - kr$ for the n'th scattering particle corresponds to the time delay associated with the incident wave as it travels to the scatterer and then back to the observation point.

Now (5.60) can be written as

(5.61)
$$p_s(r{:}t) = \frac{p_{im}}{r} \frac{\sqrt{\sigma_b}}{E[V_s]} \left\{ \cos(\omega t) \sum_{n=1}^{N} V_n^s \cos[\phi_n] - \sin(\omega t) \sum_{n=1}^{N} V_n^s \sin[\phi_n] \right\}.$$

The above equation for the pressure at the observation point for a given realization can be rewritten as

(5.62)
$$\begin{aligned} p_s(r{:}t) &= \frac{p_{im}}{r} \frac{\sqrt{\sigma_b}}{E[V_s]} \{ A_1 \cos(\omega t) - A_2 \sin(\omega t) \} \\ &= \frac{p_{im}}{r} \frac{\sqrt{\sigma_b}}{E[V_s]} \sqrt{A_1^2 + A_2^2} \cos(\omega t - \Theta) \end{aligned}$$

where A_1 and A_2 are uncorrelated random variables and $\tan \Theta = -A_2/A_1$. Let us suppose that the random variables V_n^s, and ϕ_n in (5.61) are statistically independent and ϕ is uniformly distributed over the range $(-\pi, \pi)$. According to the Central Limit theorem [49, pp. 194–200], if N is very large the amplitude factors A_1 and A_2 will have a zero-mean Gaussian distribution, i.e., their probability density function (PDF) is

$$PDF(A) = \frac{1}{\xi\sqrt{2\pi}} e^{-A^2/(2\xi^2)},$$

where ξ^2 is the variance (square of the standard deviation). To determine ξ^2 it is first necessary to find the statistical properties of the components that are being summed, namely $V_n^s \cos(\phi_n)$ or $V_n^s \sin(\phi_n)$. Let us consider just the first term. Because ϕ is uniformly distributed, it can be shown that $PDF(\cos\phi) = \left(\pi\sqrt{1 - \cos^2\phi}\right)^{-1}$, and as a result $E[\cos\phi] = 0$ and $\mathrm{var}(\cos\phi) = 0.5$. It can also be shown that because $E[\cos\phi] = 0$, the variance of the product $V_s\cos\phi$ is given by $\mathrm{var}(V_s\cos\phi) = \mathrm{var}(\cos\phi)\{\mathrm{var}(V_s) + E^2[V_s]\} = 0.5E[V_s^2]$. This enables the variance of A_1 to be expressed as

$$\xi^2 = 0.5NE[V_s^2],$$

and a similar expression can be obtained for A_2. But[15] $E^2[A_1^2] = \xi^2$, and $E^2[A_2^2] = \xi^2$ so that

$$E^2[A_1^2 + A_2^2] = 2\xi^2 = NE[V_s^2].$$

We can now return to the problem of finding the backscattering coefficient as defined by (5.59b). From (5.62) the expected value of the time-averaged backscattered square of the pressure at unit distance from the scatterers can be written as

$$E[\overline{p_1^2}] = p_{im}^2 \frac{\sigma_b N}{E^2[V_s]} \frac{E[(A_1^2 + A_2^2)]}{2} = p_{im}^2 \frac{\sigma_b N}{2} \frac{E[V_s^2]}{E^2[V_s]}.$$

By substituting this into (5.59b), the backscattering coefficient can be expressed as

(5.63)
$$\sigma_{BSC} = \frac{\sigma_b N}{V} \frac{E[V_s^2]}{E^2[V_s]} = \sigma_b n_\rho \frac{E[V_s^2]}{E^2[V_s]}$$
(a)

where $n_\rho = N/V$ is the number density of scatterers. Alternatively, this can be expressed in terms of the hematocrit. By definition, $H \equiv \mathrm{Hct}$ is the fractional

---

15. If $y = Kx^2$, and $g(x)$ is a zero mean Gaussian function, then [49, p. 125]:

$$E[y] = \int_{-\infty}^{\infty} Kx^2 g(x)dx, \quad E[y^2] = \int_{-\infty}^{\infty} K^2 x^4 g(x)dx \quad \text{and} \quad \mathrm{var}(y) = E[y^2] - E^2[y].$$

In fact, the distribution function for y is given by [48, p. 133]:

$$PDF(y) = \frac{1}{\xi\sqrt{2\pi Ky}} e^{-y/(2K\xi^2)}.$$

volume occupied by the scatterers, i.e., $H = n_\rho E[V_s]$ so that (5.63a) can be written as

$$(5.63) \qquad \sigma_{BSC} = \sigma_b \frac{H}{E[V_s]} \frac{E[V_s^2]}{E^2[V_s]} = \sigma_b \frac{H}{E[V_s]} \left\{ \frac{\text{var}(V_s)}{E^2[V_s]} + 1 \right\} \qquad \text{(b)}$$

Thus, for very small hematocrits the backscattering coefficient is directly proportional to the Hct and increases with the variance of V_s. Equation (5.63) is equivalent to that previously derived [50] for a packing factor of unity (corresponding to a pair correlation coefficient of zero, as defined in the next subsection).

5.9.4 Backscattering by Blood

Blood is a suspension of formed elements in plasma. The formed elements consist of erythrocytes (RBCs, Fig. 5.18a), leukocytes (white blood cells), and thrombocytes (platelets). In $1\,\text{mm}^3$ of normal human blood there will be approximately 5×10^6 RBCs (vol. ~$95\,\mu\text{m}^3$), ~6000 white blood cells (vol. ~$300\,\mu\text{m}^3$), and ~300,000 platelets (vol. ~$15\,\mu\text{m}^3$). Plasma contains a multiplicity of molecules, including some large-molecular-weight proteins, one of which (fibrinogen) is believed to be primarily responsible for causing RBCs to clump together under low shear conditions (see Fig. 5.18b). Compared to the effects of RBCs, the contribution to scattering by white blood cells and platelets can be neglected, in the case of white blood cells due to their small number, and in the case of platelets due to their small scattering volume.

Detailed publications in the German literature by Fahrbach [56] in 1969/70 focused on the nature of the Doppler ultrasound signal (see Chapter 9). These indicate that he was likely the first[16] to theoretically and experimentally study the stochastic nature of the backscattered signal from a random distribution of moving scatterers. Subsequently, Sigelmann and Reid [55] developed a model that enabled the backscattering coefficient to be calculated from experimental data. A report by Brody [57] in 1971 and a subsequent publication make it clear that the backscattered signal was due to constructive/destructive interference effects. He derived an expression for its autocovariance function based on several assumptions, including that the RBCs were independent point scatterers. Independent work by Atkinson and Berry [58] presented in 1974 also recognized the stochastic nature of the backscattered signal. Their work was motivated by their observations on the character of the backscattered signal due to the transmission of a short quasi-sinusoidal signal in blood. Specifically, as illustrated in Fig. 5.19, they transmitted a short $2\,\text{MHz}$ burst and noted that the received signal consisted of quasi-random groups separated by about $2.5\,\text{mm}$ in the axial direction. They also noted that when the transducer was displaced laterally and the rectified envelope was recorded at a fixed time

---

16. An historical sketch of the development of ultrasound scattering theories for blood is presented in Table 2 of reference [21].

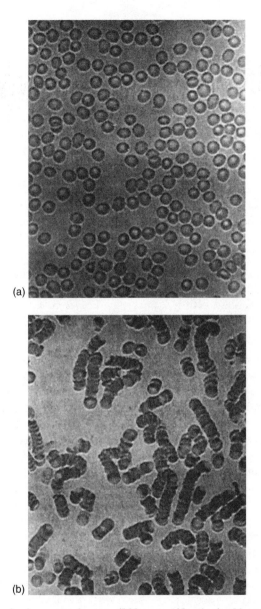

(a)

(b)

Figure 5.18 Optical microscope images (200× magnification) of human RBCs. (a) Blood in which aggregation was suppressed, (b) normal whole blood under static conditions. (Reprinted by permission of Elsevier from van der Heiden et al. [51], *Ultrasound Med. Biol.*, © 1995 World Federation of Ultrasound in Medicine and Biology.)

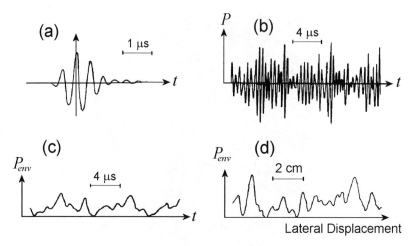

Figure 5.19 Backscattered signal from whole blood. (a) Transmitted pulse that has a 2-MHz center frequency. (b) Received signal. (c) Rectified envelope of (b). (d) Rectified envelope at a fixed time when the transducer is displaced laterally. (Reproduced with permission of IOP Publishing Ltd., from Atkinson and Berry [58], *J. Phys. A. Math. Nucl. Gen.*, © 1998 Institute of Physics.)

(see Fig. 5.19c), a similar behavior was seen, but with a scale of around 10 mm. Atkinson and Berry pointed out that the quasi-random changes of the returned signal could not arise from any physical structure, since all components were much less than a wavelength, and proposed that they arose from changes in the local density of RBC scatterers. The statistical diffraction theory that they developed to account for their observations has served as a basis for many subsequent investigations, particularly for Doppler ultrasound and image speckle analysis.

In the previous subsection, the Hct was assumed to be sufficiently small so that the position of a given scatterer was independent of the location of any other scatterer (i.e., no correlation exists between the various scatterer positions). With increasing Hct, the positions of the scatterers can no longer be chosen at random. If we consider the problem of randomly placing a finite-sized scatterer in a volume that has already achieved a high degree of occupancy, it can be readily appreciated that because many of the chosen positions are either occupied by a scatterer or have insufficient room for the placement of a new scatterer, the final placement position can be expected to have some degree of correlation with the surrounding scatterers. This must be taken into account when determining the total mean squared scattered pressure. The scattering of ultrasound by suspensions of RBCs has been the subject of several reviews that also contain comprehensive reference listings. In particular, the reader is referred to Mo and Cobbold [21], published in 1993, and to Cloutier and Qin [52], published late in 1997.

The two classical approaches used for analyzing the scattering from a suspension of small scatterers are the particle approach (used in the previous subsection for a sparse medium) and the continuum approach. In the particle approach it is recognized that RBCs are weak scatterers and that geometric ray theory can be applied to sum the scattering contributions. On the other hand, the continuum approach makes use of the fact that the resolution volume associated with the incident wave will typically contain a very large number of scatterers. For example, at a normal Hct of ~45% and for a resolution volume $1\,mm^3$, there will be approximately 5×10^6 RBCs. This suggests that the medium can be treated as a continuum with local fluctuations that represent the statistical variations in the RBC number density. In addition, a hybrid approach has also been developed that combines the strengths of both the continuum and particle methods, and this is described below.

A Hybrid Method

In the hybrid method developed by Mo [21,53], the sample volume is first divided into a large number of elementary volumes (voxels), each of which has a maximum dimension much less than a wavelength (e.g., $<\lambda/10$). Such a small dimension ensures that the incident wave has almost the same phase as it strikes each scatterer in a given voxel. As illustrated by the 2-D representation of Fig. 5.20, at any given instant of time the number of scatterers in each

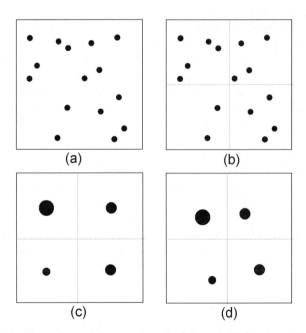

Figure 5.20 2-D illustration of the voxel method for calculating the backscattering coefficient of a distribution of identical scatterers. (a) Original particle distribution; (b) subdivision into voxels; (c) equivalent scatterers placed at voxel geometric centers; (d) more accurate representation in which an equivalent scatterer is placed at the voxel center of mass. (Adapted from Lim et al. [54]).

voxel will differ depending on the distribution of scatterers throughout the sample volume, and therefore the scattered waves contributed by each voxel can differ both in magnitude and phase. The scattered wave produced by a given voxel can be quite accurately represented by a single equivalent scatterer placed at the center of the voxel (see Fig. 5.20c) with a volume equal to the sum of all the individual scatterer volumes contained in that voxel. Consequently, the backscattering from a given sample volume can be calculated by replacing all voxels with a lattice of equivalent particles placed at the center[17] of each voxel. The total backscattered signal can then be found by simply summing the contributions in much the same way as described in the previous subsection.

It will be shown that the backscattering coefficient is directly proportional to average variance in the scatterer number density throughout the sample volume. In carrying out numerical simulations of the scattered wave produced by a dense suspension, this method has an important computational advantage. Instead of having to account for the contributions from each scatterer, it is only necessary to sum the contributions from the equivalent particles placed at the center of each voxel. For a 3-D computer simulation of scattering by RBCs at normal hematocrits, it has been shown that this can result in several orders of magnitude reduction in computation time [54]. This reference also discusses the accuracy of the voxel approach and uses a wideband Gaussian-shaped transmit pulse.

We shall assume that the sample volume V is equally divided into N_x voxels of volume V_v whose maximum dimension is much less than a wavelength. It is also assumed that the sample volume contains identical non-aggregating RBCs, each of which has volume V_s. At any given instant of time t, the number of scatterers within a voxel is a random variable, so that for the i'th voxel the number of scatterers can be expressed as the sum of the expected value $E[N_v]$ and a fluctuation term $n_i(t)$, i.e.,

$$(5.64) \qquad N_i^v(t) = E[N_v] + n_i(t),$$

in which that $E[n_i(t)] = 0$. The backscattered signal produced by the i'th voxel, which contains $N_i^v(t)$ scatterers of backscattering cross-sections σ_b, can be obtained with the help of Fig. 5.21. As indicated, the center of the voxel is taken to be at $\mathbf{r}_i$ relative to the observation point and the n'th scatterer is located at $\Delta\mathbf{r}_n$ relative to the center. If the observation point is in the far field, then, for an incident plane wave with a wave vector $\mathbf{k}$, the backscattered pressure at the observation point due to all N_i^v scatterers can be obtained from (5.60) and Fig. 5.21 as

$$p_i(t) = p_{im} \frac{\sqrt{\sigma_b}}{r_i} \sum_{n=1}^{N_i^v} \cos(\omega t + \phi_n)$$

17. If the equivalent scatterers are placed at the center of mass (see Fig. 5.20d) of each voxel rather than at the center, a more accurate representation can be achieved [54,61].

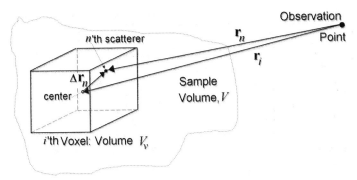

Figure 5.21 Calculating the backscattering produced by a plane incident wave at a far distant point from a small voxel that contains N_i^v scatterers.

where $\phi_n = 2\mathbf{k} \cdot (\mathbf{r}_i + \Delta \mathbf{r}_n)$. But because $(\Delta r_n)_{max} \ll \lambda \ll r_i$, it follows that $\phi_n \approx 2\mathbf{k} \cdot \mathbf{r}_i \equiv \phi$, so that the pressure from the i'th voxel simplifies to

$$(5.65) \qquad p_i(t) = p_{im} \frac{\sqrt{\sigma_b}}{r_i} N_i^v(t) \cos(\omega t + \phi_i).$$

This equation simply states that the backscattered pressure contribution of a given voxel can be found by assuming a single scatterer placed at the voxel center with a volume equal to the sum of all the scatterer volumes present in the voxel.

The total backscattered pressure waveform can be found by summing over all voxels in the sample volume. By substituting (5.64) into (5.65) the pressure due to all N_x voxels in the sample volume can be written as

$$(5.66) \qquad p(t) = \sum_{i=1}^{N_{vx}} p_i(t) = p_{im} \frac{\sqrt{\sigma_b}}{r} \left\{ E[N] \sum_{i=1}^{N_x} \cos(\omega t + \phi_i) + \sum_{i=1}^{N_x} n_i(t - t_i) \cos(\omega t + \phi_i) \right\},$$

Crystallographic   Fluctuation
Term   Term

where $E[N] = E[N_v]$ is the expected number of RBCs in any voxel and t_i is the transit time from the i'th voxel to the observation point.

The two components in the above equation are illustrated in Fig. 5.22 for a 2-D distribution. The first component represents the sum of the scattered signals from N_x regularly spaced scatterers with the same scattering strength. This has been called the *crystallographic* contribution [53]. Assuming that the sample volume is considerably larger than a wavelength, the real part of this term gives rise to a phase shift that should be nearly uniformly distributed over $(-\pi, \pi)$ and therefore should approach the average value of a cosine wave, which is zero. The second term, arising from the random fluctuations in the local Hct, is called the *fluctuation term*: hence the notion of *fluctuation scattering*, a term that was used by Atkinson and Berry [58] and subsequently by Angelsen [59] in their analysis of the Doppler signal from a suspension of RBCs. For the fluctuation signal that has a time average of zero, negative

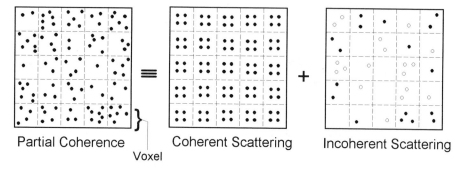

Partial Coherence   Coherent Scattering   Incoherent Scattering

Voxel

Figure 5.22 2-D representation of the backscattered signal components using the voxel approach. The sample volume is divided into voxels, each of which contains a variable number of RBCs. The partially coherent ultrasonic backscattered signal can be represented as the sum of a coherent and an incoherent part. In this example there is an average of 4 RBCs per voxel, so that the coherent part of the backscattered signal is that due to a regular pattern of 4 RBCs in each voxel. The incoherent part consists of voxel scattering by either RBCs or by negative RBC concentrations (represented by unfilled circles). (Reproduced, with permission, from Mo and Cobbold [53], *IEEE Trans. Biomed. Eng.*, 41, 29–33, © 1992 IEEE.)

values correspond to negative RBC concentrations. In the following analysis it will be assumed that the crystallographic term can be neglected.

A straightforward method for calculating the backscattering coefficient is through the *autocorrelation function* $R(t_1, t_2)$ of the process, rather than by proceeding in the manner of subsection 5.9.3. It is reasonable to assume that the n_i's in (5.66) are independent random variables that are identically distributed. For the process defined by these random variables, it follows from the Central Limit theorem that the backscattered signal is a Gaussian process with zero mean. It can be shown that such a process is completely characterized by its autocorrelation function. For a real random variable $x(t)$, the autocorrelation function is defined as $R(t_1, t_2) = E[x(t_1)x(t_2)]$. For the special case of $t_1 = t_2 = t$, then $R(t, t) = E[x^2(t)]$, which is the average power of $x(t)$. Moreover, by taking the Fourier transform of the autocorrelation function, the spectral density of the process can be determined. It therefore follows that the autocorrelation function provides valuable information for characterizing the process.

By ignoring the crystallographic term, it can be readily shown from (5.66) that the scattered pressure autocorrelation function is given by

$$R_p(t_1, t_2) = E[p(t_1)p(t_2)]$$

$$= p_{im}^2 \frac{\sigma_b}{r^2} E\left[\sum_{i=1}^{N_x} n_i(t_1 - t_i)\cos(\omega t_1 + \phi_i) \sum_{j=1}^{N_x} n_j(t_2 - t_j)\cos(\omega t_2 + \phi_j)\right]$$

$$= p_{im}^2 \frac{\sigma_b}{r^2} \sum_{i=1}^{N_x} \sum_{j=1}^{N_x} E[n_i(t_1 - t_i)n_j(t_2 - t_j)]\cos(\omega t_1 + \phi_i)\cos(\omega t_2 + \phi_j).$$

To reduce this expression to a single summation, we shall assume that in the interval $(t_1 - t_2)$ all the RBCs in a given voxel are simply replaced by those in another, thereby producing a new representation. Consequently, out of the N_x^2 terms there will be N_x pairs such that $n_i(t_1 - t_i) = n_j(t_2 - t_j)$ and $\omega_i = \omega_j$ (which implies that $\phi_i = \phi_j$). Furthermore, the $N_v(1 - N_v)$ remaining terms should approach zero, since the voxel contributions have zero mean and are statistically independent. In addition, the variance of the number of RBCs in a voxel will be denoted by $\mathrm{var}(n) = E[\{N_v - E[N_v]\}^2]$, which we have assumed to be spatially independent throughout the sample volume. In view of the above and noting that $\mathrm{var}(n) = E[n_i^2(t_1 - t_i)]$, the autocorrelation function for the scattered pressure reduces to

$$R_p(t_1, t_2) = p_{im}^2 \frac{\sigma_b}{r^2} \mathrm{var}(n) \sum_{i=1}^{N_x} \cos(\omega t_1 + \phi_i)\cos(\omega t_2 + \phi_i).$$

But for the stationary (wide-sense) process considered, the autocorrelation function depends only on $t_1 - t_2 = \tau$. Consequently, the above equation, with the help of a trigonometric relation, can be written as

$$R_p(\tau) = p_{im}^2 \frac{\sigma_b}{r^2} \mathrm{var}(n)\left\{ \frac{N_x}{2}\cos 2(\omega\tau) + \frac{1}{2}\sum_{i=1}^{N_x}\cos[\omega(t_1 + t_2 + 2\phi_i)] \right\}$$

If the sample volume dimensions are much greater than a wavelength so that the total number of voxels (N_x) will be large, the summation term will approach zero, and as a result

(5.67)
$$R_p(0) = p_{im}^2 \frac{\sigma_b N_x}{2r^2} \mathrm{var}(n).$$

Noting that for a stationary process $E[x^2(\tau)] = R(0)$ and that the backscattering coefficient, as expressed by (5.59b), is in terms of the mean square pressure at a unit distance away from a unit scattering volume, the BSC can be written as $\sigma_{BSC} = 2r^2 R_p(0)/(Vp_{im}^2)$, where V is the sample volume. Substituting (5.67) into this equation yields

(5.68)
$$\boxed{\sigma_{BSC} = \frac{\sigma_b N_x \mathrm{var}(n)}{V} = \frac{\sigma_b \mathrm{var}(n)}{V_v}},$$

where the voxel volume is given by $V_v = V/N_x$. Thus, the backscattering coefficient is directly proportional to the concentration variance of RBCs in the voxels, a result originally obtained by Angelsen [59] by using the continuum approach.

To theoretically predict how the BSC depends on the hematocrit (H) an expression for the dependence of the variance of the scatterer concentration is needed. This can be achieved by obtaining an expression for the *packing factor*[18] W and relating it to the variance. Physically, the packing factor can be viewed as a measure of the orderliness in the spatial arrangement of the RBCs. It is a measure of the amount of empty space (sometimes referred to as elbow room) between the scatterers. It can be shown [60,61] that the variance of the scatterer concentration is related to W by

(5.69) $$\text{var}(n) = V_v \varepsilon_\rho W,$$

where $\varepsilon_\rho (=N/V)$ is the average concentration of scatterers (number per unit volume) in the sample volume. The packing factor is given by [61]

(5.70) $$W = 1 - \varepsilon_\rho V_v + \frac{1}{\varepsilon_\rho V_v} \iint_{V_v} d^3\mathbf{r}_i \, d^3\mathbf{r}_j \, P(\mathbf{r}_i, \mathbf{r}_j),$$

in which $P(\mathbf{r}_i, \mathbf{r}_j)d^3\mathbf{r}_i d^3\mathbf{r}_j$ is the pair correlation function. The latter is the probability of finding the i'th and j'th scatterer in two distinct volumes $d^3\mathbf{r}_i$ and $d^3\mathbf{r}_j$, respectively. By substituting (5.69) into (5.68) and noting that the Hct can be expressed in terms of the RBC volume V_s by $H = NV_s/V = \varepsilon_\rho V_s$, the BSC can be written as

(5.71) $$\boxed{\sigma_{BSC} = \frac{\sigma_b HW}{V_s}}$$

At very low hematocrits, when the RBC positions are completely random, W approaches unity, so that the BSC is directly proportional to the Hct. As H increases, W gradually decays to zero, since closer packing inevitably leads to a more orderly arrangement. In the limit as $H \to 1$, the free space (elbow room) approaches zero ($W \to 0$), and as a result $\sigma_{BSC} \to 0$.

Deriving an explicit expression for the packing factor is a fairly difficult task. Based on the Percus-Yevick pair correlation function, Twersky [60,62] has shown that W can be expressed in terms of a parameter m [61] and the hematocrit H by

(5.72) $$W(m) = \frac{(1-H)^{m+1}}{[1+H(m-1)]^{m-1}},$$

in which $m = 1$, 2, and 3, corresponding to the packing of hard slabs (1-D), cylinders (2-D), and spheres (3-D). To account for the fractal nature of the packing of real scatterers whose geometry and symmetry may not be properly represented by simple integer values, it has been proposed that m can take on non-integer (fractal) values. It is partially for this reason that m has been called a *packing dimension* [61]. From (5.72), it follows that the packing factor W can take on a continuous range of values, depending on the scatterer symmetries and the manner in which they are packed.

---

18. The concept of the packing factor has been adapted from the statistical theory of liquids.

It can be shown that an approximate expression for the scattering cross-section of the three simple geometric forms can be written as

(5.73)
$$\sigma_{bm'} = \left(\pi\beta_{m'} R^{m'}\right)^2 \left(\frac{k}{2\pi}\right)^{m'+1} \left[\frac{\kappa_v - \kappa_o}{\kappa_o} + \frac{\rho_o - \rho_v}{\rho_v}\right]^2,$$

where m' is the *particle dimension* whose value is 1, 2, or 3, for slabs, cylinders and spheres, respectively. In addition, R is a characteristic dimension (thickness of a slab, radii of a cylinder or sphere) and $\beta_1 = 2$, $\beta_2 = \pi$, $\beta_3 = 4\pi/3$. For the case of a sphere (σ_{b3}), this equation is identical to that derived using the Born approximation, i.e. (5.39). By substituting (5.72) and (5.73) into (5.71), the BSC can then be expressed in terms of m and the Hct. The normalized results, shown in Fig. 5.23, clearly demonstrate the asymmetry of the curves, with a peak value occurring at Hct considerably less than 50%. As the fractal-packing dimension is increased from 1 to 3, i.e., as the degree of packing symmetry is increased, the peak for the curve decreases in magnitude and shifts to lower hematocrits. For example, if $m = 3.0$, the peak occurs at 13%; for $m = 1.0$, it is at 33%. As discussed in the next subsection, various flow conditions, such as turbulence and RBC aggregation, can cause local changes in the scatterer number density: these can be represented by changes in the packing dimension m and therefore in the backscattered power.

Comparison With Measurements

Comparison of the theoretical predictions with experimental measurements on blood provides a means for testing the validity of the assumptions and

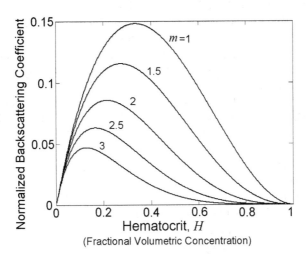

Figure 5.23 Variation of the backscattering coefficient versus hematocrit. The backscattering coefficient has been normalized by dividing by $\sigma_{bm'}/V_{sm'}$. (Reproduced, with permission, from Bascom and Cobbold [61], *J. Acoust. Soc. Am.*, 98, 3040–3049, 1995, © 1995 Acoustical Society of America.)

underlying approach. Good evidence has been presented that the BSC varies nearly as the fourth power of the frequency over a wide frequency range (2–30 MHz) [35,66] for both laminar and stirred flow conditions, and over a range of hematocrits from a few percent to normal physiological values [67]. The dependence of the BSC on the square of the average RBC volume has also been confirmed [68,69] by using RBCs obtained from a variety of species. Many experimental results have been reported describing the dependence of the BSC on Hct, starting with the first publication by Shung et al. [70]. In Fig. 5.24a we show the results reported by Mo et al. [63], obtained at a frequency of 7.5 MHz, using gently stirred porcine RBCs suspended in 0.83% saline to prevent aggregation. Comparison of these results with the fitted theoretical results obtained from (5.72), (5.73), and (5.71) with $m' = 3$ shows good agreement over a wide range of hematocrits and a theoretical peak response at about 16% Hct.

Beginning with the initial studies by Shung et al. [64], it was realized that the backscattering coefficient for blood generally depends on the flow conditions (see Fig. 5.24b). One reason for this dependence arises from the formation of aggregates, a dynamic process that is dependent on the fluid velocity gradient (shear rate). For example, if the backscattered power is measured from whole blood subsequent to flow stoppage, it is found that substantial increases in the backscattered power can subsequently occur [71,72]. At low shears or in the absence of any shear, aggregation will occur, and as a result there will be a distribution of scatterer sizes ranging from single RBCs to doublets, triplets, and so forth. At higher shear rates, the tendency of RBCs to aggregate is dominated by the disruptive effects of the shear stress. At first it might be thought that at higher hematocrits the presence of some doublets, for example, in a voxel, should have no influence on the BSC since it has been assumed that the size of a voxel is much less than a wavelength. The flaw in this argument is that the scattering is thought to be proportional to the scatterer concentration, which remains fixed for a given Hct. The correct view is to consider the influence of aggregation on var(n) instead. Suppose that all the RBCs in the sample volume were in the form of doublets; then, because the changes in a voxel must take place through two RBCs at a time, it is apparent that var(n) will be greater than when the scatterers are all single RBCs, resulting in a higher BSC [53]. More recently, the relation between the state of aggregation, the packing factor, and the backscattered signal has been explored by using computer simulations of simple aggregate distributions [74].

Experimental measurements have shown that under turbulent flow conditions the BSC from blood and RBC suspensions is also increased [64,67]. It is found that with increasing Hct, the BSC becomes greater and reaches a maximum at a higher Hct than when the flow is laminar. These effects are illustrated by the measurements on bovine RBCs shown in Fig. 5.24b. It should be noted that the packing dimension needed to achieve a best fit to the experimental results is reduced under turbulent conditions to $m = 2.17$. Measurements reported by Bascom et al. [73] for fixed human RBCs suspended in physiological saline (to prevent aggregation) at 4% Hct showed no change in

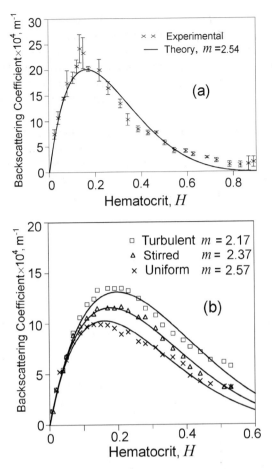

Figure 5.24 Comparison of experimental measurements for the backscattering coefficient σ_{BSC} versus hematocrit with theoretical predictions obtained from (5.72), (5.73), and (5.71) with $m' = 3$. (a) For porcine RBCs suspended in 0.85% saline. The theoretical curve was obtained by using the following measured values: $\kappa_v = 0.3496\,\text{GPa}^{-1}$, $\kappa_o = 0.443\,\text{GPa}^{-1}$, $\rho_v = 1078\,\text{kg/m}^3$, $\rho_o = 1005\,\text{kg/m}^3$, $V_s = 68\,\mu\text{m}^3$, and adjusting the parameter m to obtain a best fit to the experimental results reported by Mo et al. [63] at 7.5 MHz. (b) Measurements are those reported by Shung et al. [5.64] for bovine RBCs suspended in saline and the best fit theoretical results using: $\kappa_v = 0.357\,\text{GPa}^{-1}$, $\kappa_o = 0.443\,\text{GPa}^{-1}$, $\rho_v = 1099\,\text{kg/m}^3$, $\rho_o = 1005\,\text{kg/m}^3$, $V_s = 53\,\mu\text{m}^3$. A correction factor of 0.66 has been used, see [65]. (Reproduced, with permission, from Bascom and Cobbold [61], *J. Acoust. Soc. Am.*, 98, 3040–3049, 1995, © 1995 Acoustical Society of America.)

the BSC when the flow became turbulent. On the other hand, they reported substantial increases for human RBCs suspended in physiological saline at 41% Hct.

An explanation for these results can be found in the fractal model described earlier in this section. In brief, it is known that turbulent flow is characterized by turbulent structures such as vortices. In the presence of particles such as RBCs, it is reasonable to expect that such structures will tend to cause localized rearrangements of RBCs between the voxels, thereby increasing var(n), with a corresponding reduction in the packing dimension m. As shown in Fig. 5.23, a reduction in m also leads to an increase in the Hct at which the BSC reaches a maximum, which is in agreement with the measurements shown in Fig. 5.24b.

Under pulsatile flow conditions similar to those present in vivo, the backscattered signal has been found to vary in a cyclic manner. In part, this may be due to the time-dependent aggregation process [75,76], but it has also been observed that if turbulence is present over part of the cycle, this has an important influence on the backscattered power [77].

Problems

P1. a. Show that $\nabla^2 p - \dfrac{1}{c_o^2}\dfrac{\partial^2 p}{\partial t^2} = \dfrac{1}{c_o^2}\dfrac{\partial^2 p}{\partial t^2}\left[\dfrac{\kappa_v - \kappa_o}{\kappa_o}\right] + \nabla\cdot\left[\dfrac{\rho_v - \rho_o}{\rho_v}\nabla p\right]$ can be

   expressed as $\nabla^2 p - \dfrac{1}{c_o^2}\dfrac{\partial^2 p}{\partial t^2} = \dfrac{1}{c_o^2}\dfrac{\partial^2 p}{\partial t^2}\left[\dfrac{\kappa_v - \kappa_o}{\kappa_o} + \dfrac{\rho_v - \rho_o}{\rho_v}\right] +$

   $\nabla\left[\dfrac{\rho_v - \rho_o}{\rho_v}\right]\cdot\nabla p$ if the source scattering term is small.

   b. If the wave propagation speed is given by $c = c_o + \Delta c$, where $\Delta c/c_o \ll 1$, show that the above equation can be expressed as

   $$\nabla^2 p - \frac{1}{c_o^2}\frac{\partial^2 p}{\partial t^2} \approx -\frac{2\Delta c}{c_o^3}\frac{\partial^2 p}{\partial t^2} + \frac{1}{\rho_o}\nabla\rho_v\cdot\nabla p.$$

P2. A pulse-echo system consists of coincident and identical transmitter and receiver transducers and a scatterer consisting of a small immobile sphere of radius a whose density is the same as the suspending medium but whose compressibility differs. If it can also be assumed that $w_r^\delta(t) = A\delta(t)$, $w_i^\delta(t) = B\partial\delta(t)/\partial t$, show that the received signal is given by

   $$e_o(t) = -AB\frac{4\pi a^3\rho_o}{3c_o^2}\left[\frac{\kappa_o - \kappa_v}{\kappa_v}\right]\frac{\partial^4 e_i(t)}{\partial t^4} * h_t(\mathbf{r}_o:t) * h_t(\mathbf{r}_o:t).$$

References

1. Strutt, J.W. (Rayleigh, J.W.S.), Investigation of the disturbance produced by a spherical obstacle on the waves of sound, *Proc. London Math. Soc.*, 4, 233–283, 1872.
2. Rayleigh, J.W.S., *The Theory of Sound*, Vol. 2 (2nd edn., 1894) republished, Dover Publications, New York, 1945.
3. Shung, K.K., and Thieme, G.A. (eds.), *Ultrasonic Scattering in Biological Tissues*, CRC Press, Boca Raton, FL, 1993.

4. Morse, P.M., and Ingard, K.U., *Theoretical Acoustics*, McGraw-Hill, New York, 1968.

5. Skudrzyk, E., *The Foundations of Acoustics*, Springer-Verlag, New York, 1971.

6. Malecki, I., *Physical Foundations of Technical Acoustics*, Pergamon Press, Oxford, 1969.

7. Bowman, J.J., Senior, T.B.A., and Uslenghi, P.L.E. (eds.), *Electromagnetic and Acoustic Scattering by Simple Shapes*, North-Holland, Amsterdam, 1969.

8. Varadan, V.V., Ma, Y., Varadan, V.K., and Lakhtakia, A., Scattering of waves by spheres and cylinders, Chapter 5, pp. 211–324, in: *Field Representations and Introduction to Scattering*, Vol. 1, V.V. Varadan, A. Lakhtakia, and V.K. Varadan (eds.), North-Holland, Amsterdam, 1991.

9. Spence, R.D., and Granger, S., The scattering of sound from a prolate spheroid, *J. Acoust. Soc. Am.*, 23, 701–706, 1951.

10. Strutt, J.W. (Rayleigh, J.W.S.), On the light from the sky, its polarization and colour, *Phil. Mag.*, 41, 107–120 and 274–279, 1871.

11. Sewell, C.J.T., The extinction of sound in a viscous atmosphere by small obstacles of cylindrical and spherical form, *Phil. Trans. R. Soc.*, A210, 239–270, 1910.

12. Lamb, H., *Hydrodynamics*, pp. 511–516, 529–531, 657–659, 6th edn., Cambridge University Press, Cambridge, 1932.

13. Urick, R.J., A sound velocity method for determining the compressibility of finely divided substances, *J. Appl. Physics*, 18, 983–987, 1947.

14. Faran, J.J., Sound scattering by solid cylinders and spheres, *J. Acoust. Soc. Am.*, 23, 405–418, 1951.

15. Hickling, R., Analysis of echoes from a solid elastic sphere in water, *J. Acoust. Soc. Am.*, 34, 1582–1592, 1962.

16. Neubauer, W.G., Vogt, R.H., and Dragonette, L.R., Acoustic reflection from elastic spheres. I. Steady-state signals, *J. Acoust. Soc. Am.*, 55, 1123–1129, 1962.

17. Dragonette, L.R., Vogt, R.H., Flax, L., and Neubauer, W.G., Acoustic reflection from elastic spheres and rigid spheres and spheroids. II. Transient analysis, *J. Acoust. Soc. Am.*, 55, 1130–1137, 1962.

18. Lin, W.H., and Raptis, A.C., Acoustic scattering by elastic solid cylinders and spheres in viscous fluids, *J. Acoust. Soc. Am.*, 73, 736–749, 1982.

19. Numrich, S.K., and Uberall, H., Scattering of sound pulses and the ringing of target resonances, pp. 235–318 in: *High Frequency and Pulse Scattering*, A.D. Pierce and R.N. Thurston (eds.), Vol. 21, *Physical Acoustics*, Academic Press, New York, 1992.

20. Hackman, R.H., Acoustic Scattering from elastic solids, pp. 2–194 in: *Underwater Scattering and Radiation*, A.D. Pierce and R.N. Thurston (eds.), Vol. 22, *Physical Acoustics*, Academic Press, New York, 1993.

21. Mo, L.Y.L., and Cobbold, R.S.C., Theoretical models of ultrasonic scattering in blood, Chapter 5, pp. 125–170 in: *Ultrasonic Scattering in Biological Tissues*, K.K. Shung and G.A. Thieme (eds.), CRC Press, Boca Raton, FL, 1993.

22. Lin, W.H., and Raptis, A.C., Sound scattering from a thin rod in a viscous medium, *J. Acoust. Soc. Am.*, 79, 1693–1701, 1986.

23. Flax, L., Varadan, V.K., and Varadan, V.V., Scattering of an obliquely incident acoustic wave by an infinite cylinder, *J. Acoust. Soc. Am.*, 68, 1832–1835, 1980.

24. Li, T-B., and Ueda, M., Sound scattering of a plane wave obliquely incident on a cylinder, *J. Acoust. Soc. Am.*, 100, 2363–2368, 1989.

25. Honarvar, F., and Sinclair, A.N., Acoustic wave scattering from transversely isotropic cylinders, *J. Acoust. Soc. Am.*, 86, 57–63, 1996.

26. Wear, K.A., Frequency dependence of ultrasonic backscatter from human trabecular bone: theory and experiment, *J. Acoust. Soc. Am.*, 106, 3659–3664, 1999.

27. Chernov, L.A., *Wave Propagation in a Random Medium*, McGraw-Hill, New York, 1960.
28. Nicholas, D., An introduction to the theory of acoustic scattering by biological tissues, Chapter 1, pp. 1–28 in: *Recent Advances in Ultrasound in Biomedicine*, Vol. 1, D.N. White (ed.), Research Studies Press, Forest Grove, OR, 1977.
29. Insana, M.F., and Brown, D.G., Acoustic scattering theory applied to soft biological tissues, Chapter 4, pp. 75–124 in: *Ultrasonic Scattering in Biological Tissues*, K.K. Shung and G.A. Thieme (eds.), CRC Press, Boca Raton, FL, 1993.
30. Waterman, P.C., New formulation of acoustic scattering, *J. Acoust. Soc. Am.*, 45, 1417–1429, 1969.
31. Waterman, P.C., Matrix theory of elastic wave scattering, *J. Acoust. Soc. Am.*, 60, 567–580, 1976.
32. Varatharajulu, V., and Pao, Y-H., Scattering matrix for elastic waves, *J. Acoust. Soc. Am.*, 60, 556–566, 1976.
33. Peterson, B., and Strom, S., Matrix formulation of acoustic scattering from an arbitrary number of scatterers, *J. Acoust. Soc. Am.*, 56, 771–780, 1974.
34. Koc, S., and Chew, W.C., Calculation of acoustical scattering from a cluster of scatterers, *J. Acoust. Soc. Am.*, 103, 721–734, 1998.
35. Kuo, I.Y., and Shung, K.K., High frequency ultrasonic backscatter from erythrocyte suspension, *IEEE Trans. Biomed. Eng.*, 41, 29–33, 1994.
36. Gore, J.C., and Leeman, S., Ultrasonic backscattering from human tissue: a realistic model, *Phys. Med. Biol.*, 22, 317–326, 1977.
37. Fatemi, M., and Kak, A.C., Ultrasonic B-scan imaging: theory of image formation and a technique for restoration, *Ultrasonic Imaging*, 2, 1–47, 1980.
38. Stepanishen, P.R., Pulsed transmit/receive response of ultrasonic piezoelectric transducers, *J. Acoust. Soc. Am.*, 69, 1815–1827, 1981.
39. Dickinson, R.J., and Nassiri, D., Reflection and scattering, Chapter 6 in: *Physical Principles of Medical Ultrasonics*, 2nd edn., C.R. Hill, J.C. Bamber, and G.R. ter Haar (eds.), Wiley, Chichester, UK, 2004.
40. Jensen, J.J., A model for the propagation and scattering of ultrasound in tissue, *J. Acoust. Soc. Am.*, 89, 182–190, 1991.
41. Morse, P.M., and Feshbach, H., *Methods of Theoretical Physics*, p. 843, Vol. 1, McGraw-Hill, New York, 1953.
42. Bamber, J.C., and Dickinson, R.J., Ultrasonic B-scanning: a computer simulation, *Phys. Med. Biol.*, 25, 463–479, 1980.
43. Wright, H., Impulse response function corresponding to reflection from a region of continuous impedance change, *J. Acoust. Soc. Am.*, 53, 1356–1359, 1973.
44. Jones, J.P., Ultrasonic impediography and its applications to tissue characterization, Chapter 6, pp. 131–156 in *Recent Advances in Ultrasound in Biomedicine*, Vol. 1., D.N. White (ed.), Research Studies Press, Forest Grove, OR, 1977.
45. Kak, A.C., Fry, F.J., and Jones, J.P., Acoustic impedance profiling, Chapter 8, pp. 495–537 in Part 1 of *Ultrasound: Its Applications in Medicine and Biology*, F.J. Fry (ed.), Elsevier, Amsterdam, 1978.
46. Leeman, S., The impediography equations, pp. 517–525 in *Acoustical Imaging*, Vol. 8, D.F. Metherell (ed.), Plenum Press, New York, 1979.
47. Foldy, L.L., The multiple scattering of waves. I. General theory of isotropic scattering by randomly distributed scatterers, *Phys. Rev.*, 67, 107–119, 1945.
48. Papoulis, A., and Pillai, S.U., *Probability, Random Variables and Stochastic Processes*, 4nd edn., McGraw-Hill, New York, 2002.

49. O'Flynn, M., *Probabilities, Random Variables, and Random Processes*, Harper & Row, New York, 1982.

50. Mo, L.Y-L., and Cobbold, R.S.C., A stochastic model of the backscattered Doppler ultrasound from blood, *IEEE Trans. Biomed. Eng.*, BME-33, 20–27, 1986.

51. van der Heiden, M.S., De Kroon, M.G.M., Bom, N., and Borst, C., Ultrasound backscatter at 30 MHz from human blood: influence of rouleau size affected by blood modification and shear rate, *Ultrasound Med. Biol.*, 21, 817–826, 1995.

52. Cloutier, G., and Qin, Z., Ultrasound backscattering from non-aggregating and aggregating erythrocytes: a review, *Biorheology*, 34, 443–470, 1997.

53. Mo, L.Y-L., and Cobbold, R.S.C., A unified approach to modelling the backscattered Doppler ultrasound from blood, *IEEE Trans. Biomed. Eng.*, 39, 450–461, 1992.

54. Lim, B., Bascom, P.A.J., and Cobbold, R.S.C., Particle and voxel approaches for simulating ultrasound backscattering from tissue, *Ultrasound Med. Biol.*, 22, 1237–1247, 1996.

55. Sigelmann, R.A., and Reid, J.A., Analysis and measurement of ultrasound backscattering from an ensemble of scatterers excited by sine-wave bursts, *J. Acoust. Soc. Am.*, 53, 1351–1355, 1973.

56. Fahrbach, K., Ein beitrag zur blutgeschwindigkeitsmessung unter anwendungdes Dopplereffektes [A major contribution to blood speed measurement using the Doppler effect], *Elektromedizin*, 14, 233–246, 1969 and 15, 26–36, 1970.

57. Brody, W.R., Theoretical analysis of the ultrasonic flowmeter, PhD thesis, Dept. Elect. Eng., Stanford University, 1971 (Technical report # 4958-1). See also: Brody, M.R., and Meindl, Theoretical analysis of the CW ultrasonic flowmeter, *IEEE Trans. Biomed. Eng.*, 21, 183–192, 1974.

58. Atkinson, P., and Berry, M. V., Random noise in ultrasonic echoes diffracted by blood, *J. Phys. A. Math. Nucl. Gen.*, 7, 1293–1302, 1974.

59. Angelsen, B.A.J., A theoretical study of the scattering of ultrasound from blood, *IEEE Trans. Biomed. Eng.*, BME-27, 61–67, 1980.

60. Twersky, V., Transparency of pair-correlated, random distributions of small scatterers, with applications to the cornea, *J. Opt. Soc. Am.*, 68, 524–530, 1975.

61. Bascom, P.A.J., and Cobbold, R.S.C., On a fractal packing approach for understanding ultrasonic backscattering from blood, *J. Acoust. Soc. Am.*, 98, 3040–3049, 1995.

62. Twersky, V., Acoustic bulk parameters in distributions of pair-correlated scatterers, *J. Acoust. Soc. Am.*, 64, 1710–1719, 1978.

63. Mo, L.Y.L., Kuo, I-Y., Shung, K.K., Ceresne, L., and Cobbold, R.S.C., Ultrasound scattering from blood with hematocrits up to 100%, *IEEE Trans. Biomed. Eng.*, 41, 91–95, 1994.

64. Shung, K.K., Yuan, Y.W., Fei, D.Y., and Tarbell, J.M., Effect of flow disturbance on ultrasonic backscatter from blood, *J. Acoust. Soc. Am.*, 75, 1265–1272, 1984.

65. Lucas, R.J., and Twersky, V., Inversion of ultrasonic scattering data for red blood cell suspensions under different flow conditions, *J. Acoust. Soc. Am.*, 82, 794–799, 1987.

66. Wang, S-H., and Shung, K.K., An approach for measuring ultrasonic backscattering from biological tissues with focused transducers, *IEEE Trans. Biomed. Eng.*, 44, 549–554, 1997.

67. Yuan, Y.W., and Shung, K.K., Ultrasonic backscatter from flowing whole blood. II: Dependence on frequency and fibrinogen concentration, *J. Acoust. Soc. Am.*, 84, 1195–1200, 1988.

68. Borders, S.E., Fronek, A., Kemper, W.S., and Franklin, D., Ultrasonic energy backscattered from blood, *Ann. Biomed. Engng.*, 6, 83–92, 1978.
69. Shung, K.K., Kuo, I.Y., and Cloutier, G., Ultrasonic scattering properties of blood, pp. 119–139 in *Intravascular Ultrasound*, J. Roelandt, E.J. Gussenhoven, and N. Bom (eds.), Kluwer Academic Pub., Dordrechet, Holland, 1993.
70. Shung, K.K., Sigelmann, R.A., and Reid, J.M., Scattering of ultrasound by blood, *IEEE Trans. Biomed. Eng.*, 23, 460, 1976.
71. Yuan, Y.W., and Shung, K.K., Echoicity of whole blood. *J. Ultrasound Med.*, 8, 425–434, 1989.
72. Shehada, R.E.N., Cobbold, R.S.C., and Bascom P.A.J., Ultrasound methods for investigating the non-Newtonian characteristics of whole blood, *IEEE Trans. Ultrason. Ferroelec. Freq. Contr.*, 41, 96–104, 1994.
73. Bascom, P.A.J., Cobbold, R.S.C., Routh, H.F., and Johnston, K.W., On the Doppler signal from a steady flow asymmetric stenosis model: effects of turbulence, *Ultrasound Med. Biol.*, 19, 197–210, 1993.
74. Lim, B., and Cobbold, R.S.C., On the relation between aggregation, packing and the backscattered signal for whole blood, *Ultrasound Med. Biol.*, 25, 1395–1405, 1999.
75. Cloutier, G., and Shung, K.K., Study of red cell aggregation in pulsatile flow from ultrasonic Doppler power measurements, *Biorheology*, 30, 443–461, 1993.
76. Cloutier, G., and Shung, K.K., Cyclic variation of the power of ultrasonic Doppler signals backscattered by polystyrene microspheres and porcine erythrocyte suspensions, *IEEE Trans. Biomed. Eng.*, 40, 953–962, 1993.
77. Bascom, P.A.J., Johnston, K.W., Cobbold, R.S.C., and Ojha, M., Relation of the flow field distal to a moderate stenosis to the Doppler power, *Ultrasound Med. Biol.*, 23, 25–39, 1997.

6

Ultrasound Transducers

The history of transducer development for medical imaging and therapeutic applications is closely coupled with the invention of transduction mechanisms and the development of transducer materials. Six transduction mechanisms can be identified as originating in the 19th century:

1. *Electromagnetic*: In the presence of a static or quasi-static magnetic field, a current flowing in a conducting wire or plane results in a Lorentz force. This causes a displacement of the conducting surface. The inverse effect corresponds to an *emf* being induced in a conducting wire or plane that moves in a static or quasi-static magnetic field. Faraday in the United Kingdom and Henry in the United States discovered this around the same time (1831). Both the normal and inverse effects were made use of by Alexander Graham Bell [1] and described in his celebrated paper of 1876 on "Researches in Telephony."
2. *Electrostatic*: A time-varying Coulomb force acting on a pair of conducting planes is produced by a time-varying electric field. The inverse effect corresponds to a change in voltage (at a constant charge) or charge (at a constant voltage) between conducting planes caused by a displacement of one plane with respect to the other. The background and recent progress and are considered in Section 6.10.
3. *Magnetostrictive Effect*: That the dimensions of certain classes of materials change in the presence of a magnetic field was investigated by James Prescott Joule in 1842 and subsequently reported [2]. The inverse of this effect, i.e., when a mechanical stress is applied to certain materials there is an associated change in magnetization, was first reported by Villari [3] in 1864.

4. *Electric Spark*: The oscillatory spark discharge between two electrodes resulting in the production of ultrasonic waves (1890s; see Graff [4]).

5. *Radiant Energy*: In 1880 Alexander Graham Bell disclosed the discovery that pulses of optical energy could create an audible signal. The following year he stated [5], "In my Boston paper the discovery was announced that thin disks of very many different substances *emitted sounds* when exposed to the action of a rapidly-interrupted beam of sunlight."

6. *Piezoelectric Effect*: The historical background and developments are given starting in section 6.1.1.

All of the above mechanisms have found application for ultrasound transduction in the 20th century, and some have only relatively recently been used for medical diagnostic and therapeutic applications. For example, the spark discharge has been used as the basis of a certain commercial version of lithotripsy system for stone disintegration in which a shock wave is produced by the focusing action of an elliptical reflector. A second example is the 1963 discovery that radiant energy in the form of a pulsed laser beam is an effective means of generating very-high-frequency ultrasound pulses in the incident medium [6], and this has found useful application in flaw detection [7]. More recently, using laser pulses of very short durations, ultrasound pulses with frequencies greater than 10^{12} Hz and wavelengths approaching interatomic distances have been produced. Moreover, starting around 1990 there was considerable research aimed at developing efficient capacitive (electrostatic) transducers that can be used for ultrasound imaging. Because these transducers make use of silicon microfabrication technology, they have the potential for much lower production costs.

However, it is the transmission and detection methods based on the piezoelectric effect that have had major impact on the successful development of ultrasound imaging systems. This chapter emphasizes transducers based on the piezoelectric effect, though it concludes with a brief discussion of electrostatic transducers.

6.1 The Direct and Inverse Piezoelectric Effect

In 1880 [8] the Curie brothers (Pierre and Jacques) discovered that the application of a pressure on certain classes of crystals caused a potential difference to be generated between two conducting surfaces that contacted the crystal. This was subsequently named the *piezoelectric effect*. Less than a year later, based on thermodynamic principles, Lippman predicted the *inverse piezoelectric effect*, in which an applied electric field resulted in a change in crystal dimensions, an effect that was verified shortly thereafter by the Curie brothers [9]. As illustrated in Fig. 6.1, piezoelectric transducers convert energy from one form to another. Thus, in the piezoelectric effect the mechanical work done by an applied force displaces electrical charge, causing energy to be stored in the form of polar charge. By definition, a piezoelectric medium must

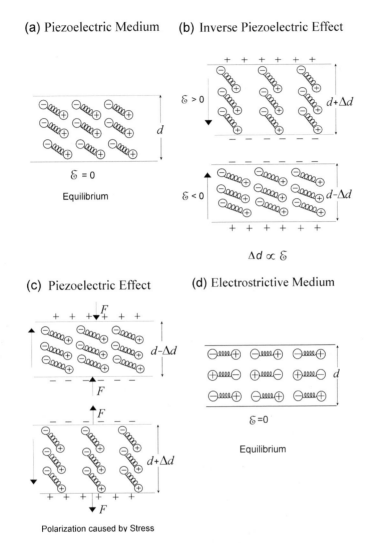

(a) Piezoelectric Medium   **(b)** Inverse Piezoelectric Effect

$\mathscr{E} = 0$

Equilibrium

$\mathscr{E} > 0$ $d + \Delta d$

$\mathscr{E} < 0$ $d - \Delta d$

$\Delta d \propto \mathscr{E}$

(c) Piezoelectric Effect   **(d)** Electrostrictive Medium

$d - \Delta d$

$d + \Delta d$

$\mathscr{E} = 0$

Equilibrium

Polarization caused by Stress

Figure 6.1 Simplified illustration of (a) a piezoelectric medium and (d) an electrostrictive medium under the action of an electric field or a strain. In (a) the dipoles represent a medium that lacks central symmetry. (b) Inverse piezoelectric effect: an applied electric field results in a rotation of the dipoles. (c) The piezoelectric effect in which the force F causes a strain: the resulting dipole rotation causes polarization of the medium. (e) Electrostrictive effect: the displacement is proportional to the square of the field. (f) A compressive force F causes a strain but no net dipole moment results from this change, i.e., the medium is not piezoelectric.

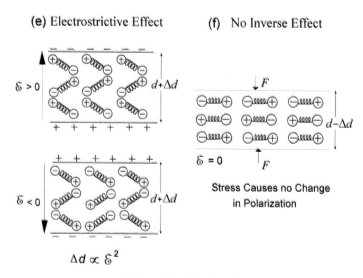

(e) Electrostrictive Effect   **(f)** No Inverse Effect

$$\Delta d \propto \mathcal{E}^2$$

Figure 6.1 *Continued*

possess both the piezoelectric and inverse piezoelectric properties. According to the definition of the direct effect given by Cady [10], "piezoelectricity is an electrical polarization produced by mechanical strain...the polarization being proportional to the strain, and changing sign with it."

Confusion sometimes exists with the *electrostrictive effect*, which, as its name suggests, concerns a change in dimensions with electric field. However, the electrostrictive effect is generally defined as one for which the dimensional changes are proportional to the *square* of the electric field, i.e., a reversal of the field does not change the direction of the strain. It is a smaller effect that arises from the nonlinear properties of the medium as opposed to the piezoelectric effect, which is linear in origin. It is present in virtually all dielectric media.

As stated by Auld [11], "The nature of piezoelectricity is intimately connected with crystal symmetry and, in fact, cannot exist in a completely isotropic material." In fact, it can be shown that any medium whose crystal structure has central symmetry *cannot* be piezoelectric. Of the 32 crystallographic classes, 21 lack central symmetry, and of these 20 are piezoelectric [12]. To illustrate why a centro-symmetric medium is not piezoelectric, consider the 2-D arrangement of electric dipoles shown in Fig. 6.1d, which are used to represent an ionic medium with central symmetry. Part (e) shows that an electric field causes a net change in dimensions, while (f) illustrates that a compressive force causes no polarization. Thus, according to the definition given earlier, the medium is not piezoelectric but is electrostrictive.

6.1.1 Piezoelectric Material Development

Single Crystal Piezoelectrics

Langevin, as part of the effort to develop a means for submarine detection during World War I, used quartz (SiO_2) transducers [13] to generate intense

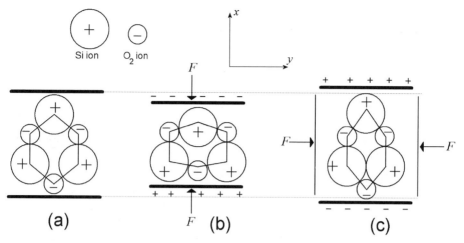

Figure 6.2 Piezoelectric effect in quartz: simplified structure showing the effect of a stress on the polarization. (a) Ion arrangement in the neutral cell. (b) Effect of compression in the x-direction. (c) Effect of compression along in the y-direction. (Reproduced, with permission, from Neubert [14], "Instrument Transducers" © 1963 Oxford University Press.)

fields in water at frequencies of around 100 kHz (see [4], p. 31). This was probably the first reported use of a piezoelectric medium for generating ultrasound. The unit cell of quartz consists of three Si atoms, each of which has +4q charges, and six O_2 atoms, each with −2q. Using the simplified 2-D representation shown in Fig. 6.2, the piezoelectric behavior can be readily understood. The charge generated by the compressive force in (a) results from the relative displacement of the Si and O_2 ions. In (c) it can be seen that a compressive force along the y-axis results in a polarization in the x-direction. Because the structure has central symmetry in the z-direction, forces in this direction produce no polarization.

Of the 20 crystal classes exhibiting piezoelectricity, 10 are *pyroelectric*, i.e., they exhibit a spontaneous polarization that changes with temperature. Conduction through the crystal will cause the free charges on the surface to be gradually neutralized, but by changing the temperature and measuring the charge that flows in a wire connecting a pair of electrodes on the surfaces, the presence of a spontaneous dipole moment can be observed. A pyroelectric medium whose polarization can be changed by an externally applied electric field is defined to be *ferroelectric*. Thus, all ferroelectrics[1] are both piezoelectric and pyroelectric. Ferroelectrics are characterized by a spontaneous dipole

---

1. The name ferroelectric is, perhaps, somewhat misleading since it suggests a mechanism similar to ferromagnetism and a connection to iron. While the mechanism is quite different, ferroelectric media do exhibit domain behavior and properties that are analogous to magnetic domains.

moment that can be redirected by an external electric field. They also have a transition temperature (the Curie point) at which a phase transition occurs and the crystal structure can change to a crystallographic class for which piezo-electricity ceases.

Piezoelectric Ceramics

Before the end of World War II the most common piezoelectric materials were quartz, Rochelle salt ($NaKC_4H_4O_6 \cdot 4H_2O$), and ammonium dihydrogen phosphate ($NH_4H_2PO_4$). Both the salt and the phosphate are ferroelectric. Independent publications in 1945 and 1946 from groups in the former USSR and the United States [9] revealed a new type of ferroelectric material consisting of ($BaTiO_3$) in a polycrystalline ceramic form. It was created by making a suitably balanced mixture that included an appropriate binder, followed by pressing and then firing at a high temperature. Regions (domains) of the same polarization direction are formed within the polycrystallites, and these are bounded by other domains with different polar directions.[2] Overall, because the domains are randomly orientated, the macroscopic behavior of the poly-crystalline ceramic is approximately isotropic. By applying a high DC electric field at a temperature close to the Curie point (120°C for barium titanate) and with the field present when the temperature is lowered, many of the domains become aligned with the applied field and some grow in volume, causing the piezoelectric properties to be greatly enhanced. This process is called *poling*. Piezoceramics have the important advantages that they can be fabricated into a variety of shapes and that the direction of polarization can be controlled.

Subsequent to these developments, in 1954 Jaffe et al. [16] reported strong piezoelectric effects in lead zirconate and lead titanate solid solutions. This led to the development of a wide variety of polycrystalline lead-zirconate-titanate $\{Pb(Zr_{1-x}, Ti_x)O_3\}$ ceramics that are generally referred to as PZT. These have major advantages over barium titanate ceramics [17–19], and as a result they began to dominate the piezoceramic commercial market. Nonetheless, barium titanate ceramics can be made with better reproducibility and have a higher speed of propagation, which gives advantages in specialized applications [27].

Relaxor-Based Piezoelectrics

The discoveries and investigations by Russian scientists of a variety of relaxor-based[3] ferroelectric materials also occurred in the 1950s. In the ceramic form,

---

2. The relation between the grain size and domain size for certain ceramic ferroelectrics has been examined by Cao and Randall [15]. For PZT they found the domain size to be proportional to the square root of the grain size for grain sizes in the range 1 to 10μm. For example, for an average grain size of 2.3μm, they found the median domain size to be 0.053μm.

3. The name originates from their dielectric relaxation properties: their permittivities and loss factors are fairly strong functions of frequency.

they appear to have little or no advantages over PZT for ultrasound transducers. However, they can be grown in single crystal form to a sufficiently large
size for fabricating arrays. Attempts to do the same with PZT have so far been
unsuccessful. In 1981 Kuwata et al. [20] reported that single crystals of the solid
solution of lead-zinc-niobate and lead titanate $\{0.91Pb(Zn_{1/3}Nbi_{2/3})O_3$-
$0.09PbTiO_3\}$ (abbreviated PZN-PT) possessed an *piezoelectric coupling factor*
(or electromechanical coupling factor, see 6.2.2) of greater than 0.9. For
improving the sensitivity, resolution, and efficiency of medical ultrasound
imaging transducers, the piezoelectric coupling factor, permittivity, and
acoustic impedance are of particular importance [21]. The coupling factor,
which is of fundamental importance, is a measure of the efficiency with which
electrical energy is converted into mechanical energy and vice versa. Because
the highest value is typically around 0.75 for PZT ceramics, the value of above
0.9 attained in single crystal relaxors represents a major improvement.

About 1992, the potential advantages of using single crystal relaxors for
ultrasound imaging arrays were recognized, as evidenced by a patent application assigned to Toshiba [22]. Since then, interest has grown rapidly. Other
single crystal relaxor-based ferroelectrics such as the solid solutions of lead-
zirconium-niobate/lead titanate and lead-magnesium-niobate/lead titanate
(PMN-PT) also exhibit piezoelectric coupling factors of greater than 0.9 [23].

Composites

Starting in the 1970s it began to be appreciated that the performance of ultrasonic transducers could be improved through the use of composite arrangements of piezoelectric and non-piezoelectric materials, rather than by using
simple piezoelectric plates. Piezoelectric composites often consist of a matrix
of elements made from a suitable piezoceramic, e.g., PZT, in a suitable
polymer. One example is a sequence of evenly spaced PZT plates separated
by an epoxy. The advantage of such an arrangement is that it combines the
superior piezoelectric properties of the chosen ceramic with the much lower
acoustic impedance of the polymer, resulting in an effective impedance that is
better matched to water. By the early 1980s research publications clearly indicated the advantages of using composites in a wide range of transducers. Subsequent commercial and manufacturing development in the 1980s led to their
use in a variety of transducers such as imaging arrays. The properties, development, and commercialization of ceramic composites have been described in
a number of reviews [25–28] and will be discussed in more detail in section
6.4.1. More recently, relaxor-based single crystal PZN-PT composites have
been described [21,24]. While these are at an early stage in their development,
they indicate promise of significant performance improvements.

6.1.2 High-Frequency Materials

Two other important aspects of piezoelectric materials that are pertinent to
medical ultrasound also occurred during the latter part of the 20th century:

the discovery that certain types of polymer possess useful piezoelectric properties and the development of thin film piezoelectric transducers capable of generating ultrasound at frequencies well beyond 100 MHz. In 1969 Kawai [29] reported the discovery that a plastic polymer, polyvinylidene fluoride (PVDF), exhibited ferroelectric properties and therefore was piezoelectric. It is a semicrystalline polymer with long molecular chains and looks, to all intent and purpose, like the plastic used for wrapping food. Sheets of different thickness can be economically produced, enabling broad-band transducers to be made that are effective into the 10- to 100-MHz range. Their price, efficiency, and ability to conform to a variety of shapes have resulted in a very wide range of uses in consumer products [30,31]. In addition, PVDF has enabled effective transducers to be fabricated for hydrophones, high-frequency imaging [32], and ultrasound biomicroscopy [33].

For the purpose of generating and detecting ultrasound at very high frequencies, well beyond that considered possible with piezoceramics, considerable effort was devoted in the early 1960s to developing techniques for vacuum deposition of thin piezoelectric films [34–36]. Much of the early research centered around polycrystalline CdS and ZnO, both of which exhibit useful piezoelectric properties. More recently, significant improvements in the piezoelectric properties were achieved by RF magnetron sputtering onto a properly orientated substrate so as to obtain a nearly epitaxial layer. Using this technique, Ito et al. [37] fabricated a 32-element ultrasonic linear array with a center frequency of 100 MHz. It should also be pointed out that for the intermediate frequency range of 50 to 200 MHz, single crystal lithium niobate (36-degree Y-cut) has useful piezoelectric properties and can be mechanically lapped to a thickness sufficient to achieve a resonant frequency of 200 MHz [38–40]. Moreover, unlike piezoceramics, whose grain size can constrain the minimum thickness, no such limitation is present with single crystal lithium niobate.

6.2 Characteristic Piezoelectric Equations

In developing equations that characterize the electromechanical properties of piezoelectric materials, we first note that a perfectly isotropic medium cannot be piezoelectric. This makes the task a good deal more complex, because now account must be taken of the differing electrical, mechanical, and piezoelectric properties in different directions. What we aim to do is obtain equations relating the mechanical variables (stress $\mathbf{T}$ and strain $\mathbf{S}$) to the electrical variables (electric displacement $\mathbf{D}$ and the electric field $\mathcal{E}$).

We shall start by considering the relations between the mechanical stress and strain. Suppose that force $\mathbf{F}$ is acting on one of the faces of the elementary cube shown in Fig. 6.3. Such a force can always be resolved into components along the Cartesian coordinate directions, which we shall denote by x_1, x_2, and x_3, corresponding to the usual x-, y- and z-directions. This force will give rise to stress components on the various faces. For example, on the face whose normal is in the x_1-direction, the stress will be

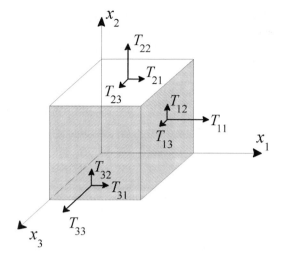

Figure 6.3 Stress components acting on an elementary cube. For the sign convention chosen, T_{11}, T_{22}, and T_{33} will be positive if the stresses are tensile and negative if compressive.

$$\mathbf{T}_1 = T_{11}\tilde{x}_1 + T_{12}\tilde{x}_2 + T_{13}\tilde{x}_3,$$

where the first subscript refers to the face whose normal component is in the 1-direction and the second subscript refers to the direction in which the stress points. Thus, T_{11} is a normal stress component in the x_1-direction (if $T_{11} > 0$ it is a traction force; otherwise it is compressive) and the other two stress components are shear stresses in the 2- and 3-directions. Similarly, on the other two faces the stresses are:

$$\mathbf{T}_2 = T_{21}\tilde{x}_1 + T_{22}\tilde{x}_2 + T_{23}\tilde{x}_3$$
$$\mathbf{T}_3 = T_{31}\tilde{x}_1 + T_{32}\tilde{x}_2 + T_{33}\tilde{x}_3 .$$

Because the cube is assumed to be in equilibrium, the stress components on the other three faces will be equal and opposite of those shown. Thus, a total of nine stress components can be identified and they form a tensor of the second rank, which can be represented by the 3×3 matrix given by[4]

$$[T_{ij}] = \begin{bmatrix} T_{11} & T_{12} & T_{13} \\ T_{21} & T_{22} & T_{23} \\ T_{31} & T_{32} & T_{33} \end{bmatrix}.$$

The components T_{11}, T_{22}, and T_{33} are the normal stress components and T_{12}, etc. are the shear stress components. For a homogeneous medium in

---

4. An excellent introduction to the use of tensors and matrices for characterizing the physical properties of crystals, including the piezoelectric crystals, is that written by Nye [41]. In what follows, we shall be using the matrix representation.

equilibrium there will be no rotation, which requires that $T_{12} = T_{21}$, $T_{13} = T_{31}$, $T_{32} = T_{23}$, and as a result of the nine components only six are independent. To simplify the notation a single index can be used and the six independent components can be written as:

$$T_1 = T_{11}, T_2 = T_{22}, T_3 = T_{33}: \qquad normal\ stress\ components$$
$$T_4 = T_{32} = T_{23}, T_5 = T_{13} = T_{31}, T_6 = T_{12} = T_{21}: \qquad shear\ stress\ components.$$

Thus, the stress can be expressed as a six-element column vector that, for purpose of compactness, can be written as

$$\mathbf{T} = \begin{bmatrix} T_1 & T_2 & T_3 & T_4 & T_5 & T_6 \end{bmatrix}^t,$$

where the superscript t stands for transpose.

The strain is also a symmetric tensor $[S_{ij}]$ and can be represented by a symmetric 3×3 matrix. Using a single index the strain can also be written as a six-element column vector:

$$\mathbf{S} = \begin{bmatrix} S_1 & S_2 & S_3 & S_4 & S_5 & S_6 \end{bmatrix}^t.$$

It can be shown that the strain components are related to the normal and shear strains by:

$$\mathbf{S} \equiv \begin{bmatrix} S_1 \\ S_2 \\ S_3 \\ S_4 \\ S_5 \\ S_6 \end{bmatrix} \equiv \begin{bmatrix} S_{11} & S_{12} & S_{13} \\ S_{12} & S_{22} & S_{23} \\ S_{13} & S_{23} & S_{33} \end{bmatrix}$$

$$= \begin{bmatrix} \dfrac{\partial \xi_{x_1}}{\partial x_1} & \dfrac{1}{2}\left(\dfrac{\partial \xi_{x_1}}{\partial x_2} + \dfrac{\partial \xi_{x_2}}{\partial x_1}\right) & \dfrac{1}{2}\left(\dfrac{\partial \xi_{x_1}}{\partial x_3} + \dfrac{\partial \xi_{x_3}}{\partial x_1}\right) \\ \dfrac{1}{2}\left(\dfrac{\partial \xi_{x_1}}{\partial x_2} + \dfrac{\partial \xi_{x_2}}{\partial x_1}\right) & \dfrac{\partial \xi_{x_2}}{\partial x_2} & \dfrac{1}{2}\left(\dfrac{\partial \xi_{x_2}}{\partial x_3} + \dfrac{\partial \xi_{x_3}}{\partial x_2}\right) \\ \dfrac{1}{2}\left(\dfrac{\partial \xi_{x_1}}{\partial x_3} + \dfrac{\partial \xi_{x_3}}{\partial x_1}\right) & \dfrac{1}{2}\left(\dfrac{\partial \xi_{x_2}}{\partial x_3} + \dfrac{\partial \xi_{x_3}}{\partial x_2}\right) & \dfrac{\partial \xi_{x_3}}{\partial x_3} \end{bmatrix},$$

where ξ_{x_1}, ξ_{x_2}, and ξ_{x_3} are displacements along the x_1, x_2, and x_3 directions. The diagonal components corresponding to S_1, S_2, and S_3, are *tensile* strains, while the other components are pure shear strains.

The electric field and electric displacement are simple three-element vectors whose components lie along the 1, 2, and 3 directions, and can therefore be written as

$$\mathbf{\mathcal{E}} = \begin{bmatrix} \mathcal{E}_1 & \mathcal{E}_2 & \mathcal{E}_3 \end{bmatrix}^t \text{ and } \mathbf{D} = \begin{bmatrix} D_1 & D_2 & D_3 \end{bmatrix}^t.$$

In a dielectric medium the presence of an electric field will cause the electrical dipoles to be partially orientated in the direction of the field. A polarization vector $\mathbf{P}$, which is defined as the dipole moment per unit volume

(Coulombs/m^3), can account for their effects. The electric displacement vector is related to the polarization by

(6.1) $$\mathbf{D} = \varepsilon_o \mathscr{E} + \mathbf{P},$$

where ε_o is the permittivity of free space (8.854×10^{-12} F/m). Moreover, the free charge density (C/m^3) is equal to the divergence of $\mathbf{D}$, i.e., $\nabla \cdot \mathbf{D} = \rho_f$, which is one of Maxwell's equations. But within a piezoelectric dielectric medium there should be no free charges (all charges are bound dipolar charges); consequently

(6.2) $$\nabla \cdot \mathbf{D} = 0.$$

Another of Maxwell's equations enables the rate of change of the electric displacement to be related to the displacement current density[5] $\mathbf{J}_{disp}$:

(6.3) $$\frac{\partial \mathbf{D}}{\partial t} = \mathbf{J}_{disp}$$

The above relations will be important in relating the electrical and mechanical properties of piezoelectric transducers.

6.2.1 Constitutive Relations

Let us assume that a piezoelectric medium is subjected to an elastic deformation that is sufficiently small so that nonlinear effects can be ignored. The stress components will be a linear function of the strain components S and electric field components $\mathscr{E}$. For example, T_1 can be expressed as[6]

$$T_1 = c_{11}^{\mathscr{E}} S_1 + c_{12}^{\mathscr{E}} S_2 + c_{13}^{\mathscr{E}} S_3 + c_{14}^{\mathscr{E}} S_4 + c_{15}^{\mathscr{E}} S_5 + c_{16}^{\mathscr{E}} S_6 - e_{11}\mathscr{E}_1 - e_{21}\mathscr{E}_2 - e_{31}\mathscr{E}_3,$$

where $c_{ij}^{\mathscr{E}}$-coefficients are various elastic stiffness constants measured with the electric field held constant (the superscript $\mathscr{E}$ indicates this) and the e-coefficients relate the mechanical and electrical properties. Equations for the other stress components can be similarly written down, and as a result the stress can be expressed in matrix form as

$$T = \begin{bmatrix} c_{11}^{\mathscr{E}} & c_{12}^{\mathscr{E}} & c_{13}^{\mathscr{E}} & c_{14}^{\mathscr{E}} & c_{15}^{\mathscr{E}} & c_{16}^{\mathscr{E}} \\ c_{21}^{\mathscr{E}} & c_{22}^{\mathscr{E}} & c_{23}^{\mathscr{E}} & c_{24}^{\mathscr{E}} & c_{25}^{\mathscr{E}} & c_{26}^{\mathscr{E}} \\ c_{31}^{\mathscr{E}} & c_{32}^{\mathscr{E}} & c_{33}^{\mathscr{E}} & c_{34}^{\mathscr{E}} & c_{35}^{\mathscr{E}} & c_{36}^{\mathscr{E}} \\ c_{41}^{\mathscr{E}} & c_{42}^{\mathscr{E}} & c_{43}^{\mathscr{E}} & c_{44}^{\mathscr{E}} & c_{45}^{\mathscr{E}} & c_{46}^{\mathscr{E}} \\ c_{51}^{\mathscr{E}} & c_{52}^{\mathscr{E}} & c_{53}^{\mathscr{E}} & c_{54}^{\mathscr{E}} & c_{55}^{\mathscr{E}} & c_{56}^{\mathscr{E}} \\ c_{61}^{\mathscr{E}} & c_{62}^{\mathscr{E}} & c_{63}^{\mathscr{E}} & c_{64}^{\mathscr{E}} & c_{65}^{\mathscr{E}} & c_{66}^{\mathscr{E}} \end{bmatrix} \begin{bmatrix} S_1 \\ S_2 \\ S_3 \\ S_4 \\ S_5 \\ S_6 \end{bmatrix} - \begin{bmatrix} e_{11} & e_{21} & e_{31} \\ e_{12} & e_{22} & e_{32} \\ e_{13} & e_{23} & e_{33} \\ e_{14} & e_{24} & e_{34} \\ e_{15} & e_{25} & e_{35} \\ e_{16} & e_{26} & e_{36} \end{bmatrix} \begin{bmatrix} \mathscr{E}_1 \\ \mathscr{E}_2 \\ \mathscr{E}_3 \end{bmatrix},$$

5. Strictly speaking, the presence of a changing electric field implies the presence of a magnetic field, but since the speed of propagation of acoustic waves is many orders of magnitude less than the speed of electromagnetic waves, the effects of the magnetic field can be ignored.

6. Except for the use of a different font for the electric field, the notation used is that given in the IEEE Standard [42].

or in abbreviated form as

(6.4) $$[T]=[c^{\varepsilon}][S]-[e]'[\mathcal{E}],$$ (a)

where $[e]'$ is the transpose of $[e]$. We shall call $[c]$ the *stiffness matrix* and $[e]$ the *piezoelectric stress matrix*. Normally, the e-coefficients are defined as a 3×6 matrix that is written as:

(6.5) $$[e]=\begin{bmatrix} e_{11} & e_{12} & e_{13} & e_{14} & e_{15} & e_{16} \\ e_{21} & e_{22} & e_{23} & e_{24} & e_{25} & e_{26} \\ e_{31} & e_{32} & e_{33} & e_{34} & e_{35} & e_{36} \end{bmatrix}.$$ (a)

The stress matrix is so named because if the specimen is clamped so as to make all the strain components zero, then the e-coefficients relate the stress components directly to the applied electric field components, e.g., $T_3 = -e_{33}\mathcal{E}_3$ if $\mathcal{E}_1 = \mathcal{E}_2 = 0$.

In a similar way, the electric displacement can be expressed in terms of the strain and electric field as

(6.4) $$[D]=[e][S]+[\varepsilon^{S}][\mathcal{E}],$$ (b)

where $[\varepsilon^S]$ is a constant strain (clamped) 3×3 *permittivity matrix*, i.e.,

$$[\varepsilon^{S}]\equiv\begin{bmatrix} \varepsilon_{11}^{S} & \varepsilon_{12}^{S} & \varepsilon_{13}^{S} \\ \varepsilon_{21}^{S} & \varepsilon_{22}^{S} & \varepsilon_{23}^{S} \\ \varepsilon_{13}^{S} & \varepsilon_{23}^{S} & \varepsilon_{33}^{S} \end{bmatrix}.$$

It should be noted that the constant strain permittivity coefficients, $[\varepsilon^S]$, can differ substantially from those measured under constant stress conditions, $[\varepsilon^T]$. Measurement of the permittivity under conditions of constant strain requires that the specimen be clamped in such a way that no displacement can occur. Since this is very difficult to achieve in practice, the constant stress permittivity is generally measured and the constant strain values are calculated using relations with ε^T and other measurable constants.

The pair of equations given by (6.4) are but one of the four sets of equations that relate the variables $T, S, D,$ and $\mathcal{E}$, and these can be written as

(6.4) $[T]=[c^{\varepsilon}][S]-[e]'[\mathcal{E}],$ (a); $[D]=[e][S]+[\varepsilon^{S}][\mathcal{E}]$:   (b)

(6.6) $[S]=[s^{\varepsilon}][T]+[d]'[\mathcal{E}],$ (a); $[D]=[d][T]+[\varepsilon^{T}][\mathcal{E}]$:   (b)

(6.7) $[S]=[s^{D}][T]+[g]'[D],$ (a); $[\mathcal{E}]=-[g][T]+[\beta^{T}][D]$:   (b)

(6.8) $[T]=[c^{D}][S]-[h]'[D],$ (a); $[\mathcal{E}]=-[h][S]+[\beta^{S}][D]$.   (b)

In the above equations additional coefficients have been introduced. The forms of the matrices for $d, e, g,$ and h are 3×6, those for ε and β are 3×3, and those for c and s are 6×6. In the four sets of constitutive equations the coefficients $c^D, c^{\varepsilon}, s^D, s^{\varepsilon}, d, g, e, h, \varepsilon^T, \varepsilon^S, \beta^T$ and β^S are related by:

$$[s^D]=[c^D]^{-1}, \quad [s^{\mathcal{E}}]=[c^{\mathcal{E}}]^{-1}, \quad [\varepsilon^T]=[\beta^T]^{-1}, \quad [\varepsilon^S]=[\beta^S]^{-1}, \qquad (a)$$

$$[d]=[\varepsilon^T][g]=[e][s^{\mathcal{E}}], \quad [e]=[d][c^{\mathcal{E}}]=[\varepsilon^S][h], \qquad (b)$$

$$(6.9) \qquad [g]=[h][s^D]=[\beta^T][d], \quad [h]=[\beta^S][e]=[g][c^D], \qquad (c)$$

$$[s^{\mathcal{E}}]-[s^D]=[g]^t[d]=[d]^t[g], \quad [c^D]-[c^{\mathcal{E}}]=[h]^t[e]=[e]^t[h], \qquad (d)$$

$$[\varepsilon^T]-[\varepsilon^S]=[e][d]^t=[d][e]^t, \quad [\beta^S]-[\beta^T]=[g][h]^t=[h][g]^t. \qquad (e)$$

Any set of mechanical, piezoelectric, and electrical parameters are sufficient to fully characterize the properties of the medium, and from this set, using the above relations, a different set can be obtained by using straightforward matrix algebra operations.

The SI units for the various coefficients are given in Table 6.1 and are written so as to emphasize the physical meaning. For example, from (6.6b) it can be see that if $\mathcal{E} = 0$ and d_{33} is the only non-zero coefficient, then $d_{33} = (D_3/T_3)_{\mathcal{E}=0}$. Thus, d_{33} expresses the charge produced per unit area per unit of stress under short-circuit conditions (this makes the electric field zero) corresponding to the direct piezoelectric effect. From (6.6a), it is evident that if there are no stress components ($T_k = 0, k = 1 \ldots 6$) and all d coefficients are zero except for d_{33}, then d_{33} expresses the deformation (meters/meter) for a given applied electric field (Volts/meter), corresponding to the inverse piezo-electric effect. The g-coefficient is also of considerable practical significance. For a constant electric displacement, it can be seen from (6.7b) that it expresses the change in electric field with pressure, i.e., when the transducer is used as a detector it determines the transducer output voltage sensitivity. From (6.9c) it should be noted that although d_{33} may be small, a material may still have a high g_{33} if the unclamped permittivity is small.

So far we have tacitly assumed that electrical and mechanical losses can be neglected. Electrical losses can be accounted for by assuming that the permittivity is complex. If the permittivity is written as $\varepsilon = \varepsilon' - j\varepsilon''$, where the

Table 6.1. Dimensions of Mechanical and Piezoelectric Coefficients

Coefficient	SI Units
$c^D, c^{\mathcal{E}}$	Newtons/meter^2
$s^D, s^{\mathcal{E}}$	1/(Newtons/meter^2)
d	Coulombs/Newton = 1/(Volts/meter)
e	Coulombs/meter^2
g	(Volts/meter)/ (Newtons/meter^2)
h	Volts/meter $\equiv$ Newtons/Coulomb
$\varepsilon^T, \varepsilon^S$	Farads/meter
β^T, β^S	1/(Farads/meter)

prime and double prime denote the real and imaginary parts of one of the permittivity components, then the imaginary term results in real power loss. The tangent of the material is defined by $\tan \delta = \varepsilon''/\varepsilon'$, which gives the angle by which the current through a capacitor differs from the quadrature current/voltage sinusoidal relationship of an ideal capacitor. Alternatively, the electrical Q can be used as a measure of the loss, where Q_e is the maximum energy stored over a cycle divided by the energy dissipated per cycle, and which is equal to the inverse of the loss tangent ($Q_e = \varepsilon'/\varepsilon''$). Mechanical losses can similarly be accounted for by introducing a complex elastic stiffness that accounts for viscous loss. The mechanical Q is then given by $Q_m = c'/c''$, where the prime and double prime refer to the real and imaginary parts.

6.2.2 Piezoelectric Coupling Factor

Of major importance in assessing and comparing the performance of various piezoelectric media is the *piezoelectric coupling factor*, which is a measure of the efficiency with which the crystal converts energy from mechanical to electrical or vice versa. Specifically, Berlincourt [18] expresses the material-coupling factor as

$$(6.10) \quad k = \sqrt{\frac{\text{Electrical (Mechanical) Work Done under Ideal Conditions}}{\text{Total Energy Stored from a Mechanical (Electrical) Source}}}.$$

Evidently, the choice of boundary conditions will affect the coupling factor, and so several different coupling factors can be defined, depending on the boundary conditions.

To obtain expression for the coupling factor in terms of the mechanical and piezoelectric coefficients, we shall consider a set of boundary conditions that is of particular importance and shall follow the derivation given by Berlincourt [18]. Let us suppose that a piezoelectric medium has electrodes on planes perpendicular to the 3-axis and that a compressive force is applied in the 3-direction ($T_3 \neq 0$, $T_1 = T_2 = 0$). If, as shown in Fig. 6.4a, the electrodes are shorted ($\mathscr{E}_{33} = 0$), then work will be done by the compressive force and the resulting strain component in the 3-direction can be obtained from (6.6a) as $S_{33} = s_{33}^{\mathscr{E}} T_3$, i.e., the slope of the stress-strain curve is $s_{33}^{\mathscr{E}}$. This change is shown in Fig. 6.5 as the path from ⓐ to ⓑ. If the electrodes are now open-circuited (Fig. 6.4b) and subsequently the compressive force is removed ($T_3 \rightarrow 0$), the magnitude of the strain will be reduced and the slope of the path taken in going from ⓑ to ⓒ will be that given by (6.7a) for a constant D, which is equal to s_{33}^{D}. If the electrodes are then connected to an electrical load, then, as the strain reduces to zero, energy will be delivered to the load, corresponding to the path from ⓒ to ⓓ in Fig. 6.5. The initial compression results in energy being stored, and the work done is the sum of the two crosshatched areas, denoted by ($W_1 + W_2$). When the electrical load is connected, the amount of work done is W_1, so that W_2 represents energy that is not available for transfer as elec-

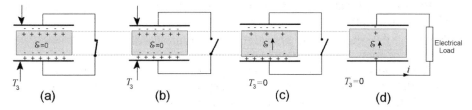

Figure 6.4 Derivation of the piezoelectric coupling factor for a piezoelectric transducer by considering a mechanical to electrical work conversion cycle for $T_1 = T_2 = 0$. It is helpful to imagine that an infinitesimally small gap exists between the electrodes and the piezoelectric medium. The charges on the surfaces of the electrodes and piezoelectric medium are indicated at the various stages. (a) After application of a compressive stress ($T_3 < 0$) with the electrodes shorted. (b) While compressed, the electrodes are open-circuited. (c) Removal of the compressive stress. Note that in going from (b) to (c) the electric displacement D_3 remains unchanged, but the electric field changes. (d) Connection of electrodes to an electrical load. The current flowing causes the charge, electric field, and strain all to reduce to zero.

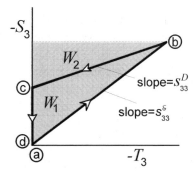

Figure 6.5 Work cycle used for calculating the coupling factor k_{33}^t. The circled letters correspond to the four parts of Fig. 6.4. The work done by the mechanical source corresponds to $W_1 + W_2$, where W_1 is the electrical work done. (Based on Berlincourt [18].)

trical output. For this ideal cycle, using the definition given by (6.10), the piezo-electric coupling factor can be written as

$$k_{33}^t = \sqrt{\frac{W_1}{W_1 + W_2}} = \sqrt{\frac{s_{33}^{\mathcal{E}} - s_{33}^D}{s_{33}^{\mathcal{E}}}},$$

But, from (6.9b) and (6.9d), $s_{33}^{\mathcal{E}} - s_{33}^D = d_{33}^2/\varepsilon_{33}^T$, so that the coupling factor can be expressed as

(6.11)
$$k_{33}^t = \frac{d_{33}}{\sqrt{s_{33}^{\mathcal{E}}\varepsilon_{33}^T}},$$

for $T_3 \neq 0$, $T_1 = T_2 = 0$.

By considering the inverse case in which a voltage source is applied to the electrodes with the specimen free from all stresses, work will be done. By subsequently determining the work done when a mechanical load is connected, the same equation can be obtained.

A second coupling factor of major practical importance is that obtained when the specimen is clamped in the lateral direction, thereby preventing any lateral strain. It can be shown [18] that this results in

$$(6.12) \qquad k_{33}^t = \frac{e_{33}}{\sqrt{c_{33}^D \varepsilon_{33}^S}},$$

for $S_3 \neq 0$, $S_1 = S_2 = 0$. Such a condition is appropriate for a piezoceramic transducer that has a small thickness compared to the lateral dimension and that is excited in the 3-direction.

6.3 Ceramic and Polymer Materials

6.3.1 Piezoceramics

Constitutive Relations

The complexity of the various matrices is greatly simplified when account is taken of the various symmetries in the crystal structure. As mentioned earlier, in the unpolarized state polycrystalline piezoelectric ceramics behave in an isotropic manner. The polycrystallites can have grain sizes that vary considerably depending on the processing and composition, and can have average dimensions in the range of 2 to 20 μm. The poling process causes the sample to become anisotropic with an axis of symmetry that coincides with the poling direction. The 3-axis is generally taken to be coincident with this direction. It is an ∞-fold axis of symmetry, so that the electrical and mechanical properties in any direction at right angles to this axis are the same. Because of the high degree of symmetry, many of the coefficients are zero, and the number of independent coefficients is drastically reduced. For example, the matrices for the elastic constants ($[c]$ and $[s]$) conditions can be shown to contain just five independent values. Thus, the elastic stiffness matrix can be written as

$$(6.13) \qquad [c^{\varepsilon}] = \begin{bmatrix} c_{11}^{\varepsilon} & c_{12}^{\varepsilon} & c_{13}^{\varepsilon} & 0 & 0 & 0 \\ c_{12}^{\varepsilon} & c_{11}^{\varepsilon} & c_{13}^{\varepsilon} & 0 & 0 & 0 \\ c_{13}^{\varepsilon} & c_{13}^{\varepsilon} & c_{33}^{\varepsilon} & 0 & 0 & 0 \\ 0 & 0 & 0 & c_{44}^{\varepsilon} & 0 & 0 \\ 0 & 0 & 0 & 0 & c_{44}^{\varepsilon} & 0 \\ 0 & 0 & 0 & 0 & 0 & c_{66}^{\varepsilon} \end{bmatrix},$$

in which $c_{66}^{\varepsilon} = \frac{1}{2}(c_{11}^{\varepsilon} - c_{12}^{\varepsilon})$. Similarly, the piezoelectric coefficients (d, e, g, h) contain three independent values so that, for example, the piezoelectric stress matrix can be expressed as

$$(6.14) \qquad [e] = \begin{bmatrix} 0 & 0 & 0 & 0 & e_{15} & 0 \\ 0 & 0 & 0 & e_{15} & 0 & 0 \\ e_{31} & e_{31} & e_{33} & 0 & 0 & 0 \end{bmatrix}.$$

Just two values are needed for the permittivity matrix, which simplifies to

$$(6.15) \qquad [\varepsilon^S] = \begin{bmatrix} \varepsilon_{11}^S & 0 & 0 \\ 0 & \varepsilon_{11}^S & 0 \\ 0 & 0 & \varepsilon_{33}^S \end{bmatrix}.$$

Thus, a total of 10 independent coefficients $(5 + 3 + 2)$ are sufficient to characterize the properties. A single matrix form can also be used to express each pair of constitutive equations. For example, the two equations in (6.6) can be written as

$$(6.16) \qquad \begin{bmatrix} S_1 \\ S_2 \\ S_3 \\ S_4 \\ S_5 \\ S_6 \\ D_1 \\ D_2 \\ D_3 \end{bmatrix} = \begin{bmatrix} s_{11}^\varepsilon & s_{12}^\varepsilon & s_{13}^\varepsilon & 0 & 0 & 0 & 0 & 0 & d_{31} \\ s_{12}^\varepsilon & s_{11}^\varepsilon & s_{13}^\varepsilon & 0 & 0 & 0 & 0 & 0 & d_{31} \\ s_{13}^\varepsilon & s_{13}^\varepsilon & s_{33}^\varepsilon & 0 & 0 & 0 & 0 & 0 & d_{33} \\ 0 & 0 & 0 & s_{44}^\varepsilon & 0 & 0 & 0 & d_{15} & 0 \\ 0 & 0 & 0 & 0 & s_{44}^\varepsilon & 0 & d_{15} & 0 & 0 \\ 0 & 0 & 0 & 0 & 0 & s_{66}^\varepsilon & 0 & 0 & 0 \\ 0 & 0 & 0 & 0 & d_{15} & 0 & \varepsilon_{11}^T & 0 & 0 \\ 0 & 0 & 0 & d_{15} & 0 & 0 & 0 & \varepsilon_{11}^T & 0 \\ d_{31} & d_{31} & d_{33} & 0 & 0 & 0 & 0 & 0 & \varepsilon_{33}^T \end{bmatrix} \begin{bmatrix} T_1 \\ T_2 \\ T_3 \\ T_4 \\ T_5 \\ T_6 \\ \mathcal{E}_1 \\ \mathcal{E}_2 \\ \mathcal{E}_3 \end{bmatrix},$$

in which $s_{66}^\varepsilon = \dfrac{1}{2}\left(s_{11}^\varepsilon - s_{12}^\varepsilon\right)$.

Properties

Some examples of the above coefficients for four piezoceramic materials are shown in Table 6.2. It will be noted that the permittivities under constant stress and strain conditions can differ substantially. For example, both PZT materials have ε_{11}^T and ε_{33}^T values that are approximately twice those for constant strain conditions. It should be noted that all four ceramics have impedances of around 30 MRayl, a value much greater than tissue (~1.5 MRayl), making it difficult to achieve a good impedance match over a wide bandwidth. Of major importance is the piezoelectric coupling factors, which as noted earlier determine the efficiency with which energy is transformed from one form to another. For transducers with lateral dimensions much greater than the thickness and operating in the thickness mode, it is the clamped coupling factor that governs the efficiency. For all the listed materials, it will be noted that the coupling factor with lateral clamping is significantly less than that with strain-free lateral conditions, i.e., $k_{33}^t < k_{33}^l$. This is especially significant when it is recalled that it is the square of the coupling factor that governs the efficiency.

For unclamped PZT-5H the efficiency is 56% ($0.75^2 \times 100$), but it reduces to 27% for clamped conditions.

The values given in Table 6.2 for the speed of propagation are those in the 3-direction under constant electric displacement conditions, as calculated from $(c_o)^D = \sqrt{c_{33}^D/\rho_o}$. Constant D conditions correspond to the situation in which the electrodes are open-circuited so that there can be no change in the surface

Table 6.2. Typical Values for Four Different Types of Piezoceramics[†]

Coefficient	Units	Barium Titanate BaTiO$_3$	Lead-Zirconate-Titanate PZT-4	Lead-Zirconate-Titanate PZT-5H	Lead Metaniobate PbNb$_2$O$_6$
s_{11}^E	10^{-12} m^2/N	8.6	12.3	16.4	17.4
s_{12}^E	10^{-12} m^2/N	−2.6	−4.1	−4.8	−4.5
s_{13}^E	10^{-12} m^2/N	−2.7	−5.3	−8.5	−5.8
s_{33}^E	10^{-12} m^2/N	9.1	15.5	20.8	14.4
s_{44}^E	10^{-12} m^2/N	22.2	39.0	43.5	35.6
d_{31}	10^{-12} C/N	−58	−123	−274	−9.5
d_{33}	10^{-12} C/N	149	289	593	85
d_{15}	10^{-12} C/N	242	495	741	90
g_{31}	10^{-3} V.m/N	−5.5	−11	−9	−3.35
g_{33}	10^{-3} V.m/N	14	25	20	30
g_{15}	10^{-3} V.m/N	21	38	27	32
$\varepsilon_{11}^T/\varepsilon_o$		1300	1475	3123	(320)
	Unitless				
$\varepsilon_{11}^S/\varepsilon_o$		1000	730	1700	(265)
$\varepsilon_{33}^T/\varepsilon_o$		1200	1300	3400	320
	Unitless				
$\varepsilon_{33}^S/\varepsilon_o$		910	635	1470	265
k_{33}^t	Unitless	0.48	0.68	0.75	0.46
k_{33}^t	Unitless	0.38	0.51	0.49	0.42
Z_o	MRayl	31.3	34.0	34.6	28.8
*$(c_o)^D$	m/s	5630	4530	4620	4880
ρ_o	kg/m^3	5550	7500	7500	5900
tan δ	Unitless	0.006	0.004	0.020	0.009
Q_m	Unitless	400	500	65	15
Curie Point	°C	115	328	193	570

[†] Values are those given in, or calculated from, Table I of [43], which references manufacturers' data sheets as the primary source.
* The wave speed in the polarization direction is the stiffened compressional speed calculated from the stiffened elastic constant using $(c_o)^D = \sqrt{c_{33}^D/\rho_o}$.

charge density on the electrodes. Values for the mechanical and electrical losses are also given in the table. For most piezoceramics these are relatively small and can be neglected for approximate design purposes.

6.3.2 Piezoelectric Polymer Materials

Since the discovery of a strong piezoelectric effect in PVDF by Kawai [29] in 1969, there has been considerable effort to measure and improve its properties as well as to develop alternative polymer-based piezoelectric films. PVDF consists of long-chain polar molecules embedded in an amorphous phase matrix. It has a semicrystalline form. It is first crystallized from the melt in the form of a thin sheet. The film is disordered and displays no macroscopic piezoelectric properties. By stretching it either uniaxially or biaxially to many times its original length at a temperature of around 62°C, the film is converted it to a non-centro-symmetric crystalline structure that is polar. Following annealing at around 120°C, the film is poled normal to the surface. This can be achieved by using a high electric field at temperatures of around 100°C for several hours, which causes partial alignment of the polar chains that on cooling become locked in place, thereby giving the film a permanent polarization.

Constitutive Relations

Unlike piezoceramics, for which there is complete rotational symmetry, the stretching process causes asymmetry about the polarization axis, and as a result the number of independent mechanical, electrical, and piezoelectric coefficients is greater. It can be shown that for piezoelectric polymers, (6.16) must be replaced by

$$
(6.17) \quad
\begin{bmatrix}
S_1 \\
S_2 \\
S_3 \\
S_4 \\
S_5 \\
S_6 \\
D_1 \\
D_2 \\
D_3
\end{bmatrix}
=
\begin{bmatrix}
s_{11}^{\mathcal{E}} & s_{12}^{\mathcal{E}} & s_{13}^{\mathcal{E}} & 0 & 0 & 0 & 0 & 0 & d_{31} \\
s_{12}^{\mathcal{E}} & s_{22}^{\mathcal{E}} & s_{23}^{\mathcal{E}} & 0 & 0 & 0 & 0 & 0 & d_{32} \\
s_{13}^{\mathcal{E}} & s_{23}^{\mathcal{E}} & s_{33}^{\mathcal{E}} & 0 & 0 & 0 & 0 & 0 & d_{33} \\
0 & 0 & 0 & s_{44}^{\mathcal{E}} & 0 & 0 & 0 & d_{24} & 0 \\
0 & 0 & 0 & 0 & s_{55}^{\mathcal{E}} & 0 & d_{15} & 0 & 0 \\
0 & 0 & 0 & 0 & 0 & s_{66}^{\mathcal{E}} & 0 & 0 & 0 \\
0 & 0 & 0 & 0 & d_{15} & 0 & \varepsilon_{11}^{T} & 0 & 0 \\
0 & 0 & 0 & d_{24} & 0 & 0 & 0 & \varepsilon_{22}^{T} & 0 \\
d_{31} & d_{32} & d_{33} & 0 & 0 & 0 & 0 & 0 & \varepsilon_{33}^{T}
\end{bmatrix}
\begin{bmatrix}
T_1 \\
T_2 \\
T_3 \\
T_4 \\
T_5 \\
T_6 \\
\mathcal{E}_1 \\
\mathcal{E}_2 \\
\mathcal{E}_3
\end{bmatrix},
$$

which contains the same number of zeros, but now there are 17 independent coefficients: 9 elastic, 5 piezoelectric, and 3 permittivities. This should be compared to the nine independent coefficients needed to characterize the electromechanical properties of piezoceramics.

Properties

Table 6.3 lists a set of values for one type of piezopolymer material together with some physical parameters; a much more complete set of data for the elastic, dielectric, and piezoelectric properties, together with details of the measurement methods, have been presented by Roh et al. [46]. It will be observed that the loss tangent for PVDF is roughly an order of magnitude greater than that for PZT-5H. Moreover, it should be noted that the loss tangent and permittivity are fairly strong functions of frequency, as is illustrated by the results shown in Fig. 6.6.

Foster et al. [32] have provided a useful table that compares some of the important properties of two types of ferroelectric polymer with PZT-5A ceramic; this is reproduced as Table 6.4.

Table 6.3. Representative Parameters for a Piezoelectric Polymer Material

Coefficient	c_{11}^D	c_{12}^D	c_{13}^D	c_{22}^D	c_{23}^D	c_{33}^D	c_{44}^D	c_{55}^D	c_{66}^D
PVDF[†]	3.61	1.61	1.42	3.13	1.31	1.63	0.55	0.59	0.69
Units					GN/m^2				
Coefficient	d_{31}	d_{32}	d_{33}	d_{24}	d_{15}	$\varepsilon_{11}^T/\varepsilon_o$	$\varepsilon_{22}^T/\varepsilon_o$	$\varepsilon_{33}^T/\varepsilon_o$
PVDF[†]	14.3	2.02	−31	−20.6	−19.6	6.9	8.6	7.6
Units			10^{-12} C/N				None	
Coefficient	k_{33}^t	Z_o	$\tan\delta$	Q_m	Speed of Sound	ρ_o		
PVDF[‡]	~0.15	~2–3	~0.3	~10	1500–2000 m/s	~1800 kg/m³		
Units	None	MRayl	None	None				

[†] Values are those given in, or calculated from [44, 45] for PVDF samples that were uniaxially stretched in the x_1-direction and supplied by Raytheon Corp.
[‡] These values vary greatly depending on the manufacturer.

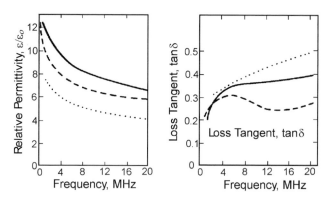

Figure 6.6 Summary of experimental results from three investigations showing the frequency dependence of the permittivity and loss tangent for PVDF. (Reproduced, with permission, from Hunt et al. [47], *IEEE Trans. Biomed. Eng.*, 30, 453–481, © 1983 IEEE.)

Table 6.4. Comparison of Properties for PVDF, P(VDF-TrFE), and PZT5A

Parameter	PVDF	P(VDF-TrFE)	PZT5A
Speed of sound, m/s	2200	2400	4350
Density, kg/m^3	1780	1880	7750
Z_o, MRayl	3.9	4.5	33.7
Relative permittivity	6.0	5.0	1200
Mechanical Q, Q_m	10	25	75
Coupling factor, k_{33}^t	0.15–0.20	0.3	0.49
Mechanical flexibility	Outstanding	Satisfactory	Poor

Reproduced, with permission, from Foster et al. [32], *IEEE Trans. Ultrason., Ferroelect., Freq. Contr.*, 47, 1363–1371, © 2000 IEEE.

6.4 Methods for Enhancing the Performance

6.4.1 Composite Materials

In the discussion of piezoceramics, two important drawbacks were noted. The first concerns the large impedance mismatch with tissue (30 MRayl vs. 1.5 MRayl), making it difficult to achieve efficient energy transfer over a wide bandwidth. Although the use of one or more impedance matching layers can enable impedance matching to be achieved, such layers, by their nature, can be effective only over a limited bandwidth. Modern pulse-echo systems often use very short pulses with fractional bandwidths exceeding 100%, and this requires a transducer with a comparable bandwidth.

A second aspect concerns the coupling factor. It was pointed out that the appropriate coupling factor for a single element transducer was k^t rather than k^l, whose value is appreciably greater. The reason that the clamped k is appropriate can be understood by examining the behavior of a small volume whose thickness is equal to that of the ceramic plate. Such a volume is surrounded on its sides by ceramic regions that prevent lateral movement, thereby making $S_1 = S_2 = 0$. If the ceramic were divided into small volumes with lateral dimensions less than a wavelength and the regions between each volume were filled with a fairly compliant medium that would permit lateral movement, then the higher value unclamped coupling factor would then be appropriate. In replacing some of the ceramic by a softer inert material, the question arises as to whether the improved efficiency would be sufficient to compensate for the decreased volume of piezoelectric active material and result in an overall improvement in performance. As will be seen, this can be achieved with the proper design.

Composite piezoceramics generally consist of ceramic elements embedded in a polymer matrix. To classify possible structural arrangements of the different phases, the concept of *connectivity* was initially used by Newnham et al. [48]. In a two-phase system, e.g., ceramic and polymer, there are 10 possible

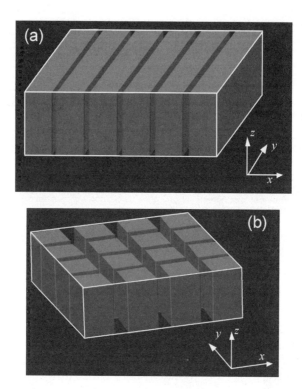

Figure 6.7 Examples of composite two-phase structures used to illustrate how the connectivity can be determined. The shaded regions correspond to the ceramic whose polarization is assumed to be in the z-direction. The unfilled regions consist of a polymer. (a) Ceramic slabs, 2-2. (b) Ceramic pillars, 1-3. (c) Ceramic and polymer pillars, 1-1. (d) Particles of ceramic, 0-3.

connectivities, of which only a few are of practical interest for transducer fabrication. The connectivity of a particular 3-D arrangement can be found by determining whether a line can be drawn through the matrix parallel to the x-axis without leaving the phase in which it started, and then repeating this process for the y- and z-axes. By repeating the entire process for the other phase and then counting the number of successes for each phase, the connectivity is obtained. This process is illustrated in Fig. 6.7 for four structures, the first (2-2) and second (1-3) of which are most commonly used in practice.

Generally, the method of fabrication for the 2-2 and 1-3 structures starts with a wafer of the polarized piezoceramic that is somewhat thicker than that required for the transducer. For a 1-3 structure the wafer is partially cut through by means of a diamond saw so as to produce kerfs in the x- and y-directions. This process results in a matrix of ceramic pillars that are still attached to the uncut part of the ceramic wafer. The kerfs are then filled with an appropriate polymer, and finally the ceramic base and the excess polymer on the surface can then be removed by lapping.

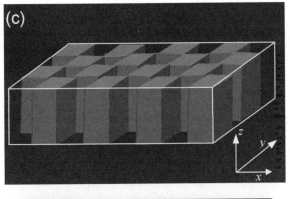

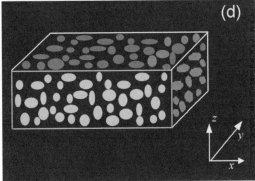

Figure 6.7 *Continued*

The smallest cut width is limited to about 20 μm by the thinness of the saw blade and the structural strength of the ceramic. This presents potential difficulties when constructing high-frequency transducer arrays. As discussed in Chapter 7, for a phased array it is desirable that the pitch (repetition distance) be less than half the wavelength. For instance, a 40-MHz array would require a pitch of 19 μm so that to avoid serious loss in sensitivity, the kerfs should be less than 10 μm. Ritter et al. [49] have reviewed some of the methods proposed for overcoming these problems.[7] For example, Lukacs et al. [51] showed that laser micromachining could be used. By fabricating linear and annular array structures from PZT and lithium niobate, they achieved kerf widths of less than 20 μm. A similar method was used Farlow et al. [52], who demonstrated kerf widths of 13 μm for a 1-3 piezocomposite transducer with a thickness of 170 μm and pillars with a pitch of 65 μm. The grain size of piezoceramics imposes a limitation on the smallest dimensions that can be used without

---

7. Using a piezoelectric actuator to displace an array in small steps, e.g., $\lambda/4$, and a synthetic aperture reconstruction scheme, much wider elements and kerfs can be used to achieve high lateral resolution, though with some loss in temporal resolution (see subsection 8.9.1 and [50]).

suffering a significant reduction in performance. With single crystal materials, such as relaxor-based ferroelectrics (see subsection 6.1.1), this is no longer a problem. In fact, lower-frequency (~5 MHz) single-element transducers have been fabricated and tested [21,24] using PZN-PT-polymer with connectivities of 1-3 and 2-2. When compared to PZT composite transducers, major improvements were obtained in terms of bandwidth and insertion loss.

The question as to the dimensions of the pillars and width of the kerfs, as well as the properties of the polymer, involves certain tradeoffs. Some of these will now be examined on the basis of the assumption that the behavior of the composite structure can be treated as homogeneous with effective parameters. Such a treatment assumes that detailed structure is small enough compared to the appropriate wavelength so that details of the complex wave motion in the structure can be ignored. Based on this assumption, Smith and Auld [53] developed effective constitutive relations for thickness mode oscillations. These enable effective mechanical, piezoelectric, and electrical coefficients to be expressed in terms of the volume fraction of the ceramic and the coefficients for the ceramic and polymer.

Effective Properties

The effective longitudinal speed is plotted in Fig. 6.8a as a function of the fractional volume of ceramic for three different types of polymer. It will be noted that at 0%, the effective speed is that of pure polymer (1950 m/s for the soft polymer), while at 100% it corresponds to the speed in the PZT5 ceramic (4325 m/s). As expected, the effective density (not shown) varies linearly between the two extremes, and as a result the characteristic impedance (Fig. 6.8b) for the composite using soft polymer varies from 1.75 MRayl at zero volume percent to 33.5 MRayl at 100%.

For the effective coupling factor (Fig. 6.8c), it can be seen that there is a wide plateau region over which the composite has a coupling factor that is significantly higher than the clamped coupling factor for the ceramic $(R_{33}^t = 0.49)$. For the soft polymer the effective coupling factor in the plateau region approaches the free coupling factor for the ceramic($k_{33}^t = 0.7$). This can be understood by noting that the presence of the soft polymer will tend to allow lateral movement of the individual ceramic posts, whereas, as explained earlier, the absence of any polymer will cause the ceramic to behave in a laterally clamped manner.

The final graph (Fig. 6.8d) shows the tradeoff between the effective characteristic impedance and coupling factor. The graph indicates that by using the soft polymer, effective characteristic impedances in the range of 5 to 10 MRayl can be achieved without causing a significant reduction in the coupling factor. For a composite designed to have an impedance in this range, the problems associated with achieving a proper match of the characteristic impedance to tissue is simplified, enabling a single matching layer to be used. However, there are other tradeoff problems. One concerns the reduction in the effective

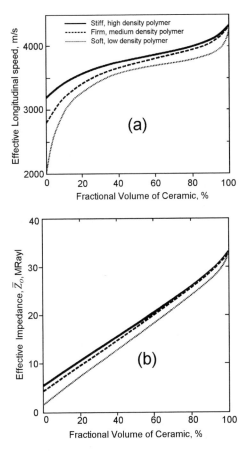

Figure 6.8 Predicted characteristics of a 1-3 composite structure based on a simplified theory developed by Smith and Auld [53]. In all four graphs the ceramic was assumed to be PZT5 and the dotted line corresponds to a soft polymer, the dashed line to a firm polymer, and the solid line to a stiff polymer. Effective (a) longitudinal speed, (b) characteristic impedance, (c) piezoelectric coupling factor. (d) Tradeoff between the piezoelectric coupling factor and the characteristic impedance. (Reproduced, with permission, from Smith and Auld [53], *IEEE Trans. Ultrason., Ferroelect., Freq. Contr.*, 38, 40–47, © 1991 IEEE.)

permittivity. As the fractional volume of ceramic is reduced, there is a nearly linear reduction in the effective permittivity from ~2000ε_o at 100% to ~20ε_o at 0%. For a given transducer cross-sectional area and thickness, a reduction in permittivity decreases the transducer capacitance, resulting in an increased electrical impedance. On transmission, impedance matching problems to the excitation source make it difficult to efficiently deliver the power to the transducer. On reception, the higher impedance may present difficulties when the output is to be transmitted to the system electronics via a relatively long

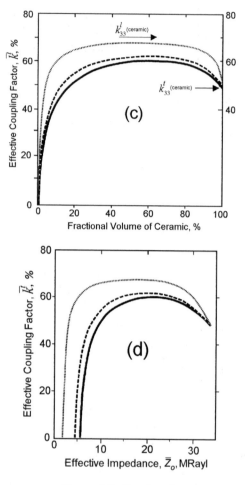

Figure 6.8 *Continued*

transmission line, which could be a miniature coaxial cable with a character-istic impedance of less than 125 Ω. For transducers or transducer elements having a very small cross-sectional area, such as those used in 2-D phased arrays, the reduction in the clamped permittivity presents serious difficulties in achieving a good signal-to-noise ratio (SNR) [54] unless a preamplifier is used adjacent to the transducer. These aspects will be clarified following a dis-cussion of some transducer models.

Effects of Lateral Modes

In the approach described above it was assumed that the lateral dimensions of the matrix elements were sufficiently far removed from the appropriate lateral wavelength so that the composite could be treated as though it were

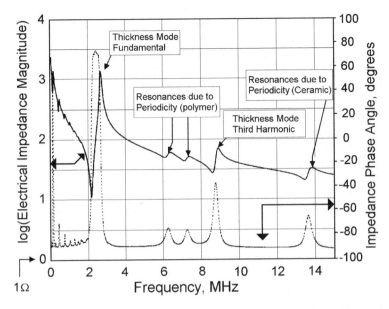

Figure 6.9 Electrical impedance graph for a 2-2 composite transducer illustrating the influence of lateral modes resulting from the structural periodicity. Note the left log scale and that zero corresponds to an impedance magnitude of 1 Ω. (Reprinted by permission of Elsevier from Papadakis et al. [28], Chapter 2, in: "Physical Acoustics: Principles and Methods", Vol. 24, Academic Press, © 1991 Academic Press.)

homogeneous. If the lateral dimensions are much larger than the thickness, then the resonant frequencies associated with the lateral dimensions will be smaller than the uncoupled fundamental thickness mode resonant frequency given by $f_p = c_o/(2\ell)$, where ℓ is the plate thickness. In a homogeneous ceramic plate, as the lateral dimension are reduced and become comparable to the thickness, the lateral modes become more strongly coupled to the thickness modes [55]. For a composite plate, this coupling is reduced.

In general, Lamb waves will be produced when a composite transducer is electrically excited, and because these are propagated in a lattice with a periodic structure, strong reflections can occur when the wavelength is equal to the lattice spacing [26,56,57]. This acoustic phenomenon is analogous to that discovered by the Braggs (father and son) in their investigation of diffraction of X-rays by a periodic crystal lattice. A Brillouin-type theory of elastic wave propagation in periodic composite materials was initially presented by Auld et al. [58,59]. Associated with the propagation of Lamb waves will be stop and pass bands. If the periodicity of the structure is designed so that the thickness mode resonant frequency is at the center of the first stop band, the laterally propagating waves will be highly attenuated. Some aspects of the above effects are illustrated by the results given in Fig. 6.9 [28]. Both the magnitude and phase of the measured electrical impedance are shown as a function of frequency for a 2-2 composite whose structure is similar to that illustrated in Fig. 6.7a. Below the fundamental thickness mode resonant frequency (~2.8 MHz), there is some evidence of minor lateral mode effects. Above the resonant frequency, the effects of periodicity of the structure are clearly evident, though for this particular design they occur well above the thickness mode resonant frequency.

The complex structure of composite transducers makes it difficult to use simple 1-D models to accurately predict their electroacoustic behavior. A 2-D analytical method for modeling multifrequency 2-2 composites has been described by Lamberti et al. [60]. A number of numerical analyses have also been presented that make use of 2-D and 3-D finite element techniques to compute the behavior of composites with various connectivities. In addition to the more general descriptions of the application of finite element methods for piezoelectric media given in [61,62], specific application of these methods to composite structures are given in [63–65].

6.4.2 Multilayer Transducers

Piezoelectric Ceramics

As mentioned in the last subsection, a difficulty with the use of composite piezoelectric media for transducers with a very small cross-sectional area, e.g., the elements in a 1-D or 2-D imaging array, arises from the reduction in permittivity, which, in combination with the small area, gives rise to a high impedance. For a given cross-sectional area, the capacitance can be substantially increased by using a structure that consists of piezoelectric ceramic layers that are acoustically in series but are electrically connected in parallel. Such an arrangement is illustrated in Fig. 6.10. It will be noted that the polarization direction in alternate layers reverses, so that the application of a voltage to the electrodes causes a field to be generated that is either in the polarization direction of all the regions or opposite to them. As a result, each region expands or contracts in phase with the others. While this method of decreasing the electrical impedance has been known for some considerable time and has been widely used for improving the performance of hydrophones [66; 67, p. 237], the application of this technique for pulse-echo ultrasound transducers using either piezopolymers [68,71] or piezoceramics [54,69,72,73] is more recent. But, as with composite transducer structures, the fabrication costs for multilayer transducers are significantly higher than for single-element devices.

If a transducer thickness of l is required then, for a *single* ceramic element of cross-sectional area A and clamped permittivity ε^T, the capacitance is given by $C_T = \varepsilon^T A / \ell$, provided that fringing effects can be ignored. If N layers of the same medium are used to achieve the same thickness, then the capacitance will be $N \times \varepsilon^T A / (\ell/N) = N^2 C_T$. Consequently, the electrical impedance decreases as the square of the number of elements, enabling better matching to be achieved into a low-impedance load or source. Goldberg et al. [70] have used finite element analysis to predict the electromechanical performance.

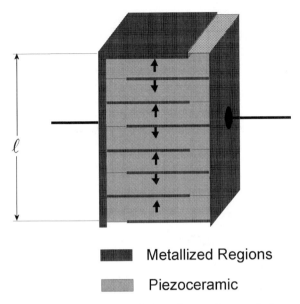

Metallized Regions

Piezoceramic

Figure 6.10 Sketch of a transducer consisting of seven layers of piezoceramic that are polarized in opposite directions (arrows indicate the polarization). The electrical capacitance is increased since the elements are electrically connected in parallel, and for the pattern shown each element has a thickness of $\ell/7$. Acoustically, the transducer behaves as if the layers are in series. (Based on Goldberg and Smith [54].)

Piezoelectric Polymers

The pulse-echo sensitivity of piezopolymers used in a conventional manner is substantially inferior to that using piezoceramics. Nonetheless, an important advantage of piezopolymers is that their characteristic impedance is much closer to tissue, enabling very wide bandwidths to be achieved. This important advantage has spurred efforts to find means of overcoming the disadvantages. Multilayer piezoelectric polymer structures can be made by folding the plastic in alternate directions to achieve polarization directions that alternate. As a result, the transducer capacitance is substantially increased and the voltage required to produce a given output power is greatly diminished. This enables the pulse-echo sensitivity to be greatly improved [68], although, because of the increased stack thickness, the bandwidth is reduced. To predict the performance and to compare with conventional single-element PZT designs, Zhang et al. [74] have developed a 1-D model of such a structure.

Barker Coded Structures

In pulse-echo systems the SNR can be improved by increasing the transmitter peak power, and increasing the bandwidth can enhance the axial resolution. The limitations imposed by the peak transmitted power were first addressed in radar and, stimulated by a 1953 monograph by Woodward [75], methods were developed for overcoming it.[8] It was shown that by transmitting a suitably encoded signal over a longer time duration and using a receiver that incorporated a matched filter (one whose response was the time-reversed form of the transmitted signal), a time-compressed form of the transmitted signal could be produced. By spreading the transmitted signal over a longer duration, a higher total energy can be transmitted without exceeding the peak power limitation, and as a result, the depth of penetration and the SNR can be increased, e.g., [77]. For ultrasound systems, issues such as the permitted diagnostic levels and nonlinear effects limit the peak power that can be transmitted. Major SNR improvements can be achieved by using coded excitation techniques and, as discussed in Chapter 7, a variety of methods are available, some of which have been developed for medical ultrasound imaging. In this subsection we shall consider just those aspects related to transducer design.

For example, let us denote the transmitted signal waveform by $e_t(t)$. If this is sent to a receiver system whose impulse response is $h_r(t) = ke_t(-t)$, where k is a matched filter constant, then the output from the receiver will be given by

$$e_{out}(t) = e_t(t) * h_r(t) = ke_t(t) * e_t(-t)$$
$$= k \int_{-\infty}^{\infty} e_t(\tau)e_t(\tau-t)d\tau = k \int_{-\infty}^{\infty} e_t(\tau)e_t(\tau+t)d\tau,$$

which is the autocorrelation function[9] of $e_t(t)$. In the frequency domain, the relation between the receiver matched filter transfer function $H(\omega)$ and the input signal $E(\omega)$ is: $H(\omega) = kE^*(\omega)$, i.e., it is the complex conjugate of the input signal.

For a digitally based compression system, a good choice for $e_t(t)$ is a Barker code sequence [77]. Binary Barker codes can be written as finite sequences of 1's and 0's, and they have the special property that their autocorrelation function can contain only three possible values: 0, 1, and N, where N is the number of bits in the code. Only nine Barker code sequences are known, of which the longest has $N = 13$. Consider, for example, Fig. 6.11, which shows the 7-bit Barker code sequence, and suppose that the transmitted signal is such that each bit has a duration of 1 second. It can be readily shown that the autocorrelation function consists of a central lobe of 2 seconds' duration and a peak amplitude that is seven times larger than the side lobes. As the code sequence length is increased, the side lobes are reduced relative to the peak. Piezoceramic and PVDF transducers configured to make use of the Barker pulse compression scheme were originally described by Sung [72] and Platte [71,78], and subsequently discussed by others [74].

---

8. The basic ideas appear to have been developed during the World War II, though they were not developed until considerably later (see 76, particularly Chapter 1).

9. See Appendix B for the definition.

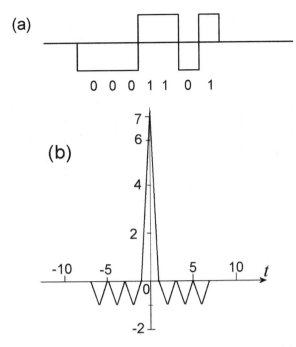

0 0 0 1 1 0 1

Figure 6.11 Barker code (a) represented as a +1 −1 sequence, and (b) its autocorrelation function.

To generate a seven-bit Barker code, the stack arrangement shown in Fig. 6.12 can be used [74,78]. Because the polarization direction corresponds to the Barker code, when a step function of voltage is applied, a Barker code stress pattern is instantaneously generated. If we assume that the propagation medium has the same density and speed of propagation as the transducer and is perfectly matched at both ends to the surrounding medium, then this stress pattern will propagate with a speed of c_o out from each end of the transducer. Consequently, the time variation of the stress pattern observed a short distance away from the transducer surface will also be the Barker code. If the receiving transducer has a polarization pattern that is the reverse of the transmitter, then the output voltage will be the autocorrelation function of the Barker code. As can be seen from Fig. 6.12c, the transmitted signal is compressed from a total duration of ℓ/c_o to a half-height duration of $\ell/(7c_o)$. To eliminate the need for a separate receiving transducer, so that a single transducer can operate in a pulse-echo mode, Zhang et al. [74] have described a switching scheme that on transmission behaves as in Fig. 6.12a and on reception as in Fig. 6.12b. They have also provided a 1-D analysis and have compared the pulse-echo performance of Barker-coded PVDF transducers with single-element PZT transducers.

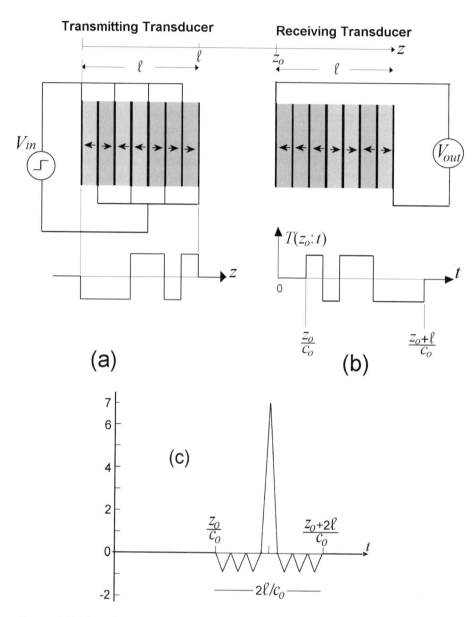

Figure 6.12 Transducer configuration used to generate a 7-bit Barker code. For simplicity it has been assumed that perfect matching exists and that the speed of sound is the same throughout. (a) Transmitting transducer in which the layers are electrically in parallel. A snapshot of the spatial distribution of the stress pattern is shown below at a time immediately following occurrence of a step voltage. (b) Receiving transducer with a polarization pattern that is the reverse of the transmitter pattern. Also shown is time variation of the stress pattern at the transducer entrance port ($z = z_o$). (c) Relative open-circuit output voltage from the receiving transducer. The central peak of the autocorrelation function occurs at $t = (z_o + \ell)/c_o$ and has a half-height duration of $\ell/(7c_o)$.

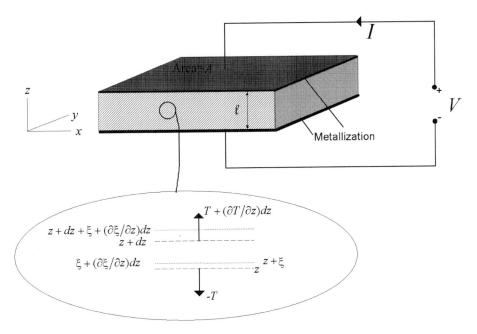

Figure 6.13 Analysis of a piezoelectric plate polarized in the z-direction.

6.5 One-Dimensional Transducer Models

One-dimensional models provide a useful starting point for predicting the behavior of transducers and optimizing their performance. The basis of such models is a solution to the 1-D wave equation for propagation in the direction of polarization. Such a solution assumes that the lateral transducer dimensions are much larger than the thickness and that the behavior is linear. In addition, losses are generally assumed to be negligible, though, as will be seen, these can be readily accounted for by straightforward extensions to the model.

6.5.1 Analysis

For the metallized piezoelectric plate of cross-sectional area A shown in Fig. 6.13, we shall assume the electrodes are sufficiently thin so that their influence on wave propagation through the piezoelectric medium can be ignored.[10] It will also be assumed that the piezoelectric medium is polarized in the z-direction and that there are no lateral strains ($S_1 = S_2 = 0$). The coordinate axes are as shown in the figure, with the plane $z = 0$ coincident with the bottom surface and the plane $z = \ell$ coincident with the top. It should be noted that the transducer can be represented as a three-port device: one electrical port

---

10. Derivations are given, for example, in [12,79,80].

and two acoustic ports. The electrical port parameters consist of the current and voltage between the two metallized surfaces, while the acoustic port parameters consist of the force and particle velocity on each surface.

Consider the elementary volume illustrated in Fig. 6.13, consisting of a plane slice parallel to the electrodes located at z and having a thickness dz. For a wave propagating in the z-direction, the stress[11] in the piezoelectric medium is a function of both z and time, i.e., $T(z:t)$. As indicated in the figure, at a given instant of time the displacement of the plane at z is denoted by ξ and that for the plane at $z + dz$ is $\xi + (\partial\xi/\partial z)dz$. Consequently, a first-order approximation for the strain within the elementary volume between these two planes is given by

$$(6.18) \qquad\qquad S \approx \frac{\partial\xi}{\partial z}dz/dz = \partial\xi/\partial z.$$

Now the force acting on the elementary volume is $A(\partial T/\partial z)dz$, and since its mass is $\rho_o A dz$, it follows from Newton's second law that $A\dfrac{\partial T}{\partial z}dz = \rho_o A dz\dfrac{\partial^2\xi}{\partial t^2}$, which simplifies to

$$(6.19) \qquad\qquad \frac{\partial T}{\partial z} = \rho_o\frac{\partial^2\xi}{\partial t^2}.$$

With the help of one of the constitutive relations, specifically (6.8a), the stress in this 1-D model can be written as

$$(6.20) \qquad\qquad T = c^D S - hD$$

and its spatial derivative as

$$\frac{\partial T}{\partial z} = c^D\frac{\partial S}{\partial z} - h\frac{\partial D}{\partial z}.$$

In the absence of free charges in the piezoelectric medium, (6.2) gives $\partial D/\partial z = 0$, so that by substituting the above equation into (6.19) and making use of (6.18), the differential equation for the displacement is

$$(6.21) \qquad\qquad \boxed{c^D\frac{\partial^2\xi}{\partial z^2} = \rho_o\frac{\partial^2\xi}{\partial t^2}}.$$

As will be shown, equations relating the electrical and mechanical transducer properties at the three ports can be obtained by solving this equation using appropriate boundary conditions.

In Fig. 6.14a, the forces on the two surfaces are defined to be positive when acting into the surfaces. Consequently, with the help of Fig. 6.13 it can be seen that these forces are related to the stresses (force/unit area) by $F_1 = -AT(0)$

---

11. For notational simplicity in this 1-D analysis we shall omit the use of the 3- or 33-subscripts.

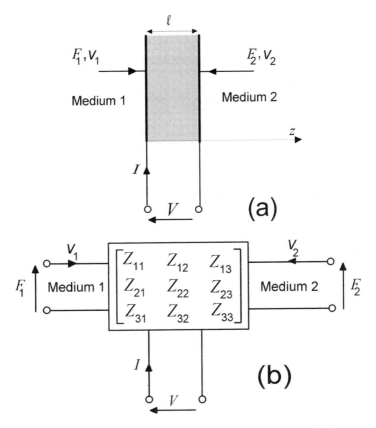

Figure 6.14 1-D model showing the sign conventions normally used. There are two acoustic ports and one electrical port. In (a) both the forces and the surface velocities are defined as being positive into the piezoelectric surfaces. Thus $v_1 = v(0)$, $v_2 = -v(\ell)$, and $F_1 = -AT(0)$, $F_2 = -AT(\ell)$. (b) Equivalent circuit with one electrical port and two mechanical (acoustic) ports.

and $F_2 = -AT(\ell)$. Similarly, the velocities of the two surfaces are given by $v_1 = v(0)$ and $v_2 = -v(\ell)$.

If the wave number (propagation constant) is denoted by[12] $\beta = \omega/c_o^D = \omega/\sqrt{c^D/\rho_o}$, then the harmonic solution to (6.21) can readily be shown to be

$$\xi(z;t) = B_1 e^{j(\omega t - \beta z)} + B_2 e^{j(\omega t + \beta z)},$$

which consists of two traveling waves moving in opposite directions. This equation can be transformed to a more convenient form by using some elementary trigonometric relations, yielding

12. To avoid confusion with the piezoelectric coupling factor, we have temporarily used β instead of k to denote the wave number.

(6.22) $$\xi(z{:}t) = e^{j\omega t}[B_3 \sin(\beta z) + B_4 \cos(\beta z)].$$

The constants B_3 and B_4 in this equation can be expressed in terms of the particle velocities on the two boundaries as follows. At $z = 0$ the velocity is $v_1 = v(0) = (\partial \xi / \partial t)_{z=0} = j\omega B_4 e^{j\omega t}$, so that the velocity phasor is given by

(6.23) $$\underline{v}_1 = j\omega B_4 \qquad\qquad\text{(a)}$$

In addition, at $z = \ell$

(6.23) $$\underline{v}_2 = -v(\ell) = -j\omega[B_3 \sin(\beta \ell) + B_4 \cos(\beta \ell)]. \qquad\text{(b)}$$

Equations for the forces acting on the transducer surfaces can be obtained with the help of Fig. 6.14a, (6.20), and (6.22) and can expressed as:

(6.24)
$$F_1 = -AT(0) = -A[c^D S - hD]_{z=0} = A\left[hD - c^D \frac{\partial \xi}{\partial z}\bigg|_{z=0}\right]$$
$$= A[h\underline{D} - \beta c^D B_3]e^{j\omega t}, \qquad\qquad\text{(a)}$$

and

(6.24)
$$F_2 = -AT(\ell) = -A[c^D S - hD]_{z=\ell} = A\left[hD - c^D \frac{\partial \xi}{\partial z}\bigg|_{z=\ell}\right]$$
$$= A[h\underline{D} - \beta c^D B_3 \cos(\beta \ell) + \beta c^D B_4 \sin(\beta \ell)]e^{j\omega t}. \qquad\text{(b)}$$

In addition, from (6.3) the electric displacement phasor can be expressed in terms of the current phasor by $\underline{D} = \underline{I}/j\omega A$. Substituting this into the two equations of (6.24) and using (6.23) to express the constants B_3 and B_4 in terms of the boundary velocities, the force equations simplify to

(6.25)
$$\underline{F}_1 = -j[Z_a \cot(\beta \ell)\underline{v}_1 + Z_a \mathrm{cosec}(\beta \ell)\underline{v}_2 + h\underline{I}/\omega]$$
$$\underline{F}_2 = -j[Z_a \mathrm{cosec}(\beta \ell)\underline{v}_1 + Z_a \cot(\beta \ell)\underline{v}_2 + h\underline{I}/\omega]{,}$$

where $Z_a = AZ_o = A\rho_o\sqrt{c^D/\rho_o} = A\sqrt{c^D \rho_o}$ is the *acoustic impedance*, with units of Rayl·m². It is important to note that we have used the subscript a to distinguish the *acoustic impedance* from the *characteristic acoustic impedance* Z_o, whose units are Rayl.

The final equation relates the applied voltage V to the forces and current. This can be obtained by observing that the potential difference between two points A and B is defined as the work done in taking a unit positive test charge from B to A in the presence of an electric field $\mathcal{E}$. It can be written as the line integral

$$V_{AB} = -\int_B^A \mathcal{E} \cdot \mathbf{dL}.$$

Applying this definition to Fig. 6.14a and using (6.8b), it can be seen that

$$V = \int_0^\ell \mathcal{E}dz = \int_0^\ell -hS + (D/\varepsilon^S)dz$$
$$= \frac{D\ell}{\varepsilon^S} - h\int_0^\ell \frac{\partial \xi}{\partial z}dz = \frac{D\ell}{\varepsilon^S} - h\left[B_3 \sin(\beta z) + B_4 \cos(\beta z)\right]_0^\ell$$

in which (6.22) has been used in the final step. Now (6.23) enables B_3 and B_4 to be written in terms of the surface velocities, so that the voltage phasor can be expressed as

(6.26) $$\underline{V} = -\frac{j}{\omega}\left[\frac{\underline{I}\ell}{A\varepsilon^S} + h(\underline{v}_1 + \underline{v}_2)\right] = -\frac{j}{\omega}(h\underline{v}_1 + h\underline{v}_2 + \underline{I}/C_o),$$

where $C_o = A\varepsilon^S/\ell$ is the clamped capacitance of the piezoelectric medium.

Equations (6.25) and (6.26) can now be rewritten in the compact matrix form:

(6.27) $$\begin{bmatrix} \underline{F}_1 \\ \underline{F}_2 \\ \underline{V} \end{bmatrix} = -j\begin{bmatrix} Z_a\cot(\beta\ell) & Z_a\mathrm{cosec}(\beta\ell) & h/\omega \\ Z_a\mathrm{cosec}(\beta\ell) & Z_a\cot(\beta\ell) & h/\omega \\ h/\omega & h/\omega & 1/(\omega C_o) \end{bmatrix}\begin{bmatrix} \underline{v}_1 \\ \underline{v}_2 \\ \underline{I} \end{bmatrix}.$$

This characterizes the terminal behavior of the three-port transducer model shown in Fig. 6.14a and enables the impedance elements shown in Fig. 6.14b to be identified, e.g., $Z_{33} = -j/(\omega C_o)$. Additional equations that arise from the source and load impedances external to the transducer should also be noted. For example, if the transducer is used as a transmitter of acoustic energy and is excited by a voltage source V_S whose impedance is Z_S, then the acoustic impedances of the transmission and backing media can be written as $Z_B = -\underline{F}_1/\underline{v}_1$ and $Z_T = -\underline{F}_2/\underline{v}_2$, respectively, and the source impedance by $Z_S = -(\underline{V} - \underline{V}_S)/\underline{I}$. These relations, when used in (6.27), result in three equations with three unknowns. However, from a design standpoint these equations by themselves are not helpful in providing an intuitive grasp of the processes involved. What would be helpful is a model (or models) whose elements are related to the transduction mechanism, and some of these will be described in the next subsection.

Finally, it should be noted that propagation losses can be accounted for by assuming a propagation constant, a complex quantity given by $\gamma = \alpha + j\beta$, where α is the attenuation constant (Nepers/m) and $\beta = 2\pi/\lambda$. In addition, the dielectric loss can be accounted for by assuming the permittivity to be complex, though a useful approximation is to represent the loss by a resistor R_s in series with an ideal capacitor. Although both α and R_s are normally frequency-dependent quantities, it is often reasonable to use center frequency values over the transducer bandwidth. With these approximations, a more general form of (6.27) is

(6.28) $$\begin{bmatrix} \underline{F}_1 \\ \underline{F}_2 \\ \underline{V} \end{bmatrix} = -j\begin{bmatrix} Z_a\cot(\gamma\ell) & Z_a\mathrm{cosec}(\gamma\ell) & h/\omega \\ Z_a\mathrm{cosec}(\gamma\ell) & Z_a\cot(\gamma\ell) & h/\omega \\ h/\omega & h/\omega & jR_s + 1/(\omega C_o) \end{bmatrix}\begin{bmatrix} \underline{v}_1 \\ \underline{v}_2 \\ \underline{I} \end{bmatrix}.$$

6.5.2 Four Transducer Models

Exact Models of Mason, Redwood, and KLM

In 1948 Mason [82] proposed the circuit model shown in Fig. 6.15, whose terminal equations are identical to those given by (6.27).[13]

---

13. An interesting historical account of the development of circuit models is given in the paper by Ballato [81].

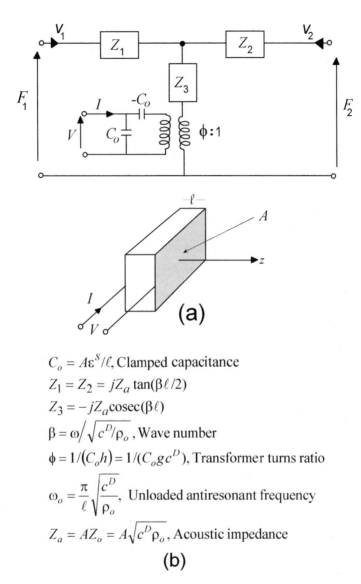

(a)

$C_o = A\varepsilon^S/\ell$, Clamped capacitance

$Z_1 = Z_2 = jZ_a \tan(\beta\ell/2)$

$Z_3 = -jZ_a\csc(\beta\ell)$

$\beta = \omega/\sqrt{c^D/\rho_o}$, Wave number

$\phi = 1/(C_o h) = 1/(C_o g c^D)$, Transformer turns ratio

$\omega_o = \dfrac{\pi}{\ell}\sqrt{\dfrac{c^D}{\rho_o}}$, Unloaded antiresonant frequency

$Z_a = AZ_o = A\sqrt{c^D\rho_o}$, Acoustic impedance

(b)

Figure 6.15 Mason 1-D model of a piezoelectric plate excited in the thickness expansion mode. (a) Circuit model. (b) Equations describing parameters of the model, which satisfies (6.27). The transformer turns ratio has MKS units of volts/Newton.

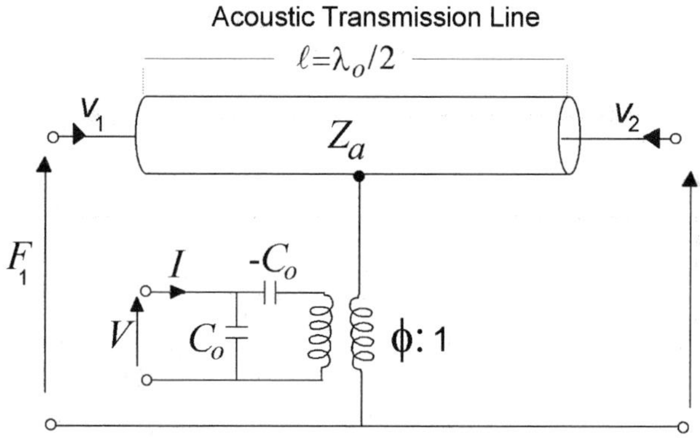

Acoustic Transmission Line

Figure 6.16 The Redwood model. This model can be obtained from the Mason model by simply replacing the T-network of Fig. 6.15 by an equivalent acoustic transmission line of length ℓ and acoustic impedance $Z_a = AZ_o$. The parameters of this model are the same as the Mason model given in Fig. 6.15.

Subsequently, Redwood [83] developed a transmission line model[14] (Fig. 6.16) that is more amenable for transient analysis and physical interpretation. Using this model, he determined the transducer transient acoustic response when a step of voltage was applied and also determined the electrical response when a step function of force was applied. A different model, illustrated in Fig. 6.17, is that proposed in 1970 by Krimholtz et al. [85,86] and which is commonly referred to as the KLM model. By straightforward analysis [80], it can be shown that the equations governing the terminal properties of all three models are identical to (6.27), and consequently they are all exact 1-D models for longitudinal thickness mode wave motion in a piezoelectric disk whose lateral dimensions are large compared to the thickness. Equations that express the circuit element properties in terms of the transducer material properties are also given.

In examining all three models, it will be noted that the transformer ratio is a dimensioned parameter. This is because the transformer acts as an interface between the electrical and mechanical parts of the circuit. For the Mason and Redwood models, the transformer turns ratios are independent of frequency, whereas for the KLM model this is not the case. It is reasonable to expect that the piezoelectric medium should behave as a distributed acoustic delay line that is excited throughout its thickness by the time-varying electric field. For the Mason model, Z_1, Z_2, and Z_3 are frequency-dependent impedances whose physical interpretation is not immediately evident. In the Redwood model, an acoustic transmission line whose length is half the resonant wavelength ($\lambda_o/2$) has replaced these three impedances. It should be noted that the transformer

14. Closely related to the Redwood model is one proposed in 1983 by Banah et al. [84], which models the acoustic properties by a reentrant acoustic transmission line.

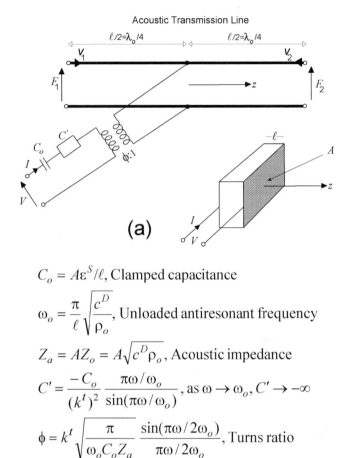

$C_o = A\varepsilon^S/\ell$, Clamped capacitance

$\omega_o = \dfrac{\pi}{\ell}\sqrt{\dfrac{c^D}{\rho_o}}$, Unloaded antiresonant frequency

$Z_a = AZ_o = A\sqrt{c^D\rho_o}$, Acoustic impedance

$C' = \dfrac{-C_o}{(k^t)^2}\,\dfrac{\pi\omega/\omega_o}{\sin(\pi\omega/\omega_o)}$, as $\omega \to \omega_o$, $C' \to -\infty$

$\phi = k^t\sqrt{\dfrac{\pi}{\omega_o C_o Z_a}}\,\dfrac{\sin(\pi\omega/2\omega_o)}{\pi\omega/2\omega_o}$, Turns ratio

(b)

Figure 6.17 The KLM model of a disk transducer operating in the thickness. (a) Circuit model. (b) Equations for the circuit parameters. Note that the "capacitor" C' has an impedance of $Z_{C'} = \dfrac{1}{j\omega C'} = \dfrac{j(k^t)^2}{\omega C_o}\,\dfrac{\sin(\pi\omega/\omega_o)}{\pi\omega/\omega_o}$ whose reactance is positive for $\omega < \omega_o$ and zero when $\omega = \omega_o$. The transformer turns ratio has MKS units of $[(\text{Ohms/Newton})(\text{m/s})]^{1/2}$.

output drives this transmission line on the common (shield) connection, and consequently the transformer output appears as two sources, one at each end of the transmission line. We shall make use of this model in section 6.7.1 for discussing the impulse response.

The KLM model shown in Fig. 6.17 contains two quarter-wave acoustic transmission lines with their common terminals connected to the transformer. As discussed by Desiltes et al. [87], the KLM model replaces the distributed nature of the coupling by a single coupling point, and the difference between this approximation and the distributed coupling is included through the frequency-dependent transformer turns ratio and a series reactance. From a design standpoint, the KLM model more readily allows the effects of various termination conditions at the two acoustic ports to be interpreted and allows an intuitive approach to be used in optimizing the transducer performance. At the electrical port, there are two capacitors in series: the clamped capacitor and one whose capacitance is negative for $\omega < \omega_o$ and that approaches $-\infty$ as $\omega \to \omega_o$, i.e., at the resonant frequency. In the neighborhood of the resonant frequency, $|C'| \gg C_o$ so that C' can be regarded as a short circuit.

Approximate Model of Van Dyke

In 1925 Van Dyke [88,89] showed[15] how the simple electrical model shown in Fig. 6.18 could be obtained from the equations describing the vibration of a lightly loaded piezoelectric transducer feeding *acoustic* transmission and backing impedances denoted by Z_T and Z_B, respectively. It will be noted that this model contains a series branch consisting of L, C, and R that will have a series resonant frequency f_s, and a parallel branch with an unloaded anti-resonant frequency[16] of f_p. By comparison with the KLM model and assuming $\omega \to 0$, it can be seen that $C'_o = C_o - C$. The validity of this approximate model[17] is limited to a lightly loaded transducer close to the resonant frequency, and it can be helpful in designing appropriate electrical matching to a source or load.

As an example, we consider a 5 mm-diameter ($A = 19.6 \times 10^{-6} \text{m}^2$) PZT-5H disk that has a resonant frequency of 5 MHz and that is immersed in water. Consequently, the load acoustic impedances are given by $Z_T = Z_B = 19.6 \times 10^{-6} \times 1.5 \times 10^6 = 29.4 \text{ Rayl.m}^2$. From Table 6.2 it can be seen that the relevant transducer material properties are $k^t = 0.49$, $(c_o)^D = 4620 \text{ m/s}$, and $\varepsilon^S = 1470\varepsilon_o$. Now the transducer thickness required for an unloaded antiresonant

---

15. Although the discovery of this circuit model is sometimes attributed to Van Dyke, it should be noted that in 1914/15 Butterworth [90] proposed an electrical model for a mechanically vibrating system with several degrees of freedom. He showed that in the region of the resonant frequency, it consists of a capacitor in parallel with the series combination of an inductor resistor and capacitor. Although no mention is made of its applicability to piezoelectric resonators and no reference is made by Van Dyke to this earlier work, many refer to the circuit model as the *Butterworth-Van Dyke* model. It should also be noted that Dye [91] independently arrived at the same model for a quartz crystal: his work was published shortly after Van Dyke's brief report.

16. As noted in [92], these two resonant frequencies are variously referred to in the literature. Thus, the series resonant frequency $= f_s =$ frequency of maximum conductance, $f_m =$ frequency of minimum impedance, $f_r =$ resonant frequency = frequency of zero susceptance and, $f_m = f_s = f_r$ (lossless), $f_m < f_s < f_r$ (lossy). Also, the parallel resonant frequency $= f_p =$ frequency of maximum resistance, $f_a =$ anti-resonant frequency = frequency of zero reactance, $f_n =$ frequency of maximum impedance and, in general, $f_a = f_p = f_n$ (lossless), $f_a < f_p < f_n$ (lossy).

17. It should be noted that a more accurate representation is obtained if ω_s is replaced by ω_p in the expression given in Fig. 6.18 for the series resistance R [93].

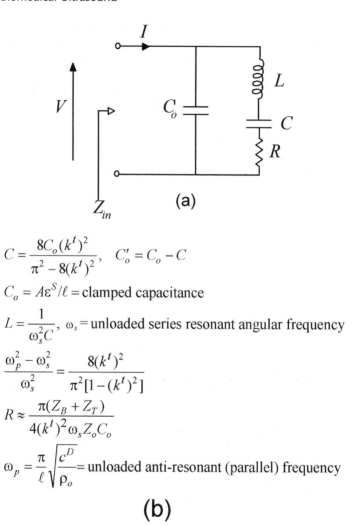

$$C = \frac{8C_o(k^t)^2}{\pi^2 - 8(k^t)^2}, \quad C'_o = C_o - C$$

$$C_o = A\varepsilon^S/\ell = \text{clamped capacitance}$$

$$L = \frac{1}{\omega_s^2 C}, \quad \omega_s = \text{unloaded series resonant angular frequency}$$

$$\frac{\omega_p^2 - \omega_s^2}{\omega_s^2} = \frac{8(k^t)^2}{\pi^2[1-(k^t)^2]}$$

$$R \approx \frac{\pi(Z_B + Z_T)}{4(k^t)^2 \omega_s Z_o C_o}$$

$$\omega_p = \frac{\pi}{\ell}\sqrt{\frac{c^D}{\rho_o}} = \text{unloaded anti-resonant (parallel) frequency}$$

(b)

Figure 6.18 Approximate 1-D circuit model of a lightly loaded transducer in the vicinity of the resonant frequency. (a) Circuit model. (b) Circuit parameters defining the model.

frequency of 5 MHz can be found from $\ell = (c_o)^D/(2f_o)$, yielding $\ell = 4620/(2 \times 5 \times 10^6) = 0.462$ mm, so that the clamped capacitance is $C_o = A\varepsilon^S\varepsilon_o/\ell = 553$ pF. Using these in the equations of Fig. 6.18, the circuit element values can be calculated as $R = 22.7\,\Omega$, $L = 11.8\,\mu\text{H}$, $C = 108$ pF, and $C' = 445$ pF. The input impedance can be obtained by straightforward circuit analysis as

$$1/Z_{in} = \underline{I}/\underline{V} = j\omega C' + j\omega L + \frac{1}{j\omega C} + R,$$

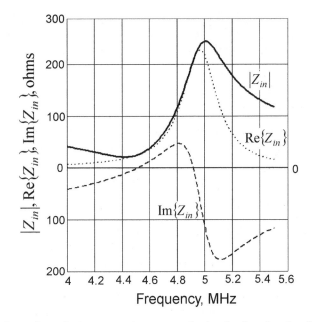

Figure 6.19 Input impedance versus frequency obtained using the simplified model of Fig. 6.18. The magnitude and real and imaginary parts are shown for a 5-mm-diameter, 5 MHz PZT-5H disk transducer that has no acoustic matching layers and that is immersed in water.

and the results are plotted in Fig. 6.19. As will be shown, these results are quite close to those obtained using the exact 1-D model equations. It should be noted that $|Z_{in}|$ is a maximum at a frequency f_p that is slightly less than the unloaded antiresonant frequency of $f_o = 5\,\text{MHz}$; also, the series resonant frequency of $f_s = 4.46\,\text{MHz}$ corresponds approximately to the minimum value of $|Z_{in}|$. For a lossless unloaded transducer, as $f \to f_o = f_p$, $|Z_{in}| \to \infty$ and as $f \to f_s$, $|Z_{in}| \to 0$. Transducer losses are not accounted for in this model, though an additional fixed resistance in series with R would be a reasonable approximation.

6.5.3 Matrix Computation Methods

By formulating the frequency domain characteristics of transducers in terms of matrices, direct use can be made of the built-in matrix operations that are an integral part of many software packages. This approach makes use of well-known techniques for characterizing electrical two-port networks that are well described in many textbooks [94,95]. Sittig [35,96,97] was one of the first to discuss its application and to provide a clear description of the method used for computing both the transmit and receive frequency domain response. He obtained the *transmission matrix* (often called the T-matrix) for the piezo-electric layer from (6.27) and represented the electrode layer and matching layer(s) by individual matrices. Subsequently, using a similar approach,

Selfridge and Gehlbach [98] represented each element of the KLM model as an individual matrix component, thereby providing the computational model with a more direct physical interpretation.[18] This approach will be used in the following analysis.

Transmission Matrix

If the back port sees an acoustic impedance of Z_B, then by substituting $v_1 = -F_1/Z_B$ into (6.27), the electrical and acoustical port parameters can be written in the form

$$\begin{bmatrix} V \\ I \end{bmatrix} = \begin{bmatrix} A_{11} & A_{12} \\ A_{21} & A_{22} \end{bmatrix} \begin{bmatrix} F_2 \\ -v_2 \end{bmatrix},$$

in which, for notational simplicity, the underscore on phasor quantities has been omitted. The parameters of $[A]$ are complex quantities that characterize the transfer from one port to the other, and because of this the matrix is often called a *transmission matrix* and the elements are referred to as the *transmission parameters*. It should be noted that I and v_2 are defined to be positive when pointing into the transducer, thus $-v_2$ is positive when pointing out of the acoustic port. It can be shown [94,95] that the determinant of $\mathbf{A}$ is unity (det $\mathbf{A} = A_{11}A_{22} - A_{12}A_{21} = 1$) and consequently the network possesses reciprocal properties.[19] When an ideal rigid reflector is used to reflect a plane wave transmitted from a transducer with reciprocal properties, the form of the transmit/receive transfer function is considerably simplified [110].

As illustrated in Fig. 6.20 and subsequently discussed in subsection 6.6.4, one or more matching layers consisting of non-piezoelectric media are generally used to improve the bandwidth and efficiency. The transmission properties of each layer can be represented as a two-port network, which in turn can be characterized by its 2×2 transmission matrix. For the nth lossless layer of a medium of thickness ℓ_n, propagation constant β_n, and acoustic impedance Z_n, the acoustic input and output can be obtained by putting $h = 0$ into (6.27); after some algebraic manipulations, this yields

(6.29) $$\begin{bmatrix} F_n \\ V_n \end{bmatrix} = \begin{bmatrix} \cos(\beta_n \ell_n) & jZ_n \sin(\beta_n \ell_n) \\ \dfrac{j\sin(\beta_n \ell_n)}{Z_n} & \cos(\beta_n \ell_n) \end{bmatrix} \begin{bmatrix} F_{n+1} \\ -V_{n+1} \end{bmatrix} = [A_n] \begin{bmatrix} F_{n+1} \\ -V_{n+1} \end{bmatrix},$$

where the matrix parameters characterize the transmission acoustic properties of the layer and the matrix $\mathbf{A}_n$ has reciprocal properties. Here again, the

---

18. A useful discussion of the changes needed to achieve consistency between the various models and to correct for a small number of errors present in the literature has been given by Whitworth [93].

19. For a reciprocal network, if a current I_s is applied to the electrical port and produces a particle velocity v_2 when an acoustical short exists ($Z_T = 0$) at the output, then the ratio of the open-circuit output voltage to a force F_2 applied to the acoustic port is given by $V_o/F_2 = v_2/I_s$.

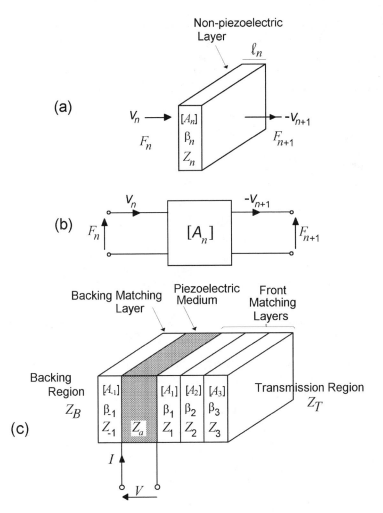

Figure 6.20 Accounting for the presence of matching layers. (a) Non-piezoelectric layer with an acoustic impedance of Z_n and a thickness of ℓ_n. (b) Two-port representation; the front port particle velocity is now defined to be positive out from the port. (c) Transducer with multiple transmission and backing layers.

sign of the particle velocity from port 2 should be noted.[20] By defining the transmission matrix in this way, it can be shown that for N cascaded layers (Fig. 6.20c), the equation governing the input and output parameters takes the form

$$\begin{bmatrix} F_1 \\ V_1 \end{bmatrix} = \prod_{n=1}^{N} [A_n] \begin{bmatrix} F_{N+1} \\ -V_{N+1} \end{bmatrix},$$

20. By putting $\ell_n = 0$ in (6.29), it can be seen that $v_n = -v_{n+1}$, so that on the output side if the velocity is negative, its direction will be positive out of the surface.

where for the $(N + 1)$th region, e.g., the transmission medium, $Z_T = -F_{N+1}/V_{N+1}$ and the overall transmission matrix consists of the matrix for each layer post-multiplied by the matrices of succeeding layers. Single electrical or acoustic elements can be readily incorporated into the overall matrix by writing down their transmission properties. For example, in the case of a series impedance Z_{ser}, the transmission matrix is $\begin{bmatrix} 1 & Z_{ser} \\ 0 & 1 \end{bmatrix}$ and that for a shunt impedance Z_{sht} is $\begin{bmatrix} 1 & 0 \\ 1/Z_{sht} & 1 \end{bmatrix}$.

Losses in the medium can be accounted for by making the propagation constant a complex quantity, and as a result the transmission matrix then takes the form

$$[A_n] = \begin{bmatrix} \cosh(\gamma_n \ell_n) & Z_n \sinh(\gamma_n \ell_n) \\ \dfrac{\sinh(\gamma_n \ell_n)}{Z_n} & \cosh(\gamma_n \ell_n) \end{bmatrix},$$

where $\gamma = \alpha + j\beta$, in which α is the attenuation constant (Nepers/m) and $\beta = 2\pi/\lambda$.

Transmit and Receive Response

Calculation of both the transmission and reception response will be illustrated by considering the simplified schematics shown in Fig. 6.21, in which single front and back matching layers are assumed. The excitation source has an output impedance of Z_s and is connected via a coaxial cable to an electrical

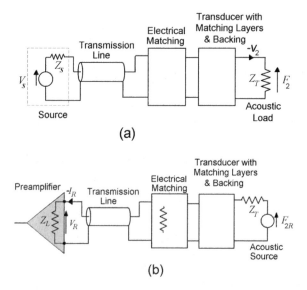

Figure 6.21 Simplified models of (a) a transmission circuit and (b) a reception circuit.

matching network and then to the transducer, whose front port is loaded by the transmission medium with an acoustic impedance of Z_T. In Fig. 6.22 the transmission line and matching network are represented by matrix $\mathbf{A}^{elt}$, and the other matrices are obtained from the KLM model and matching layer

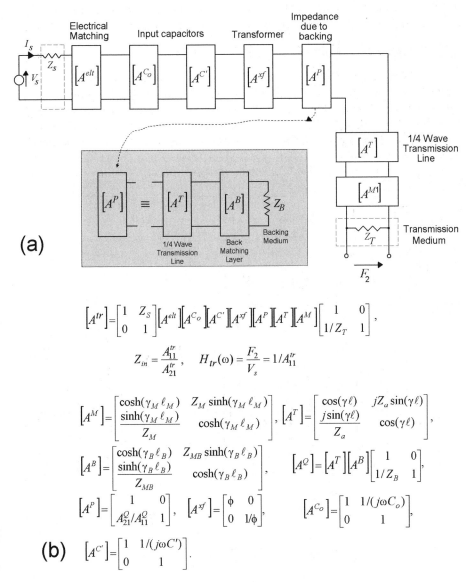

(a)

(b)

$$[A^{tr}] = \begin{bmatrix} 1 & Z_S \\ 0 & 1 \end{bmatrix} [A^{elt}][A^{C_o}][A^{C'}][A^{xf}][A^P][A^T][A^M] \begin{bmatrix} 1 & 0 \\ 1/Z_T & 1 \end{bmatrix},$$

$$Z_{in} = \frac{A_{11}^{tr}}{A_{21}^{tr}}, \quad H_{tr}(\omega) = \frac{F_2}{V_s} = 1/A_{11}^{tr}$$

$$[A^M] = \begin{bmatrix} \cosh(\gamma_M \ell_M) & Z_M \sinh(\gamma_M \ell_M) \\ \dfrac{\sinh(\gamma_M \ell_M)}{Z_M} & \cosh(\gamma_M \ell_M) \end{bmatrix}, \quad [A^T] = \begin{bmatrix} \cos(\gamma \ell) & jZ_a \sin(\gamma \ell) \\ \dfrac{j\sin(\gamma \ell)}{Z_a} & \cos(\gamma \ell) \end{bmatrix},$$

$$[A^B] = \begin{bmatrix} \cosh(\gamma_B \ell_B) & Z_{MB} \sinh(\gamma_B \ell_B) \\ \dfrac{\sinh(\gamma_B \ell_B)}{Z_{MB}} & \cosh(\gamma_B \ell_B) \end{bmatrix}, \quad [A^Q] = [A^T][A^B] \begin{bmatrix} 1 & 0 \\ 1/Z_B & 1 \end{bmatrix},$$

$$[A^P] = \begin{bmatrix} 1 & 0 \\ A_{21}^Q/A_{11}^Q & 1 \end{bmatrix}, \quad [A^{xf}] = \begin{bmatrix} \phi & 0 \\ 0 & 1/\phi \end{bmatrix}, \quad [A^{C_o}] = \begin{bmatrix} 1 & 1/(j\omega C_o) \\ 0 & 1 \end{bmatrix},$$

$$[A^{C'}] = \begin{bmatrix} 1 & 1/(j\omega C') \\ 0 & 1 \end{bmatrix}.$$

Figure 6.22 Transmission matrix method for calculating the acoustic transmission response using the KLM transducer model. The transducer is assumed to have single matching layers at the front and back and to be excited by a voltage source of impedance Z_S. (a) Signal flow path. The transfer characteristics of each block are represented by a matrix. (b) The total transformation matrix is given together with the input impedance, transmitted force/voltage transfer function, and values for the matrix elements.

properties previously described. The effects of the backing region are represented by a shunt impedance of A_{11}^Q/A_{21}^Q, whose value can be obtained from the matrix $\mathbf{A}^P$. Expressions for the impedance seen by the voltage source and the transfer function are also given. It should be noted that the series source impedance and the shunt load impedance have been included in the overall matrix, and consequently the input current and the output force and velocity

can be found from $\begin{bmatrix} V_s \\ I_s \end{bmatrix} = [A''] \begin{bmatrix} F_2 \\ 0 \end{bmatrix}$ and $v_2 = -F_2/Z_T$.

For the arrangement shown in Fig. 6.21b, the transducer is used as a receiver and the electrical port is connected via a coaxial cable to a preamplifier whose input impedance is Z_L. The matrix representation of this circuit is given in Fig. 6.23, together with equations for the overall transmission matrix and the transfer function. To calculate the transmit/receive (two-way) transfer function, it can be assumed that an ideal reflector is placed sufficiently close to the acoustic port that the effects of diffraction can be ignored. When the returned pressure

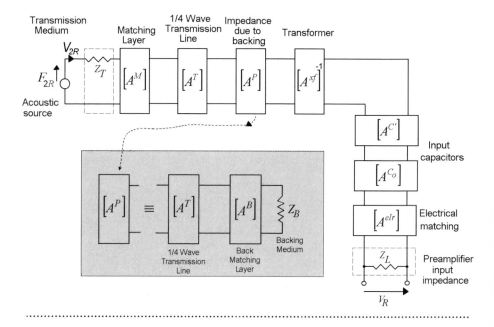

$$\left[A^{rec}\right] = \begin{bmatrix} 1 & Z_T \\ 0 & 1 \end{bmatrix} \left[A^M\right] \left[A^T\right] \left[A^P\right] \left[A^{xf}\right]^{-1} \left[A^{C'}\right] \left[A^{C_o}\right] \left[A^{elr}\right] \begin{bmatrix} 1 & 0 \\ 1/Z_L & 1 \end{bmatrix} \ , \ H_{rec}(\omega) = \frac{V_R}{F_{2R}} = 1/A_{11}^{rec}$$

Figure 6.23 Matrix method based on the KLM transducer model for calculating the voltage response at the input of a preamplifier due to an acoustic force. Single front and back matching layers are assumed. The transmission matrix is given together with the received voltage/force transfer function. All matrices are specified in Fig. 6.22b.

wave is incident on a rigid acoustic port of unit area, the resulting force will be twice that of the incident pressure. Thus, if the same transducer is used for both transmission and reception, the received force will be given by $F_{2R} = 2F_2$, which then enables the overall (two-way) transfer function (V_R/V_s) to be obtained. In fact, because the transducer behaves as a linear reciprocal device, the transmit and receive transfer functions, apart from a scaling term, have the same functional dependence on frequency, and this simplifies determination of the overall transfer function.

A convenient way of expressing the transmit/receive response is in terms of the insertion loss. The insertion loss of a network is generally defined as the ratio of the power delivered into a load by a source in the absence of the network, to the power delivered by the same source to the same load with the network present, and the result is expressed in dB. If both the receiver input impedance and the excitation source impedance are real quantities (R_L and R_s, respectively), then the insertion loss is given by

$$IL = 20\log\left\{\frac{R_L}{R_L + R_S} \frac{\left|A_{11}^{tr} A_{11}^{rec}\right|}{2}\right\}, \tag{a}$$

(6.30)

where the matrix elements are given in Figs. 6.22 and 6.23. For the special case in which $R_s = R_L$, this simplifies to

$$IL = 20\log\left\{\frac{\left|A_{11}^{tr} A_{11}^{rec}\right|}{4}\right\}$$

(6.30)

$$= 20\log\left\{\frac{Z_T\left|A_{11}^{tr}\right|^2}{4R_L}\right\} = 20\log\left\{\frac{R_L\left|A_{11}^{rec}\right|^2}{4Z_T}\right\}. \tag{b}$$

6.6 Application of the KLM Model

In applying the KLM model, it is helpful to make use of a well-known equation for the input impedance of a lossless acoustic transmission line that is characterized by an impedance Z_c. For a line of length ℓ terminated by a load impedance Z_r, the input impedance can be found by first post-multiplying the matrix $[A_n]$, given by (6.29), by the matrix for a shunt load. If the propagation constant is expressed in terms of the wavelength λ, by using $\beta = 2\pi/\lambda$ and omitting the subscripts n, the new matrix can be written as

$$[A'] = \begin{bmatrix} \cos(2\pi\ell/\lambda) & jZ_c\sin(2\pi\ell/\lambda) \\ \dfrac{j\sin(2\pi\ell/\lambda)}{Z_c} & \cos(2\pi\ell/\lambda) \end{bmatrix} \begin{bmatrix} 1 & 0 \\ 1/Z_r & 1 \end{bmatrix}.$$

The input impedance can then be found from $Z_i = A'_{11}/A'_{21}$, yielding

$$Z_i = Z_c \frac{Z_r + jZ_c\tan(2\pi\ell/\lambda)}{Z_c + jZ_r\tan(2\pi\ell/\lambda)}. \tag{6.31}$$

(6.31)

We shall briefly examine the implications of this equation for some specific conditions. If the line has a length of $\lambda/4$ and is terminated with an impedance of Z_r, then the input impedance is $Z_i(\lambda/4) = (Z_c)^2/Z_r$. If the line is shorted $(Z_r = 0)$, then $Z_i(\lambda/4) = \infty$. For a line of any length that is terminated by its characteristic impedance $(Z_r = Z_c)$, then $Z_i(\ell) = Z_c$. And finally, if the load is an open circuit, then $Z_i(\ell) = -jZ_c\cot(2\pi\ell/\lambda)$.

Consider the elementary conditions illustrated in Fig. 6.24a, in which the transducer sees a backing acoustic impedance of Z_B and a transmission acoustic impedance of Z_T, both regions being semi-infinite in extent. At the resonant frequency, the acoustic impedance seen by the mechanical side of the transformer consists of Z_a^2/Z_B in parallel with Z_a^2/Z_T, and this combination, when transformed to the electrical side, results in a *radiation resistance* given by

$$(6.32) \qquad R_{ao} = \frac{2(k')^2}{\pi^2 f_o C_o} \frac{Z_a}{Z_B + Z_T}.$$

Thus, as shown in Fig. 6.24c, the electrical input impedance at resonance consists of the clamped capacitance of C_o in series with the radiation resistance. Evidently, if $Z_B = Z_T = 0$, the radiation resistance will be infinite. It should also be noted that the radiation resistance is inversely proportional to the transducer cross-sectional area.

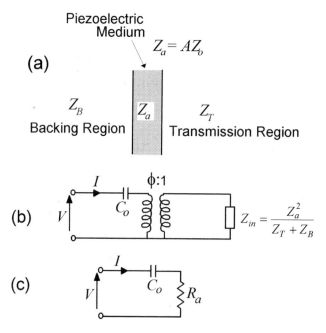

Figure 6.24 An acoustic transducer of cross-sectional area A with backing and transmission regions that have acoustic impedances of Z_B and Z_T, respectively. (a) Physical arrangement. (b) Equivalent transformer load at the resonant frequency. (c) Obtaining the radiation resistance.

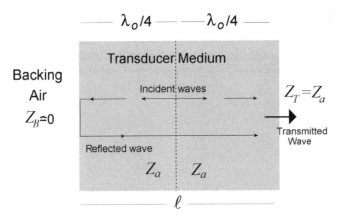

Figure 6.25 A transducer excited at its resonant frequency with stress waves originating from the center propagating toward each surface. The backward wave gets reflected and inverted at the backing interface and arrives back at the center with exactly the right time delay to cause reinforcement of the wave propagating to the right.

The KLM model provides some useful insights as to the conditions that occur at resonance. According to this model, the effective source of the waves is the center plane of the transducer medium. As illustrated in Fig. 6.25, waves from this plane progress in both directions. For an air-backed transducer with perfect matching of the front surface, the reflected wave from the back interface causes the stress wave emitted from the front surface to have twice the amplitude of that when the reflection is absent.

6.6.1 Quarter-Wave Matched and Air-Backed

As a second example, we consider the situation shown in Fig. 6.26. Here the backing side of the transducer is air ($Z_o^{Air}/Z_o^{PZT} \approx 10^{-5}$) and the transmission side

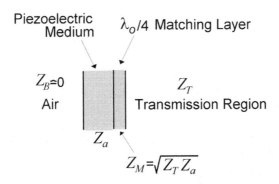

Figure 6.26 An air-backed transducer with a $\lambda/4$ matching layer that gives an exact impedance match for the front surface, though only at the resonant frequency.

is acoustically matched to water by means of a matching layer that is quarter-wave thick at the transducer resonant frequency ($\omega = \omega_o$). The acoustic imped-ance of such a layer will be given by $Z_M = \sqrt{Z_a Z_T}$ (see subsection 1.6.1). Because the input impedance of a shorted quarter-wave transmission line is infinite ($Z_B \approx 0$) and $Z_T = Z_a$, then from (6.32) the radiation resistance at the resonant frequency simplifies to

(6.33)
$$R_{ao} = \frac{2(k^t)^2}{\pi^2 f_o C_o}.$$

As an example, we consider a 5-MHz air-backed PZT-5H disk of 5 mm diameter. The relevant material properties are $k^t = 0.49$, $(c_o)^D = 4620$ m/s, and $\varepsilon^S = 1470\varepsilon_o$. Now the transducer resonant thickness is given by $\ell = 4620/(2 \times 5 \times 10^6) = 0.462$ mm, so that the clamped capacitance is $C_o = A\varepsilon^S\varepsilon_o/\ell = 553$ pF. Substituting these values into (6.33) yields a radiation resistance of 17.6 Ω.

6.6.2 Unloaded Input Impedance

In the absence of any load on the transducer, the impedance seen on the acoustic side of the transformer can be obtained by noting that in the KLM model the impedances arising from each surface are in parallel and their values are given by the transmission line equation of (6.31). This yields

$$Z_{tr}^{acoust} = (jZ_a/2)\tan(2\pi\ell/\lambda) = (jZ_a/2)\tan(\pi\omega/2\omega_o),$$

which, when reflected to the electrical side, becomes

$$Z_{tr}^{elect} = \frac{2j(k^t)^2}{C_o \pi\omega^2/\omega_o} \sin^2(\pi\omega/2\omega_o)\tan(\pi\omega/2\omega_o).$$

This impedance is in series with the capacitors C_o and C' of the KLM model, and consequently, with the help of the expression for C' in Fig. 6.17, the total electrical input impedance is given by

(6.34)
$$Z_{in} = \underline{V}/\underline{I} = \frac{1}{j\omega C_o}\left[1 - \frac{(k^t)^2}{(\pi\omega/2\omega_o)}\tan(\pi\omega/2\omega_o)\right].$$

By rewriting this as $Z_{in} = (1/j\omega C_o) + Z_m$, Z_m can be identified as the additional input impedance caused by the acoustic motion and is generally called the *motional acoustic impedance*. Three additional features of (6.34) should also be noted. The first is that if $\omega \to \omega_o(2n + 1)$, where $n = 0,1,2..$, then $|Z_{in}| \to \infty$, i.e., antiresonances occur when the transducer thickness is an odd number of half wavelengths. Specifically, the value $n = 0$ corresponds to the fundamental (half wavelength) antiresonant (parallel) frequency ($\omega_p \equiv \omega_o$).

The second feature of (6.34) is that $|Z_{in}| = 0$ when the term in brackets is zero, i.e., when

$$\pi\omega/2\omega_o = (k^t)^2 \tan(\pi\omega/2\omega_o).$$

The solution to this equation gives the series resonant frequency, which will differ from the value obtained in the absence of electromechanical coupling. It can be readily shown that in the absence of any coupling ($k^t = 0$), $\omega = \omega_o$; in addition, as the coupling approaches unity ($k^t \rightarrow 1$), $\omega \rightarrow 0$. For example, if $k^t = 0.49$, and $f_o = 5 \times 10^6$ MHz, then the series resonant frequency is $f_s = 4.46 \times 10^6$ Hz, which is precisely the value obtained for the example given with the simplified circuit model of Fig. 6.18 in the absence of loading ($Z_B = Z_T = 0$, $R = 0$). As pointed out and experimentally verified by Onoe et al. [108], the shift in series resonant frequency can be attributed to the influence of the electromechanical coupling.

Finally, it can be readily shown from (6.34) that the series and parallel resonance frequencies are related by

$$k_t = \sqrt{(\pi\omega_s/2\omega_p)}\tan[\pi(\omega_p - \omega_s)/2\omega_p].$$

Thus, by measuring the two resonant frequencies for an unloaded transducer, the coupling factor can be determined [42,108].

6.6.3 Loaded Input Impedance

Of considerable practical importance is the input impedance for any load or backing impedances. This can be obtained either directly from (6.27) by putting $Z_B = -\underline{F}_1/\underline{v}_1$ and $Z_T = -\underline{F}_2/\underline{v}_2$, and then solving for $Z_{in} = \underline{V}/\underline{I}$, or by direct use of either the Mason or KLM models. For this more general case,

(6.35)
$$Z_{in} = \frac{V}{I} = \frac{1}{j\omega C_o} + Z_m,$$
(a)

where the motional acoustic impedance is given by [80]

(6.35)
$$Z_m = \frac{(k^t)^2\{jZ_a(Z_B + Z_T)\sin(\pi\omega/\omega_o) - 2Z_a^2[1 - \cos(\pi\omega/\omega_o)]\}}{j\omega C_o(\pi\omega/\omega_o)[(Z_a^2 + Z_B Z_T)\sin(\pi\omega/\omega_o) - jZ_a(Z_B + Z_T)\cos(\pi\omega/\omega_o)]}.$$
(b)

As expected, when the transducer is unloaded ($Z_B = Z_T = 0$), the input impedance reduces to that given by (6.34).

6.6.4 Power Transfer Efficiency

For pulse-echo transducers, the conversion efficiency of power from an electrical source into an acoustic load and power from an acoustic source to an electrical load are generally important design factors. In efficiently delivering energy from an electrical source to an acoustic load, both the electrical matching between the source and transducer and the acoustic matching conditions at the front and back ports should be carefully considered. Similar considerations apply when the transducer is used as a detector. For pulse-echo applications, the bandwidth and associated phase delay are of major importance. A wide bandwidth will not necessarily give good pulse-echo response unless it is accompanied by a fairly linear change in phase over the passband. For example, if the skirts of the bandpass characteristics are too steep or there is a high ripple in the pass band, the associated nonlinear phase shift can extend the duration of the impulse response (sometimes called ringdown). On transmission, this increases the effective pulse duration, which can degrade the axial resolution of a pulse-echo system.

The first paper to systematically study the electrical and acoustic conditions needed to optimize the performance was that published by Kossoff [99] in 1966. He discussed the effects of backing, matching of the front face, and phase shift. This work was extended by subsequent studies of Goll and Auld [100,101] and Desiltes et al. [87] and in an important review by Hunt et al. [47]. Because of the large number of variable parameters, the problem of determining an optimal design has often been approached using computer-based optimization methods either in the time domain [102] or frequency domain [103]. More recently, Rhyne [104] has described the development of a computer-based optimization approach in which the properties of the various acoustic matching layers are adjusted to achieve a best match to an appropriately selected target transfer function. Using classic filter theory and accounting for losses, he showed that within the passband, the system transfer function has an all-pole characteristic and can be optimized by using a steepest descent algorithm to achieve a best match to an all-pole target transfer function.

Electrical Matching

If the transducer is assumed to be lossless, then it is relatively straightforward to calculate the power delivered to the acoustic load and to express this in terms of the power delivered by the source. By using an electrical matching network between the source and transducer, the power transfer efficiency can be optimized. The network design is based on the well-known fact that that maximum power transfer is achieved when the load impedance is equal to the complex conjugate of the source impedance, i.e., $Z_s = Z_L^*$. As indicated in Fig. 6.27a, for a source whose output impedance is real, this network should cancel out the imaginary part of the load impedance. Thus, if the transducer is represented as the series combination of an acoustic radiation resistance $R_a(\omega)$ and a reactance $X(\omega)$, the input impedance of the network when loaded by the transducer should be equal to the source resistance R_s over the entire frequency range of practical interest. Simple networks can achieve this only over a limited frequency range; more complex networks are needed for wide-band matching.

The power transfer efficiency to both acoustic ports can be defined by

$$(6.36) \quad \eta = \frac{\text{Total Acoustic Output Power (at both Ports)}}{\text{Maximum (matched) Electrical Power Delivered}}$$

$$= \frac{W}{|V_s|^2/(8R_s)},$$

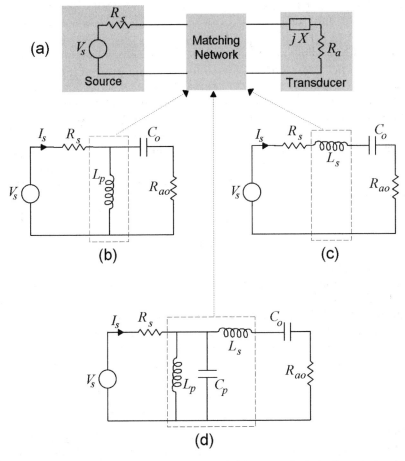

Figure 6.27 Some electrical matching networks. (a) General block diagram in which the transducer is represented by a radiation resistance and a reactance X. (b) Shunt and (c) series inductance matching networks. (d) More complex network according to the design discussed by Selfridge et al. [102]. The above three networks are shown with the transducer at its antiresonant frequency.

in which W is the total acoustic power and $|V_s|^2/(8R_s)$ is the maximum power delivered by the source.[21] When power is being emitted from both ports, the transfer efficiency for the front port is reduced from the overall efficiency by the factor $Z_T/(Z_T + Z_B)$ and can be found from

(6.37)
$$\eta_F = \eta \frac{Z_T}{Z_T + Z_B} = \frac{8R_s P Z_T}{|V_s|^2(Z_T + Z_B)},$$

21. Note that we are working in terms of sinusoidal phasor amplitudes: had we been using RMS values, the numerical factor would be 4 rather than 8.

where P is the total acoustic power from both ports. Consequently, for equally loaded ports the transfer efficiency for one of the ports will be $-3\,dB$ ($= 10\log0.5$) less than the overall efficiency.

In the block diagram of Fig. 6.27a, the transducer input impedance is modeled by the series combination of an acoustic radiation resistance R_a and a reactance X. The general optimization problem consists of finding the electrical matching network that will maximize the power transfer over the required bandwidth. We shall consider the simpler case in which the transducer is excited at its antiresonant frequency and the matching network simply consists of either a shunt inductor or a series inductor as shown in (b) and (c), where R_{ao} is given by (6.32). It is evident that if $L = 1/(\omega_o C_o)$, the input impedance seen by the source will be purely resistive, and if the inductor is ideal, it will equal R_{ao}. Under these circumstances the power transfer efficiency is

$$\eta = \frac{W}{|V_s|^2/(8R_s)} = \frac{4R_{ao}R_s}{(R_{ao}+R_s)^2},$$

which, as expected, is unity when $R_{ao} = R_s$.

In the general off-resonance case, the input impedance of the transducer will be given by $Z_{in}(\omega) = R_a(\omega) + jX(\omega)$ and the acoustic power can be found from $W = \mathrm{Re}\{\underline{V}\underline{I}^*/2\}$, where $\underline{V}$ and $\underline{I}$ are the voltage and current phasors at the transducer terminals and the star denotes the complex conjugate. Application of this equation to the circuit of Fig. 6.27a, with a matching network consisting of a series inductance of $L = 1/(\omega_o^2 C_o)$, results in an efficiency of

$$\eta(\omega) = \frac{4R_a R_s}{(R_a+R_s)^2 + \left[\omega/(\omega_o^2 C_o) + X(\omega)\right]^2},$$

which reduces to the previous equation for the particular case of $\omega = \omega_o$.

To illustrate the effects of including a series inductance on the impedance characteristics and the effects of impedance mismatch, we shall again consider a 5-MHz PZT-5H air-backed disk transducer with a 5-mm diameter. The relevant properties are $k^t = 0.49$, $(c_o)^D = 4620\,m/s$, $\varepsilon^S = 1470\varepsilon_o$, $\ell = 0.462\,mm$, and $C_o = 553\,pF$. From Fig. 6.28a, it can be seen that the real part of the transducer input impedance is $\sim18\,\Omega$ at 5.0MHz. At this frequency the presence of the series inductor will cause the load seen by the source to be real and to be equal to $18\,\Omega$, resulting in a power transfer efficiency of unity. The impedance graph also shows the imaginary part of the input impedance of an inductor in series with the transducer, which, as expected, is exactly zero at 5.0MHz.

The transmission power loss[22] characteristics shown in Fig. 6.28b indicate that the series inductor decreases the power loss, though with some reduction ($\sim17\%$) in the -3-dB bandwidth. In accord with the observations of Hunt

---

22. The power loss or gain in dB's is defined by:

$$\overline{W}_{dB} = 10\log\left(\frac{\text{Power at Observation Point}}{\text{Electrical Power Delivered to the Transducer}}\right)$$

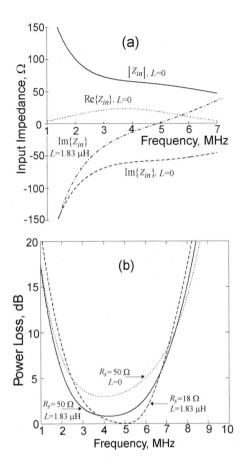

Figure 6.28 Effect of electrical matching using a series inductance on the characteristics of an air-backed 5 MHz PZT-5H disk transducer with a diameter of 5 mm. For simplicity, it was assumed that the front face was perfectly matched to the propagation medium at all frequencies. (a) Input impedance characteristics of the transducer. The imaginary part is shown with and without the tuning inductor. (b) Transmission power loss for (i) no tuning inductor and $R_s = 50\,\Omega$; an ideal series inductor with (ii) $R_s = 50\,\Omega$ and (iii) $R_s = 18\,\Omega$. Note that the real part of the transducer input impedance at 5.0 MHz is ~18 Ω.

et al. [47], it can be seen that the power loss characteristic is fairly insensitive to the mismatch between the source impedance and load. Specifically, at 5 MHz with the tuning inductor, when the source resistance is decreased by almost a factor of three (50 Ω to 18 Ω), the power loss increases by less than 1.2 dB. A further feature of this graph is that the frequency of minimum transmission loss for the untuned transducer is significantly lower than the half-wave resonant frequency, as noted by Kossoff [99].

The use of the simple shunt inductor circuit of Fig. 6.27b can similarly be examined. As shown by Hunt et al. [47], its use results in a higher impedance near the center frequency, which can make it easier to achieve better matching to a 50-Ω source. More complex electrical networks, such as that shown in Fig. 6.27d, have also been devised to obtain better matching over a wider range of frequencies [105,106].

Acoustic Matching

It is noted in Fig. 6.26 that the proper choice for the thickness and characteristic impedance of a matching layer enables the impedance seen by a piezoelectric medium to be perfectly matched to the transmission medium at the frequency where the matching layer thickness is exactly $\lambda/4$. However, at other frequencies a mismatch will occur, with a consequent reduction in transmitted power. As shown by Collin [107, pp. 345–346], if the acoustic impedance of the matching layer is $Z_M = \sqrt{Z_a Z_{T1}}$, where Z_{T1} is the acoustic impedance of the propagation medium, and R_m is the maximum reflection coefficient that can be tolerated over the angular frequency range of $\Delta\omega$, then the fractional range is given by

$$\frac{\Delta\omega}{\omega_o} = 2 - \frac{4}{\pi}\arccos\left|\frac{2R_m\sqrt{Z_a Z_{T1}}}{(Z_{T1} - Z_a)\sqrt{1 - R_m^2}}\right|.$$

The bandwidth is zero for $R_m = 0$ and increases with the maximum reflection that can be tolerated.

To calculate the electrical input impedance and power loss characteristics, we shall assume an air-backed transducer with a single matching layer of $Z_M = \sqrt{Z_a Z_{T1}}$. The impedance seen by port 2 of the transducer looking toward the transmission medium can be found from (6.31). Consequently, the load seen by port 2 per unit transducer area will be

$$Z_i(\omega) = \sqrt{Z_a Z_{T1}} \frac{Z_{T1} + j\sqrt{Z_a Z_{T1}}\tan(a_m\omega/\omega_o)}{\sqrt{Z_a Z_{T1}} + jZ_{T1}\tan(a_m\omega/\omega_o)},$$

where $a_m = \alpha\pi/2$ and α is unity[23] if the layer is exactly $\lambda/4$ thick at ω_o. By replacing Z_T in (6.35b) by the above expression for $Z_i(\omega)$, the electrical input impedance characteristics of the acoustically matched transducer can be calculated by substituting the result into (6.35a).

As an example, we consider the same 5-MHz PZT-5H disk transducer as previously assumed and will calculate the input impedance and transmission power loss characteristics. For both of the series tuned power loss curves shown in Fig. 6.29b, it can be seen that the ripple in the passband is significantly reduced compared to the untuned case. Comparison of the power loss characteristics with those for perfect matching over the entire frequency range

---

23. Goll [101] has shown that increasing the thickness of the quarter-wave plate, e.g., 4% to 10%, partially compensates for the frequency dependence of the KLM model transformer turns ratio, thereby making the response flatter in the passband [87].

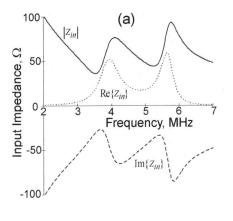
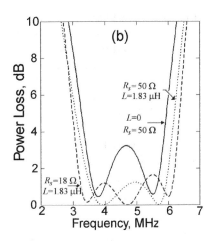

Figure 6.29 Air-backed 5-mm-diameter, 5-MHz PZT-5H disk transducer with a single $1.1\lambda_o/4$ acoustic matching of the front face to water and a series tuning inductor. The factor of 1.1 was chosen to reduce the ripple in the passband. (a) Input impedance of transducer. (b) Transmission power loss with and without a tuning inductor.

Table 6.5. Double Matching Layer Design for a Backed Transducer

Characteristic Acoustic Impedance	Formulae	Values for $Z_{T1} = 1.5$ MRayl and $Z_{ae} = 18.54$ MRayl
1st Layer	$Z_{M1} = Z_{ae}^{4/7} Z$	6.31 MRayl
2nd Layer	$Z_{M2} = Z_{ae}^{1/7} Z$	2.15 MRayl

Based on McKeighen [92].

(Fig. 6.28b) shows that use of the matching layer results in a reduction in the −3-dB bandwidth and steeper skirts.

To further improve the gain-bandwidth product, multiple matching layers can be used to advantage, though the problem of optimization is considerably more complex [87,101,109]. Desiltes et al. [87] examined the use of two quarter-wave matching layers and, assuming the transducer to be air-backed, derived the formulae given in Table 6.5. When the piezoelectric ceramic is backed by a medium with an acoustic impedance approaching the ceramic, as is typically used for generating a pulse with a short ringdown time, McKeighen [92] has shown that it is better to use an effective impedance Z_{ae} (seen looking into the piezoceramic, averaged over the bandwidth) in the formulae rather than the acoustic impedance of the bulk ceramic. For a ceramic of 33.4 MRayl with a backing impedance of 3 MRayl, he finds that $Z_{ae} = 18.54$ MRayl, which yields the two impedance values given in the right column.

To illustrate the potential advantages of a three-layer arrangement, the theoretical and measured responses for the transducer whose design parameters are listed in Table 6.6 are shown in Fig. 6.30. By placing an aluminum reflector close to the transducer surface and assuming that attenuation and beam spreading could be neglected in the intervening distance, the ratio of the transmitted power from a 50-Ω source to the received power in a 50-Ω load was determined. From this value the two-way insertion loss [35,110] was calculated. The authors reported that the measured two-way (−6 dB) bandwidth was 88% of the 4.02-MHz center frequency. In the passband, the experimentally observed losses are ~3 dB greater than those calculated. This could be due to the losses in the tuning inductor and transducer that were ignored in the calculations. By taking the inverse Fourier transform of the round-trip transfer function, the calculated impulse response was obtained this is compared to the measured response in Fig. 6.30b.

6.6.5 Effect of Backing

As previously noted, the backing layer acoustic impedance has a major effect on the power transfer efficiency and bandwidth. Specifically, it was noted that if the transducer is air-backed ($Z_B \sim 0$), almost no power is lost through the backing, while if it has the same acoustic impedance as the transducer, power will be lost to the backing both in transmission and reception. In the next subsection we shall examine the transfer efficiency for the latter condition in the absence of a matching network, though with an optimized source resistance. To produce a pulse with a short ringdown but to retain good efficiency, a compromise must be made in the backing impedance. In such a case, the backing medium will typically have an impedance in the range 3 to 7 MRayl. Often, polymer resins are used for both the front and back layers. The backing might consist of an epoxy loaded with powders of aluminum oxide, tungsten, and its oxides to produce sufficient attenuation so that echoes are on the order of −100 dB below the primary pulse [92].

Transfer Efficiency for $Z_B = Z_T = Z_o$

Let us consider the transfer efficiency to the front port at the resonant frequency from a source that has a resistive (R_s) impedance and that can be optimized to give the smallest loss. At the resonant frequency, the acoustic impedance is simply R_{ao} in series with C_o (Fig. 6.27c), so the acoustic power delivered to either port can be expressed as

$$W(\omega_o) = \frac{|V_s|^2 R_{ao}/2}{\left(R_{ao} + R_s\right)^2 + 1/\left(\omega_o C_o\right)^2}.$$

By substituting this into (6.37) and putting $Z_B = Z_T$, the power transfer efficiency becomes

$$\eta_F = \frac{2R_s R_{ao}}{\left(R_{ao} + R_s\right)^2 + 1/\left(\omega C_o\right)^2}.$$

Table 6.6. Values for a Triple Matching Layer Air-Backed Transducer

Piezoelectric ceramic (air-backed)	PbTiO₃
Diameter	15.0 mm
Thickness	0.625 mm
Effective coupling coefficient	0.53
Effective stiffened acoustic velocity	5034 m/s
Effective characteristic acoustic impedance	34.9 MRayl
Effective permittivity	145 ε₀
Series inductor (resonant at 0.87f₀)	4.6 μH
Matching layer 1 (light borosilicate glass)	
Characteristic acoustic impedance	14.2 MRayl
Speed of sound	5360 m/s
Matching layer 2 (glass-epoxy composite)	
Characteristic acoustic impedance	4.12 MRayl
Speed of sound	2800 m/s
Matching layer 3 (urethane resin)	
Characteristic acoustic impedance	1.92 MRayl
Speed of sound	1750 m/s
Thickness coefficient for all matching layers, α	1.18

Data from Inoue et al. [109].

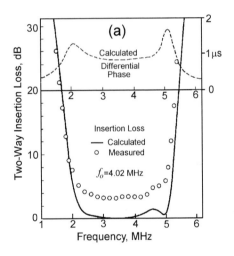
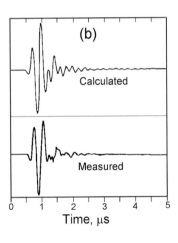

Figure 6.30 Measured and calculated characteristics of a triple matched, propagating into water, air-backed transducer whose parameters are given in Table 6.6. (a) Two-way CW insertion loss and differential phase delay. (b) Pulse-echo response. (Reproduced, with permission, from Inoue et al. [109], *IEEE Trans. Ultrason., Ferroelect., Freq. Contr.*, 34, 8–16, © 1987 IEEE.)

If this expression is differentiated with respect to R_s and equated to zero, the source resistance for maximum power transfer efficiency can be found as $R_s = R_{ao}\sqrt{1+1/(\omega C_o R_{ao})^2}$. By substituting this into the above equation and using (6.32) for the radiation resistance, the optimal transfer efficiency can be expressed as

$$(6.38) \qquad \eta_F^{opt} = \frac{1}{1+\sqrt{1+\pi^2/(k^t\sqrt{2})^4}},$$

which has a maximum value of 0.39 (–4.6 dB) when $k_t = 1$. If $k_t = 0.49$, then $\eta_F^{opt} = 0.131$ corresponding to –8.8 dB, which means that two-way insertion loss will be 17.6 dB. This should be compared to the air-backed case, for which the two-way transfer efficiency with tuning at the resonant frequency is 0 dB and 7 dB without tuning.[24]

6.7 Transient Response

A simple approach for determining the response for a given excitation wave-form is to multiply the frequency spectrum of the waveform by the transducer transfer function and to then to perform an inverse Fourier transform. Alternatively, an exact expression for the impulse response can be obtained, and this can then be convolved with the excitation waveform. For example, Kohler [112] has obtained an exact expression for the impulse response of a piezo-electric layer, assuming the backing and transmission media to be identical. While these methods provide direct quantitative results, physical insight is provided through the Redwood model of Fig. 6.16.

6.7.1 Impulse Response

The Redwood model [83] provides a convenient means for qualitatively estimating the response to an impulse of voltage for various termination conditions of practical interest [80, pp. 47–50]. Redwood simplified his model [111] by assuming that the effect of the negative capacitance could be ignored, i.e., it behaves like a short circuit, and that the voltage source was ideal. This source, together with C_o, can now be placed on the acoustic side of the transformer (Fig. 6.31). With the help of this model, Redwood showed that a voltage impulse will cause a stress to be immediately generated at each surface, and as a result waves will be propagated from both surfaces in both directions.

For the first termination condition illustrated in Fig. 6.31a, both ports are assumed to be perfectly matched to the piezoelectric medium. If the source is a positive voltage impulse at $t = 0$, then a positive stress impulse will be present on both surfaces at $t = 0$, and the acoustic "voltage" will be equally divided between the load and the coaxial line impedance, i.e., $F_1(t) = F_1(t) = V/(2\phi)$. On examining the figure it can be seen that the voltage pulse across the coaxial

---

24. For this case it can be shown that $\eta_F^{opt} = 2/\left[1+\sqrt{1+\pi^2/(2k^t)^4}\right]$.

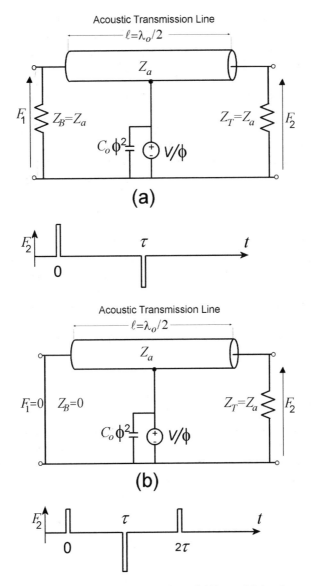

Figure 6.31 An approximate form of the Redwood 1-D model for determining the voltage impulse response. (a) Both the back and front ports exactly matched. (b) Back port shorted ($Z_B = 0$) and front port matched. The acoustic waveforms at the front port for both conditions are shown for a voltage impulse. The pulses are sketched as short-duration, finite-amplitude pulses.

line (center conductor to sheath) is inverted with a value of $-V/(2\phi)$, so that the pulse originating from the surface of the back port will arrive at the front port after a time equal to the transit time τ through the piezoelectric medium; this therefore results in a negative stress pulse on the front face.

For the second termination condition shown in Fig. 6.31b, the backing is assumed to be a short circuit with the front surface matched. In this case, the coaxial line will have the full voltage across it $(-V/\phi)$ at the backing port, and as a result a negative stress will occur at $t = \tau$ on the front surface, which is double the stress that occurred at $t = 0$. The negative wave progressing from the front port to the left will be reflected and inverted at the backing port and will arrive back at the front port after a delay of 2τ, giving the third pulse shown in the bottom half of the figure. This extended time duration of the impulse response corresponds to a reduction in bandwidth as compared to the matched backing case.

Additional reflected pulses can occur in both cases due to imperfect matching, and these further extend the duration of the acoustic response to a short-duration excitation. Experimental measurements have shown qualitative agreement with the above model [80, pp. 47–50; 111], and these provide some justification for ignoring the effects of the negative capacitor.

From the above discussion it would seem better to match the back port to a highly absorbing medium. However, as noted earlier, the loss of energy from the backing port causes a large increase in the two-way insertion loss.

6.7.2 Differential Phase Delay

Both the insertion loss and phase characteristics provide useful indications of the transient response characteristics. While the insertion loss provides information on the bandwidth, the phase characteristics provides information concerning distortion that arises from the nonlinear frequency dependence of the phase shift. The delay associated with the change in phase with frequency is determined by

$$\tau(\omega) = \frac{d\theta}{d\omega},$$

where θ is the phase expressed in radians. Now, the phase shift can readily be determined by making use of the matrix method described in section 6.5.3; specifically, θ can be found from $\theta(\omega) = \arg(A_{11}^{tr} A_{11}^{rec})$, where the matrix components are given in Figs. 6.22 and 6.23.

To illustrate these results, we consider the same air-backed 5-MHz PZT-5H disk transducer as previously assumed (see Fig. 6.29). The two-way insertion loss and input/output phase characteristics are shown in Fig. 6.32. Also shown is the slope of the phase shift, which provides a measure of the time-domain characteristics. It is evident that the series tuned transducer response has reduced ripple in the passband and therefore should have a transient response with less distortion. For the three-layer structure previously considered in

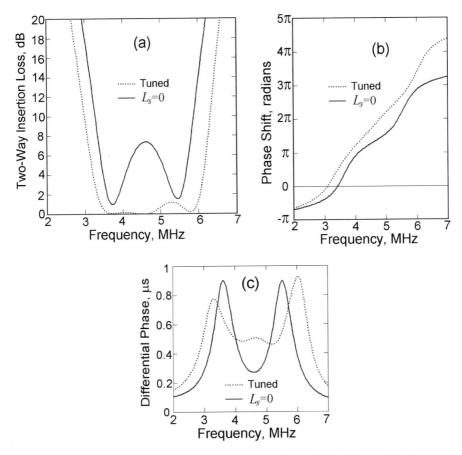

Figure 6.32 Two-way (a) insertion loss, (b) phase shift, and (c) differential phase delay for an air-backed transducer with a single matching layer to a water load. Each graph shows the influence of a simple series tuning inductor. An excitation source resistance of $R_s = 18\,\Omega$ and a receiving preamplifier load of $R_L = 50\,\Omega$ were assumed. The two-way insertion loss was calculated from (6.30).

Fig. 6.30, the differential phase delay exhibits a much flatter response in the passband.

6.8 Protection Circuits

In pulse-echo systems in which the same transducer acts as both an acoustic source and detector, a means must be provided to isolate the preamplifier from the large excitation voltage used during transmission and to prevent the relatively small received signal from being partially attenuated by the transmission circuit. Typically, the excitation pulse may be many tens of volts, which, if allowed to enter the sensitive receiving preamplifier, could cause permanent damage. Even if damage does not result, saturation of the preamplifier can result and a long recovery time before linear operation is restored may occur. During the reception phase, it is important that the transmitter circuit be isolated from the transducer. If some of the available received power from the transducer is dissipated in the transmitter, the sensitivity would be reduced, and in addition the noise contributed by the transmitter circuits might degrade the SNR. Protection circuits are generally used to achieve these aims, and some examples are described below.

6.8.1 Low-Frequency Protection Circuits

Follett and Atkinson [113] have described one approach to achieving good isolation, and a modified version of their circuit is shown in Fig. 6.33a. The back-to-back diode pairs D_1, D_2, and D_3 act as limiters that prevent the voltage

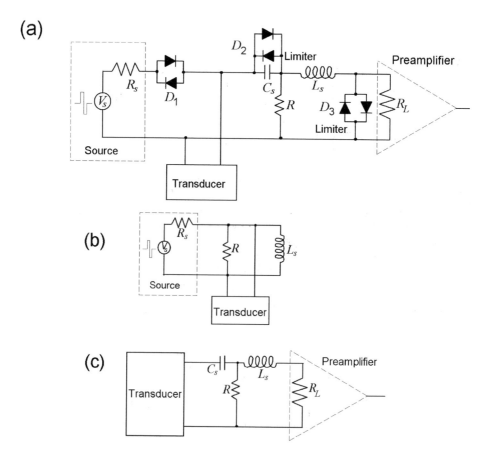

Figure 6.33 Transmit/receive protection circuit in which the transducer "box" is assumed to contain electrical matching. (a) Complete circuit: the diode pair D_1 is sometimes called an expander. If the diodes are assumed to be ideal, the circuit simplifies to (b) during transmission and to (c) during reception.

across them from exceeding some small value, e.g., ±0.7 V. For simplicity we assume that the transducer is tuned and matched to both R_s and R_L $(R_s = R_L)$ and that $R \gg R_L$. During the excitation pulse, all three diode limiters can be approximated as short circuits, so that the circuit simplifies to that of Fig. 6.33b, in which the voltage across the transducer terminals is the same as that across the inductor L_s. During reception, because the voltage generated by the transducer will be small, all three diode pairs act as open circuits, so that the amplifier and capacitor C_s are activated and the transmission source is disconnected, enabling the circuit to be reduced to Fig. 6.33c. By choosing the series combination of L_s and C_s to satisfy $\omega_o = 1/\sqrt{L_sC_s}$, the transducer will be matched to the amplifier input impedance at the transducer antiresonant frequency. If L_s is chosen so that its reactance is much larger than R_L, (e.g., $\omega_oL_s = 5R_L$: for example, if $R_L = 50\,\Omega$ and $f_o = 5\,MHz$, then $L_s = 8.0\,\mu H$ and $C_s = 127$ pF) then, during the transmission period, most of the available source energy is delivered to the transducer. The inclusion of resistor R, e.g., $500\,\Omega$, results in a reduction in the time needed to eliminate the stored energy and therefore in a reduced amplifier dead time.

A second and rather simpler approach is that shown in Fig. 6.34. Resistors R_1, R_2, and R_3 are all chosen to be much greater than R_L and are such that in combination with the voltage $-V$, both diodes D_2 are conducting during the reception phase. For this phase the incremental resistance of both diodes is in series with R_L, thereby causing some signal loss and a decrease in SNR. During the transmit phase, one of these diodes will be reverse biased, thereby preventing most of the signal from reaching the preamplifier. The diode pair D_3 will limit what reaches the preamplifier.

For ultrasound imaging systems that use a large number of transducer elements for steering and focusing, the problem of protection can be circumvented if the processes of acoustic field generation and reception use separate array elements. For 2-D arrays, as used for 3-D real-time imaging, many hundreds (perhaps several thousand) individual elements may be needed. To reduce the need for a large number of transmission lines and to avoid difficulties associated with the power dissipation in the transducer casing, separation of the two functions becomes particularly important [69].

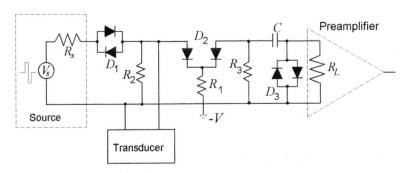

Figure 6.34 An alternative form of a transmit/receive protection circuit (courtesy Mike Fife and Dr. Clyde Oakley, Tetrad Corp., Englewood, CO).

6.8.2 High-Frequency Protection Circuits

If the connections between the transducer to the transmitter and receiver to the transducer are much less than a wavelength, then transmission line effects can be ignored. For example, suppose that a coaxial cable is used to connect the transmitter and receiver to a 20-MHz transducer. A typical small-diameter coaxial cable[25] may have a propagation speed of around 0.6 of the speed of light, and consequently, at 10 MHz, one wavelength would correspond to 18 m. For cable lengths of less than about 1 m, the influence of the cable can be approximately represented by its lumped capacitance. At higher frequencies or with longer transmission lines, the impedance properties, which depend on the termination conditions, need to be accounted for. In fact, transmission lines of the proper lengths and appropriate termination conditions can be used to obtain nearly perfect matching (at a single frequency) of the transducer to a source or a load.

Long transmission lines and high-frequency transducers are needed in certain medical applications, such as catheter- and endoscope-based imaging systems. Lockwood et al. [116] have described how protection of the preamplifier can be achieved along with a good pulse-echo response by proper choice of the transmission line lengths between the excitation source, transducer, and receiver. Their method made use of a computer search in which the line lengths were varied to determine the combination needed to maximize the pulse-echo amplitude response. Subsequently, using a transmission matrix approach (see section 6.5.3), Lockwood and Foster [117] made use of a time-domain "badness" criterion previously introduced by Selfridge et al. [102] to choose the best transmission line electrical matching network. The "badness" criterion consists of a function that incorporates the effects of both the pulse-echo amplitude and its duration, so that optimization of the electrical matching network was achieved by searching for a combination of transmission line properties that minimize this function.

One of the designs given by Lockwood et al. [116] is shown in Fig. 6.35. A 45- to 50-MHz transducer is assumed to be at the end of a 100-cm catheter and is connected via a 50-Ω transmission line to the catheter entrance. The preamplifier input and excitation source are also connected via 50-Ω

---

25. Although the means by which the probe is connected to the transmitter and receiver are somewhat beyond the scope of this book, nonetheless it does present some interesting practical challenges. For transducer arrays with a large number of elements that must be individually addressed, e.g., 256, the weight and flexibility associated with the use of coaxial cables can be a serious problem. In addition, for an intravascular imaging array transducer, because the connections need to be passed down a catheter, the maximum diameter is limited to a few millimeters. For both of these applications, the use of miniature coaxial cables with impedances of around 75 Ω and signal isolations of around 60 dB may not be practical. An interesting scheme that enables a fairly large number, e.g., 50, of coaxial-like cables to be packed together is described by Buck and Olson [114]. Ribbon-based cables [115] provide an alternate means. Typically, they have characteristic impedances of 120 Ω, and the isolation between conductors is in the range of 30 to 40 dB.

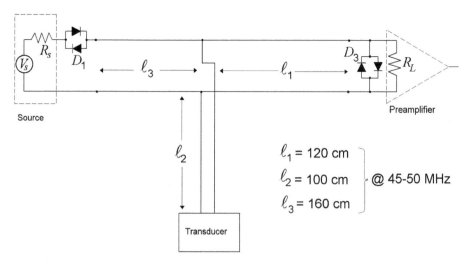

Source

Preamplifier

$\ell_1 = 120$ cm
$\ell_2 = 100$ cm   @ 45-50 MHz
$\ell_3 = 160$ cm

Transducer

Figure 6.35 Use of transmission lines (coaxial cables) to achieve the best pulse-echo response for a high-frequency transducer at the end of a 100-cm catheter. (Based on Lockwood et al. [116].)

transmission lines and join the transducer transmission line at the T-junction located near the catheter entrance. During transmission, diodes D_3 appear as a short circuit, so that if $\ell_1 = \lambda_o/4$, the line appears as an open circuit at the T-junction (though only at the center frequency). Consequently, the excitation signal is transmitted to the transducer with little loss of energy. During reception, line ℓ_1 is assumed to be matched to the amplifier input resistance. However, line ℓ_3, which is open-circuited, has an important influence, depending on its length. Assuming that ℓ_2 is fixed by the length of the catheter, the best values for ℓ_1 and ℓ_3 were determined by computer simulations, and these are given in the figure. It should be noted that the value chosen for ℓ_1 is somewhat greater than a quarter-wavelength length (100 cm).

Poulsen [118] has also discussed the issue of wideband protection at high frequencies and has shown that by inserting a wideband small-signal transformer at the preamplifier end of ℓ_1, the signal loss on reception can be significantly reduced.

6.9 Noise Considerations

One approach for improving the SNR of a pulse-echo system, thereby enabling weak echoes to be detected, is to increase the transmitted power. However, limitations imposed by the effects of nonlinear propagation, power dissipation in the transducer and/or the transducer housing, breakdown voltage limits, and regulatory safety issues may not make this possible. If a limitation is imposed on the maximum transmitted power or voltage, then one method to enable echoes from deeper-lying structures to be detected can be achieved by reducing the system noise. This requires that noise properties of the piezoelectric medium, amplifier, connecting cable, and electrical matching elements be included in the overall system model so that the SNR can be optimized.

A number of papers have addressed these issues. Some have addressed the problem of optimizing hydrophone sensitivity to obtain the best SNR [119–122], and others have been concerned with the problem of optimizing the performance of ultrasound imaging arrays [69,123,124].

In the approach used by Rhyne [125], the transmission and reception properties are separately accounted for. He shows that the transmission properties can be characterized by the *radiation efficiency* spectrum, which is defined as the ratio of the acoustic power delivered to the transmission medium, to the maximum power that can be withdrawn from the excitation source. It is an absolute measure of the performance and has an upper bound of 0 dB, corresponding to all the available power from the source being delivered to the acoustic load. The radiation efficiency accounts for any impedance mismatch as well as power losses in the transducer and connecting transmission line, and has the advantage of being *independent* of the excitation source impedance.

Rhyne [125] shows how the transmission and reception properties are affected by the design by considering two transducers whose properties are listed in Table 6.7. To illustrate the effects of electrical matching to a 50-Ω transmission line, transducer A uses a matching transformer and the second transducer (B) is mismatched. Both transducers are assumed to be air-backed and have two front acoustic matching layers. Transducer A has a Butterworth

Table 6.7. Properties of Transducers A and B (see Fig. 6.36)

Property	A—Butterworth	B—Chebyshev
Area	1.1 mm^2	1.1 mm^2
Z_T	1.54 MRayl	1.54 MRayl
Z_B	400 Rayl	400 Rayl
Z_o	32 MRayl	32 MRayl
f_o	5.89 MHz	4.918 MHz
Z_1	6.90 MRayl	7.71 MRayl
f_1	4.83 MHz	4.78 MHz
Z_2	2.10 MRayl	2.31 MRayl
f_2	4.98 MHz	4.96 MHz
Matching transformer turns-ratio	3.83	N/A
$|Z_{in}|$ @ 5 MHz	*54.9 Ω	637 Ω
arg(Z_{in}) @ 5 MHz	−30.9°	−36.1°
−3 dB bandwidth	70%	70%

Data from Rhyne [125].
* As seen from the transmission line side of the matching transformer.

transfer function and an input impedance magnitude of 55 Ω, as seen via a 3.83 (turns ratio) transformer. The second transducer has a Chebyshev transfer function, no matching transformer, and an input impedance magnitude of 637 Ω. It can be seen from Fig. 6.36a that the radiation efficiency over the passband for transducer A is close to −0.9 dB, while for transducer B, which is severely mismatched to a lossless 50-Ω transmission line, there is a loss of approximately 7 dB. To illustrate the influence of transmission line losses, Rhyne assumed that the 50-Ω transmission line was 2.0 m long and that the losses arose from its series resistance of 3 Ω/m. He found that the passband loss for transducer A is increased by approximately 0.6 dB.

To characterize the properties of the reception system, the noise contributed by the various parts must be considered. Four sources of noise that contribute to the total noise at the output of the preamplifier can be readily identified: (i) acoustic thermal noise from the radiation resistance, (ii) noise

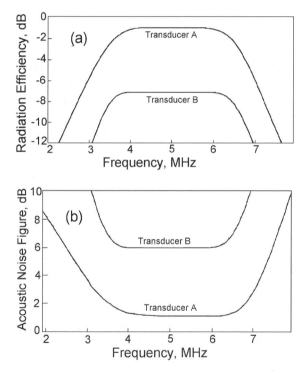

Figure 6.36 For transducers A and B listed in Table 6.7: (a) radiation efficiency spectrum assuming a lossless 50-Ω transmission line, (b) acoustic noise figure spectrum assuming a lossless noise-matched 50-Ω transmission line and a preamplifier with an input resistance 50 Ω, an optimal noise source resistance of 50 Ω, and a noise figure 1.2 dB. From (a) it can be seen that both transducers have a −3 dB bandwidth of 3.5 MHz centered at 5 MHz. (Reproduced, with permission, from Rhyne [125], *IEEE Trans. Ultrason., Ferroelect., Freq. Contr.*, 45, 559–566, © 1998 IEEE.)

arising from electrical and mechanical losses in the transducer, (iii) noise due to losses in the transmission line and matching elements, and (iv) noise contributed by the preamplifier.

Because the thermal noise power arising from the radiation resistance is inherent to the system, Rhyne [125] points out that it makes good sense to characterize the reception sensitivity by means of the acoustic noise factor $F(\omega)$ or noise figure, $F_{dB}(\omega) = 10 \log F(\omega)$. These provide a direct measure of the degradation of the preamplifier output by the noise arising from the transducer, transmission line, and preamplifier. If the acoustic noise factor is defined by:

$$F(\omega) = \frac{\text{SNR at preamplifier input due to acoustic radiation noise}}{\text{SNR at preamplifier input due to acoustic radiation}}\text{,}$$
$$\text{plus all other noise sources}$$

then the amount by which the noise figure is below 0 dB is an absolute measure of the noise contributed by the transducer, transmission line, and preamplifier.

The piezoelectric transducer can contribute to the noise through mechanical and electrical loss mechanisms. Mechanical losses can be accounted for by including an attenuation coefficient (a complex wavenumber), and electrical losses through the inclusion of a series resistance. Both of these are accounted for in the matrix equation given by (6.28). A coaxial cable connecting the transducer to the amplifier can also contribute to noise through the thermal noise arising from its series resistance and dielectric loss. In addition, the loss resistance of an inductor used for tuning and a matching transformer (if used) will also contribute. Finally, the noise characteristics of the preamplifier and the impedance conditions existing at its input must be included.

The overall acoustic noise figure is the sum of the transducer and preamplifier noise figures. The contribution due to the transducer is unaffected by the loading presented by the preamplifier. On the other hand, the source impedance affects the noise figure contributed by the preamplifier. It can be shown that the best noise performance occurs when the real part of the transducer input impedance is equal to the optimal noise source resistance of the preamplifier. A good deal of flexibility exists in preamplifier design, enabling a fairly wide range of optimal noise source resistances to be achieved without increasing the amplifier noise figure. As an example, Rhyne [125] selected a preamplifier with a noise figure of 1.2 dB, an input resistance of 50 Ω, and an optimal noise resistance of the same value. Consequently, a 50-Ω transmission line was chosen for linking the transducer (or matching transformer) and preamplifier. The calculated noise figure spectra for the two designs are illustrated in Fig. 6.36b. It can be seen that transducer A, which is well matched to the optimal noise resistance, has a noise figure close to that of the preamplifier, while transducer B, which is severely mismatched, has an acoustic noise figure of about 6 dB.

6.10 Capacitive Transducers

The idea of using the force between different charges on a conducting membrane and a closely spaced metal plate was initially proposed and used as a means of generating sound waves around the 1880s. In a paragraph summarizing some earlier work, *La Lumiere Electrique* [126] referred to earlier work proposing the use of a capacitor as a means of generating sound as well as for detecting it. Dolbear in 1880 and 1881 filed two U.S. patent applications [127,128] that clearly described the use of electrostatic attraction between two plates as a means for both generating and detecting sound. These events took place a few years subsequent to the invention of the moving coil (electromagnetic) method of generating sound in the mid-1870s. Subsequently, there were a number of reports [129,130], including a U.S. patent[26] filed in 1929 [131], for producing sound by electrostatic means. Many of these have been described in Hunt's authoritative book [132] on electroacoustics, which includes a carefully researched chapter on the history, together with many original source references. The 1916 report by Langevin and Chilowski [133] appears to be the first to discuss the generation of ultrasound by using a capacitor structure. In their early experiments for developing a method of underwater submarine detection, they used a thin sheet of mica on an insulated metal plate. The water in which this structure was immersed formed the other plate of the capacitor. With this design they generated ultrasonic waves at frequencies of around 100 kHz, though with intensities considerably below that needed for successful application for submarine detection. They appreciated the need for very high electric fields (on the order of 10^6 V/cm) to generate intense pressure waves; however, electrical breakdown severely limited what they could achieve. In the years up to 1985, occasional reports have appeared [134,135] describing electrostatic ultrasonic transducers. More recently, with the development of silicon-based microfabrication technology, there has been a revival of interest in electrostatic transducers for both air and fluid applications.

We consider first the simple parallel plate structure illustrated in Fig. 6.37, in which the moveable upper plate is supported by a spring. For an applied voltage of V, the attractive electrostatic force between the plates can be found from the change in stored energy for an incremental change in plate separation. For a medium of thickness ℓ and permittivity ε separating the plates, the force can be found from

(6.39)
$$F_C = -\frac{\partial W}{\partial z} = -\frac{\partial}{\partial z}\left(\frac{1}{2}CV^2\right) = -\frac{1}{2}V^2\frac{\partial}{\partial z}\left(\frac{\varepsilon A}{\ell - z}\right)$$
$$= \frac{\varepsilon A V^2}{(\ell - z)^2}$$

---

26. The patent described an electrostatic speaker composed of many small sections able to radiate sound without magnets or cones or baffles. The first commercial full-range electrostatic loudspeaker (Quad ESL) was based on this patent and was marketed in 1957.

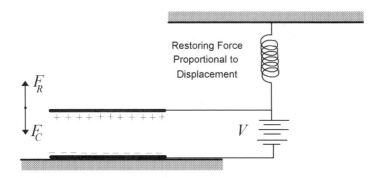

Figure 6.37 Simplified model of an electrostatic transducer consisting of two parallel plates: a fixed bottom plate and a moveable upper plate attached to a spring.

where A is the plate area and C is the capacitance. From this it can be seen that the attractive force is independent of the sign of V. Consequently, in the absence of any DC bias, the application of a sinusoidal source of $V_{ac}\sin(\omega t)$ will result in $0.5V_{ac}[1-\cos(2\omega t)]$, corresponding to a DC and a second harmonic component. In the presence of a polarizing voltage V_p, we have $V = V_p + V_{ac}\sin(\omega t)$, so that the force is given by

$$F_C = \frac{\varepsilon A[V_p + V_{ac}\sin(\omega t)]^2}{(\ell - z)^2} \approx \frac{\varepsilon A[V_p^2 + 2V_pV_{ac}\sin(\omega t)]}{(\ell - z)^2},$$

provided $V_{ac} \ll V_p$. Consequently, by applying a polarizing voltage or by incorporating a medium with a permanent polarization, i.e., an electret, the fundamental component can be retained.

Assuming a restoring force proportional to the plate displacement, equilibrium requires that $F_C = F_R = kz$, where k is a "spring" constant. Consequently, by making use of (6.39), the equation describing the equilibrium position is given by

(6.40) $$kz = \frac{\varepsilon A V^2}{(\ell - z)^2}.$$

It should be noted that as the voltage is increased, a z-location is reached at which the electrostatic force can no longer be balanced by the spring restoring force. At this location, an increment in the applied voltage will cause a catastrophic collapse of the moveable plate to the underlying one. The approximate critical voltage (V_c) at which this occurs can be found by first determining the z-location from (6.40) by using the condition $\partial z/\partial V = \infty$. This yields $z_c = \ell/3$, which, when substituted back into (6.40), enables V_c to be found as

(6.41) $$V_c = \sqrt{\frac{8k\ell^3}{27\varepsilon A}}.$$

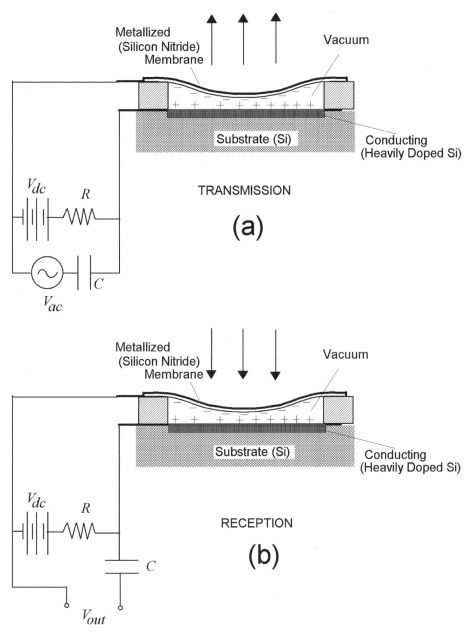

Figure 6.38 Principles of an electrostatic transducer used for (a) transmission and (b) reception. For both, a polarizing voltage V_{dc} is used.

As this critical voltage is approached, the sensitivity to an incident pressure signal on the membrane displacement increases. In fact, Hunt [132] has shown that the electromechanical coupling factor (defined in the same way as the piezoelectric coupling factor, see (6.10)) approaches unity as $V \to V_c$ and has reported measured values as high as 0.7.

In practice, the rim of the membrane will be clamped and the electrostatic force will vary over the membrane surface, depending on the distance to the substrate. This makes the analysis considerably more complex. A more realistic configuration is sketched in Fig. 6.38. Here, the application of a polarizing voltage causes the membrane to be attracted toward the substrate, its equilibrium position being determined by its elastic and geometric characteristics, the gap, the applied voltage, and the pressure difference. If an AC signal is superimposed on the polarizing voltage, the membrane will vibrate and a pressure wave will be propagated, as illustrated in (a). In a similar way, if a pressure wave is incident on the membrane, as shown in (b), the membrane–substrate gap will change and, because R is assumed to be large, a displacement current will flow, creating an AC output voltage.

For generating and detecting acoustic waves at higher frequencies, the mechanical resonant frequency is of major importance. This can be decreased by reducing the area. To compensate for the decreased sensitivity, a multiplicity of small elements connected in parallel must be used, as originally described in Kellogg's patent [131].

The development of silicon microfabrication technology, starting around the 1970s, provided the basis for making very small electrostatic devices for detecting and generating ultrasound. An early proposal is that of Higuchi et al. [136,137], who described the use of silicon micromachining technology for fabricating a linear array consisting of seven elements on the same chip and operating in the 100-kHz range. Anisotropic etching was used to make many small pyramidal holes in the underlying silicon and a metallized 12-μm polyester film was stretched over the surface to form a membrane for each element. The reproducibility of this type of membrane construction cannot be expected to be satisfactory. However, major improvements resulted from the use of silicon nitride membrane formed on a separate chip and subsequently bonded to the chip with the substrate holes. Holm and Hess [138] were the first to describe the use of this method for fabricating a subminiature condenser microphone. To maintain control over the stresses in the silicon nitride membrane, two silicon slices were used. One was used as the substrate and formed the fixed electrode; the second was processed to form a thin metallized silicon nitride membrane with a thickness of 150 nm. By bonding the two structures together, a microphone was formed. Relatively large-area ($0.8 \times 0.8\,\text{mm}^2$) structures were made in this manner.

Micromachined electrostatic transducers with silicon nitride membranes designed for transmission and reception in fluids were described in 1996 by Soh et al. [139]. These used a single wafer fabrication technique in which an underlying (sacrificial) layer was etched away to form the membrane. A multiplicity of individual elements were formed and connected in parallel to achieve a large effective area. As illustrated in Fig. 6.38, if the cavity is evacuated, the fluid pressure will cause the membrane to bend. Superimposed on this will be the added bending caused by the electrostatic polarizing force.

When immersed in water, the silicon nitride membrane is heavily damped, and as a result very wide fractional bandwidths can be achieved. This and the ease of manufacture and potentially high electromechanical conversion efficiency make micromachined electrostatic transducers an attractive possibility for 2-D and 3-D ultrasonic imaging. In fact, a 1-D array consisting of 128 elements, with each element containing 750 cells connected in parallel, has been used to obtain images of a test phantom immersed in vegetable oil [140]. More recent work with a 2-D array consisting of 0.4 × 0.4 mm elements, each containing 76 cells, has been used to demonstrate 3-D imaging [141].

References

1. Bell, A.G., Researches in telephony, *Proc. Am. Acad. Arts. Sci.*, 12, 1–10, 187 (Reproduced in: *Acoustic Transducers*, I.D. Groves (Ed.), Hutchinson Ross Pub. Co., Stroudsburg, PA, 1981.)
2. Joule, J.P., On the effect of magnetism upon dimensions of iron and steel bars, *Phil. Mag.*, 30, 76–87 and 225–241, 1847.
3. Villari, E., Intorno alle modificazioni del momento magnetico di una verga di fero e di acciaio, prodotte par la trazione della medesima e pel passaggio di una corrente attraverso la stressa, *Il Nuovo Cimento*, 20, 317–362, 1864. See also: Uber die Anderungen des Magnetischen Moments, welche der Zug un das Hindurchleiten eines Galvanischen Stroms in einem Stabe von Stahl oder Eisen Hervorbringen, *Annalen der Physik und Chemiue*, 126, 87–122, 1865.
4. Graff, K.F., A history of ultrasonics, Chapter 1, pp. 1–97, in: *Physical Acoustics*, Vol. 15, W.P. Mason, and R.N. Thurston (Eds.), Academic Press, New York, 1981.
5. Bell, A.G., Upon the production of sound by radiant energy, *Phil. Mag.*, 11, 510–528, 1881.
6. Hutchins, D.A., Ultrasonic generation by pulsed lasers, Ch. 2, pp. 21–123, in: *Physical Acoustics*, Vol. 18, W.P. Mason, and R.N. Thurston (Eds.), Academic Press, New York, 1988.
7. Scruby, C.B., and Drain, L.E., *Laser Ultrasonics, Techniques and Applications*, Adam Hilger, Bristol, UK, 1990.
8. Curie, P., and Curie, J., Développement par pression de l'électricité polaire dans les cristaux hémièdres à faces enclinées, *Compt. Rendus*, 91, 383, 1880.
9. Mason, W.P., Piezoelectricity, its history and applications, *J. Acoust. Soc. Am.*, 70, 1561–1566, 1981.
10. Cady, W.G., *Piezoelectricity* (p. 4), McGraw-Hill, New York, 1946.
11. Auld, B.A., Wave propagation and resonance in piezoelectric materials, *J. Acoust. Soc. Am.*, 70, 1577–1585, 1981.
12. Ristic, V.M., *Principles of Acoustic Devices*, Wiley, New York, 1983.
13. Langevin, P., Procédé et appareils d'émission et de réception des ondes élastiques sous-marines à l'aide des propriétés pièzo-électriques du quartz (Brevet francais, No 505703, Sept. 17, 1918), pp. 538–542, in: *Oevres Scientifiques de Paul Langevin*, CNRS, Paris, 1950.

14. Neubert, H.K.P., *Instrument Transducers* (p. 305), Oxford University Press, New York, 1963.

15. Cao, W., and Randall, C.A., Grain size and domain size relations in bulk ceramic ferroelectric materials, *J. Phys. Chem Solids*, 57, 1499–1505, 1996.

16. Jaffe, B., Roth, R.S., and Marzullo, S., Piezoelectric properties of lead zirconate-lead titanate solid solution ceramic ware, *J. Appl. Phys.*, 25, 809–810, 1954.

17. Jaffe, H., and Berlincourt, D.A., Piezoelectric transducer materials, *Proc. IEEE.*, 53, 1372–1386, 1965.

18. Berlincourt, D.A., Piezoelectric crystals and ceramics, Ch. 2, pp. 63–124, in: *Ultrasonic Transducer Materials*, O.E. Mattiat (Ed.), Plenum Press, New York, 1971.

19. Jaffe, B., Cook, W.R., and Jaffe, H., *Piezoelectric Ceramics*, Academic Press, New York, 1971.

20. Kuwata, J., Uchino, K., and Nomura, S., Phase transitions in the $0.91Pb(Zn_{1/3}Nbi_{2/3})O_3–0.09PbTiO_3$ system, *Ferroelectrics*, 37, 579–582, 1981. Also: Dielectric and piezoelectric properties of $0.91Pb(Zn_{1/3}Nbi_{2/3})O_3–0.09PbTiO_3$ single crystals, *Jpn. J. Appl. Phys.*, 21, 1298–1302, 1982.

21. Oakley, C.G., and Zipparo, M.J., Single crystal piezoelectrics: a revolutionary development for transducers, pp. 1157–1167, in: *2000 IEEE Ultrasonics Symp. Proc.*, 2000.

22. Saitoh, S., Izumi, M., Shimanuki, S., et al., Ultrasonic probe, US patent: 5,295,487, March 22, 1994 (filed Feb. 9, 1993).

23. Park, S-E., and Shrout, T.R., Characteristics of relaxor-based piezoelectric single crystals for ultrasonic transducers, *IEEE Trans. Ultrason., Ferroelect., Freq. Contr.*, 4, 1140–1147, 1997.

24. Ritter, T., Geng, X., Shung, K.K., et al., Single crystal ZN/PT-polymer composites for ultrasound transducer applications, *IEEE Trans Ultrason., Ferroelect., Freq. Contr.*, 47, 792–800, 2000.

25. Smith, W.A., Shaulov, A.A., and Singer, B.M., Properties of composite piezoelectric materials for ultrasonic transducers, pp. 539–544, in: *1984 IEEE Ultrasonics Symp. Proc.*, 1984.

26. Smith, W.A., The role of piezocomposites in ultrasonic transducers, pp. 755–766, in: *1989 IEEE Ultrasonics Symp. Proc.*, 1989.

27. Smith, W.A., New opportunities in ultrasonic transducers emerging from innovations in piezoelectric materials, pp. 3–26, in SPIE, Vol. 1733, 1992.

28. Papadakis, E.P., Oakley, C.G., Selfridge, A.R., and Maxfield, B., Fabrication and characterization of transducers, Ch. 2, pp. 43–134, in: *Ultrasonic Instruments and Devices II*, E.P. Papadakis (Ed.), Vol. 24 of: *Physical Acoustics: Principles and Methods*, R.N. Thurston, and A.D. Pierce (Eds.), Academic Press, New York, 1999.

29. Kawai, H., The piezoelectricity of poly(vinylidene) fluoride, *Jap. J. Appl. Phys.*, 8, 975–976, 1969.

30. Sessler, G.M., Piezoelectricity in polyvinylidenefluoride, *J. Acoust. Soc. Am.*, 70, 1596–1608, 1981.

31. Fukada, E., History and recent progress in piezoelectric polymers, *IEEE Trans. Ultrason., Ferroelect., Freq. Contr.*, 47, 1277–1290, 2000.

32. Foster, F.S., Harasiewicz, K.A., and Sherar, M.D., A history of medical and biological imaging with polyvinylidene fluoride (PVDF) transducers, *IEEE Trans. Ultrason., Ferroelect., Freq. Contr.*, 47, 1363–1371, 2000.

33. Foster, F.S., Pavlin, C.J., Harasiewicz, K.A., et al., Advances in ultrasound biomicroscopy, *Ultrasound Med. Biol.*, 26, 1–27, 2000.

34. Meitzler, A.H., Piezoelectric transducer materials and techniques for ultrasonic devices operating above 100 MHz, Ch. 3, pp. 125–182, in: *Ultrasonic Transducer Materials*, O.E. Mattiat (Ed.), Plenum Press, New York, 1971.

35. Sitting, E.K., Design and technology of piezoelectric transducers for frequencies above 100 MHz, Ch. 5, pp. 221–275, in: *Physical Acoustics*, Vol. 9, W.P. Mason, and R.N. Thurston (Eds.), Academic Press, New York, 1972.

36. Foster, N.F., Piezoelectricity in thin film materials, *J. Acoust. Soc. Am.*, 70, 1609–1614, 1981.

37. Ito, Y. Kushida, K., Sugawara, K., and Takeuchi, H., A 100-MHz ultrasonic transducer array using ZnO thin films, *IEEE Trans. Ultrason., Ferroelect., Freq. Contr.*, 42, 316–324, 1995.

38. Knapik, D.A., Starkoski, B., Pavlin, C.J., and Foster, F.S., A real-time 200 MHz ultrasound B-scan imager, pp. 1457–1460, in: *1997 IEEE Ultrasonics Symp. Proc.*, 1997.

39. Knapik, D.A., Starkoski, B., Pavlin, C.J., and Foster, F.S., A 100–200 MHz ultrasound biomicroscope, *IEEE Trans. Ultrason. Ferroelect. Freq. Contr.*, 47, 1540–1549, 2000.

40. Cannata, J.M., Ritter, T.A., Chen, W-H., and Shung, K.K., Design of focused single element (50–100 MHz) transducers using lithium niobate, pp. 28–35, in: *Ultrasonic Imaging and Asignal Processing*, M.F. Insana, and K.K. Shung (Eds.), Proc. SPIE Vol. 4325, Medical Imaging, 2001.

41. Nye, J.F., *Physical Properties of Crystals: Their Representation by Tensors and Matrices*, 2nd ed., Oxford Univ. Press, Oxford, 1985.

42. ANSI/IEEE Standard 176–1987, IEEE Standard on Piezoelectricity, Inst. Elect. Electron. Engrs., Piscathway, NJ, 1988.

43. Hayward, G., Bennett, J., and Hamilton, R., A theoretical study on the influence of some constituent material properties on the behavior of 1-3 connectivity composite transducers, *J. Acoust. Soc. Am.*, 98, 2187–2196, 1995.

44. Varadan, V.V., Roh, Y.R., Varadan, V.K., and Tancrell, R.H., Measurement of all the elastic constants of poled PVDF films, pp. 727–730, in: *1989 IEEE Ultrasonics Symp. Proc.*, 1989.

45. Roh, Yongrae, Development of local/global SAW sensors for measurement of wall shear stress in laminar and turbulent flows, PhD thesis, Pennsylvania State Univ., 1990.

46. Roh, Y., Varadan, V.V., and Varadan, V.K., Characterization of all the elastic, dielectric, and piezoelectric constants of uniaxially orientated poled PVDF films, *IEEE Trans. Ultrason., Ferroelect., Freq. Contr.*, 49, 836–847, 2002.

47. Hunt, J.W., Arditi, A., and Foster, F.S., Ultrasound transducers for pulse-echo medical imaging *IEEE Trans. Biomed. Eng.*, BME-30, 453–481, 1983.

48. Newnham, R.E., Skinner, D.P., and Cross, L.E., Connectivity and piezoelectric-pyroelectric composites, *Mat. Res. Bull.*, 13, 525–536, 1978.

49. Ritter, T.A., Shrout, T.R., and Shung, K.K., Development of high-frequency medical ultrasound arrays, pp. 1127–1133, in: *2001 IEEE Ultrasonics Symp. Proc.*, 2001.

50. Tutwiler, R.L., Stitt, J.P., Ritter, T.A., et al., Precision mechanically scanned HF ultrasound arrays, pp. 873–876, in: *2003 IEEE Ultrasonics Symp. Proc.*, 2003.

51. Lukacs, M., Sayer, M., Lockwood, G., and Foster, S., Laser micromachined high frequency ultrasound arrays, pp. 1209–1212, in: *1999 IEEE Ultrasonics Symp. Proc.*, 1999.

52. Farlow, R., Galbraith, W., Knowles, M., and Hayward, G., Micromachining of a piezocomposite transducer using a copper vapor laser, *IEEE Trans. Ultrason., Ferroelect., Freq. Contr.*, 48, 639–640, 2001.

53. Smith, W.A., and Auld, B.A., Modeling 1-3 composite piezoelectrics: thickness-mode oscillations, *IEEE Trans. Ultrason., Ferroelect., Freq. Contr.*, 38, 40–47, 1991.

54. Goldberg, R.L., and Smith, S.W., Multilayer piezoelectric ceramics for two-dimensional array transducers, *IEEE Trans. Ultrason., Ferroelect., Freq. Contr.*, 41, 761–771, 1994.

55. Sato, J., Kawabuchi, M., and Fukumoto, A., Dependence of the electromechanical coupling coefficient on the width-to-thickness ratio of plank-shaped piezoelectric transducers used for electronically scanned ultrasound diagnostic system, *J. Acoust. Soc. Am.*, 67, 1609–1611, 1979.

56. Gururaja, T.R., Schulze, W.A., Cross, L.E., et al., Piezoelectric composite materials for ultrasonic transducer applications. Part I: Resonant modes of vibration of PZT rod-polymer composites, *IEEE Trans. on Sonics and Ultrasonics*, SU-32, 481–498, 1985.

57. Certon, D., Casula, O., Patat, F., and Royer, D., Theoretical and experimental investigations of lateral modes in 1-3 piezocomposites, *IEEE Trans. Ultrason., Ferroelect., Freq. Contr.*, 44, 643–651, 1997.

58. Auld, B.A., Kunkel, H.A., Shui, Y.A., and Wang, Y., Dynamic behavior of periodic piezoelectric composites, pp. 554–558, in: *1983 IEEE Ultrasonics Symp. Proc.*, 1983.

59. Auld, B.A., Shui, Y.A., and Wang, Y., Elastic wave propagation in three-dimensional periodic composite materials, *J. Phisique*, 45, 159–163, 1984.

60. Lamberti, N., Montero de Espinosa, F.R., Iula, F.R., and Carotenuto, R., Two-dimensional modelling of multifrequency piezocomposites, *Ultrasonics*, 37, 577–583, 2000.

61. Allik, H, and Hughes, T.J.R., Finite element method for piezoelectric vibration, *Int. J. Numerical Methods for Engineering*, 2, 151–157, 1970.

62. Lerch, R., Simulation of piezoelectric devices by two- and three-dimensional finite elements, *IEEE Trans. Ultrason., Ferroelect., Freq. Contr.*, 37, 233–247, 1990.

63. Hashimoto, K.Y., and Yamaguchi, M., Elastic, piezoelectric and dielectric properties of composite materials, pp. 697–702, in: *1986 IEEE Ultras. Symp. Proc.*, 198.

64. Hossack, J.A., and Hayward, G., Finite element analysis of 1-3 composite transducers, *IEEE Trans. Ultrason., Ferroelect., Freq. Contr.*, 38, 618–629, 1991.

65. Hayward, G., Bennett, J., and Hamilton, R., A theoretical study on the influence of some constituent material properties on the behavior of 1-3 connectivity composite transducers, *J. Acoust. Soc. Am.*, 98, 2187–2196, 1995.

66. Cady, W.G., A theory of the crystal transducer for plane waves, *J. Acoust. Soc. Am.*, 21, 65–73, 1949.

67. Bobber, R.J., *Underwater Electroacoustic Measurements*, Naval Research Laboratory, Washington, D.C., 1970.

68. Swartz, R.D., and Plummer, J.D., On the generation of high-frequency acoustic energy with polyvinylidene fluoride, *IEEE Trans. Sonics Ultrason.*, SU-44, 295–303, 1980.

69. Goldberg, R.L., Emery, C.D., and Smith, S.W., Hybrid multi/single layer array transducers for increased signal-to-noise ratio, *IEEE Trans. Ultrason., Ferroelect., Freq. Contr.*, 44, 315–325, 1997.

70. Goldberg, R.L., Jergens, M.J., Mills, D.M., et al., Modeling of piezoelectric multilayer ceramics using finite element analysis, *IEEE Trans. Ultrason., Ferroelect., Freq. Contr.*, 44, 1204–1214, 1997.

71. Platte, M., Barker-coded multilayer transducers of polyvinylidenefluoride for use in the ultrasonic pulse-echo technique, *Acustica*, 56, 29–33, 1984.

72. Sung, K.M., Piezoelectric multilayer transducers for ultrasonic pulse compression, *Ultrasonics*, 22, 61–68, 1984.

73. Izumi, S.M., Saitoh and Abe, K., A low-impedance ultrasonic probe using a multilayer piezoceramic, *Japan J. Appl. Phys.*, 28, 54–56, 1989.

74. Zhang, Q., Lewin, P.A., and Bloomfield, P.E., PVDF transducers: a performance comparison of single-layer and multilayer structures, *IEEE Trans. Ultrason., Ferroelect., Freq. Contr.*, 44, 1148–1155, 1997.

75. Woodward, P.M., *Probability and Information Theory, with Applications to Radar*, Pergamon Press, London, 1953.

76. Cook, C.E., and Bernfeld, M., *Radar Signals: an Introduction to Theory and Application*, Artech House, Boston, 1993 (originally published 1967 by Academic Press).

77. Peebles, P.Z., *Radar Principles*, Ch. 7, Pulse Compression with Radar Signals, Wiley, New York, 1998.

78. Platte, M., PVDF ultrasonic transducers, *Ferroelectrics*, 75, 327–337, 1987.

79. Katz, H.W. (Ed.), Ch. 3 in: *Solid State Magnetic and Dielectric Devices*, Wiley, New York, 1959.

80. Kino, S., *Acoustic Waves: Devices, Imaging and Analog Signal Processing*, Prentice-Hall, 1986.

81. Ballato, A., Modeling piezoelectric and piezomagnetic devices and structures via equivalent networks, *IEEE Trans. Ultrason., Ferroelect., Freq. Contr.*, 48, 1189–1240, 2001.

82. Mason, W.D., *Electromechanical Transducers and Wave Filters*, Van Nostrand, Princeton, NJ, 1948.

83. Redwood, M., Transient performance of a piezoelectric transducer, *J. Acoust. Soc. Am.*, 33, 527–536, 1961.

84. Banah, A.H., Korpel, A., and Vogel, R.F., Feynman diagram analysis of transducer impulse response, *J. Acoust. Soc. Am.*, 73, 677–687, 1983.

85. Krimholtz, R., Leedom, D., and Matthaei, G., New equivalent circuits for elementary piezoelectric transducers, *Elect. Lett.*, 6, 398–399, 1970.

86. Leedom, D., Krimholtz, R., and Matthaei, G., Equivalent circuits for transducers having arbitrary even-or-odd symmetry, *IEEE Trans. Sonics Ultrasonics*, SU-18, 128–41, 1971.

87. DeSilets, C.S., Fraser, J.D., and Kino, G.S., The design of efficient broadband piezoelectric transducers, *IEEE Trans. Sonics Ultrasonics*, SU-25, 115–125, 1978.

88. Van Dyke, K.S., The electrical network equivalent of a piezo-electric resonator, *Phys. Rev.*, 25, 895, 1925 (abstract of presentation at Am. Phys. Soc. Meeting, April 1925).

89. Van Dyke, K.S., The piezo-electric resonator and its equivalent circuit, *Proc. IRE*, 16, 742–764, 1928.

90. Butterworth, S., On a null method of testing vibration galvanometers, *Proc. Phys. Soc. London*, 26, 264–273, 1914. On electrically-maintained vibrations, *Proc. Phys. Soc. London*, 27, 410–424, 1915.

91. Dye, D.W., The piezo-electric quartz resonator and its equivalent circuit, *Proc. Phys. Soc. London*, 38, 399–458, 1925–26.

92. McKeighen, R.E., Design guidelines for medical ultrasonic arrays, pp. 2–18, in: *Ultrasonic Transducer Engineering*, K.K. Shung (Ed.), Proc. SPIE Vol. 3341, Medical Imaging, 1998.

93. Whitworth, G., Discussion of one-D piezoelectric transducer models with loss, *IEEE Trans. Ultrason., Ferroelect., Freq. Contr.*, 48, 844–846, 2001.

94. Kraus, A.D., *Circuit Analysis*, Ch. 18, pp. 653–709, West Pub. Co., St Paul, MN, 1991.

95. Huelsman, L.P., *Basic Circuit Theory*, Ch. 11, pp. 582–648, 3rd ed., Prentice Hall, Englewood Cliffs, NJ, 1991.

96. Sittig, E.K., Transmission parameters of thickness-driven piezoelectric transducers arranged as multilayer configurations, *IEEE Trans. Sonics Ultrasonics*, SU-14, 167–174, 1967.

97. Sittig, E.K., Effects of bonding and electrode layers on the transmission parameters of piezoelectric transducers used in ultrasonic digital delay lines, *IEEE Trans. Sonics Ultrasonics*, SU-16, 2–10, 1969.

98. Selfridge, A.R., and Gehlbach, S., KLM transducer model implementation using transfer matrices, pp. 875–877, in: *1985 IEEE Ultrasonics Symp. Proc.*, 1985.

99. Kossoff G. The effects of backing and matching on the performance of piezoelectric ceramic transducers, *IEEE Trans. Sonics Ultrasonics*, SU-13, 20–30, 1966.

100. Goll, J.H., and Auld, B.A., Multilayer impedance matching schemes for broadbanding of water loaded piezoelectric transducers and high Q electric resonators, *IEEE Trans. Sonics Ultrasonics*, SU-22, 52–53, 1975.

101. Goll, J.H., The design of broad-band fluid-loaded ultrasonic transducers, *IEEE Trans. Sonics Ultrasonics*, SU-26, 385–393, 1979.

102. Selfridge, A.R., Baer, R., Khuri-Yakub, B.T., and Kino, G.S., Computer-optimized design of quarter-wave acoustic matching and electrical matching networks for acoustic transducers, pp. 644–648 in: *1981 IEEE Ultrasonics Symp. Proc.*, 1981.

103. Van Combruge, M., and Thompson, W., Optimization of the transmitting characteristics of a Tonplitz-type transducer by proper choice of impedance matching layers, *J. Acoust. Soc. Am.*, 77, 747–752, 1985.

104. Rhyne, T.L., Computer optimization of transducer transfer functions using constraints on bandwidth, ripple and loss, *IEEE Trans. Ultrason., Ferroelect., Freq. Contr.*, 43, 1136–1149, 1996.

105. Anderson, J., and Wilkins, L., The design of optimum lumped broadband equalizers for ultrasonic transducers, pp. 422–427, in: *1977 IEEE Ultrasonics Symp. Proc.*, 1977.

106. Augustine, L.J., and Anderson, J., An algorithm for the design of broadband equalizers for ultrasonic transducers, *J. Acoust. Soc. Am.*, 66, 629–635, 1979.

107. Collin, R.E., *Foundations for Microwave Engineering*, 2nd ed., McGraw-Hill, New York, 1992.

108. Onoe, M., Tiersten, H.E., and Meitzler, A.H., Shift in the location of resonant frequencies caused by large electromechanical coupling in thickness-mode resonators, *J. Acoust. Soc. Am.*, 35, 36–42, 1963.

109. Inoue, T., Ohta, M., and Takahashi, S., Design of ultrasonic transducers with multiple acoustic matching layers for medical application, *IEEE Trans. Ultrason., Ferroelect., Freq. Contr.*, 34, 8–16, 1987.

110. Sitting, E.K., Definitions relating to conversion losses in piezoelectric transducers, *IEEE Trans. Sonics Ultrasonics*, SU-18, 231–234, 1971.

111. Redwood, M., A study of waveforms in the generation and detection of short ultrasonic pulses, *Appl. Mater. Res.*, 2, 76–84, 1963.

112. Kohler, B., Impulse response of a piezoelectric layer, *Acustica*, 73, 144–152, 1991.

113. Follett, D.H., and Atkinson, P., Ultrasonic pulse-echo system design: transmitter-receiver matching, *Ultrasound Med. Biol.*, 2, 326, 1976.

114. Buck, G.A., and Olson, R.A., Ultrasound imaging probe assembly, US Patent 6,030,346, Feb. 29, 2000 (filed April 20, 1998).

115. Griffith, J., and Lebender, R., Electrical characteristics of ribbon-based probe cables, pp. 1085–1090, in: *1999 IEEE Ultrasonics Symp. Proc.*, 1999.

116. Lockwood, G.R., Hunt, J.W., and Foster, F.S., The design of protection circuitry for high-frequency ultrasound imaging systems, *IEEE Trans. Ultrason., Ferroelect., Freq. Contr.*, 38, 48–55, 1991.

117. Lockwood, G.R., and Foster, F.S., Modeling and optimization of high-frequency ultrasound transducers, *IEEE Trans. Ultrason., Ferroelect., Freq. Contr.*, 41, 225–230, 1994.

118. Poulsen, J.K., Low loss wideband protection circuit for high frequency ultrasound, pp. 823–826, in: *1999 IEEE Ultrasonics Symp. Proc.*, 1999.

119. Young, J.W., Optimization of acoustic receiver noise performance, *J. Acoust. Soc. Am.*, 61, 1471–1476, 1970.

120. Rhyne, T.L., and Panda, S., Design implications of using transducer noise figure as the basis of sensitivity, pp. 1167–1170, in: *1993 IEEE Ultrasonics Symp. Proc.*, 1993.

121. Boltz, E.S., and Fortunko, C.M., Absolute sensitivity limits of various ultrasonic transducers, pp. 951–954, in: *1995 IEEE Ultrasonics Symp. Proc.*, 1995.

122. Farlow, R., and Hayward, G., The absolute sensitivity of a piezocomposite transducer, pp. 911–914, in: *1997 IEEE Ultrasonics Symp. Proc.*, 1997.

123. Goldberg, R.L., and Smith, S.W., Optimization of signal-to-noise ratio for multilayer PZT transducers, *Ultrasonic Imaging*, 17, 95–115, 1995.

124. Oakley, C.G., Calculation of ultrasonic transducer signal-to-noise ratios using the KLM model, *IEEE Trans. Ultrason., Ferroelect., Freq. Contr.*, 44, 1018–1026, 1997.

125. Rhyne, T.L., Characterizing ultrasonic transducers using radiation efficiency and reception noise figure, *IEEE Trans. Ultrason., Ferroelect., Freq. Contr.*, 45, 559–566, 1998.

126. *La Lumiere Electrique*, 3, 286, 1881.

127. Dolbear, A.E., Apparatus for transmitting sound by electricity, US Patent 239,742, April 1881 (filed October 1880).

128. Dolbear, A.E., Mode of transmitting sound by electricity, US Patent 240,578, April 1881 (filed February 1881).

129. Wente, E.C., A condenser transmitter as a uniformly sensitive instrument for the absolute measurement of sound intensity, *Phys. Rev.*, 10, 39–63, 1917.

130. Sell, H., Eine neue kapazitive methode zur umwandlung mechanisher schwingungen in elektrische und umgekehrt (A new capacitive method for converting mechanical oscillations into electrical and vice-versa), *Zeit. Tech. Physik*, 18, 3–10, 1937.

131. Kellogg, E.W., Production of sound, US Patent 1,983,377 Dec. 4, 1934 (filed Sept. 17, 1929). (It describes an electrostatic speaker composed of many small sections able to radiate sound without magnets or cones or baffles. This patent, as well as the 1932 British patents of Hans Vogt, influenced Peter Walker to build the Quad ESL flat panel speaker in 1957, versions of which continue to be commercially available).

132. Hunt, F.V., *Electroacoustics: The Analysis of Transduction and its Historical Background* (see Chapter 5, Electrostatic Transducer systems) Harvard Univ. Press, Cambridge, MA, 1954.

133. Langevin, P. (in collaboration with M.C. Chilowsky), Procédé et appareils pour la production de signaux sous-marins diriges et pour la localisation a distance d'ob-

stacles sous-marins (Brevet francais, No 502913, May 29, 1916), pp. 527–537, in: *Oevres Scientifiques de Paul Langevin*, CNRS, Paris, 1950. See also: Chilowsky, M.C., and Langevin, P., Echo ranging with electrostatic transducer, French Patent 502,913, published May 29, 1920 (applied for May 29, 1916).

134. Khul, W., Schodder, G.R., and Schodder, F.K., Condenser transmitter and microphones with solid dielectric for airborne ultrasonics, *Acoustica*, 4, 520–532, 1954.

135. Cantrell, J.H., Heyman, J.S., Yost, W.T., et al., Broadband electrostatic transducer for ultrasonic measurements in liquids, *Rev. Sci. Instrum.*, 50, 31–33, 1979.

136. Higuchi, K., Suzuki, K., and Tanigawa, H., Ultrasonic phased array transducer for acoustic imaging in air, pp. 559–562 in: *1986 IEEE Ultrasonics Symp. Proc.*, 1986.

137. Suzuki, K., Higuchi, K., and Tanigawa, H., A silicon electrostatic ultrasonic transducer, *IEEE Trans. Ultrason., Ferroelect., Freq. Contr.*, 36, 620–627, 1989.

138. Holm, D., and Hess, G., A subminiature condenser microphone with silicon nitride membrane and silicon back plate, *J. Acoust. Soc. Am.*, 85, 476–480, 1989.

139. Soh, H.T., Ladabaum, I., Atalar, A., et al., Silicon micromachined ultrasonic immersion transducers, *Appl. Phys. Lett.*, 69, 3674–3676, 1996.

140. Oralkan, O., Ergun, A.S., Johnson, J.A., et al., Capacitive micromachined ultrasonic transducers: next generation arrays for acoustic imaging? *IEEE Trans. Ultrason., Ferroelect., Freq. Contr.*, 49, 11596–11610, 2002.

141. Oralkan, O., Ergun, A.S., Cheng, C-H., et al., Volumetric imaging using 2D capacitive micromachined ultrasonic transducer arrays (CMUTs): initial results, pp. 1083–1086, in: *2002 IEEE Ultrasonics Symp. Proc.*, 2002.

7

Ultrasound Imaging Arrays

Ultrasound images differ from their optical counterpart in that they map the local acoustic properties of the medium such as the density and compressibility as opposed to the optical properties. They are subject to distortion from a variety of sources, including diffraction, attenuation, dispersion, and inhomogeneities in the medium. Imaging arrays enable acoustic images to be obtained without the need for mechanical scanning of single-element transducers, and they can do so at a sufficiently high frame rate that avoids significant motion distortion caused by fast-moving structures such as those in the heart. Developments in transducers and array design, together with new signal-processing techniques, have enabled major improvements to be made in ultrasound contrast, resolution, dynamic range, frame rate, and signal-to-noise ratios (SNR).

This chapter[1] is the first of two concerned with the theory, design, and application of arrays for 2-D and 3-D imaging. It begins with a brief historical overview[2] that describes how ultrasound imaging evolved from pulse-echo metal flaw detectors and was influenced by the techniques developed for radar during World War II. Simple CW excited 1-D arrays consisting of point source elements will first be examined. This leads to the concepts of beam focusing and steering using pulse-excited array elements of finite size. Sparse arrays and

---

1. The comprehensive chapter of Goldstein and Powis [1] was particularly helpful in preparing this chapter.

2. Accounts of the development of diagnostic ultrasound imaging by Edler and Lindstrom [2], Levi [3], and Woo [4], along with an excellent review by Goldberg and Kimmelman [5], should be useful to the reader interested in obtaining further details.

arrays of higher dimensionality are then examined, followed by a discussion of 3-D imaging. The final section turns from matters associated with array analysis to the problem of array synthesis.

7.1 Historical Background

Before outlining the sequence of developments that led to 2-D ultrasonic imaging, it may be helpful to define certain terms concerning the manner in which the information is displayed. The term "A-scan," which originates from the early radar days, refers to the display of a pulse-echo signal on an oscilloscope (A-scope) as an amplitude-versus-time (or distance) graph. We shall interpret A as amplitude and therefore *A-mode* as *Amplitude mode*. An alternative means of display is one in which a single line is drawn on an oscilloscope but with brightness that is related to the echo signal amplitude. This form of scan has often been referred to in the past as a B-scan, and when displayed on an oscilloscope, it is referred to as a B-scope image, where B stands for brightness. If the echo information from a sequence of scan lines is displayed in this manner, the 2-D image so formed will be referred to as a *B-mode* gray-scale image. The number of gray-scale levels that can be successfully distinguished by eye in a CRT display is quite limited e.g., 10, which was a problem in earlier B-mode systems that lacked modern digital processing techniques. Examples of A- and B-mode recordings are shown in Fig. 7.1. The C-scope display refers to a second form of 2-D intensity-modulated display, but one in which the image is formed perpendicular to the plane of a B-mode scan. It is sometimes referred to as a *C-mode* or a *Constant depth mode* image.

7.1.1 A- and B-Mode Systems

The development and use of pulse-echo A-mode for medical diagnosis can be considered a logical outcome of the invention and development of pulse-echo

━━━━━━━━━━━━━━━━━━━━━━━━━━━━━━━━━━━━━━▶

Figure 7.1 A- and B-mode recordings. (a) A- and B-mode recordings made in the late 1970s using a linear array transducer with 71 crystal elements. Time/depth is from left to right. The B-mode image presented in (ii) clearly shows the fetal skull, placenta, and umbilical cord. The horizontal white marker line shows the position of the A-mode recording presented in (i). Echoes from both sides of the skull, together with an echo from the midline, are clearly evident. The caliper lines enable the biparietal diameter to be measured (28 mm). (Reproduced, with minor changes, from a brochure describing the Roche Abdoscan 5 real-time ultrasound system.) (b) Gray-scale image of a fetal spine made with a GE system (late 1990s) and a curvilinear array with a center frequency of near 3.5 MHz. The enlarged portion is approximately 27×27 mm^2, the image depth is 10 cm, and there are four transmit focal zones, marked by triangles. The short dashes are separated by 1 cm. (Reproduced, with permission, from GE Health Care website.)

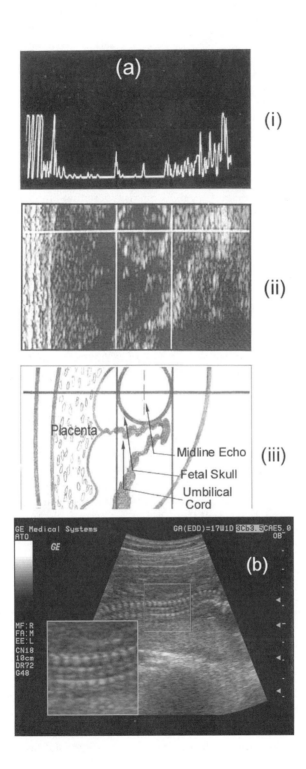

techniques for detecting flaws in metal castings, a technique of special importance in the production of armaments. Firestone [6–8] in the United States and Sproule [9] in England were primarily responsible for these inventions, many of which were kept secret until the end of World War II. The original idea of using ultrasound for flaw detection had been proposed much earlier (1929) by Sokolov [10] while working in Leningrad (now St. Petersburg) and 2 years later by Muhlhauser [11] in Germany. However, unlike the pulse-echo methods of Firestone and Sproule, these proposals used CW excitation and detected the presence of a flaw by measuring the changes in the signal transmitted through the specimen. A subsequent U.S. patent application by Sokolov in 1937 [12] is particularly important since it also suggests a method for obtaining a 2-D map of the transmission through a test material, much like the method used for forming an x-ray picture.

The first paper suggesting that ultrasound could be used for diagnostic purposes was a 1942 publication in German by K. T. Dussik [13], who indicated that he had been working in this area since 1937. He and his brother (F. Dussik) developed a transmission method for measuring the absorption of CW ultrasound through the head. Using separate transmission and reception transducers, with the latter being in line with the transmitter on the opposite side of the head, they produced a 2-D image that they called a "hyperphonogram." They interpreted the image as a transmission absorption image, much like that of an x-ray, and suggested that a rough image of the ventricles had been obtained.[3] Since geometric distortion of the ventricles can provide an indication of the presence of a tumor, it was expected that this technique would be of diagnostic value. In a 1947 paper the Dussik brothers and Wyt [14] provided further details of their method. Hueter and Bolt in the United States, who were aware of the Dussiks' work, approached the problem of designing a system for visualizing the ventricles in a much more systematic manner. Their system used strips of barium titanate for transmission and measured the attenuation through the head at a transmission frequency of about 2.5 MHz. In a 1951 paper they showed a preliminary 2-D cross-sectional image that they called an ultrasonogram, which they claimed gave an outline of the ventricles. Even though subsequent investigations [15] showed that their images as well as those of the Dussik brothers arose from fortuitous artifacts caused by the transmission properties of the skull, their work served to emphasize the importance and potential of ultrasound for diagnostic imaging.

Subsequent to World War II a number of investigators explored the possible use of A-mode systems, often making use of commercial metal flaw detectors and surplus wartime radar and ultrasound equipment. The earlier investigators included Ludwig and Struthers [16], who used ultrasound for detecting gallstones, French et al. [17] for localizing brain tumors, Wild [18[4],19] for measuring the properties of biologic tissue using 15 MHz pulsed ultra-

---

3. The ventricles are structures that occupy the central portion of the brain.

4. This paper also contains the first suggestion that measurements could be made from within body cavities, specifically the bowel.

sound, Wild and Neal [20] for breast tumor diagnosis, and Mundt and Hughes [21] for ocular diagnosis. Of major importance was the development of 2-D cross-sectional imaging system by Wild and Reid [22]. Their seminal publication in the February 1952 issue of *Science* showed how a cross-sectional ultrasound image could be obtained and how such an image could be much more readily interpreted in terms of the underlying anatomy. Indeed, it was the complexity of the A-mode signal and the difficulty of relating it to the anatomy that spurred the development of B-mode imaging. The method described how a 15 MHz pulse-echo transducer was mechanically rotated through an angle to produce a sector scan. In their paper they stated that the echo signals were displayed "as spots of varying intensity on the face of the television screen . . . the brightness of which varies according the strength of the echoes returning." From this quotation it is clear that a pseudo gray-scale display was used. A further important feature of their system was the compensation for attenuation effects [23]. Received signals arising from increasing depth (or increasing time) suffer more attenuation, and as a result the signal amplitude rapidly diminishes. To partially compensate for this they caused the receiver gain to increase with time, a well-known radar technique for reducing the signal amplitude caused by close-in structures and increasing those from distant targets. Known as sensitivity time control (STC) but often called *swept gain* or *time-gain compensation* (TGC), it can result in dramatic improvements in the image quality. In 1952 Wild and Reid [24] described the results from a pilot clinical study of their system for detecting breast tumors, and this was followed by the results of a more comprehensive study [25] in 1954.

Several months after the Wild and Reid's publication in *Science*, Howry and Bliss [26] described a mechanically scanned imaging system of somewhat similar design that had been independently developed, and also presented cross-sectional images of tissue structures and a forearm. The development of this system and that of Wild and Reid was aided by the earlier (wartime) developments in radar, particularly Plan Position Indicators (PPI) that displayed the reflected signals from aircraft on a long persistence cathode ray tube, from which their position could be determined. An important subsequent development by the Howry group was the first description of 3-D ultrasound imaging, which they described briefly in a 1954 publication [27] and more fully in 1956 [28]. The latter publication presented a schematic of their system (Fig. 7.2a) and showed it was capable of imaging projections of a 3-D wire mesh test object system. They also showed a pair of stereoscopic images of a forearm. That same year, Kikuichi et al. [30] described[5] a B-mode imaging system that, like the 3-D Howry system, used the linear (as opposed to sector) scanning scheme illustrated in Fig. 7.2b. They provided examples of its clinical use as part of a preliminary investigation into the potential use of ultrasound in cancer diagnosis.

Subsequently, there was gradual acceptance and application of this new imaging modality to various medical fields, such as ophthalmology [31,32],

5. First presented at the International Congress on Acoustics, June 1956.

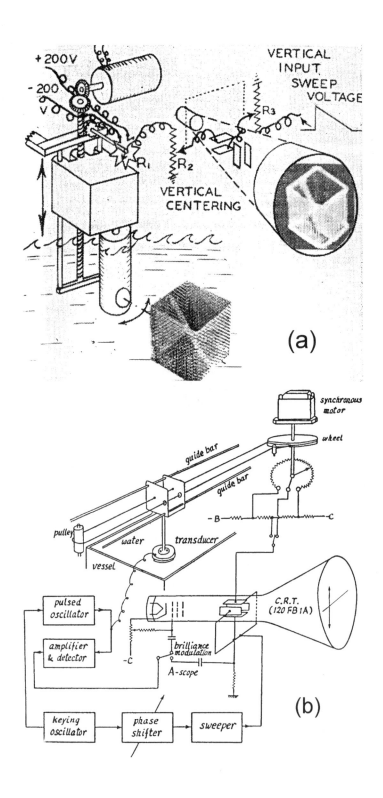

Figure 7.2 Examples of some early ultrasound imaging systems. (a) Imaging system to enable 3-D projections to be obtained. The transducer (immersed in water) is moved mechanically in a 2-D scanning motion. A wire mesh (1.5 inches high) test object is shown, and the result of one image is shown on the face of the cathode ray tube. (Used, with permission, from Howry et al. [28], *J. Appl. Physiol.*, 9, 304–306, © 1956 American Physiological Society.) (b) B-mode imaging system (Ultrasono-tomograph) developed in Japan around 1955/6 and used for some preliminary clinical tests. (Reproduced, with permission, from Kikuchi et al. [30], *J. Acoust. Soc. Am.*, 29, 824–833, © 1957 Acoustical Society of America.)

◀ ───

abdominal examination [35], and obstetrics and gynecology[6] [34]. Taking this new technology to commercialization and developing it to the stage where it could be used in routine clinical diagnosis was a comparatively slow process. By the late 1950s and early 1960s, manually controlled contact scanners became available. Probably the best of these[7] was one invented and designed by Brown in collaboration with Donald[8] that was described in 1959 [36]. The system used separate transmit and receive 2.5 MHz crystals mounted in the same probe housing, which could be moved by hand over the skin surface, using olive oil to ensure good acoustic coupling of the transducers to the skin. Prior diagnostic ultrasound systems used a probe that followed a prescribed scanning path and that made acoustic contact to the patient via a water bath, which often resulted in reverberation artifacts. A second important advance made by Brown [38] in designing this system was the ability to superimpose a rocking motion on the probe motion as it was guided by hand over the skin surface. Interfaces that are not normal to the incident beam give a greatly reduced echo. In fact, Kossoff et al. [39] have pointed out that soft tissue boundaries typically show a decrease of −20 dB for every 6-degree decrease in angle. Thus, as illustrated in Fig. 7.3a, the effect of the rocking motion described by Brown is to produce a substantially increased echo amplitude from interfaces not parallel to the skin surface, a process known as *compound scanning*.[9] A third and

6. For a valuable historical review of the developments in obstetric ultrasound from 1957 to 1997, see [33].

7. According to Brown [see quotation in 37, p. 511], about 1,500 units of an improved version of this scanner were sold throughout Europe.

8. Ian Donald, who was appointed to the Chair of Midwifery at the University of Glasgow in 1954, is considered to be the pioneer in developing the application of ultrasound diagnostic methods to obstetrics and gynecology.

9. In 1964 Howry and Gordon [40] stated that the principle of compound scanning was originally proposed in 1952 by Howry. While this may be true, neither of Howry's 1952 journal publications mentions this. The essence of the idea may have been proposed in 1954, when mention is made of the problem arising from media behind a strongly reflecting surface. Holmes et al. [27] wrote, "This problem was solved . . . by obtaining a combination of four pictures with the scanning device placed in four different quadrants." In 1958, Holmes and Howry [29] wrote, "By scanning both horizontally and in a circular manner around the part to be examined, the bright spots can be compounded to give the appearance of an anatomical picture on the oscilloscope screen." Based on these facts, it seems reasonable to attribute to Brown, Holmes, and Howry co-discovery of compound scanning.

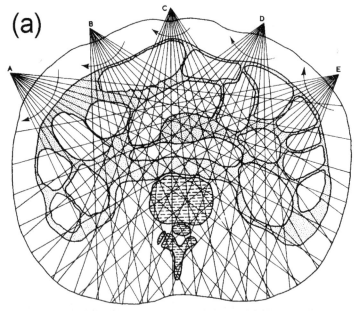

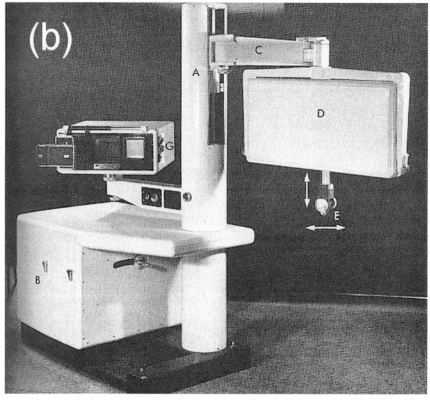

Figure 7.3 Compound scanning. (a) Illustration published in 1959 displaying the basic principles of compound scanning. An abdominal region is shown in which the probe contacts the skin and is manually moved over the surface with a superimposed rocking motion. The prototype system that was developed by Tom Brown at Kelvin and Hughes Ltd., Glasgow, in collaboration with Professor Ian Donald, operated at 2.5 MHz. It took several minutes to record a complete gray-scale scan on photographic film. (Reproduced, with permission of the International Federation for Medical & Biological Engineering, from Brown [36], © 1960 IFMBE.) (b) Photograph of the Diasonograph, a second-generation commercial version of the original system developed in Glasgow. This particular model was custom-designed for Sunden [41] and used three different PZT probes operating at 1.5, 2.5, and 5 MHz. The probe (E) could be rocked by means of knurled knobs (for compound scanning), and its angle was determined by sine/cosine potentiometers mounted on the shaft. As indicated by the two arrows, the probe could also be moved vertically and along one horizontal axis, its position being determined by two linear potentiometers. Two oscilloscopes are on the assembly (G). The one on the left had a short-persistence phosphor and is shown with a camera mounted in front for recording the B-mode, and the right-hand one had a long-persistence phosphor for visually monitoring the B-mode image and viewing A-mode traces. (Reproduced, with permission of Munksgaard Int. Publ. from Sunden [41], *Acta Obstet. Gynecol. Scand.* (Suppl. 6), 43, 1–191, © 1964.)

◄───

vital aspect concerned the ability of the system to display a very wide range in scattered signal amplitudes from different depths in the form of a continuous range of gray-scale levels, ranging from white to black. As noted earlier, attenuation causes the returned signal amplitude to diminish rapidly with increasing depth, and mostly because of this, the useful received signal amplitude might vary by as much as 100 dB. Displaying and recording echoes that covered such a wide range presented serious difficulties for the technology available at that time. By using swept gain,[10] Brown showed how a wide range in signal amplitudes could be accommodated and recorded on film as gray-scale[11] images. These were incorporated in a second-generation commercial B-mode imaging system (Fig. 7.3b) whose operation and features were fully described by Sunden [41].

10. Holmes et al. [27] may also have used swept gain. They wrote, "By constructing a gain compensator we have corrected for the absorption of sound in tissue in such a way that objects on the surface of the body appear on the screen as of the same size and density as those deep within the structures." However, Reid and Wild [23] seem to have prior claim on the first use of swept gain in ultrasound B-mode imaging.

11. With regard to the invention of gray-scale imaging, Brown [38] has written, "Much has since been made by others, years later, about the 'invention' of grey-scale imaging. The reality is that the display in the machines developed in Glasgow in the mid-1950's was a grey-scale one from the outset. The function of the signal processor was two-fold. In the first case it provided a degree of time-domain pulse shaping, in an attempt to separate echoes arriving closely-spaced in time. Secondly, and this is probably the most important function, it was to enable the display to record the very large dynamic range of signals which were received, without going into 'hard limiting' at the top end, or suppression of small echoes at the bottom end. When we say 'very large' we mean at least 60 dB."

Improvements to the gray-scale imaging technique were described by Kossoff et al. [42], and these involved the use of both swept gain and logarithmic amplification. At a fixed depth, the gain controlled by the swept gain amplifier will be fixed, but the scattered signal arising at this depth might, for example, vary over a 30-dB range, depending on the nature of the scatterer. Since a display system may enable only 6 to 10 levels of gray scale to be discriminated, some signal compression is needed to avoid loss of information, and this can be provided by a logarithmic amplifier. Such an amplifier provides high gain for small signals and reduced gain for large signals, thereby compressing the signal range. By this and other means, the group working with Kossoff made a number of significant improvements to the image quality that were described in their classic paper of 1976 [39], thereby substantially enhancing the value of B-mode ultrasound as a diagnostic imaging modality.

By the mid-1960s, a wide variety of imaging systems had become commercially available. Amongst these was the Vidoson, which was manufactured around 1965/6 by Siemens in Germany and which was developed by Krause and Soldner [43–45]. An important advance made by this system was the ability to form real-time images of moving structures. It used two transducers mounted on opposite ends of a rotating cylinder that was at the focus of a parabolic mirror, all of which was immersed in a water bag. Using a center frequency of 2.5 MHz, it provided a linear scan consisting of about 140 lines at about 15 frames/s.

7.1.2 Dynamic Range Issues

Of major concern in the design of gray-scale B-mode imaging systems is the need to ensure that the very large range of echo amplitudes can be accommodated within the imitations of the amplification, digitization, and display/recording subsystems. To illustrate these problems we consider a 3 MHz center frequency system designed for abdominal imaging. If the system is capable of imaging to a depth of 20 cm and the attenuation is 0.7 dB/(cm·MHz), then the range in signal amplitudes due to attenuation alone will be 84 dB (2×20 cm $\times 3 \times 0.7$ db/cm). Moreover, at a given depth, depending on the scattering target and the angle of incidence, the received signal could easily differ by more than 40 dB. The analog methods initially available for processing and displaying information were limited in their ability to cope with such a wide range. Early systems generally used a preamplifier followed by a TGC amplifier with a range of 60 dB and a log amplifier that could compress a 40-dB range into 10 or 20 gray-scale levels.

7.1.3 C-Mode Imaging

As mentioned earlier, a C-mode image is one formed in a plane normal to a B-mode image; in this regard, it is more akin to a classic x-ray image. It appears that several groups realized that this type of display could enable images to be produced that had superior resolution to those produced by standard B-mode methods.[12] To obtain a C-mode image, it is necessary to use a gate that selects data from a specific depth from an A-mode line and then to complete the image by a 2-D scanning movement of the transducer so that the entire region to be measured is sampled. von Ardenne et al. [46,47] used a strongly focused transducer and a gate in the form of a slit so as to display only those signals that arose from reflections close to the focus. By synchronizing the movement of the slit with the movement of the transducer, they were able to obtain C-mode images. Thurstone et al. [48] also realized the importance of using a highly focused transducer to obtain improved lateral resolution. They used a time gate to select the signals corresponding to the focus and provided a clear explanation of their C-mode recording system. Using a 2.25 MHz pulse, they claimed a resolution of better than 1 mm in all three spatial directions. They were able to obtain a complete image in 8 to 10 minutes and provided as an example an in vitro C-mode image of a coronal section of the brain.

One of the difficulties with the proposed methods was the length of time required to complete a scan using a rectilinear scanning pattern that necessitated stopping and reversing the mechanism. Following a suggestion by Brown [50] for 3-D ultrasound imaging, McCready and Hill [49] proposed that by using a spiral scan, discontinuities in the transducer movement would be avoided, enabling the scan time to be reduced. By this means they estimated that an area of $100 \, cm^2$ could be scanned in around 10 seconds.

7.1.4 M-Mode Recording

Another major ultrasound achievement was the development of a method for noninvasive cardiac diagnosis by Edler and Hertz [51,52] in 1954. By transmitting ultrasound pulses in quick succession along the same path toward various cardiac structures and recording the received waveform, they were able to map the spatial variation of a given scattering region as a function of time. They first achieved this in 1953 by using a commercially available A-mode ultrasonic flaw detector together with a specially designed camera system in which the film was moved at a constant rate past a slit. In the past, such records were sometimes called a time-motion (TM) record, but now they are more generally known as *M-mode* (motion). The resulting image enabled the movement, and hence the velocity, of specific cardiac structures to be determined. Clinical investigations by Edler over the first 5 years after the initial announcement, together with improvements in the technique, details of the methodology, and its verification, are presented in [53].

Edler and Hertz initially obtained M-mode recordings of cardiac motions by means of the system illustrated in Fig. 7.4a. With a conventional A-mode

12. Possibly the earliest C-mode images were those obtained and developed for NDE. Details of the system and the images obtained in 1956 at the Automation Instruments Power Plant Inspection Division test laboratory in Paramount, California, have been recorded on the website, http://www.uxr.com/histndt2.htm, run by UXR, 67 West Easy Street, Unit 118, Simi Valley, CA 93065, USA.

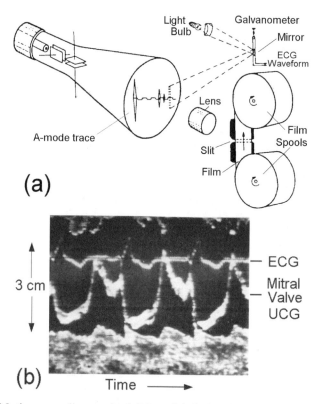

Figure 7.4 Motion recording method (M-mode) devised by Edler and Hertz in 1953/4. As shown in (a), a film is moved at a constant velocity past a slit to record a horizontal sample of the A-mode waveform displayed on the CRT. (b) Portion of an M-mode photographic recording from a normal mitral valve. The UCG (UltrasoundCardioGram) trace of the anterior mitral valve leaflet shows the position of the leaflet, which is approximately 6 to 8 cm from the chest wall. The rising portion represents movement toward the chest wall and vice versa. The peak of the UCG waveform corresponds to the maximal opening of the valve. (Reprinted by permission of Elsevier from Howry and Gordon [40], Ch. 13 in *Ultrasound as a Diagnostic and Surgical Tool*, E & S Livingstone Ltd. © 1964.)

display and a reasonably high pulse repetition rate, they used a lens to focus the CRT image onto a slit that was in close proximity to the film. The slit served to select a horizontal sample of the CRT image so that only the portion of the reflected signal whose amplitude was above a certain threshold was recorded on film. Those signals from stationary reflecting objects would therefore be recorded as straight lines, and those that were moving would result in curves. Edler and Hertz realized the importance of being able to relate their recordings to the electrocardiogram (ECG), so they also provided a means whereby the ECG waveform could be simultaneously recorded. To do so, the ECG waveform from an amplifier was applied to a galvanometer whose mirror

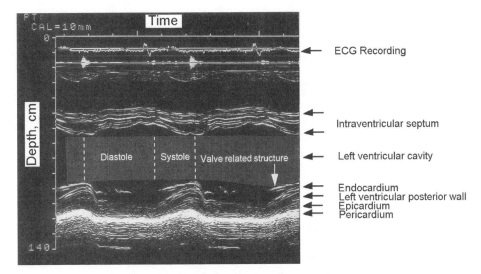

Figure 7.5 M-mode cardiac image showing the left ventricular posterior wall and intraventricular septum. (Reprinted by permission of Elsevier from Fleming et al. [54], *Ultrasound Med. Biol.*, 22, 573–581, © 1996 World Federation of Ultrasound in Medicine and Biology.)

caused a spot of light to be horizontally displaced on the face of the CRT, and this was recorded on the moving film. A much more recent M-mode cardiac image is shown in Fig. 7.5.

7.1.5 Imaging Arrays

The development of ultrasound imaging arrays was in large measure due to the much earlier invention and development of radiofrequency antenna arrays that began at the end of the 1800s. The patents granted to Brown (1899) and Stone (1901) marked the beginning of a sequence of publications that were referenced in Foster's well-known 1926 paper [55] on antenna arrays. It appears that Walter [56] in 1908, based on some controversial suggestions by Artom [57] two years earlier, first showed how it was possible to achieve beam steering by changing the phase of the signal applied to the antenna. A great deal of effort was expended on the development of 1-D and 2-D antenna array systems, using periodic and aperiodic arrangements that incorporated beam steering and focusing. Their use in radar and communication systems was especially important during World War II and in the years following.

In the audible frequency range, the development of acoustic arrays, including the use of beam steering, can also be traced back many years. Some of the very early publications are referenced in Stenzel's 1927 paper [58] on the directional characteristics of arrays of point sources; in addition, the theory and experimental results for loudspeaker arrays are given in a 1930 publication by Wolff and Malter [59]. Some of the first publications concerning the

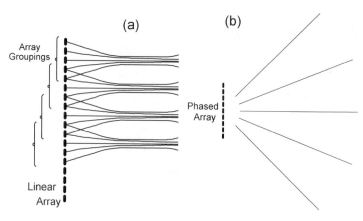

Figure 7.6 Simple array scanning methods. (a) A sequential linear scan transducer in which an adjacent group of elements is used to generate a beam. The scan starts by using the top group of elements for transmission and reception. Repeating this process for successive crystal element groups produces a rectilinear scan. (b) Sector scan in which all array elements contribute to the transmitted beam, and phasing is used to produce beam steering.

design and use of *ultrasonic* arrays originated from Tucker's group [60,61] at the University of Birmingham (UK). In the 1950s they developed a sector scanner (Fig. 7.6b) for underwater echo-ranging applications. Subsequently, the same group described an improved imaging system that used thirty 500 kHz array elements, had a sector scan of ±15 degrees, and displayed the underwater image on a long persistence CRT [62].

The first publication of an electronic sequential scanning system for medical applications appears to be the 10-element ultrasonic array described by Bushman in 1965 [63] that was used for imaging the eye. The transducer elements were mounted on a concave surface that approximately matched the curvature of the eye, and each was excited in turn to enable a complete frame of echo information to be obtained and displayed. A somewhat similar system was reported in 1971 by Bom et al. [64,65]. Their transducer consisted of a ~7-cm-long array of 20 rectangular elements that were resonant at ~3 MHz and that were individually excited to create 20 scan lines. Initial clinical results for cardiac imaging were reported in 1973 [66]. At about the same time (1971) as the initial publication of Bom et al., Uchida et al. [67] described a sequential linear array system in which each line was formed from 20 overlapping groups of elements within a 200-element linear array.[13] As illustrated in Fig. 7.6a, each group of elements was used for both transmission and reception. Each element had a width of 0.5 mm, a height of 12 mm, a center–center spacing of 0.7 mm, and a thickness of 1 mm, corresponding to a resonant frequency of 2 MHz. The transducer array was incorporated into a commercial-

---

13. See also the description of a 1.5 MHz linear array transducer consisting of PZT bars 0.4 mm wide and 20 mm high together with an image of a sponge [68].

quality diagnostic system that was capable of ~17 frames/s: it offered the advantage of much improved lateral resolution as compared to transducers that use a single element, in which the beam displacement is governed by the element width.

Of major significance in the development and use of arrays for medical imaging was the work of Somer [69,70]. In his 1968 publications he pointed out the potential advantages of electronically scanned arrays for producing real-time images of rapidly moving structures and described a sector scan (Fig. 7.6b) system that could be steered over a 90-degree sector at 30 frames/s. The transducer consisted of 21 elements with a resonant frequency of 1.3 MHz and a spacing of just under $\lambda/2$. Moreover, the small size of the array ($1.0 \times 1.1 \, cm^2$), compared to that developed by Bom et al., made this scheme much more appropriate for cardiac imaging.[14] The subsequent contributions of von Ramm and Thurstone [71–73], which included an account of the clinical application of sector scanning for cardiac imaging [74], were important influences on the development of commercial clinical diagnostic systems.

7.2 Properties of Imaging Arrays

The field produced by an ultrasonic array in the far field is very similar to that developed by an array of antennae, the theory of which has been summarized in the chapter by Cheston and Frank [75] and in the frequently referenced book by Steinberg [76]. The presentation of this section is partially based is a theoretical description of ultrasound imaging arrays by Macovski [77] and a much earlier paper by Tucker [78]. In addition, Ziomek [79, Chapter 7] provides a useful discussion of array theory, particularly in relation to underwater applications, and the classic text of Skudrzyk [80, Chapter 26] also contains a helpful account.

Arrays of individual transducer elements, when used for generating an ultrasound beam or for detecting a source, can be both focused and steered. They can be classified as either *linear arrays* or *plane arrays*. Linear (1-D) arrays consist of elements arranged so that their center of symmetry lies on a line as illustrated in Fig. 7.7a. On the other hand, plane arrays consist of elements arranged in a 2-D pattern (Fig. 7.7c). The elements of an array can be either *periodic* or *aperiodic*. For a periodic array the elements have a periodic spacing, but this can lead to the generation of grating lobes (see section 7.2.1) within the field of view if the element spacing is not sufficiently small e.g., $<\lambda/2$. If they are aperiodic, the elements can be arranged either in a deterministic but nonperiodic manner or in a random manner [76]. If the elements are chosen by a random process to lie anywhere within a given length (or area), such an array is called a *random array*. An aperiodic array can also be

---

14. The barriers presented by the ribcage and gas-filled lungs severely restrict ultrasonic access to the heart, and as a result a small-footprint transducer that uses sector scanning is needed.

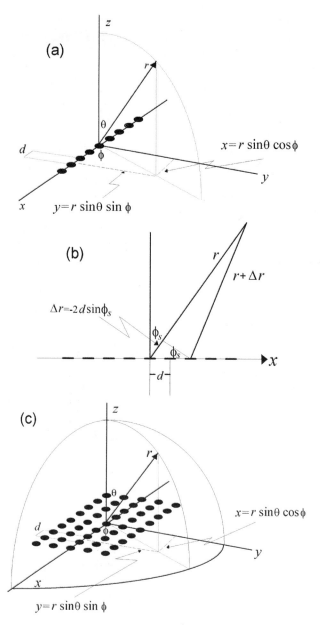

Figure 7.7 Point source arrays. (a) 1-D periodic array of omnidirectional point sources. (b) Cross-sectional view. The difference in path lengths to the observation point results in a phase shift. (c) 2-D periodic array that enables the beam to be steered in both the azimuthal (ϕ) and elevation directions (θ). The angular direction of an observation point can be specified by means of the direction cosines $u_x = \sin\theta\cos\phi$ and $u_y = \sin\theta\sin\phi$.

constructed by fully populating a periodic array and then removing a specified fraction of elements by a random process. Such an array is sometimes
referred to as a *statistical array*, or as a *sparse periodic array*.

7.2.1 Steering and Focusing: A Geometric Approach

The ability to steer and focus an array both in transmission and reception is
vital for obtaining real-time high-quality images. Early systems generally
relied on analog circuits, such as tapped delay lines, for achieving these functions. Subsequently, with the availability of high-speed A/D converters and
processors, digital systems have generally been used and as such are generally
referred to as digital beamformers [81,82]. We shall discuss beamformers in
terms of their application to transmission and reception and will initially
assume that the array elements are point sources.

Transmission

Consider N point sources (for convenience, N is assumed to be odd) arranged
as a 1-D array with a center–center spacing of d, and suppose that each source
is excited with the same amplitude. If, as shown in Fig. 7.8a, the waveform to
each element is delayed by a constant amount (equivalent to a change of phase
for CW excitation), the transmitted wavefront will propagate at an angle ϕ_s
(the azimuthal steering angle), proportional to the delay. Specifically, the
required inter-element delay for an azimuthal angle of ϕ_s is given by $\Delta\tau = (d/c_o)\sin\phi_s$. Focusing can be achieved by introducing the time delays indicated
in Fig. 7.8b. With the help of Fig. 7.9a, the delay required for the n'th element
can be expressed as [83]

$$\tau_n = \frac{1}{c_o}\left[\sqrt{R_F^2 + (N-1)^2 d^2/4} - \sqrt{R_F^2 + (nd)^2}\right],$$

where $-(N-1)/2 \le n \le (N-1)/2$, the z-axis focal point is denoted by R_F, and
the index n is referenced to the central element. From this expression it can
be seen that the required delay for the two outer elements is zero, and that
for the central element ($n = 0$) it is the maximum. In the presence of both
steering and focusing, the delays to each element can also be found from
Fig. 7.9a as [83]

(7.1)
$$\tau_n = \frac{1}{c_o}\left[\sqrt{R_F^2 + (N-1)^2 d^2/4 + (N-1)R_F d\sin|\phi_s|}\right.$$
$$\left. - \sqrt{R_F^2 + (nd)^2 - 2nR_F d\sin\phi_s}\right].$$

For a given array, the first term of this expression is a constant that is equal to
the delay needed to ensure that all delays are positive for $-N \le n \le N$ and
$-\pi/2 < \phi < \pi/2$. If the second square root term is expanded to a second order
in (nd/R_F), then

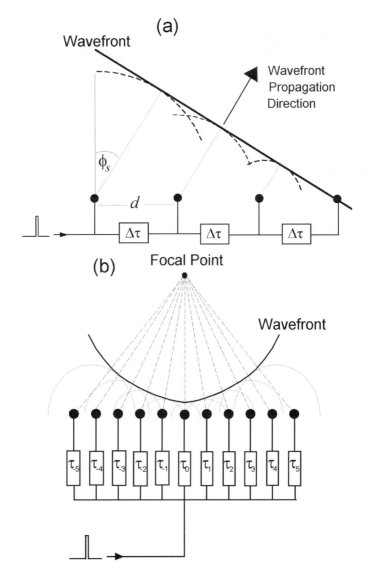

Figure 7.8 Beam steering and focusing on transmission by means of time delay elements. (a) The steered wavefront propagates in a direction determined by the magnitude of the time delays $\Delta\tau$. This sketch represents a snapshot of the wavefront at $t = 3\Delta\tau$ when the excitation consists of an impulse at $t = 0$. (b) Focusing is achieved by means of delays that vary as the square of the element position.

$$\sqrt{R_F^2 + (nd)^2 - 2nR_Fd\sin\phi_s} \approx R_F - nd\sin\phi_s + \left[(nd)^2 \Big/ (2R_F)\right]\cos^2\phi_s.$$

This enables a useful approximation for larger f-numbers ($R_F/(2Nd) > 2$) to be written as [95, p. 233; 96]

$$(7.2) \qquad \tau_n \approx \frac{nd\sin\phi_s}{c_o} - \frac{(nd)^2\cos^2\phi_s}{2c_oR_F} - \tau_0,$$

in which the linear first term accounts for the beam steering angle, the quadratic second term accounts for the beam focusing, and the final term is a constant delay.

The required delay times can be illustrated by means of a 33-element array that has an inter-element spacing of 0.15 mm ($\lambda/2$, for 5 MHz: $D \sim 5$ mm) and that is focused at a point 3 cm away from the central transducer element. From Fig. 7.9b it should be noted that relatively small delays are needed for focusing, compared to that needed for large angle deflections (Fig. 7.9c), and these delays are functions of both the steering angle and focal point. Errors in the time delay requirements arise from the fact that the actual delays that can be provided in a digital system are discrete approximation to the ideal computed values. These quantization errors can cause appreciable degradation of the side lobe response, as was appreciated in the earlier stages of array development [83,84], when limitations in digital processing speeds required the use of relatively large time increments, e.g., 0.125 μs for a 2.25 MHz system. To avoid significant focusing errors, modern systems require delay quantization errors corresponding to about $\lambda/32$ [85] or less. Holm and Kristoffersen have given a worst-case example as to how quantization errors affect the side lobe level for various focal depths [86].

A second source of focusing error arises from variations in the speed of propagation over the region to be imaged. Ultrasound is used clinically under conditions where the sound speed variations throughout the image can be more than 150 m/s (see Fig. 1.11), corresponding to ±5%. Such variations can produce large increases in the lateral beam width (300%) and can be responsible for significant reductions in the pulse-echo amplitude, e.g., 10 dB, as was demonstrated by Anderson et al. [87] using sound speed errors of ±8% with a commercial ultrasound scanner.

Reception: Dynamic Focusing

Steering and focusing in reception can be accomplished by delaying and summing the received signal. Focusing in transmission is restricted to a fixed point per excitation and therefore cannot be changed once the transducer elements have been excited. On the other hand, in reception the focal point can be changed, provided the delays are changed before arrival of the wavefront at the elements, and this makes it possible to track a source, provided its path is known. Thus, the basic idea of dynamic focusing on reception is to change the focal length of the aperture so that as each scattered wave arrives at the

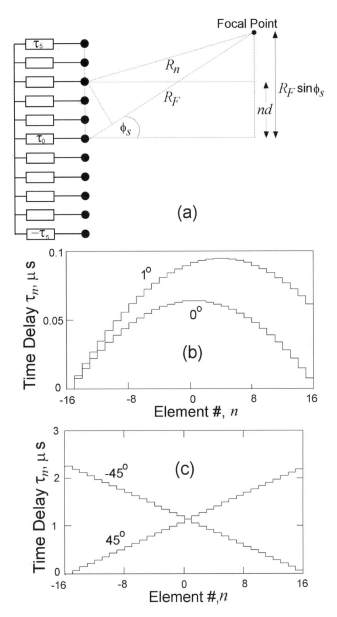

Figure 7.9 Beam steering and focusing using an array with spacing of 0.15 mm and focused at 3.0 cm from the central element. The delays are shown for a 33-element array and transmission in a medium with $c_o = 1,500$ m/s. (a) Geometry used for calculating the required delays. (b) Delays needed for 0-degree and 1-degree deflections with focusing. (c) Delays needed for plus and minus 45-degree deflections, but no focusing.

receive aperture, the signal detected by each element is delayed by exactly the amount needed to focus the receive aperture to the point where the signal originated. For simplicity, we shall assume that the transmitted pulse is propagating along the z-axis in an ideal manner. As illustrated in Fig. 7.10, the pulse arrives at the scatterer at position z_1 and produces a spherical wave that arrives at the transmit/receive aperture after a time $2z_1/c_o$. The received signal produced by each element is delayed to correct for the difference in arrival times and then is summed to produce the focused signal from z_1. Similarly, the scattered signal produced by the scatterer at z_2 is delayed and summed.

The use of dynamic focusing on reception for ultrasound appears to have been originally suggested in 1957 by Schuck [89][15] and was mentioned by Reid and Wild [88] in relation to proposals and analysis of annular arrays for ultrasound imaging. However, the technical challenges of implementing this idea were considerable, and the idea seems to have been laid to rest until the 1970s. At that time various schemes for producing the controlled delays needed for dynamic focusing were examined that included digitally controlled delay lines [71] and the use of charge-coupled devices (CCDs) [90] in which the clock frequency could be varied by means of a voltage-controlled oscillator. In the imaging system developed at Duke University, a PDP 11–20 computer[16] was used to control tapped analog delay lines and to make rapid changes in the delay for each receive channel of the 16-element phased array [73]. One of the problems with switched delay lines was the noise injected into the received signal when they were switched. In 1977 Maslek [92] filed a patent application for a scheme in which the RF signal was multiplied (mixed) with a local oscillator frequency, enabling fine delays to be varied by simply changing the local oscillator phase, thereby avoiding the need for switching. Burkhardt et al. [93] used a similar scheme in their 32-element sector scanner and pointed out that the basic idea had been proposed and used much earlier by Tucker et al. [60] for underwater (sonar) phased-array imaging. An alternative scheme that used quadrature sampling[17] was proposed by Powers et al. [94], who used it in their 4-element, 5 MHz annular-array B-mode scanner.

With significant advances in A/D converter technology and a number of newly proposed dynamic delay schemes,[18] digital beamforming schemes became more widely used. To avoid significant degradation of the image quality obtained with a 5 MHz system, the delays should be accurate to about 5 ns, corresponding to ~$\lambda/32$. Some of the commercial systems available in the

15. I am grateful to Dr. J. Reid for help in tracking this down (Jan. 20, 2001). Schuck's patent, which was filed in September 1957 and granted in May 1963: it was assigned to Minneapolis-Honeywell.

16. It is perhaps of interest to note that one of the first examples of real-time use of a dedicated digital computer to control the scanning, signal acquisition, and display of ultrasound images was that described by Fry et al. [91] in 1968. The system was used for brain scanning and included a means of displaying C-mode images.

17. In quadrature sampling, two samples are taken 90 degrees apart with respect to the center frequency, every sampling interval [94]. The minimum sampling rate required for a 60% bandwidth system is 0.6 of the center frequency.

18. See [96] for a useful review and reference listing.

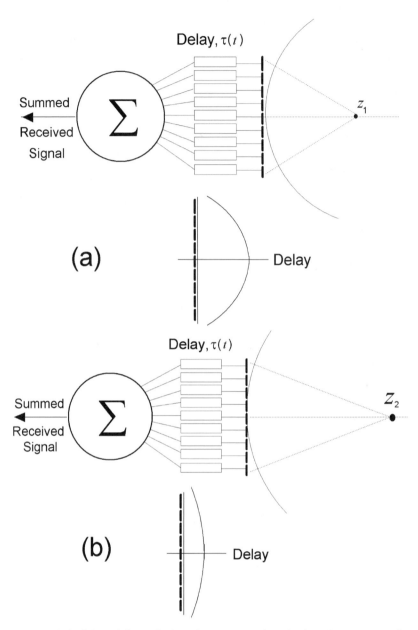

Figure 7.10 Principles of dynamic focusing on reception. A nine-element array is shown, and the wavefronts from scatterers at locations z_1 and z_2 are shown in (a) and (b) respectively, as they arrive at the aperture. The delays for the signals detected by each element are time-dependent. As the transmitted wave progresses along the z-axis, the required delays are reduced.

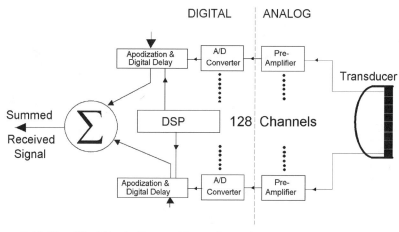

Figure 7.11 Simplified block diagram illustrating a digital beamforming receiver system that uses a low-noise preamplifier, a high-speed (40 MHz) A/D converter (≥12 bit), and a digital delay (shift register) controlled by a digital signal processor (DSP).

1990s used 128 channels and had a reception architecture similar to that illustrated in Fig. 7.11.

For the purpose of describing the process of beamforming both in transmission and reception, it is helpful to consider a far-field expression for the received signal. Let us consider an array with N elements that are used for both transmission and reception, and suppose that the transmitted waveform is denoted by $V_T(t)$ and $\xi_{X,j}$ is the transmit apodization function. The waveform seen at the focal point will be proportional to $\sum_{j=0}^{N} \xi_{T,j} V_T\left(t - \tau_{T,j} + R_{fp}/c_o\right)$, where R_{fp} is the distance to the focal point and $\tau_{T,j}$ is the transmit delay for the j'th element. If reception involves dynamic focusing, then we must incorporate a time-dependent delay of $\tau_{R,i}(t)$ and a time-dependent aperture function $\tau_{R,i}(t)$. Generally, the latter is increased in time so as to maintain a nearly constant f-number and therefore the same lateral resolution. The received signal from an ideal scatterer can be written as

$$V_R(t) = \sum_{i=0}^{N} \xi_{R,i}(t) \sum_{j=0}^{N} \xi_{T,j} V_T\left(t - \tau_{R,i}(t) - \tau_{T,j} + 2R_{fp}(t)/c_o\right),$$

where the outer summation index i refers to the receive elements. This result is sometimes referred to as the beamformer equation [81].

An important problem associated with the simple scheme shown in Fig. 7.11 arises from the different arrival times of the signals at the A/D from each array element. Because of limitations in A/D sampling rate in combination with a sufficient dynamic range,[19] the delayed samples may differ from those required

19. In the mid to late 1990s, commercial A/D converters were available with 10 to 12 bits of sampling at 20 to 40 MHz (see [102] for a listing).

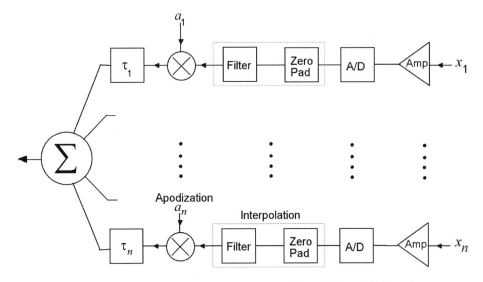

Figure 7.12 Details of a time-domain beamformer. Through the addition of zeros between each sample followed by low-pass filtering, the sampling rate can be increased.

to correctly reconstruct the output signal from the summer. These delay errors can be avoided by using interpolation to substantially increase the sampling rate following the initial sampling at a rate consistent with the requirement of a large dynamic range. This process, a well-known technique in digital signal processing [97], consists of first inserting L zeros between each of the original samples, and then low-pass filtering so as to remove the aliased portions of the signal. The result is an interpolated version of the original signal, sampled at a rate equal to $(L + 1)$. In Fig. 7.12, which illustrates the modified time-domain technique, the interpolated high sample rate signal is apodized, then delayed and finally summed.

An alternative scheme for reducing the delay errors is to use an oversampling[20] A/D converter consisting of a single-bit delta-sigma ($\Delta\Sigma$) modulator [98,99]. Such schemes were first investigated for ultrasound beamforming in the early 1990s [100–102], and shortly thereafter for radar [103].

Instead of generating an entire word, consisting perhaps of 10 to 12 bits at each sample, as is done in more conventional A/D converters, a $\Delta\Sigma$ A/D converter determines only the changes in the input analog signal between samples. In its simplest form (Fig. 7.13), this can be achieved by means of an integrator and a clocked quantizer within a feedback loop that compares the current input level to the value generated by the quantizer. The scheme enables the quantizer output to track the input. Specifically, if the input increases between successive samples, then a binary one is produced; on the other hand, a zero is generated if the input decreases. As illustrated, the output

20. Oversampling implies that the sampling rate is in excess of the Nyquist rate.

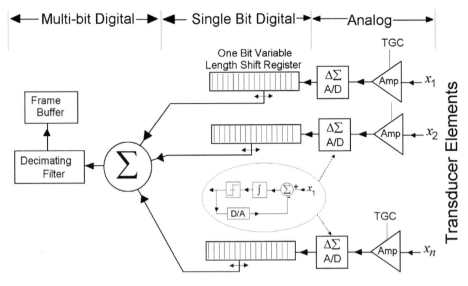

Figure 7.13 Simplified sketch of a first-order oversampling delta-sigma single-bit analog-digital converter system for a receive beamformer. By changing the tap position on the shift registers, appropriate focusing and deflection delays can be dynamically generated. (Based on Freeman et al. [101].)

of the $\Delta\Sigma$ converter is a stream of ones and zeros, which can be temporarily stored in a shift register. Typically, the shift register must have several hundred stages to accommodate the range of dynamic time delays needed for beam focusing and deflection. Because of its simplicity, a one-bit $\Delta\Sigma$ converter can sample at very high speeds, which can be well beyond the Nyquist rate for the source. For example, systems can be designed to operate at more than 32 times the center frequency, which, for a 7 MHz center frequency imaging system, would be 224 MHz. This is sufficient to avoid the sampling rate delay errors discussed earlier. The decimator/filter shown in the figure reduces the sampling rate from what might be many hundred MHz to a frequency sufficient for properly representing the time variations of the input signal. A low-pass filter is used to reduce the high-frequency quantization noise introduced by the modulator.

7.2.2 Grating and Side Lobes

Associated with the periodic structure of an array is the possible presence of *grating lobes*, a name that originates from the lobes produced by an optical diffraction grating. It is important to distinguish between grating and *side lobes*. Side lobes are subsidiary structures that are present with most simple transducers and are also present in the CW radiation pattern of arrays. Grating lobes occur in symmetric locations about the main lobe, have a similar structure to the main lobe, and can have the same amplitude. Their origin is analogous to the presence of aliased signal seen with a time-varying signal when the sampling rate is less than that given by the Nyquist criterion. In fact, the criterion that the inter-element spacing must satisfy to avoid grating lobes can be derived from the sampling theorem [79, pp. 528–532]. Specifically, to unambiguously recover the image information obtained by a spatially sampled aperture for beam steering directions from $-\pi/2$ to $\pi/2$, the spacing between the samples must be less than $\lambda/2$, where λ is the shortest wavelength present in the aperture. In practice, much smaller beam steering angles are generally used, e.g., from $-\pi/4$ to $\pi/4$, allowing the maximum spacing to be taken as approximately half the center frequency wavelength rather than the shortest wavelength.

Of major importance in the design of arrays for medical ultrasound imaging are the grating and side lobe levels relative to the main lobe, since these define the system dynamic range. One of the first groups to recognize their importance was Burckhardt et al. [104] in 1973. Typically, considerable portions of an image consist of signals that have been scattered by relatively weak scatterers. Consequently, if a side lobe encounters a strong scattering region, it can cause a scattered signal to be produced whose strength can be comparable to that returned from the main beam, thereby causing an imaging artifact. To prevent such artifacts, the transmit/receive response due to grating and side lobes should be at least 30 to 40 dB below the central lobe response.

7.2.3 Linear Point Source Arrays

A simple analytic approach for predicting the response of an array is to consider a 1-D array of point sources, such as that illustrated in Fig. 7.7a. Since the number of elements in a typical ultrasound array is quite large, e.g., 64, it makes little difference to results if the number is assumed to be even or odd. In the analysis that follows the number is taken to be odd, enabling the center element to be placed at the origin of coordinates and thereby somewhat simplifying the analysis.

Consider the two monochromatic point sources marked in Fig. 7.7b, and suppose that both are excited with the same signals. Then the pressure at an observation point r will be the sum of the two contributions and is given by

$$p(r;t) = \frac{A}{r} e^{j(\omega t - kr)} + \frac{A}{r + \Delta r} e^{j[\omega t - k(r + \Delta r)]} \approx \frac{A}{r} e^{j(\omega t - kr)}[1 + e^{-jk\Delta r}],$$

where A is the source strength expressed in (N/m), and the approximate form is valid in the far field. Note that the term in square brackets determines how the intensity varies with the observation direction angle ϕ_s and that the field distribution is independent of the elevation angle θ.

Sinusoidal Excitation

Let us consider the case for which the excitation is harmonic with an angular frequency of ω and there is no focusing, just beam steering through an angle of ϕ. This can be achieved by making the phase angle depend linearly on the source location, i.e., $\phi_n = n\Delta\phi$, where $\Delta\phi$ is the change in phase between the n'th and $n+1$ elements. At a far distant $(r \gg Nd/2)$ observation point whose spherical coordinates are (r,ϕ), the pressure is given by

$$p(r, \phi{:}t) \approx \frac{A}{r}e^{j(\omega t - kr)} \sum_{n=-(N-1)/2}^{(N-1)/2} e^{j\omega(\Delta t_n - \Delta r_n/c_0)} = \frac{A}{r}e^{j(\omega t - kr)} \sum_{n=-(N-1)/2}^{(N-1)/2} e^{-jn(kd\sin\phi - \Delta\phi)},$$

in which the time delay for the nth element is $\Delta t_n = n\Delta\phi/\omega$ and $\Delta r_n = nd\sin\phi$. By making use of the relation

(7.3)
$$\sum_{n=-(N-1)/2}^{(N-1)/2} e^{-jn\Psi} = \frac{\sin(N\Psi/2)}{\sin(\Psi/2)},$$

and letting $\Psi = kd\sin\phi - \Delta\phi$, the pressure at an observation point is given by

(7.4)
$$p(r, \phi{:}t) \approx \frac{A}{r}e^{j(\omega t - kr)} \frac{\sin\left[\dfrac{N}{2}(kd\sin\phi - \Delta\phi)\right]}{\sin\left[\dfrac{1}{2}(kd\sin\phi - \Delta\phi)\right]}.$$
(a)

Examination of this expression shows that because of the additional factor of N in the numerator, over a given span of angles, the $\sin[.]$ term in the numerator becomes zero much more often than that in the denominator. The angles for which the numerator is zero and the denominator is *non-zero* results in a pressure amplitude of zero. However, the angles for which *both* the numerator and denominator are zero (in the limit, the ratio is equal to N) correspond to the peaks of the main lobe and grating lobes (when present). It can be readily shown that the observation angles at which the main and grating lobes occur can be found from $\sin\phi = \dfrac{\lambda}{d}\left(\pm m - \dfrac{\Delta\phi}{2\pi}\right)$, where $m = 0$ corresponds to the main lobe and $m = 1, 2, 3\ldots$ correspond to the grating lobe angles. Also, in the absence of any steering, as the spacing d is increased, the first grating lobes appear at $\phi = \pm 90$ degrees when $d = \lambda$. Steering causes the main lobe to increase in width and to be displaced by an angle of $\sin^{-1}(\Delta\phi/kd)$. At the main lobe and grating lobe angles, the pressure is a maximum and is given by $p(r) \approx \dfrac{A}{r}N$. Over an observation angle of $\pm\pi/2$ and over a beam steering angle of $\pm\pi/2$, no grating lobes will be seen, provided $d < \lambda/2$.

Fig. 7.14 illustrates some of the above properties. In (a) and (b) are shown a 65-element array with a spacing of $\lambda/2$. Beam steering through 30 degrees causes some widening of the main lobe. The effects associated with a greater spacing ($d = 1.1\lambda$) are shown in (c) and (d). In the absence of steering, two grating lobes are present. Because the length of this array is more than twice that of (a) and the two have the same number of elements, both the main and side lobes are narrower.

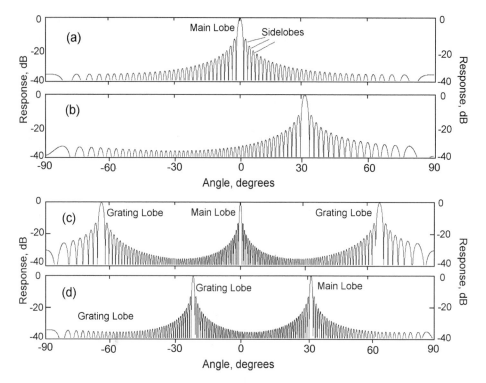

Figure 7.14 Formation of grating lobes and the effect of beam steering for a linear array consisting of 65 equally spaced point sources. The normalized far-field magnitude of the transmit pressure versus observation angle is plotted. (a) Element spacing $d = \lambda/2$, (b) beam steering 30.2 degrees: no grating lobe is seen. (c) Element spacing $d = 1.1\lambda$, showing the presence of two grating lobes. (d) Beam steering of 30.2 degrees: a strong grating lobe is seen.

It is also of interest to examine how the response is affected by the far-field approximation. By taking the observation point to be at a constant distance from the center of a 65-element array of point sources and using the exact expression for the field due to each elementary source, the field pattern shown in Fig. 7.15 can be obtained. It can be seen that close to the array the response is relatively constant over a wide range of angles, and the pattern bears little resemblance to that seen in the far field.

Pulse Excitation of Simple Arrays

In the above discussion, all the source points were assumed to be harmonically excited at the same frequency. A more realistic situation is to consider the far-field response when pulse excitation is used. We shall assume a

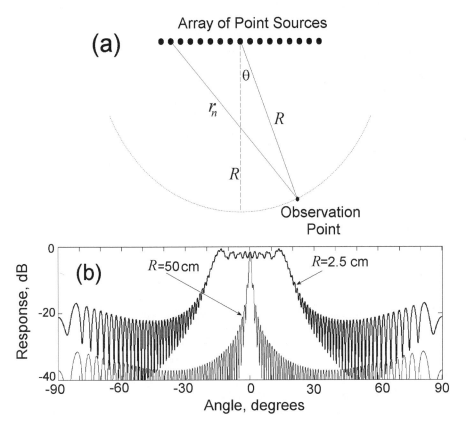

Figure 7.15 Near- and far-field response for a linear array of 65 point sources excited at 5 MHz in water. Separation distance $d = 0.25$ mm ($d = 0.833\lambda$, total length $= 1.625$ cm). (a) Geometry. (b) Near-field (2.5 cm) and far-field (50 cm) pressure response as a function of the observation angle.

Gaussian modulated sinusoidal waveform such that the complex pressure at a distance r from a point source is given by

$$p(r{:}t) = \frac{A}{r}e^{j\omega_c(t-r/c_o)}e^{-\sigma_\omega^2(t-r/c_o)^2/2},$$

where ω_c is the angular center frequency and the −6-dB bandwidth is equal to $2.36\sigma_\omega/\omega_c$. As shown in Chapter 1, subsection 1.4.1, the corresponding frequency spectrum is also Gaussian and is given by

$$\underline{p}(r{:}\omega) = \frac{A}{r}\frac{\sqrt{2\pi}}{\sigma_\omega}e^{-j\omega r/c_o}e^{-(\omega-\omega_c)^2/2\sigma_\omega^2}.$$

At a far-field point (R,θ), the waveform can be found by summing over all N elements of the array, i.e.,

$$\underline{p}(R, \theta : t) \approx \frac{A}{R} e^{j\omega_c t} \sum_{n=-(N-1)/2}^{(N-1)/2} e^{-j\omega_c r_n / c_o} e^{-\sigma_\omega^2 (t - r_n / c_o)^2 / 2},$$

where

$$r_n = \sqrt{(R \cos\theta)^2 + (nd + R \sin\theta)^2}.$$

Fig. 7.16 compares the far-field pulse and CW response for a 65-element linear array. It can be seen that the primary effect of the pulse excitation is to remove the side lobe scalloping without affecting the main lobe dimensions. The presence of a wide distribution of frequencies in the excitation waveform reduces the interference that arises from the periodic nature of the array in combination with the periodicity of the excitation.

7.2.4 Planar Point Source Arrays

A similar type of analysis can be extended to the *planar array* of point sources, such as that illustrated in Fig. 7.7c. With such an arrangement the beam can be steered in two dimensions, enabling 3-D pulse-echo ultrasound measurements to be made. In analyzing the radiation characteristics it is convenient to make use of a coordinate system [75,105] that represents the angular coordinates of a far-field observation point on a rectangular coordinate system. If a point (r, θ, ϕ) that lies on a hemisphere of unit radius $(r = 1)$ is projected onto the plane of the array, then the Cartesian coordinates of the projected point will be given by the direction cosines, $u_x = \sin\theta \cos\phi$ and $u_y = \sin\theta \sin\phi$, both of which lie in the range $-1 \leq u \leq 1$. Consequently, the far-field response can be characterized by a 3-D graph of the beam intensity at each point u_x, u_y. If the spacing in either direction is greater than $\lambda/2$, grating lobes will be created, and all of these will be seen when the field of view extends to the horizon.

7.2.5 Linear Array of Rectangular Elements

In Fig. 7.17 the elements are assumed to be identical and to have the dimensions indicated. If there are an odd number of elements N, then $D = (N - 1)d + W$. Assuming that each element is excited with the same CW signal, then the aperture function, which provides a complete 2-D description of the array geometry, is given by

$$S(x_1, y_1) = \text{rect}\left(\frac{y_1}{H}\right)\left[\left\{\text{rect}\left(\frac{x_1}{D}\right) \times \sum_{n=-\infty}^{\infty} \delta(x_1 - nd)\right\} * \text{rect}\left(\frac{x_1}{W}\right)\right],$$

where x_1 and y_1 are the coordinates on the source plane $z = 0$. As shown in Fig. 7.17b, this expression contains the product of the rect{.} and infinite sum of δ-functions, which creates a sequence of δ-functions at the center of each element. By convoluting this with rect{x_1/W}, the width of each element is replicated at the δ-function locations.

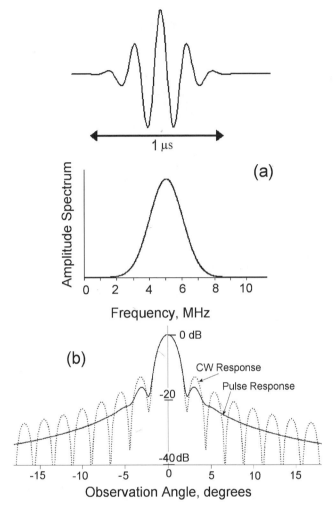

Figure 7.16 Pulse response in the far field ($R = 50\,\text{cm}$) of a 65-element point source linear array for a 5-MHz center frequency pulse with a fractional bandwidth ($-6\,\text{dB}$) of 47%. The element spacing was assumed to be $\lambda_c/2.5$. (a) Pulse waveform and its spectrum. (b) Response compared to that for CW excitation at 5 MHz. The pulse response was taken to be the maximum pressure at the observation point.

Beam steering can be achieved by requiring that the phase of the signal applied to each element vary linearly with the element position. In the above equation, this can be introduced by multiplying the summation term by $e^{j\Delta\varphi x_1/d}$, where $\Delta\varphi$ is the phase shift between successive elements governing the beam steering. In addition, apodization can also be introduced through a function $A(x_1)$ that describes the amplitude distribution to each element. Consequently, the aperture function becomes

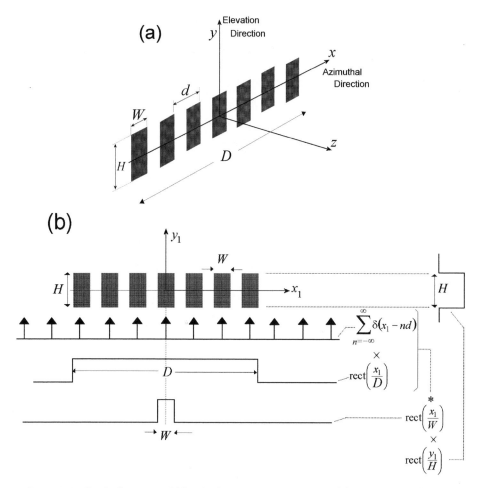

Figure 7.17 Periodic array of identical rectangular elements. (a) Geometry. (b) Generation of the aperture function by multiplication and convolution.

(7.5)

$$S(x_1, y_1) = \mathrm{rect}\left(\frac{y_1}{H}\right)\left[\left\{\mathrm{rect}\left(\frac{x_1}{D}\right) \times A(x_1)e^{j\Delta\varphi x_1/d}\sum_{n=-\infty}^{\infty}\delta(x_1 - nd)\right\} * \mathrm{rect}\left(\frac{x_1}{W}\right)\right].$$

In Chapter 3 it was shown that at a far-field (Fraunhoffer) observation point (x_o, y_o, r), the field distribution produced by an aperture on the plane can be found by taking the Fourier transform of the aperture function and evaluating it at the spatial frequencies $k_x = -kx_o/r$ and $k_y = -ky_o/r$. Specifically, the pressure distribution is given by (see [3.31])

(7.6)

$$\underline{p}(x_o, y_o : \omega) = \frac{j\omega\rho_o v_o}{2\pi r}e^{-jkr}\Im\{S(x_1, y_1)\}.$$

If the apodization function is unity, then the Fourier transform can be obtained and the pressure response becomes[21,22]

$$p(x_o, y_o:\omega) = \frac{j\omega\rho_o v_o e^{-jkr}}{2\pi r} \frac{HDW}{d} \mathrm{sinc}\left(\frac{y_o H}{\lambda r}\right) \mathrm{sinc}\left(\frac{x_o W}{\lambda r}\right)$$

(7.7)

$$\times \sum_{n=-\infty}^{\infty} \mathrm{sinc}\left[D\left(\frac{x_o}{\lambda r} - \frac{n}{d} - \frac{\Delta\varphi}{2\pi d}\right)\right].$$

For the special case in which the array consists of elements whose width is equal to the element spacing and there is no beam steering (i.e., $W = d$ and $\Delta\varphi = 0$), the array then becomes identical to that of a simple rectangular trans-ducer of area $D \times H$. By making use of a special identity,[23] it can be readily shown that (7.7) reduces to

(7.8) $$p(x_o, y_o:\omega) = \frac{j\omega\rho_o v_o}{2\pi r} e^{-jkr} HD \,\mathrm{sinc}\left(\frac{y_o H}{\lambda r}\right)\mathrm{sinc}\left(\frac{x_o D}{\lambda r}\right),$$

which is identical to the expression given in Chapter 3 (3.66) for the far-field pressure response for a simple rectangular transducer of width D and height H.

An alternative approach is to represent the array as a *finite* sequence of rect functions. If both apodization and linear phasing are assumed, then the aper-ture function is given by

$$S(x_1, y_1) = \mathrm{rect}\left(\frac{y_1}{H}\right)\left[\sum_{n=-(N-1)/2}^{(N-1)/2} A_n e^{jn\Delta\varphi} \mathrm{rect}\left(\frac{x_1 - nd}{W}\right)\right],$$

where A_n describes the apodization for the nth element and, as before, $\Delta\varphi$ is the change in phase between successive elements. Application of the shift theorem enables the Fourier transform to be obtained and evaluated at the appropriate spatial frequencies, yielding

(7.9) $$\Im\{S(x_1, y_1)\} = HW \,\mathrm{sinc}\left(\frac{y_o H}{\lambda r}\right)\mathrm{sinc}\left(\frac{x_o W}{\lambda r}\right)\sum_{n=-(N-1)/2}^{(N-1)/2} A_n e^{jn\Delta\varphi} e^{jnkdx_o/r}.$$

Further simplification is possible when the apodization is assumed to be uniform ($A_n = 1$). By making use of (7.3), it follows that the summation term in (7.9) simplifies to

---

21. Note that the definition used for the $\mathrm{sinc}(.)$ function is: $\mathrm{sinc}(\varsigma) = \sin(\pi\varsigma)/\pi\varsigma$; some authors define it by: $\mathrm{sinc}(\varsigma) = \sin(\varsigma)/\varsigma$.

22. As discussed in subsection 7.2.6, for small array elements, the far-field pressure should be multiplied by an obliquity factor of $\cos\theta$, where $\theta = \sin^{-1}(x_o/r)$, but for the moment this will be neglected.

23. $\mathrm{sinc}(K) \sum_{n=-\infty}^{n=\infty} \mathrm{sinc}[N(K-1)] = \mathrm{sinc}(KN)$, provided N is an odd positive integer.

$$\sum_{n=-(N-1)/2}^{(N-1)/2} e^{jn\Delta\varphi} e^{jndkx_o/r} = \frac{\sin\left[\dfrac{N}{2}\left(\dfrac{kdx_o}{r}+\Delta\varphi\right)\right]}{\sin\left[\dfrac{1}{2}\left(\dfrac{kdx_o}{r}+\Delta\varphi\right)\right]}.$$

Consequently, the far-field pressure can be written as

(7.10)

$$p(x_o, y_0 : \omega) = \frac{j\omega\rho_o v_o e^{-jkr}}{2\pi r} HW \, \mathrm{sinc}\left(\frac{y_o H}{\lambda r}\right) \mathrm{sinc}\left(\frac{x_o W}{\lambda r}\right)$$

$$\times \frac{\sin\left[\dfrac{N}{2}\left(\dfrac{kdx_o}{r}+\Delta\varphi\right)\right]}{\sin\left[\dfrac{1}{2}\left(\dfrac{kdx_o}{r}+\Delta\varphi\right)\right]},$$

which can be shown to yield the same result as (7.7), and for $W = d$ and $\Delta\varphi = 0$, it also reduces to (7.8). Comparison of (7.10) with (7.4b) reveals that final term is exactly the field profile of omnidirectional point sources placed at the center of each elementary area. Thus, the overall field in the x-direction is simply the product of the single-element field pattern with the field due to an array of point sources.

The above results could have been deduced from the array product theorem [79, Chapter 7], which can be derived as follows. If the aperture function for an element is denoted by $E(x)$ and the array contains N such elements positioned at $x_1 \ldots x_N$, then the overall aperture function is given by

$$E(x) * \sum_{n=1}^{N} A_n e^{j\beta x_n} \delta(x - x_n),$$

where the phase is assumed to be proportional to the source location and given by βx_n. By using the convolution theorem, the Fourier transform can be written as

$$\Im\left\{ E(x) * \sum_{n=1}^{N} A_n e^{j\beta x_n} \delta(x - x_n) \right\} = \Im\{E(x)\} \Im\left\{ \sum_{n=1}^{N} A_n e^{j\beta x_n} \delta(x - x_n) \right\}.$$

From this it follows that the far-field pattern of an array that consists of identically shaped elements with complex weighting coefficients is given by the product of the single-element directivity function and the directivity of an array of point sources that are located at the center of each element and that have the same complex weightings. Note that the theorem applies even when the spacing of elements is not constant.

As an example, Fig. 7.18 shows the pressure response for a 65-element rectangular array on the plane $y = 0$ calculated from (7.10). The responses for two different excitation frequencies are shown together with the response of a single element. At the lower frequency (5 MHz), the element spacing is sufficiently small so that grating lobes are not present over the 60-degree

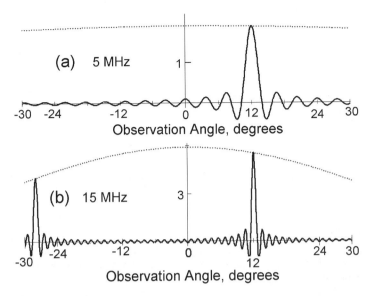

Figure 7.18 Pressure field on the plane $y = 0$ for a 65-element linear rectangular array with dimensions of $W = 100\,\mu m$ and $d = 150\,\mu m$. It is assumed that the apodization is uniform, that the observation sector is 60 degrees (±30 degrees), and that the beam is steered through 12 degrees. The dotted curve corresponds to the far-field response of a single element of width W. Excitation at (a) 5 MHz ($d = \lambda/2$) and (b) 15 MHz ($d > \lambda/2$).

observation sector. At the higher frequency of 15 MHz, a grating lobe is present, the amplitude of which is appreciably modulated by the angular variation of the single-element response.

7.2.6 Obliquity Factor

One-dimensional arrays typically use transducer elements whose width (W) can be significantly less than the thickness (ℓ) and whose height (H) is many tens of wavelengths, giving them a plank-like appearance. Strong acoustic coupling may exist between the thickness and width modes, depending on the ratio W/ℓ. Using finite element analysis, Sato et al. [106] have shown that for a certain value for W/ℓ the electromechanical coupling factor is a maximum, and that typically this occurs at around $W/\ell = 0.6$. In the far field, it is physically reasonable to expect that the directivity function should approach zero as the observation angle approaches ±90 degrees. However, this is not in agreement either with experimental measurements [107] or theoretical predictions based on the assumption that the transducer behaves as a rigid baffle. Delannoy et al. [108] drew attention to this problem when they measured the far-field angular behavior of a strip transducer ($W = 1\,mm$, $H = 20\,mm$) excited at 570 kHz and radiating into water. By assuming that the boundary behaves as

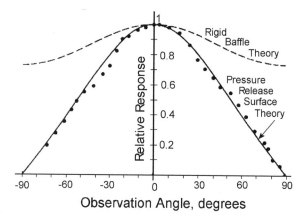

Figure 7.19 The angular response of a single plank-like element with a width of $W = 0.305\,\text{mm}$, which is radiating at 2.5 MHz into water ($\lambda = 0.75\,\text{mm}$). The theoretical response predictions are based on the assumptions of (i) a rigid baffle: $p(\theta) = p_o\,\text{sinc}(\pi W \sin\theta/\lambda)$ and (ii) a pressure release surface: $p(\theta) = p_o\,\text{sinc}(\pi W \sin\theta/\lambda)\cos\theta$. (Reproduced, with permission, from Selfridge et al. [109], *Appl. Phys. Lett.*, 37, 35–36, © 1980 Acoustical Society of America.)

a pressure release surface[24] and that the source can be taken as an infinite strip, excellent agreement was obtained with the experimental results. Subsequently, Selfridge et al. [109] reported similar experimental and theoretical results showing that the far-field directivity function differed from the rigid baffle result by $\cos\theta$, where θ is the angle that the normal to the transducer surface makes to the observation direction. This is clearly illustrated by the measurements shown in Fig. 7.19, which shows far better agreement with theory when the $\cos\theta$ obliquity term is included. More recently, laser interferometric measurements of the surface displacements of linear array elements and hydrophone radiation pattern measurements have shown similar agreement [110].

7.2.7 Sparse Arrays

It was long ago recognized that a major difficulty in the development of planar periodic arrays was the requirement that the element spacing must be sufficiently small so that grating lobes would not be present for the largest steering angles needed. This requirement means that for a given aperture size, a large number of elements must be used, and this greatly increases the system complexity and cost. One method of circumventing this is to eliminate the periodicity by removing elements at random from a periodic array until a given fraction of the original (dense) structure remain. Such an array is often

---

24. For a pressure release surface, the pressure is defined throughout the boundary; e.g., it is uniform on the transducer surface and zero elsewhere.

referred to as a *sparse* array [76, Chapter 8]. Very substantial reductions in the complexity can be achieved, though with some significant penalties associated with the side lobe levels. Unlike dense periodic arrays, for which the side lobe level decreases with the angular deviation from the main lobe, for a random periodic array the expected value of the side lobe power remains independent of angle except close to the main lobe. It can be shown [76, pp. 139–144] that the ratio of the *average* side lobe to the main lobe power is equal to $1/N$, where N is the number of radiators. For example, to achieve a ratio of $-30\,\text{dB}$ ($=10\log 0.001$), 1,000 elements would be needed. However, the *peak* power of the side lobes will be about 7 dB higher [111], resulting in a peak power ratio of $-23\,\text{dB}$.

To illustrate some features of the radiation pattern of random arrays, we shall consider a periodic linear array that, if fully populated, would contain 512 elements (a fully populated array will be referred to as a *dense* array). We shall assume that 50% and 84% of the elements have been removed at random, so that the final arrays contain 256 and 64 elements, respectively. If the elements are assumed to be omnidirectional point sources, the far-field radiation pattern will be as shown in Fig. 7.20. It is important to note that the reduction in the number of elements causes a reduction in the maximum

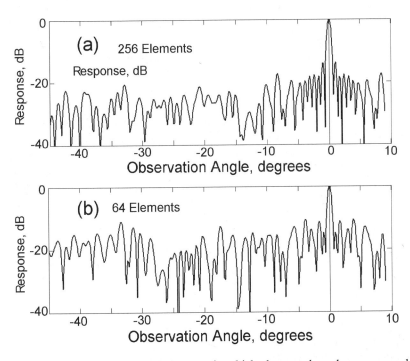

Figure 7.20 Periodic array of 512 elements in which elements have been removed at random, yielding a sparse periodic array of (a) 256 and (b) 64 elements. Each element is assumed to be a point source, and the relative magnitude of the response in the far field is shown as a function of the observation angle.

transmit pressure and in the SNR. However, the SNR can be partially restored by increasing the power delivered to each element.

For 2-D arrays, the number of elements that are required for even a relatively modest size aperture could be very large. For example, a dense 65 × 65 array would require 4,225 elements, making it a challenging task to individually address each element as transmitters and receivers. At least two means have been investigated for eliminating grating lobes and reducing the number of elements. One, as described in subsection 7.2.10, is based on using different transmit and receive apertures whose elements are spaced to make the grating lobes destructively interfere. A second method, based on earlier developments in 2-D sparse radar arrays, is that described by Turnbull and Foster [112].

In their theoretical investigations, Turnbull and Foster studied the field characteristics of a dense 65 × 65 array from which a random selection of elements had been removed and that occupied an area of 1×1 cm^2. Assuming a pulse with a center frequency of 4.5 MHz ($d = 0.45\lambda$), a −6-dB bandwidth of 2 MHz, and a transmit focus at 40 mm from the array, they determined the pulse-echo response when the elements had been reduced by factors of 4, 6, and 8. Over this range and for steering angles up to 45 degrees in both directions, they found that the main lobe shape was not significantly affected and the pulse-echo side lobes remained below −50 dB, provided the reduction was not much greater than a factor of 4. Much more substantial reductions in the number of elements can be achieved by using separate (and sparse) transmission and reception arrays, as will be discussed in subsection 7.2.10.

7.2.8 Inter-Element Cross-Coupling

It has long been realized that cross-coupling between the elements of ultrasound transducers can cause a serious degradation in performance [117]. Two types of cross-coupling have been identified and analyzed: electrical [113] and acoustic [114,118]. In the first, electrostatic and electromagnetic cross-coupling can arise from capacitive, resistive leakage, and inductive coupling between the leads connecting the elements. In the second, waves of various types can be propagated laterally between elements through the backing, through the front surface structures, or directly between the elements, and this has been recognized as a serious problem, especially when the elements are small and closely spaced. In their investigations, Kino and DeSilets [114] showed that the coupling of energy to adjacent elements causes the effective aperture of a single element to increase. In an array, such as that illustrated in Fig. 7.18, this can cause an unacceptable drop-off in the main lobe response at high steering angles [115]. In addition, Lamb wave coupling can be responsible for shifting the peak of the angular response away from 0 degrees, as was noted by Delannoy et al. [116]. An important advantage of sparse arrays arises from the increased element separation, which enables the cross-coupling to be reduced.

In some of the first commercial linear-array designs, such as that described by Dias [119] and illustrated in Fig. 7.21, the substrate consisted of a highly

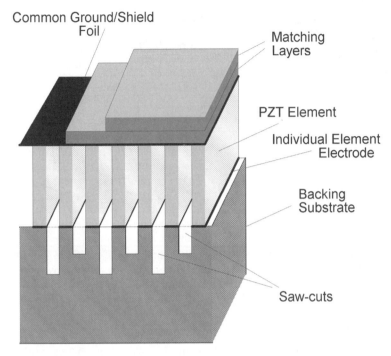

Common Ground/Shield Foil

Matching Layers

PZT Element

Individual Element Electrode

Backing Substrate

Saw-cuts

Figure 7.21 Early type of phased array construction. The piezoelectric ceramic was initially bonded to a substrate that also served as a highly attenuating backing medium. Saw-cuts through the PZT at differing depths into the substrate reduced the acoustic cross-coupling. Not shown is a cylindrical acoustic lens for focusing in the elevation direction.

absorbing medium (tungsten particles embedded in a polyvinyl matrix), and saw-cuts were made through the piezoceramic, through the lower electrode, and into the substrate. Differential saw-cut depths resulted in reduced acoustic cross-coupling.

One of the earliest reports of cross-coupling in 2-D arrays is that described by Turnbull and Foster [112], who investigated both electrical and acoustic effects in fully populated and sparse arrays. They reported that the primary effect of electrical coupling was a severe loss in gain at large steering angles, though with little change in the shape. Subsequently, using both electrical (network analyzer) and mechanical measurements (laser interferometry), Certon et al. [120] investigated the cross-coupling in 1–3 piezocomposite 2-D arrays and have shown that symmetrical Lamb waves within the composite plate are primarily responsible for the observed effects.

7.2.9 Amplitude Weighting (Apodization)

As noted earlier, apodization on transmission consists of weighting the signal amplitudes applied to each element of the array. The use of apodization for

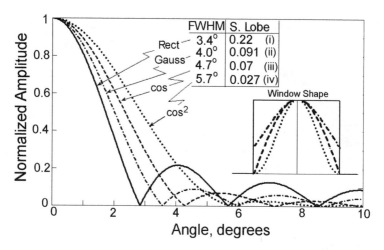

Figure 7.22 Effect of apodization on the far-field response of a 128-element linear array. (i) Rectangular window, (ii) Gaussian window, (iii) cos window, (iv) cos² window. For all four windows the main lobe angular FWHM and the first side lobe amplitude (S. Lobe) are given in the table. The window shapes are also shown.

improving the performance of an ultrasound array is a particular application of the more general signal analysis problem of choosing a window function [122] that will reduce the side lobes relative to the main lobe. However, since some increase in the angular width of the main lobes (and therefore a loss in resolution) accompanies this reduction, it is important that the tradeoff be carefully examined. In Fig. 7.22 the effects of three different apodization functions are illustrated for a 128-element linear array and are compared to a simple rectangular window whose first side lobe is just 13 dB below the peak. For example, with the cosine-squared window, the first side lobe is at –32 dB, though the width of the main lobe at the –3-dB level is increased by ~1.6.

Of considerable importance is the weighting method described in 1946 by Dolph, which, because it depends on certain properties of the Chebyshev polynomials, is generally called the Dolph-Chebyshev method. Dolph showed that a distribution function could be specified for a given permitted maximum side lobe level that would achieve a minimum beam width. For example, a Dolph-Chebyshev apodization function designed to achieve a –40-dB side lobe level would have a main lobe that was 1.35 times wider than that for a rectangular window at the –3-dB level: even at –50 dB, the widening factor is still less than 1.5. However, unlike most other apodization functions, the side lobe levels for the Dolph-Chebyshev method do not decrease.

While apodization functions have been considered in relation to array design, the same functions can also be used to obtain improved time-response characteristics from bandpass filters. For example, based on the Dolph-Chebyshev apodization function in the frequency domain, the time distribution function is given by

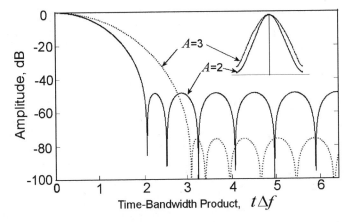

Figure 7.23 Dolph-Chebyshev time domain response for two different values of the side lobe level response. $A = 2$ corresponds to $-48.6\,dB$ and $A = 3$ to $-75.8\,dB$.

$$G(t) = \cos\left[\pi\sqrt{(t\Delta f)^2 - A^2}\right]\Big/\cosh(\pi A),$$

where Δf is the bandwidth and the parameter A, which specifies the desired side lobe level, can be determined from

$$20\log\left[1/\cosh(\pi A)\right] = \text{desired sidelobe level in dB}.$$

An example is shown in Fig. 7.23.

The well-defined side lobes seen in the above figures arose from the effects of interference caused by narrowband (CW) excitation. From subsection 7.2.5 we know that the presence of a broad spectrum of frequencies can greatly reduce the side lobe interference pattern, and consequently the ability of various apodization schemes to reduce the side lobes needs to be examined for broadband excitation. An early investigation was that reported by t'Hoen [121], who studied the influence of nine different apodization schemes for wideband excitation of a linear ultrasound array focused in the near field. For each scheme he related the FWHM (which governs the lateral resolution) and the beam width at $-25\,dB$ (which is a measure of the sensitivity to artifacts) and concluded that the cosine, Hamming[25], sinc, and 10% truncated Gaussian were close to optimal in regard to image quality. A subsequent study (1996) by Daft and Engeler [123] points out the importance of apodization, especially when the center-to-center spacing of the elements is greater than $\lambda/2$, which is sometimes the case in practice. However, they also point out that the effective aperture (see subsection 7.2.10, particularly Fig. 7.24) for a rectangular transmit/receive array is triangular (i.e., it is self-windowed), which makes the case for adding a new window function far from clear.

As noted in subsection 7.2.1, in reception the aperture size is often changed dynamically, and consequently if an apodization function is used, it too must

---

25. $W(n) = 0.54 + 0.46\cos(n\pi/m)$

also be changed dynamically. In transmission several focal zones can be used (sacrificing frame rate), and the resulting parts of the image would be stitched together. Associated with these may be different apodization functions.

7.2.10 Separate Transmit and Receive Apertures

By using separate transmit and receive elements, several advantages can be gained. In the first place, the problems that arise from interference between the transmit and receive circuits are avoided. Second, by choosing suitable element spacing for the two arrays, the locations of the transmit and receive grating lobes could be designed to achieve partial cancellation in the two-way radiation pattern. This idea seems to have been first pursued by von Ramm et al. [124], initially for 1-D arrays and subsequently for 2-D arrays [125]. For example, in one of their 2-D arrays they used 32 transmitter elements uniformly spaced on a cross (+) and 32 receiving elements uniformly spaced on a cross at an angle (×). Many different combination of transmit and receive apertures could be used, and as a result it is important to have a means of comparing the performance. Gehlbach and Alvarez [126], who introduced the concept of *effective aperture*, described such a means.

Effective Aperture

The effective aperture is a receive aperture that when used with a point source transmitter would produce an identical transmit/receive response to that produced by the particular transmit/receive array combination being examined. Thus, for the purpose of comparison the combination of two different arrays is reduced to an effective receive aperture in combination with a point source transmitter.

In the far field, we know that the radiation response is given by the Fourier transform of the aperture function. If $S_T(x_1/\lambda)$ and $S_{\Re}(x_1/\lambda)$ denote the far-field transmit and receive aperture functions, then at an observation point (R,θ), the associated radiation patterns for each aperture can be written as

$$P_T(R,\theta) = \Im[S_T(x_1/\lambda)], \quad P_{\Re}(R,\theta) = \Im[S_{\Re}(x_1/\lambda)].$$

However, the two-way (transmit/receive) field response is the product of the two field patterns, i.e.,

(7.11) $$P_{T\Re}(R,\theta) = P_T(R,\theta) \times P_{\Re}(R,\theta),$$

which, with the help of the convolution theorem and the previous two equations, can be rewritten as $P_{T\Re}(R,\theta) = \Im[S_T(x_1/\lambda) * S_{\Re}(x_1/\lambda)]$. Noting the definition of effective aperture given earlier and denoting it by $S_E(x_1/\lambda)$, we have

$$P_{T\Re}(R,\theta) = \Im[\delta(x_1/\lambda) * S_E(x_1/\lambda)] = \Im[S_E(x_1/\lambda)].$$

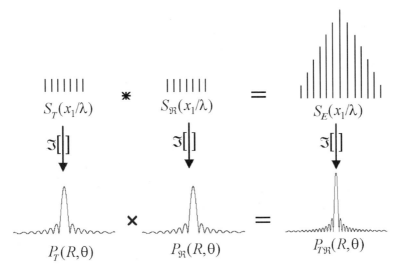

Figure 7.24 Relations between the transmit and receive apertures, and the effective aperture. Identical transmit and receive apertures are shown. The apertures are denoted by $S(x_1/\lambda)$, the field patterns by $P(R,\theta)$ and the Fourier transform by $\Im\{.\}$. (Based on Lockwood et al. [127].)

Consequently, the effective aperture can be expressed as

(7.12) $$S_E(x_1/\lambda) = S_T(x_1/\lambda) * S_\Re(x_1/\lambda).$$

To illustrate how (7.11) and (7.12) are related, Fig. 7.24 shows identical 7-element transmit and receive arrays. By convoluting the transmit and receive apertures, it can be seen that the effective array has 13 elements with triangular apodization, and that the field response of a single-element transmit aperture in combination with this 13-element receive aperture is identical to that obtained using the two 7-element transmit and receive apertures.

The above ideas can be extended to 2-D by generalizing (7.12) to

$$S_E(x_1, y_1) = S_T(x_1, y_1) ** S_\Re(x_1, y_1).$$

If the transmit and receive apertures are separable, i.e., $S_T(x_1, y_1) = S_{Tx}(x_1)S_{Ty}(y_1)$ and $S_\Re(x_1, y_1) = S_{\Re x}(x_1)S_{\Re y}(y_1)$, then the effective aperture simplifies to

$$S_E(x_1, y_1) = [S_{Tx}(x_1) * S_{\Re x}(x_1)][S_{Ty}(y_1) * S_{\Re y}(y_1)].$$

Sparse Array Design

In arriving at the best design of a sparse 1-D array, it is first necessary to specify the desired two-way radiation profile. This determines the properties of the effective aperture, including its apodization. The design task then reduces to finding what transmit and receive array combination gives the best approximation to this effective aperture. Several different combinations may yield the same effective aperture. The best choice may require that the minimum number of elements be used, or it may be a combination that yields the closest approximation. Lockwood et al. [127] have described a number of different strategies in arriving at approximate solutions and have shown that the minimum number of elements needed in each array is such that the product of the two numbers is equal to the square root of the number of elements in the effective array. As an example, they consider a dense (all elements present) 128-element linear array and show experimentally that the number of elements could be reduced by a factor of four by using 16 transmit and 16 receive elements, while maintaining the secondary lobe at least 55 dB below the main lobe. Such a reduction represents the potential for a significant decrease in the complexity and cost of a scanning array.

A variety of methods have been proposed for achieving substantial reductions in the number of active elements in 2-D arrays through the use of separate transmit and receive apertures. These include elements that are placed on concentric rings [128] and the use of vernier array designs [129,130], as described next.

The principles of the vernier method are illustrated in Fig. 7.25. In (a) a pair of vernier rulers are shown. The tick marks for the primary scale A have spacings of pd, where p is an integer and d is a distance; those for the secondary scale B are spaced by $(p - 1)d$. Thus, for the spacings shown, $p = 10$ and $d = 0.1$ mm, and the displacement of the slider is 1.25 cm. By using the vernier scale relations for the transmit and receive apertures, the effective aperture has a spacing of exactly d. This is illustrated in (b), where the transmit array is spaced by $(p - 1)d = 2d$, the receive by $pd = 3d$. By choosing d to be $\lambda/2$, the grating lobes are eliminated.

Many different 2-D vernier array patterns are possible, some of which are given in [130]. An example is shown in Fig. 7.26 for $p = 3$ with 193 transmit and 193 receive elements, together with the computed response for the conditions detailed in the figure caption.

7.2.11 Wave Distortion Due to Dynamic Focusing

As discussed in subsection 7.2.1, dynamic focusing on reception enables the array to increase its focal point with time, and this can be achieved by changing the delay associated with each array element. Maginess and Walker [131,132] have shown that for a transmit pulse with non-zero duration, such a process can cause appreciable distortion of the waveform received from targets close to the array, where the delay changes most rapidly. As will be seen, the received waveform is expanded in duration so that the spectrum will be shifted down in frequency.

Consider a point scatter at a location z on the axis of the array illustrated in Fig. 7.27a, and let us suppose that the transmitted waveform is in the form of the pulse of duration Δt shown in (b) (i). On arrival at the scatterer (ii) it gives rise to spherical waves that reach the center of the array (iii) after a time

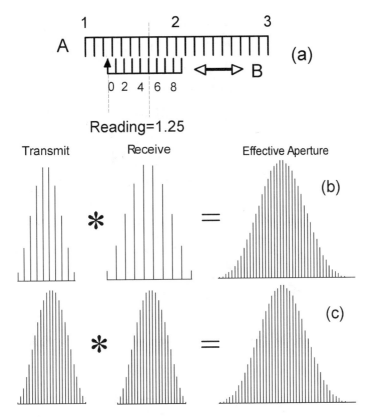

Figure 7.25 Vernier cosine squared apodized sparse 1-D arrays. (a) A simple vernier scale in which the least significant digit is determined by the mark on scale B that is aligned with the mark on scale A. (b) Vernier array pair corresponding to $p = 3$ consisting of 10 transmit and 10 receive elements, together with the effective aperture. (c) Equivalent dense arrays consisting of 24 transmit and 24 receive elements. (Based on Brunke and Lockwood [130].)

$t = z/c_o$ and reach the nth element at a time $\sqrt{z^2 + x_n^2}/c_o$. Let us suppose that the signal from the center element is subject to a fixed delay of τ_0 that is large enough to ensure that all delays are non-negative. It can be readily shown that the delay for the nth element, as indexed from the center of the array, is given by

$$\tau(x_n, t) = \tau_0 - \frac{1}{c_o}\left[\sqrt{z^2 + x_n^2} - z\right].$$

Noting that $z = c_o t$, this delay will change at a rate

$$\frac{d\tau(x_n, t)}{dt} = 1 - \frac{c_o t}{\sqrt{(c_o t)^2 + x_n^2}},$$

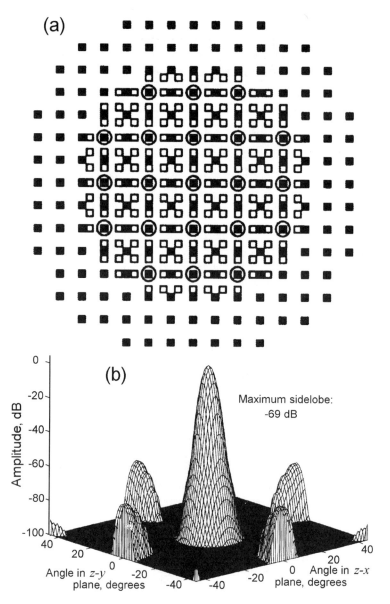

Figure 7.26 Example of 2-D vernier array ($p = 3$). (a) Array geometry: the transmit elements are the solid filled squares, the receive elements are the unfilled squares, and the elements that are shared elements are enclosed by a circle. (b) Transmit/receive response for a 35% bandwidth (−6 dB) pulse assuming a point target, no beam steering, cosine squared apodization, a focal distance of 4 × transmit aperture (*f*/4), dynamically focused receive from *f*/3 to *f*/5 in increments of 1/20 × transmit aperture width. (Reproduced, with permission, from Brunke and Lockwood [130], *IEEE Trans. Ultrason. Ferroelect. Freq. Contr.*, 44, 1101–1109, © 1997 IEEE.)

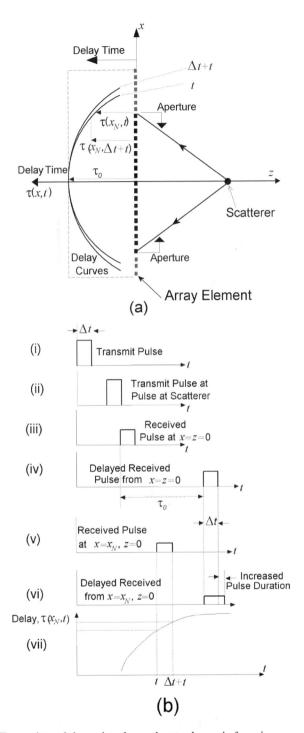

Figure 7.27 Expansion of the pulse shape due to dynamic focusing on reception. For simplicity, it is assumed that transmit pulse is rectangular with a duration of Δt and that a point scatterer is on-axis. (a) Aperture and approximate shape of delay needed for dynamic focusing at the time of arrival of the pulse at a given point on the aperture and at a time Δt later. (b) Waveforms produced by the scatterer at the center and edge of the array.

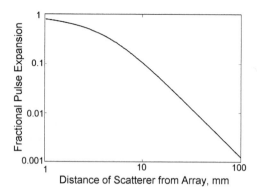

Figure 7.28 Fractional expansion of a pulse due to dynamic focusing on reception caused by an on-axis scatterer as calculated from (7.13). The array was assumed to have an aperture of 10 mm.

which is always positive or zero. Thus, over the transmit pulse duration, the delay will increase by

$$(7.13) \qquad \Delta\tau(x_n, t) \approx \left[1 - \frac{z}{\sqrt{z^2 + x_n^2}} \right] \Delta t,$$

or in other words, the contribution from the n'th array element will be expanded in time. The maximum expansion occurs for the signal at the edge of the aperture ($x = x_N$); for all other elements the expansion will be less, dropping to zero at the center element. Consequently, if the transmit waveform is a short sinusoidal pulse, the effect of dynamic focusing will be to cause a reduction in the center frequency of the received pulse, i.e., an apparent Doppler shift is produced.

For example, let us assume that the total aperture is 10 mm and that a pulse with a duration of 0.5 μs is incident on the scatterer in water ($c_o = 1500$ m/s). The graph of Fig. 7.28 shows that the fractional expansion ($\Delta\tau/\Delta t$) for a scatterer 10 mm from the center is 0.1, and for one 20 mm away it is 0.005.

7.3 Arrays for Two- and Three-Dimensional Imaging

7.3.1 One-Dimensional Arrays

It is perhaps helpful to review the most commonly referred to array structures and to compare their imaging performance. But before starting, it should be noted that some confusion can arise from the terminology.[26] In Fig. 7.29a, an array is illustrated in which a beam is formed by exciting a group of adjacent elements, e.g., 32 out of 256 elements, and a scan over the imaging area is

---

26. R.L. Powis has provided some useful ideas on this topic in a web note entitled "Transducers and Oxymorons" (www.classicalmedical.com/review/to.html).

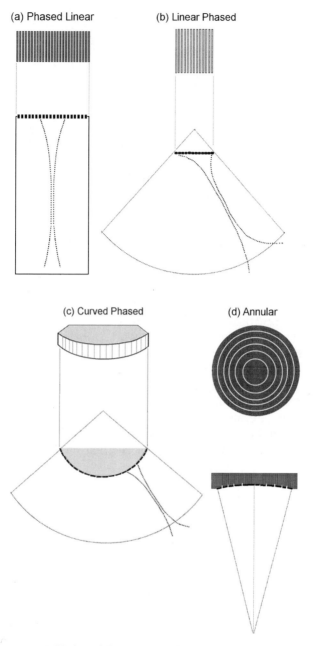

Figure 7.29 Various 1-D arrays used for real-time 2-D imaging.

achieved electronically moving the group to adjacent elements. Azimuthal steering and focusing can also be used in transmission and reception by properly phasing and apodizing the elements in the group. Since linear movement of the beam is combined with focusing, we shall refer to this as a *phased linear array*. A fixed-focus cylindrical lens is generally used to reduce the slice thickness in the elevation direction. However, as illustrated in Fig. 7.30, outside the focal region the elevation sample volume dimension is considerably increased. Moreover, the far-field first side lobe associated with an unapodized rectangular element is only 13.4 dB below the main lobe (see Fig. 7.22 or Fig 3.38). One method for increasing the depth of field in the elevation direction and to reduce the side lobe response is by apodization. By introducing a gradient in the attenuation of the lens material, various apodizations [133] can be obtained. A comparison of the −10-dB contours for an apodized and unapodized lens is presented in Fig. 7.30.

In the *linear phased array* (note the order of the words) transducer shown in (b), all elements are used to obtain the results for each scan line. The fan-like sector scan formed by this process causes the line density to decrease with depth, resulting in a possible loss in information. As with the phased linear array, when a cylindrical lens is used, the slice thickness can be reduced in the vicinity of the focal plane. Moreover, the smaller array footprint enables images to be made though limited windows, e.g., imaging the heart by using the space between the ribs.

An array with a wide field of view is the *curvilinear phased array* (also called a convex array) illustrated in (c). Such arrays use groups of elements similar to the phased linear array and provide for an increased field of view without requiring steering. Because steering inevitably results in some loss in lateral resolution, the curvilinear phased array maintains its resolution over a wide field of view. Moreover, the absence of steering enables better side lobe

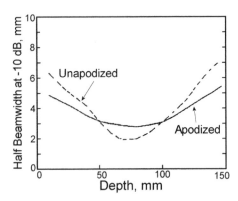

Figure 7.30 The effect of apodization on the depth of field for an elevation lens. The apodization increases the depth of field and decreases the side lobe level.
(Reproduced, with permission of the International Society for Optical Engineering, from McKeighen [133], pp. 2–18 in *Ultrasonic Transducer Engineering*, Vol. 3341, Medical Imaging, © 1998 SPIE.)

rejection to be achieved. But, as with (b), the line density decreases with depth. Such an array might consist of 128 elements with $d = 400\,\mu m$ (arc length ~5 cm), $H = 10\,mm$, and $W = 350\,\mu m$.

The *annular array* shown in (d) has the advantage of cylindrical symmetry so that the sample volume dimensions are independent of angle. Such an array was originally proposed in 1957 by Schuck [89] and discussed in [88]. In subsequent years more detailed consideration was given to the design and application of such transducers [137,138]. However, electronic steering is not feasible, and consequently high-speed mechanical rocking of the transducer is required to form a real-time image. This led to problems associated with the coupling fluid (reverberation, refraction) and decreased reliability compared to the electronically deflected arrays. Perhaps the most complete description of such an array is that contained in the papers by Foster et al. [134,135]. Their system consisted of a 3.0-cm-diameter, 12-element, 4.5 MHz array with a 6.5-cm radius of curvature. The array could be focused to a point 3.0 cm from the array where the *f*-number (focal length/diameter) was 1.0 and the beam diameter was 0.34 mm. A two-zone transmit focus scheme with cosine apodization was used. The foci were at 50 and 130 mm, and the resulting images were stitched together at 76 mm. On reception, a dynamic focusing scheme was used, similar to that described by Kim et al. [136].

Aperture Selection

As illustrated in the geometric ray sketch of Fig. 7.31, for a constant aperture size the depth of field decreases as the focal point F decreases. Consequently, for a wide-aperture, short-focal-length lens (i.e., a small *f*-number), the range of depths over which good focusing is maintained will be small. Uniform image quality can be maintained over a relatively broad range of depths by specifying that the *f*-number be held constant as the focal point moves from the near-field position to the greatest depth, and this can be achieved by increasing the aperture $\mathcal{D}$ so that $F/\mathcal{D}$ remains constant. Such a specification, in the case of a simple focused circular aperture, will ensure that the lateral FWHM on the focal plane remains constant (see (3.56)). In dynamic focusing a constant *f*-number approach means that a small aperture is used close to the transducer, and as the focal point moves away, the size is increased in proportion. Evidently, such a process can continue only to the point where no further aperture increase is possible, at which point the *f*-number will start to increase.

One of the first systems to incorporate these ideas was the "expanding-aperture" 12-element annular array described by Dietz et al. [138]. In this 4.0 cm diameter transducer, four elements were used at the minimum focal point of 1.5 cm. As the focal point was increased, so was the number of annuli, a process that was continued until the maximum of 12 annuli was reached at a focal point of 12.5 cm. Beyond this, the *f*-number could no longer be held constant.

For a 1-D linear array that uses a cylindrical lens, the elevational depth of field is determined by the *f*-number. Moreover, except in the immediate

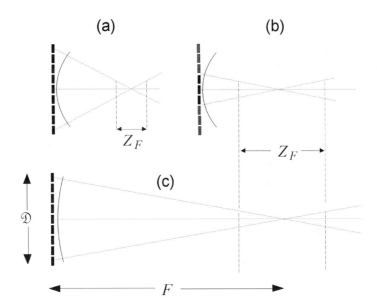

Figure 7.31 Effect of aperture and focal point F on the depth of field. For (a) and (c) which have the same aperture $\mathcal{D}$ but differing focal points, the depths of field Z_F, differ greatly. (b) Shows that the depth of field can be made the same as (c) by reducing the aperture.

vicinity of the focal point, the spatial resolution in the two directions will differ greatly.

7.3.2 Three-Dimensional Imaging

Historical Background

The idea of using a sequence of ultrasound 2-D tomographic slices to construct a 3-D image can be traced back to the original 3-D imaging proposals and demonstration by the Howry group in 1954/56 (see Fig. 7.2). The first example of the use and clinical application of 3-D ultrasound is that described by Baum and Greenwood [139] in 1961 for use in ophthalmologic diagnosis. They transferred a sequence of B-mode images of the eye taken in steps of approximately 0.5 mm onto transparent photographic plates. By stacking the plates in the proper order and with appropriate spacing, a 3-D model was formed that enabled the structure of the eye to be much more readily interpreted than was possible with a single B-mode image. As illustrated in Fig. 7.32, Baum and Greenwood used this technique to diagnose a patient with a tumor above the right eye.

In the subsequent 35 years, a variety of attempts have been made to develop systems that could produce and display 3-D clinical images, first by using an articulated-arm single-transducer system and later by translating 1-D arrays and more recently by 2-D arrays. Some of the early initiatives in 3-D

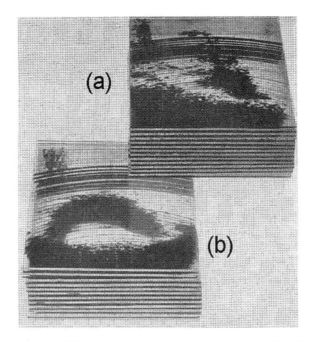

Figure 7.32 Sequence of B-mode images recorded on photographic plates taken through the right eye of a patient with a tumor. (a) This stack of plates corresponds to a 3-D image of the volume above the globe, where a tumor was identified. The upper right portion shows the lesion. (b) This stack of plates corresponds to the 3-D region below those of (a) and shows a normal globe and its orbit. (Reproduced from Baum and Greenwood [139], *NY State J. Med.*, 61, 4149–4157, 1961. Used by permission of the Medical Society of the State of New York).

ultrasound were those of Brown [50], whose work on the invention and development of the Diasonograph (see Fig. 7.3) has been previously described. In [50] Brown suggested that a spiral scan pattern would be an efficient means of acquiring 3-D data, an idea subsequently adapted in a proposed C-mode scanning system. In the early 1970s Brown [38] and his associates[27] working at Sonicaid Ltd. (Scotland) developed a 3-D ultrasound imaging system that was exhibited in 1976. Unfortunately, it was based on a "static" B-mode scanner and appeared at the time when real-time displays that used rotating transducers had been available for some time and linear arrays were entering the marketplace. This, together with the difficulty of convincing the medical profession as to its advantages, resulted in commercial failure. McDicken et al. [141] were probably the first (1972) to describe and demonstrate a method for generating a stereoscopic pair of ultrasound images. They used a fiberoptic linear array that was mechanically coupled to an A-mode transducer. They

27. A description was presented at a conference held in 1976 and summarized in the conference proceedings [140].

transferred the brightness mode A-display to the focal plane of a stereoscopic camera by using the fiberoptic array. By moving the transducer in a 3-D scanning pattern, stereo recordings were made.

One of the first to investigate the use of computers for extracting 3-D information from a sequence of 2-D scans was Robinson [142]. In a 1972 publication he demonstrated how information on planes that intersected the stored B-mode scans could be obtained. With the computer systems available at that time, this was a comparatively slow and expensive process. One of the earliest systems that made use of a real-time scanner for obtaining 2-D slices for subsequent 3-D cardiac image reconstruction was that proposed by King et al. [143] in 1975. One of the challenges was to determine the transducer alignment so that the information as to the exact plane and direction of each B-mode image could be sent to the computer along with the B-mode data. The system proposed by King et al. made use of a spark-gap position-recording apparatus. This consisted of three air spark gaps arranged in the form of a triangle and attached to the transducer handle. Excitation produces sonic waves whose arrival times at an array of microphones placed at fixed locations provides the information needed to calculate the transducer position and orientation. Beginning in the late 1970s Brinkley et al. [144,145] provided details of their spark-gap locating system and described methods for 3-D reconstruction from which organ volume information could potentially be extracted. About the same time (1982), Greenleaf [146] described a system that stored some 75 B-mode image scans that were obtained by mechanically translating a 10 MHz real-time transducer in steps of approximately 0.3 mm. The image data, which were stored on magnetic tape, were subsequently used by 3-D calculation programs to obtain sectional and perspective displays. Similar work was published that same year by Ghosh et al. [147], who used a sector scanner that was at a fixed position but was rotated through various angles to obtain the necessary B-mode image data for computer reconstruction.

Throughout the 1980s significant progress was made with the availability of more powerful computer systems and improved B-mode imaging transducers, some of which was focused on obtaining improved accuracy in volume estimation, especially for cardiology. This work has been reviewed by McCann et al. [148], who also described improved methods for obtaining and processing B-scans. They used a 5 MHz, 90-degree sector scan transducer that was rotated in small steps through 180 degrees, similar to that used by Ghosh et al., to obtain both in vitro and in vivo scans of the heart. In their studies of image display methods, they found that surface modeling techniques provided more anatomic details than with the volume display methods, and as a result they were easier to interpret.

Shortly after the development of 1-D arrays for real-time imaging, work began on the development of 2-D arrays that many realized would eventually enable 3-D imaging to be performed without incurring the difficulties associated with using 1-D arrays. A good deal of the initial work centered at Stanford University under the direction of Meindl, and some of this is described in a review paper published in 1976 [149].

Three-Dimensional Imaging Using One-Dimensional Arrays

One of the difficulties associated with 2-D ultrasound images of complex bio-logic systems is that of proper interpretation in terms of the known anatomic structure. An important advantage of 3-D imaging, along with image display software, is the ability to view, rotate, and manipulate a volume or a surface in a pseudo-3-D form [150]. Quantitative values for the size of organs can be an important aspect of accurate diagnosis as well as for judging the progress of a disease and the effects of therapy. Volume determination based on 2-D imaging is based on estimating the dimensions in three mutually perpendicu-lar directions but generally requires certain assumptions to be made concern-ing the geometry. These introduce errors that can be significantly reduced if quantitative 3-D imaging is used. Thus, an important potential advantage of 3-D imaging is the improvement in the accuracy and precision with which organ volume determinations can be made [151].

In the 1990s there was a major increase in interest in the development of 3-D imaging systems based on the use of 1-D arrays and their clinical appli-cation. These developments and results have been described in a number of review papers [152–154,156] and books [155]. Two types of systems can be identified: those that make use of mechanized scanning and freehand image acquisition systems. As illustrated in Fig. 7.33, for the mechanized systems, the transducer can be translated, rotated, or rocked in fixed increments to produce a specific number of 2-D B-mode images. An important advantage of motor-ized systems is that a predetermined number of 2-D images can be acquired at set intervals so that the volume to be imaged is uniformly sampled. In addi-tion, because of the predetermined nature of the mechanical movement, a

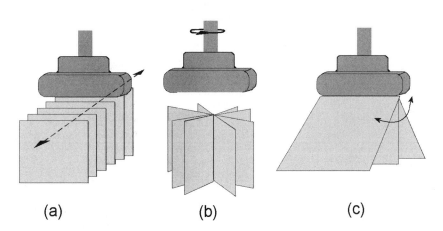

| (a) | (b) | (c) |

Figure 7.33 Examples of motorized scanning systems using a 1-D array for 3-D imaging. (a) Linear scan. (b) Rotational movement. (c) Rocking motion (fan or tilt scanning).

position registration system should not be needed for subsequent software alignment of the images.

To obtain real-time 3-D images using a mechanically rocked 1-D array, very high frame rates are needed. This requires the use of special signal-processing techniques for the beamforming such as an oversampling $\Delta\Sigma$ A/D converter (see subsection 7.2.1). In addition, by combining sparse array techniques with a synthetic aperture (see section 8.5), studies by Inerfield et al. [157] have indicated that B-mode frame rates in excess of 1,000/s are feasible.

Various scanning and image acquisition methods, along with their disadvantages, are summarized in Table 7.1.

One of the advantages of freehand systems is that the physician or sonographer has the freedom to move the probe as in a normal 2-D examination. In practice, it is likely that there is less need to obtain a 3-D image with a freehand 1-D system, and consequently the flexibility of such a system is an important advantage over the less flexible motorized systems. However, to obtain a

Table 7.1. Summary of 3-D Scanning Methods: Acquisition Methods and Disadvantages

Scanning Method	Image Acquisition Method	Disadvantages
Mechanical		
Linear	Acquired images are parallel to each other with equal spacing	Bulky device
Tilt	Acquired images are fan-like with equal angular spacing	Resolution degrades with depth
Rotational	Acquired images are propeller-like with equal angular spacing	Motion of axis of rotation results in artifacts
Free-Hand		
Acoustic	Measure time-of-flight of sound from spark gaps on transducer to microphones above patient	Line of sight required and sound velocity varies with humidity
Articulated arms	Measure angulation between movable arms	Scanning volume limited, flexing of arms
Magnetic sensor	Measure magnetic field generated by transmitter beside the patient with receiver on transducer	Ferrous metals distort magnetic field
Image correlation	Measure speckle decorrelation between adjacent images	Special computer processor required, compound motion is difficult to track
No position sensing	Distance or angle between images is assumed	Cannot measure distance
2-D Arrays		
	2-D phased array transmits a diverging pyramidal beam and returned echoes are displayed in real time as multiple planes	System cost and signal/noise

Reproduced, with permission of IOP Publishing Ltd., from Fenster et al. [156] *Phys. Med. Biol.*, 46, R67–R99, © 2001 Institute of Physics.

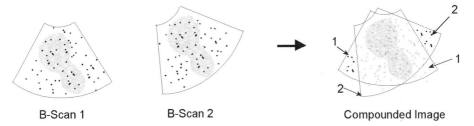

B-Scan 1   B-Scan 2   Compounded Image

Figure 7.34 Spatial compounding of two B-mode images. By accurately registering the two images and then averaging, an improved SNR can be obtained. The same principle can be applied to 3-D imaging when the scan planes intersect. (Based on Rohling et al. [158].)

good-quality 3-D image, additional skill is needed to ensure that no gaps are left and that the volume is sufficiently well sampled. It is almost inevitable that some of the scan planes will intersect, and thus the issue as to how to deal with spatial compounding must be addressed. As illustrated in Fig. 7.34, spatial compounding involves the use of intersecting B-mode images, accurate alignment, and an averaging process. Because the image speckle seen from different observation directions is only partially correlated, the averaging process increases the SNR, thereby improving the image quality.

All freehand systems require a means of accurately determining the physical relationship between each 2-D image. The problem of providing accurate registration information is a challenging one, since there are six degrees of freedom (three spatial and three angular). Moreover, the sensor must be sufficiently small and light so that when attached to the transducer handle it causes no appreciable hindrance. Relatively small alignment errors can cause smearing of the structures and thereby degrade the resulting images. Alignment errors can arise from (i) movement of the patient and changes in the volume shape over the data acquisition period; (ii) differences in the speed of propagation; (iii) errors arising from the inherent inaccuracy of the sensor and the calibration process.

Two methods have already been mentioned for position sensing: the spark scheme and the articulated arm. To these should be added devices based on electromagnetic fields and optical methods using lasers or light-emitting diodes. Sensors based on the use of AC or pulsed electromagnetic fields[28] have been incorporated into a number of commercialized systems. They use a transmitter whose position serves as a reference and that contains coils that generate a nonuniform field. The receiver contains three orthogonal coils that are used to detect the local magnetic field components produced by the transmitter. Such sensors can provide rapid sensing information (100/s) and can yield RMS positioning and angular accuracies of 0.2 mm (range, −0.7 to 0.5 mm) and 0.2 degrees (range, −0.8 to 0.9 degrees), respectively [159]. Nonetheless, the

---

28. For example, Ascension Technology, Burlington, Vermont, USA (www.ascension-tech.com); Polhemus Inc., Colchester, Vermont, USA (www.polhemus.com).

performance is not sufficient to avoid some loss in image quality. To achieve improved registration accuracy, Rohling et al. [158] used an electromagnetic sensor to provide approximate registration information and a software-based technique to make corrections. Their method involved searching for a peak in an intensity correlation function, and this required a search in six-dimensional parameter space. Their use of 3-D spatial compounding with the corrected registration process resulted in improved in vivo volume estimates of the human gallbladder.

Associated with the challenges of 3-D ultrasound are the problems of developing suitable algorithms for data processing, visualization, and display strategies. In addition, when imaging structures that undergo rapid periodic movement, the issue of how best to obtain synchronization must be addressed, whether it be through measurement and recording of the ECG or through Fourier analysis of the cardiac motion. These and other related issues have been reviewed in [154], in the book by Nelson et al. [155], and in a more recent journal by Fenster et al. [156].

7.3.3 Two-Dimensional Arrays for Two-Dimensional and Three-Dimensional Real-Time Imaging

2-D arrays provide the opportunity for generating real-time 3-D images. However, associated with increased element population can be greatly increased array fabrication and signal processing costs. An intermediate step between 1-D and 2-D arrays is one in which some control of the focus in the elevation plane is provided without requiring a large increase in the number of active elements. In fact, a variety of geometries have been proposed that provide varying degrees of control in the elevation plane. To avoid confusion over nomenclature, Wildes et al. [160] used the definitions given in Table 7.2.

1.5-D and 1.75-D Arrays

Examples of the 1.5- and 2-D arrays are shown in Fig. 7.35. The 1.5-D array at the top, consists of five rows of elements and a fixed lens to reduce the focusing delays and improve the focusing properties. The choice of the y-direction row

Table 7.2. Nomenclature Concerning Array Structures

Array	Elevation Properties
1 D	Fixed aperture and focus
1.25 D	Fixed focus but variable aperture
1.5 D	Variable apodization, focusing, and aperture, but all are symmetric about the centerline of array
1.75 D	Same as 1.5 D but no symmetry constraint
2 D	Full steering, focusing, apodization, and aperture control

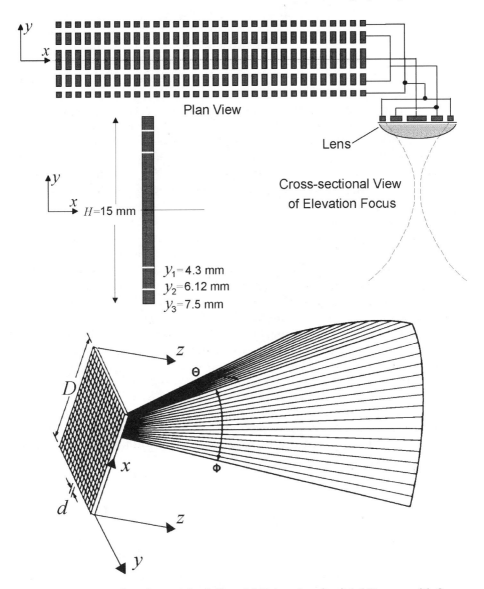

Figure 7.35 Examples of arrays for 2-D and 3-D imaging. (top) 1.5-D array with five rows. (bottom) Pyramidal measurement volume for a 2-D phased array formed from a mosaic of square elements. (Reproduced, with permission, from Smith et al. [125], *IEEE Trans. Ultrason. Ferroelect. Freq. Contr.*, 38, 100–108, © 1991 IEEE.)

boundaries has been discussed by Wildes et al. [160], who examined three possible strategies: (i) all elements have the same areas; (ii) Fresnel lens design; (iii) boundaries are chosen to minimize the time-delay errors between elements. In the Fresnel lens design illustrated in the figure, the boundaries of the elements in the y-direction are proportional to the square root of the row number [161], i.e.,

$$y_i = \frac{H}{2}\sqrt{\frac{i}{N_R}},$$

where N_R is the number of row segments ($N_R = 3$) with index i and H is the total array height. As pointed out by Wildes et al. [160], the advantage of improved elevation performance with unequal area designs can be offset by the losses that arise from electrical impedance mismatch to the smaller elements.

Comparison of the elevation resolution for 1-D and 1.5-D designs with different numbers of rows is illustrated in Fig. 7.36. This comparison [162] assumed a 32-element segment of a linear array, $W = 350\,\mu m$, $d = 400\,\mu m$, excited by a 5 MHz center frequency Gaussian pulse with a −3-dB bandwidth of 2.35 MHz. In the azimuthal direction the arrays were focused at 4.0 cm on transmit and dynamically focused on receive with $f/2$. In the elevation direction, a cylindrical lens with a fixed focus at 4.0 cm was assumed, and time delays were used in the extra rows of the 1.5-D array to provide dynamic focusing on receive. In (a) it can be seen that close to the array the elevation beam width is substantially reduced by the use of five or seven row arrays. Moreover, a slice thickness of around 1.5 mm is maintained over a wide range of z-axis locations, e.g., 2.5 to 6 cm for a five-row array.

With a 1.75-D array, limited deflection is possible in the elevation direction along with variable depth elevation focusing. One such array whose performance has been described has a center frequency of 5 MHz and a 60% bandwidth. It has 128 elements in the azimuthal direction and 10 elevation rows. The performance of this array has been evaluated by Guo et al. [163], who determined the increase in beam width when steered in the elevation direction. On the basis of their measurements and simulations, they concluded that the performance was sufficient to enable 3-D imaging to be performed within a 30-degree elevation angle.

2-D Arrays

In the early 1990s a number of papers were published describing initial steps toward developing 2-D arrays using PZT elements and demonstrating some initial images. The group at Duke University fabricated PZT 20 × 20 arrays using square PZT elements, but because of hardware limitations they initially used only 64 elements (32 for transmission and 32 for reception) [125]. In a paper published in 1991 they showed stereoscopic images of metal objects obtained with a high-speed (8 frames/s) phased-array volumetric imaging system [164] whose pyramidal measurement volume was similar to that shown in Fig. 7.35. That same year, using a 2.5 MHz 16 × 16 array [165] with 96 transmit and 32 receive elements, they presented (and published) in vivo B- and C-mode images that showed considerable promise [166]. Subsequent development by this group [167] led to the first commercially available[29] 3-D phased-array system designed primarily for use in cardiology, where the

29. Circa 1997, Volumetrics Medical Imaging.

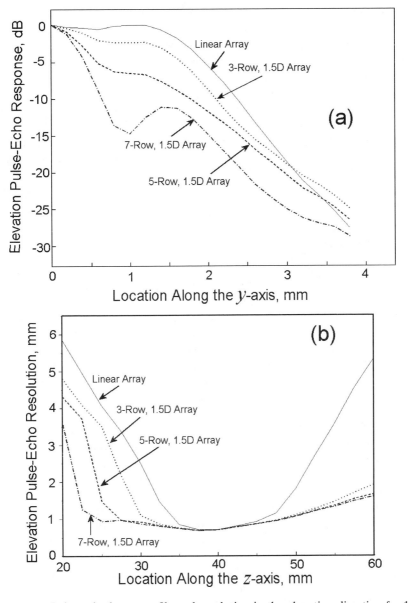

Figure 7.36 Pulse-echo beam profile and resolution in the elevation direction for 1-D and 1.5-D arrays. (a) Beam profile at $z = 25$ mm. (b) Elevation resolution (slice thickness in the y-direction, -6 dB resolution). (Reproduced, with permission, from Crombie [164].)

pyramidal measurement volume, high frame rate, and a small transducer footprint are especially important. For example, they reported the design of a sparse 2-D phased array (128 × 128 = 16,384 elements) that that used 256 transmitters and 256 receivers and formed a 65-degree pyramidal measurement volume. By using the scheme described below to produce 16 receive lines for every transmission pulse, they were able to obtain 4,096 (16 × 256) image lines at a frame rate of 30/s. The software enabled real-time viewing of multiple image planes at any desired angle, depth, and origin [168].

Other particularly important contributions to the early development of 3-D arrays was the work at the University of Toronto by Turnbull and Foster [112,170] and subsequently by Lockwood and Foster [129], some of which was discussed earlier in regard to the design and simulation of sparse arrays (see subsections 7.2.7 and 7.2.10).

Increasing the Frame Rate

A vital issue in a real-time 3-D imaging system, as well as in conventional B-mode systems that use a multiplicity of transmit focal zones, concerns the maximum rate at which each line of information can be acquired. In a conventional B-mode imaging system that images to a depth of 15 cm in tissue, the maximum pulse transmission rate would be about 5,000/s. This is governed by the need to wait for the information to be returned from the most distant location before the next pulse is transmitted. If the frame rate needed to properly capture a transient process were 30/s, then the maximum number of scan lines per frame would be about 160. Since the same limit also applies to a 3-D system, this would require that a smaller volume be sampled unless the spatial resolution or frame rate is sacrificed. A technique frequently used to improve the effective lateral resolution over the entire image depth is to use a multiplicity of focal zones. Within each zone a wide aperture/low f-number imaging is used to achieve improved resolution, and the images from each zone are then "stitched" together. An example is shown in Fig. 7.1b, which used the images from four transmit focal zones to create the overall image. Here again, frame rate is sacrificed to achieve improved lateral resolution.

One method proposed for solving the above dilemma was to form many receive lines from a single transmitted pulse. In the B-mode imaging system described by Delannoy et al. [171], a complete frame of 70 lines was formed from a single transmit pulse, which enabled imaging to be performed at 1,000 frames/s. Subsequently Shattuk et al. [172] described the performance of a 1-D array system in which four lines of data were acquired for each transmission. The first application of these ideas to a 2-D array appears to be that described by von Ramm et al. [164]. Consider the example shown in Fig. 7.37, where the −6 db transmit pulse angular response is broadened (perhaps by decreasing the aperture) so that it subtends an angle of 2 degrees. If the scattered information is processed in parallel so that seven receive beams are synthesized, each with an angular response of 0.5 degrees and uniformly spaced throughout the solid angle defined by the transmit pulse, then for a single

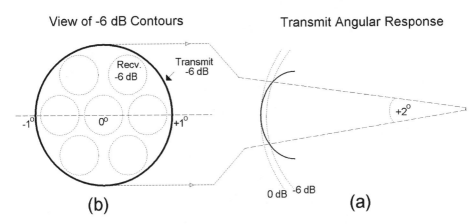

Figure 7.37 Example (not to scale) of a method for increasing the line density and/or the frame rate by using a single transmission pulse and synthesizing seven received lines. (a) Main transmit beam angular response. (b) The –6-dB contours of the synthesized receive lines.

transmission, seven scan lines can be computed from the information recorded from the receive elements. Because of the increased angular dimensions of the transmit pulse, there will be a decrease in the pulse-echo main lobe to side lobe ratio and a loss in spatial resolution. As mentioned earlier, the Duke University group used this idea in a variety of sparse 2-D array designs for their pyramidal phased array and were able to realize 16 receive lines in 4 × 4 matrix around the transmit beam.

An alternative method proposed for increasing the line density is based on using a multiplicity of transmissions at the same time [173] and from each transmission, using either the same or a different aperture, determining the received signal. In the case of a phased linear array it is possible to form two or more separate apertures and to simultaneously transmit beams from these [174]. However, for a linear phased array in which all elements are used to form each transmitted beam, separate apertures could not be used. To overcome this problem Mallart and Fink [175] proposed and experimentally demonstrated a scheme based on Fig. 7.38. If we consider pulse waveforms applied to the seven transmitter elements, it can be seen that two focused beams will be produced simultaneously that propagate in differing directions. By adding additional steered and focused waveforms, Mallart and Fink showed that eight beams could be transmitted. However, they found that as the number of transmitted beams is increased, so the side lobe levels increase. Using a 128-element, 3 MHz linear array, they showed images of a phantom that demonstrated little deterioration in image quality, provided no more than between four and six transmitted beams were used. Extending this 1-D result to a 3-D array, they suggested that between 16 and 36 simultaneous beams could be produced.

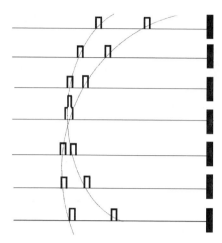

Figure 7.38 Simultaneous transmission of two beams using a phased array. The waveforms and delays needed for each element of the array to focus and steer the beams are indicated.

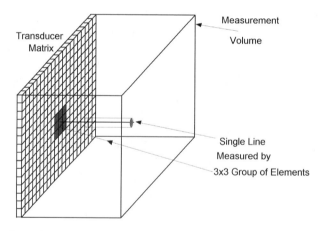

Figure 7.39 Scanning a 3-D rectilinear volume by means of a 2-D phased linear array. The group of elements is stepped along both the *x*- and *y*-directions.

Rectilinear Volumetric Arrays

The use of a motorized 1-D array to generate 3-D rectilinear images suggests that the same could be achieved by means of a 2-D array. By using the element groupings illustrated in Fig. 7.39 and moving them in an incremental manner throughout the matrix, a complete frame of information can be obtained [176]. As discussed by Yen et al. [168], a full wavelength inter-element spacing would be needed for realistic measurement volumes, along with realizable array dimensions and frame rates that are acceptable for the clinical applications. For a 5 MHz, 38.4×38.4-mm^2 array, this corresponds to 16,384 (128×128) elements. If it is assumed that eight receive lines can be computed for each transmitted beam, 2,048 transmissions per frame would be needed. Assuming a measurement volume depth of 6.0 cm and a sound speed of 1,500 m/s, this translates to a frame rate of about 6/s. As pointed out by Yen and Smith [169], a potential advantage of a rectilinear scan is that it enables a much wider field of view to be obtained compared to a sector scan, thereby improving the performance close to the skin surface. They describe the design of an array that uses a Mills cross-arrangement of elements at a center frequency of 5 MHz. With this scheme they achieved spatial resolutions in the 1- to 2-mm range, a volume image rate of 47/s, over a volume of 30 mm (azimuthal) × 8 mm (elevation) × 60 mm (depth).

7.4 Summary of Design Factors

The complexity and interrelated factors that affect the properties of a B-mode imaging system are summarized in Table 7.3. This shows the relevant engineering properties that influence the image formation and its quality.

7.5 Array Field Synthesis

One method that has been developed and used clinically for tumor destruction is to make use of localized heating produced by focused ultrasound, a technique known as ultrasound hyperthermia [178]. For many years it has been known that tumors are vulnerable to higher temperatures and that ultrasound is one technique for noninvasively raising the temperature. If a temperature in the range of 42 to 43°C is maintained in soft tissue for a sufficient length of time, destruction will result. Moreover, depending on the choice of frequency, the depth to which energy can be deposited can be varied (e.g.,[30] 0 to 3 cm for 3.5 MHz, 8 to 10 cm for 1 MHz). To achieve reasonably uniform heating over a given cross-sectional area, a multiple focus method, such as that illustrated in Fig. 7.40, can be used. In this example, a 2-D ultrasound array is used to produce a cross-sectional region that is reasonably uniform in terms of the heat production. By appropriate choice of the driving amplitude and phase to each element of the array, the geometry of energy deposition region can be controlled to make it closely match the tumor.

Several approaches can be used to determine the amplitude and phase pattern to be applied to a given array to achieve the best approximation to a specified radiation pattern. This synthesis problem is generally more difficult than the analysis task addressed in Chapters 2 and 3.

30. Labthermonics Technologies Inc., 701 Devonshire Drive, Champaign, IL 61820, USA (www.labthermics.com/sono.html).

Table 7.3. Engineering Properties That Affect Image Quality

Engineering Property	Effect on Image Quality
Size and growth of transmit and receive apertures	Large aperture size yields superior lateral spatial resolution. Variable aperture size enables f-number to remain constant with depth to provide uniform spatial resolution.
Number and position of transmit zones	Provides uniformly high spatial resolution throughout the region of interest.
Number, size, and spacing of piezoelectric elements; number of independent array channels	In the image plane: spacing elements one-half the resonant frequency wavelength suppresses grating lobes and increases gray-scale resolution. Where size is approximately equal to the spacing and the number is large, sensitivity is a maximum. Large number of elements on independent electronic channels gives high spatial resolution.
f-number	Small f-numbers yield high lateral spatial resolution and shallow depth of field, requiring many transmit foci to obtain uniform spatial resolution. For strongly focused transducers (low f-numbers), depth of focus is approximately proportional to the f-number.
Transmit and receive apodization	Weighting the center elements more than the side elements (apodization) decreases grating lobe amplitude but broadens the main lobe. Therefore apodization is a method for increasing gray-scale resolution (reducing grating lobes) at the expense of spatial resolution (broad main lobe).
Transducer bandwidth and center frequency	Spatial resolution increases with frequency (shorter pulse lengths and narrower beam widths) as depth of penetration decreases because of tissue attenuation. High bandwidths increase axial spatial resolution but decrease transducer sensitivity.
Receive sensitivity and dynamic range	In general, high receive sensitivity and dynamic range increase gray-scale resolution. If the beam properties are poor, however, gray-scale resolution can decrease as receive sensitivity and dynamic range increase.
Output power	Increasing output power increases system sensitivity until nonlinear propagation effects begin. Nonlinear effects transfer energy to high-frequency harmonics, which are preferentially attenuated in tissue and for which the system is insensitive to receive. Image quality features are marginally increased with large increases in power.
Frame rate, line density, image width and depth	High frame rate is required to avoid temporal aliasing and maximize temporal information density. High line density is required to avoid spatial aliasing and maximize spatial information density. The limited speed of sound (c_o) dictates how these parameters are traded off according to: $c_o = 2 \times$ Depth $\times$ Line Density $\times$ Frame Rate for gray-scale imaging.

Reprinted by permission of Elsevier from Insana and Hall [177].

7.5.1 Field Conjugation Method

For CW excitation, the synthesis task can be simplified if it is assumed that each array element is in the far field at the observation plane. Ibbini and Cain [179] have described a synthesis technique that makes use of the principle of reciprocity and phase conjugation. Phase conjugation [180,181] is the generation of a wavefront that is the reverse of an incident wave: it therefore describes a wave that at all points moves in exactly the opposite direction. Mathematically, it corresponds to reversing the sign of the phase term, so that using the complex representation of a sinusoidal wave, it is the complex conjugate of the incident wave. In optics, phase conjugation is of great practical importance since it provides a means for correcting the effects of wavefront distortion. Some of the techniques are also applicable in ultrasound, in particular for correcting the effects of phase distortion due to transmission through an inhomogeneous medium [182]. Nikoonahad and Pusateri [183] first reported (1989) the development of a real-time ultrasonic (300 kHz) phase conjugate "mirror" using a 1-D array.

With reference to Fig. 7.40, we shall suppose that a total of M control points are specified, which can consist of focal points or points where a reduced response is required. If a CW point source exists at the m'th focal point, then the magnitude and phase of the particle velocity at the center of each element of the array can be calculated, so that if there are N elements a vector given by $[v_{1m} \, v_{2m} \ldots v_{nm} \ldots v_{Nm}]^t$ can be constructed, where t denotes the transpose and v is the complex particle velocity. If this process is repeated for all M focal points and the amplitude of each point source is proportional to the control point response, then a complex array can be constructed given by

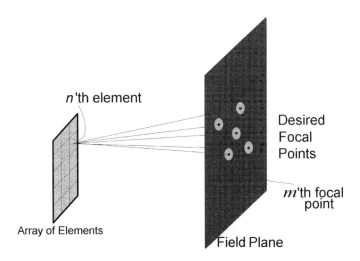

Figure 7.40 Synthesis method in which a desired set of field points, e.g., several foci, on a given plane can be obtained from appropriately excited elements of an array.

$$\mathbf{V} = \begin{bmatrix} v_{11} & \cdot & v_{1m} & \cdot & v_{1M} \\ v_{21} & \cdot & v_{2m} & \cdot & v_{2M} \\ \cdot & \cdot & \cdot & \cdot & \cdot \\ \cdot & \cdot & \cdot & \cdot & \cdot \\ v_{N1} & \cdot & v_{Nm} & \cdot & v_{NM} \end{bmatrix}.$$

By conjugating this matrix (i.e., the complex conjugate of each term), the complex excitation needed to be applied to each array element will be given by the sum of the real and imaginary parts of each row.

Many simplifications result when the far-field approximation can be assumed. Karpelson et al. [185] have shown that by using a Fresnel approximation for the radiation field produced by a rectangular element, the field conjugation method can give good accuracy up to points relatively close to the source elements, with an order of magnitude reduction in computation time compared to the more exact pseudoinverse method described in the next subsection.

As an example, we consider a $90 \times 90\,\text{mm}^2$ planar array consisting of 400 (20×20) elements and wish to synthesize an acoustic field consisting of four equal-intensity focal points at $(-10, -10)$, $(10, -10)$, $(-10, 10)$, and $(10, 10)$ mm on a plane 12 mm from the source plane at a frequency of 2.3 MHz. The amplitudes and phases of the normal component of velocity on each element were calculated using the approximate field conjugation method and, from these, the field profile shown in Fig. 7.41 was calculated using the Rayleigh integral. It can be seen that four foci at the specified locations are produced.

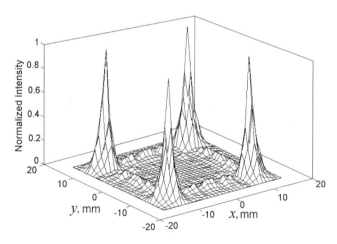

Figure 7.41 Example of a four-foci field at a distance of 12 mm from a 20×20 planar array ($90 \times 90\,\text{mm}^2$) excited at 2.3 MHz. The amplitudes and phases of signals applied to each element were calculated using the field conjugation method. (Reproduced, with permission, from Karpelson et al. [185], *IEEE Trans. Ultrason. Ferroelect. Freq. Contr.*, 42, 793–797, © 1995 IEEE.)

7.5.2 A Pseudoinverse Method

Ebbini and Cain [184] have developed a more exact synthesis method based on the Rayleigh equation as given by (2.32). Let us consider an $N \times N$ array of source elements and M control points; then the pressure at the m'th control point due to the nth array element can be obtained from (3.17) as

$$\underline{p_{mn}}(\mathbf{r}_m) = \frac{j\omega\rho_o v_{on}}{2\pi} \iint_{S_n} \frac{e^{-jk|\mathbf{r}_m - \mathbf{r}_n|}}{|\mathbf{r}_m - \mathbf{r}_n|} dS_n,$$

where $\mathbf{r}_m$ is the observation point, $\mathbf{r}_n$ is a point on an elementary area dS_n of the nth array element, and v_{on} is the normal component of velocity on that surface. Consequently, the total pressure at the mth control point is the sum of all the contributions from all N^2 elements, i.e.,

$$\underline{p_m}(\mathbf{r}_m) = \frac{j\omega\rho_o}{2\pi} \sum_{n=1}^{N^2} v_{on} \iint_{S_n} \frac{e^{-jk|\mathbf{r}_m - \mathbf{r}_n|}}{|\mathbf{r}_m - \mathbf{r}_n|} dS_n.$$

This can be expressed as

(7.14) $$\mathbf{H}\mathbf{v}_0 = \mathbf{p},$$

where $\mathbf{p} = [p(\mathbf{r}_1)\ p(\mathbf{r}_2) \ldots p(\mathbf{r}_M)]^t$, $\mathbf{v}_0 = [v_{o1}\ v_{o2} \ldots v_{oN^2}]^t$, and the matrix $\mathbf{H}$ is a propagation operator given by

$$\mathbf{H}(m, n) = \frac{j\omega\rho_o}{2\pi} \iint_{S_n} \frac{e^{-jk|\mathbf{r}_m - \mathbf{r}_n|}}{|\mathbf{r}_m - \mathbf{r}_n|} dS_n.$$

Given the values of the pressure $\mathbf{p}$ for all control points, we seek the values of the complex surface velocity $\mathbf{v}_0$ for each source array element, i.e., we seek a solution of (7.14). Ebbani and Cain [184] have shown that if the total number of array elements is greater than the number of points where the field has been specified, i.e., $N^2 > M$, then the minimum norm least-square estimate of $\mathbf{v}_0$ is given by

(7.15) $$\hat{\mathbf{v}}_0 = \mathbf{H}^{*t} \left(\mathbf{H}\,\mathbf{H}^{*t} \right)^{-1} \mathbf{p},$$

where $\mathbf{H}^{*t}$ is the conjugate transpose of $\mathbf{H}$ and represents the backward propagation operator, i.e., from the control points to the array elements. Ebbani and Cain have discussed the physical significance of the above solution and have described the methods for evaluating (7.15).

References

1. Goldstein, A., and Powis, R.L., Medical ultrasonic diagnostics, Ch. 2, pp. 43–191 in: *Ultrasonic Instruments and Devices I*, E.P. Papadakis (Ed.), Vol. 23 of: *Physical Acoustics: Principles and Methods*, R.N. Thurston, and A.D. Pierce (Eds.), Academic Press, New York, 1999.

2. Edler, I., and Lindstrom, K., The history of echocardiography, *Ultrasound Med. Biol.*, 30, 1565–1644, 2004.
3. Levi, S., The history of ultrasound in gynecolocogy 1950–1980, *Ultrasound Med. Biol.*, 23, 481–552, 1997.
4. Woo, J.S.K., A short history of the developments of ultrasound in obstetrics and gynecology (in three parts), *http://www.ob-ultrasound.net/history.html*, 1999.
5. Goldberg, B.B., and Kimmelman, B.A., *Medical Diagnostic Ultrasound: A Retrospective on its 40th Anniversary*, pp. 1–49, Eastman Kodak Health Sciences Publication, 1988.
6. Firestone, F.A., Flaw detecting device and measuring instrument, US Patent 2,280,226, 1942 (filed 1940).
7. Firestone, F.A., The supersonic reflectoscope for interior inspection, *Metal Progress*, 505–512, 1945.
8. Firestone, F.A., The supersonic reflectoscope, an instrument for inspecting the interior of solid parts by means of sound waves, *J. Acoust. Soc. Am.*, 17, 287–299, 1946.
9. Desch, C.H., Sproule, D.O., and Dawson, W.J., The detection of cracks in steel by means of supersonic waves, *Welding J.*, 36, 1s–25s (supplement in 3 sections: Section 2—Sproule, D.O., The supersonic flaw detector, 3s–12s), 1947.
10. Sokolov, S.Y., Zur Frage der Fortpflanzung ultrakustischer Schwingungen in verschiedenen Korpern [On the problem of the propagation of ultrasonic oscillations in various bodies], *Elek. Nachr. Tech.*, 6, 454–461, 1929.
11. Muhlhauser, O., Verfahren zur Zustandsbestimmung von Werkstoffen, besonders zur Ermittlung von Fehlern darin, German Patent: 569,598, 1933 (filed 1931).
12. Sokolov, S.J., Means for indicating flaws in materials, US Patent 2,164,125, 1939 (filed 1937).
13. Dussik, K.T., Uber die Moglichkeit, hochfrequente mechanische Schwingungen als diagnostisches Hilfsmittel zu verwerten [On the possibility of using ultrasound waves as a diagnostic aid], *Zeit. fur die gesamte Neurol. und Psychiat.*, 174, 153–168, 1942.
14. Dussik, K.T., Dussik, F., and Wyt, L., Auf dem Wege zur Hyperphonographie des Gehirnes [On the way towards hyperphonography of the brain], *Wiener Med. Wochenschr.*, 97, 425–430, 1947.
15. Guttner, von W., Fiedler, G., and Patzold, J., Uber Ultraschallabbildungen am menschilchen Schadel [On ultrasound images of the human cranium], *Acustica*, 2, 148–156, 1952.
16. Ludwig, D., and Struthers, F.W., Detecting gall-stones with ultrasonic, *Electronics*, 23, 172, 1950.
17. French, L.A., Wild, J.J., and Neal, D., The experimental application of ultrasonics to the localization of brain tumors: preliminary report, *J. Neurosurg.*, 8, 198–203, 1951.
18. Wild, J.J., The use of ultrasonic pulses for the measurement of biologic tissues and the detection of tissue density changes, *Surgery*, 27, 183–188, 1950.
19. Wild, J.J., The discovery of ultrasonic soft tissue reflection, *Ultrasonics International 81*, Conf. Proc. pp. 229–234, 1981.
20. Wild, J.J., and Neal, D., Use of high-frequency ultrasonic waves for detecting changes of texture of living tissues, *Lancet*, 1, 655–657, 1951.
21. Mundt, G.H., and Hughes, W.F., Ultrasonics in ocular diagnosis, *Am. J. Ophthamol.*, 41, 488–498, 1956.

22. Wild, J.J., and Reid, J.M., Application of echo-ranging techniques to the determination of the structure of biological tissues, *Science*, 115, 226–230, 1952.

23. Reid, J.M., and Wild, J.J., Ultrasonic ranging for cancer diagnosis, *Electronics*, 25, 136–138 (No. 5), 1952.

24. Wild, J.J., and Reid, J.M., Further pilot echographic studies on the histologic structure of tumors the living intact human breast, *Am. J. Pathol.*, 28, 839–861, 1952.

25. Wild, J.J., and Reid, J.M., Echographic visualization of lesions of the living human breast, *Cancer Res.*, 14, 277–283, 1954.

26. Howry, D.H., and Bliss, W.R., Ultrasonic visualization of soft tissue structures of the body, *J. Lab. Clin. Med.*, 40, 579–592, 1952.

27. Holmes, J.H., Howry, D.H., Posakony, G., and Cushman, C.R., The ultrasonic visualization of soft tissue structures in the human body, *Trans. Am. Clin. Climatological Association*, 66, 208–225, 1954.

28. Howry, D.H., Posakony, G., Cushman, C.R., and Holmes, J.H., Three-dimensional and stereoscopic observation of body structures by ultrasound, *J. Appl. Physiol.*, 9, 304–306, 1956.

29. Holmes, J.H., and Howry, D.H., Ultrasonic visualization of edema, *Trans. Am. Clin. Climatological Assoc.*, 70, 225–235, 1958.

30. Kikuchi, Y., Uchida, R., Tenaka, K., and Wagai, T., Early cancer diagnosis through ultrasonics, *J. Acoust. Soc. Am.*, 29, 824–833, 1957.

31. Baum, G., and Greenwood, I., The application of ultrasonic locating technique to opthamology, *Arch. Ophthamol.*, 60, 263–279, 1958.

32. Baum, G., and Greenwood, I., High-resolution ultrasonography and its application to clinical ophthamology, pp. 412–421 in: Proc. 3rd Int. Conf Med. Electronics, Part 3, London, 1960.

33. McNay, M., and Fleming, J.E.E., Forty years of obstetric ultrasound 1957–1997: from A-scope to three dimensions, *Ultrasound Med. Biol.*, 25, 5–55, 1999.

34. Donald, I., Sonar: a new diagnostic echo-sounding technique in obstetrics and gynecology, *Proc. Roy. Soc. Med.*, 55, 637–638, 1962.

35. Donald, I., MacVicar, J., and Brown, T.G., Investigation of abdominal masses by pulsed ultrasound, *Lancet*, 1, 1188–1194, 1958.

36. Brown, T.G., Direct contact ultrasound scanning techniques for the visualization of abdominal masses, pp. 358–366 in: *Medical Electronics* (Proc. 2nd Int. Conf. on Med. Electronics, Paris, 1959), C.N. Smyth (Ed.), Iliffe and Sons Ltd, London, 1960.

37. Levi, S., The history of ultrasound in gynecolocogy 1950–1980, *Ultrasound Med. Biol.*, 23, 481–552, 1997.

38. Brown, T.G., Development of ultrasonic scanning techniques in Scotland, 1956–1979: personal recollections, and, "Virtual reality" in ultrasonic imaging, a project out of time? *http://www.ob-ultrasound.net/brown-on-ultrasound.htlm*, 1999.

39. Kossoff, G., Garrett, W.J., Carpenter, D.A., Jellins, J., and Dadd, M.J., Principles and classification of soft tissues by grey scale echography, *Ultrasound Med. Biol.*, 2, 89–105, 1976.

40. Howry, D.H., and Gordon, D., Ultrasonic tomography, Ch. 13, pp. 113–123 in: *Ultrasound as a Diagnostic and Surgical Tool*, D. Gordon (Ed.), E & S Livingstone Ltd, Edinburgh, 1964.

41. Sunden, B., On the diagnostic value of ultrasound in obstetrics and gynaecology, *Acta Obstet. Gynecol. Scand.* (Suppl. 6), 43, 1–191, 1964.

42. Kossoff, G., Robinson, D.E., and Garrett, W.J., Design criteria for ultrasonic visualization systems, *Ultrasonics*, 2, 29–38, 1964.

43. Krause, W., and Soldner, R., Ultraschallbildverfahren (B-scan) mit hober Bildfrequenz fur medizinische Diagnostik, *Electromedica*, 35, 8–11, 1967.

44. Krause, W.E.E., and Soldner, R.E., Ultrasonic imaging technique (B-scan) with high image rate for medical diagnosis: principle and technique of the method, p. 315 in: Digest of the 7th Int. Conf. Med. Biolog. Eng., Stockholm, 1967.

45. Patzold, J., Krause, W., Kresse, H., and Soldner, R., Present state of an ultrasonic cross-section procedure with rapid image rate. *IEEE Trans Bio-Med. Eng.*, 17, 263–265, 1970.

46. von Ardenne, M., and Millner, M., The U.S. Focoscan method, *IRE Trans. Biomed. Electron.*, 9, 145–149, 1962.

47. von Ardenne, M., Grossmann, H., and Millner, M., Vergleich von Ultra-schallkopfen ohne und mit Fokussierung bei iherer Anwendung in medizinischen Ultraschall-Diagnostik-Geraten, *Acustica*, 16, 134–142, 1965.

48. Thurstone, F.L., Kjosnes, N.I., and McKinney, W.M., Ultrasonic scanning of biologic tissue by a new technique, *Science*, 149, 302–303, 1965.

49. McCready, V.R., and Hill, C.R., A constant depth ultrasonic scanner, *Br. J. Radiol.*, 44, 747–750, 1971.

50. Brown, T.G., Visualization of soft tissues in two and three dimensions: limitations and development, *Ultrasonics*, 5, 118–124, 1967.

51. Edler, I.G., Echocardiography: a historical perspective, Ch. 1, pp. 1–33, in: *Two-Dimensional Echocardiography and Cardiac Doppler*, J.N. Schapira, J.G. Harold, and C. Beeder (Eds.), 2nd Ed., Williams & Wilkins, Baltimore, 1990. See also: Edler, I.G., Early echocardiography, *Ultrasound Med. Biol.*, 17, 425–431, 1994.

52. Edler, I., and Hertz, C.H., The use of ultrasonic reflectoscope for the continuous recording of movements of heart walls, *Kungl. Fysiograf. Sallsk. Lund Forh.*, 24 (No. 5), 1–19, 1954.

53. Edler, I., Ultrasoundcardiography: *Part I*: Edler, I., The use of ultrasound as a diagnostic aid and its effect on biological tissues. Continuous recording of the movements of various heart structures using an ultrasound echo method, pp. 7–65. *Part II.*, Edler, I., Gustafson, A., Karlefors, T., and Christensson, B., Mitral and aortic valve movements recorded by an ultrasonic echo-method, pp. 67–82. *Part III*, Edler, I., Atrioventricular valve motility in the living human heart recorded by ultrasound, pp. 83–115. *Acta Med. Scand. Suppl.*, 370, 1–123, 1961.

54. Fleming, A.D., Palka, P., McDicken, W.N., Fenn, L.N., and Sutherland, G.R., Verification of cardiac Doppler tissue images using grey-scale M-mode images, *Ultrasound Med. Biol.*, 22, 573–581, 1996.

55. Foster, R.M., Directive diagrams of antenna arrays, *Bell Syst. Tech. J.*, 5, 292–307, 1926.

56. Walter, L.H., The radiation from directive aerials in wireless telegraphy, *The Electrician*, 53, 790–792, 1910.

57. Artom. Paper read to the Italian electrotechnical association in 1908. A translated version appears in *Electrical Review*, 53, p. 814, 1908.

58. Stenzel, H., Uber die Richtwirkung von Schallstrahlern [On the directional effect of sound sources], *Elektrishe Nachrichten Technik*, 4, 239–253, 1927.

59. Wolff, I., and Malter, L., Directional radiation of sound, *Bell Syst. Tech. J.*, 2, 201–241, 1930.

60. Tucker, D.G., Welsby, V.G., and Kendall, R., Electronic sector scanning, *J. Br. I.R.E.*, 18, 465–484, 1958.

61. Tucker, D.G., and Welsby, V.G., Electronic sector-scanning ASDIC: an improved fish-locator and navigational intrument, *Nature*, 185, 277–279, 1960.

62. Welsby, V.G., and Dunn, J.R., A high-resolution electronic sector-scanning sonar, *Radio and Electronic Engineer (previously, J. Brit. I.R.E.)*, 26, 205–208, 1963.

63. Bushman, W., New equipment and transducer for ophthalmic diagnosis, *Ultrasonics*, 3, 18–21, 1965.

64. Bom, N., Lancee, C.T., Honkoop, J., and Hugenholtz, P.G., Ultrasonic viewer for cross-sectional analyses of moving cardiac structures, *Bio-Med. Eng.*, 6, 500–508, 1971.

65. Bom, N., Lancee, C.T., van Zwieten, G., Kloster, F.E., and Roelandt, J., Multiscan echocardiography, I: Technical description, *Circulation*, 48, 1066–1074, 1973.

66. Kloster, F.E., Roelandt, J., ten Cate, F.J., Bom, N., and Hugenholtz, P.G., Multiscan echocardiography, II: Techniques and initial clinical results, *Circulation*, 48, 1075–1064, 1973.

67. Uchida, R., Hagiwara, Y., and Irie, T., Electro-scanning ultrasonic diagnostic equipment, *Jpn. Medical Electronics*, 58–62, 1971/72.

68. Okujima, M., and Endoh, N., Design of directional array transducer for electronic scan ultrasonic tomograph, *Jpn. Medical Ultrasonics*, 10, No. 1, 71–74, 1972.

69. Somer, J.C., Electronic sector scanning for ultrasonic diagnosis, *Ultrasonics*, 6, 153–159, 1968.

70. Somer, J.C., Instantaneous and continuous picture obtained by a new two-dimensional scan technique with a stationary transducer, pp. 234–238 in: *Proceedings in Echo-Encephalography* (Int. Symp. on Echo-encephalography, Erlangen, Germany, April 1967), E. Kazner, W. Schiefer, and K.J. Zulch (Eds.), Springer-Verlag, Berlin, 1968.

71. Thurstone, F.L., and von Ramm, O.T., A new ultrasound imaging technique employing two-dimensional electronic beam steering, pp. 249–259 in: *Acoustical Holography*, Vol. 5, P.S. Green (Ed.), Plenum Press, New York, 1974.

72. Thurstone, F.L., and von Ramm, O.T., Electronic beam scanning for ultrasonic imaging, pp. 43–48 in: *Ultrasonics in Medicine*, M. deVlieger, D.N. White, and V.R. McCready (Eds.), Exerpta Medica, Amsterdam, 1974.

73. von Ramm, O.T., and Thurstone, F.L., Cardiac imaging using a phased array ultrasound system: I. System design, *Circulation*, 53, 258–262, 1976.

74. Kisslo, J., von Ramm, O.T., and Thurstone, F.L., Cardiac imaging using a phased array ultrasound system: II. Clinical technique and application, *Circulation*, 53, 262–267, 1976.

75. Cheston, T.C., and Frank, J., Array antennas, Ch. 11, pp. 11-1 to 11-71 in: *Radar Handbook*, M.I. Skolnik (Ed.), McGraw-Hill, New York, 1970.

76. Steinberg, B.D., *Principles of Aperture and Array System Design*, Wiley, New York, 1976.

77. Macovski, A., Ultrasonic imaging using arrays, *Proc. IEEE*, 67, 484–495. 1979.

78. Tucker, D.G., Some aspects of the design of strip arrays, *Acustica*, 6, 403–411, 1956.

79. Ziomek, L.J., *Fundamentals of Acoustic Field Theory and Space-Time Signal Processing*, CRC Press, Boca Raton, Florida, 1995.

80. Skudrzyk, E., *The Foundations of Acoustics*, Springer-Verlag, New York, 1971.

81. Thomenius, K.E., Evolution of ultrasound beamformers, pp. 1615–1622 in: *1996 IEEE Ultrasonics Symp. Proc.*, 1996.

82. Tutwiler, R.L., Ultrasonic beamforming architectures, pp. 43–54 in: *Ultrasonic Transducer Engineering*, K.K. Shung (Ed.), Proc. SPIE Vol. 3341, Medical Imaging, 1998.

83. von Ramm, O.T., and Smith, S.W., Beam steering with linear arrays, *IEEE Trans. Biomed. Eng.*, 30, 438–452, 1983.

84. Magnin, P.A., von Ramm, O.T., and Thurstone, F.L., Delay quantization error in phased array images, *IEEE Trans. Sonics Ultrasonics*, 28, 305–310, 1981.

85. Peterson, D.K., and Kino, G.S., Real-time digital image reconstruction: a description of imaging hardware and an analysis of quantization errors, *IEEE Trans. Sonics Ultrasonics*, 31, 337–351, 1984.

86. Holm, S., and Kristoffersen, K., Analysis of worst-case phase quantization sidelobes in focused beamforming, *IEEE Trans. Ultrason. Ferroelect. Freq. Contr.*, 39, 593–599, 1992.

87. Anderson, M.E., McKeag, M.S., and Trahey, G.E., The impact of sound speed errors on medical ultrasound imaging, *J. Acoust. Soc. Am.*, 107, 3540–3548, 2000.

88. Reid, J.M., and Wild, J.J., Current developments in ultrasonic equipment for medical diagnosis, *Proc. Nat. Electronics Conf.*, 12, 1002–1015, 1956.

89. Schuck, O.H., Variable focus transducer, US Patent 3,090,030, May 14, 1963 (filed Sept. 9, 1957).

90. Walker, J.T., and Meindl, J.D., A digitally controlled CCD dynamically focused phased array, pp. 80–83 in: *1975 Ultrasonics Symp. Proc.*, 1975.

91. Fry, W.J., Leichner, G.H., Okuyama, D., Fry, F.J., and Fry, E.K., Ultrasonic visualization system employing new scanning and presentation methods, *J. Acoust. Soc. Am.*, 44, 1324–1338, 1968.

92. Maslak, S.H., Acoustic imaging apparatus, US Patent 4,140,022, Feb. 20, 1979 (filed Dec. 20, 1977).

93. Burkhardt, C.B., Grandchamp, P.A., Hoffman, H., and Fehr, R., A simplified ultrasound phased array sector scanner, pp. 385–393 in: *Echocardiography*, C.T. Lancee (Ed.), Martinus Nijhoff Pub., The Hague, 1979.

94. Powers, J.E., Phillips, D.J., Brandestini, M.A., and Sigelmann, R.A., Ultrasound phased array delay linesbased on quadrature sampling techniques, *IEEE Trans. Sonics Ultrason.*, 27, 287–294, 1980.

95. Kino, G.S., *Acoustic Waves: Devices, Imaging, and Analog Signal Processing*, Prentice-Hall, Englewood Cliffs, NJ, 1987.

96. Freeman, S.R., Quick, M.K., Morin, M.A., Anderson, R.C., Desilets, C.S., Linnenbrink, T.E., and O'Donnell, M., Delta-sigma oversampled ultrasound beamformer with dynamic delays, *IEEE Trans. Ultrason. Ferroelect. Freq. Contr.*, 46, 320–332, 1999.

97. Crochiere, R.E., and Rabiner, L.R., *Multirate Digital Signal Processing*, Prentice-Hall, Englewood Cliffs, NJ, 1983.

98. Norsworthy, S.R., Schreier, R., and Temes, G.C. (Eds.), *Delta-Sigma Data Converters: Theory, Design, and Simulation*, IEEE Press, Piscataway, NJ, 1997.

99. Cherry, J.A., Snelgrove, W.M., *Continuous-Time Delta-Sigma Modulators for High-Speed A/D Conversion: Theory, Practice and Fundamental Performance Limits*, Kluwer, Boston, 1999.

100. Noujaim, S.E., Garverick, S.L., and O'Donnell, M., Phased array ultrasonic beam forming using oversampled A/D converters, US Patent 5,203,335, April 20, 1993 (filed March 2, 1992).

101. Freeman, S.R., Quick, M.K., Morin, M.A., Anderson, R.C., Desilets, C.S., Linnenbrink, T.E., and O'Donnell, M., Delta-sigma oversampled ultrasound beamformer with dynamic delays, *IEEE Trans. Ultrason. Ferroelect. Freq. Contr.*, 46, 320–332, 1999.

102. Freeman, S.R., Quick, M.K., Morin, M.A., Anderson, R.C., Desilets, C.S., Linnenbrink, T.E., and O'Donnell, M., Heterodyning technique to improve performance of delta-sigma-based beamformers, *IEEE Trans. Ultrason. Ferroelect. Freq. Contr.*, 46, 771–790, 1999.

103. Dean, M., Digital beamforming array, US Patent 5,461,389, Oct. 24, 1995 (filed June 30, 1994).

104. Burckhardt, C.B., Grandchamp, P-A., and Hoffman, H., Methods for increasing the lateral resolution of B-scan, pp. 391–413 in: *Acoustical Holography and Imaging*, P.S. Green (Ed.), Plenum Press, New York, 1973.

105. von Aulock, W.H., Properties of phased arrays, *Proc. IRE*, 48, 1715–1727, 1960.

106. Sato, J., Kawabuchi, M., and Fukumoto, A., The width-to-thickness ratio of plank-shaped piezoelectric transducers used for electronically scanned ultrasound diagnostic systems, *J. Acoust. Soc. Am.*, 66, 1809–1811, 1979.

107. Sato, J., Fukukita, H., Kawabuchi, M., and Fukumoto, A., Farfield angular radiation pattern generated from arrayed piezoelectric transducers, *J. Acoust. Soc. Am.*, 67, 333–335, 1980.

108. Delannoy, B., Lasota, H., Bruneel, C., Torguet, R., and Bridoux, E., The infinite planar baffles problem in acoustic radiation and its experimental verification, *J. Appl. Phys.*, 50, 5189–5195, 1979.

109. Selfridge, A.R., Kino, G.S., and Khuri-Yakub, B.T., A theory for the radiation pattern of a narrow-strip acoustic transducer, *Appl. Phys. Lett.*, 37, 35–36, 1980.

110. Felix, N., Certon, D., Lacaze, E., Lethiecq, M., and Patat, F., Experimental investigation of cross-coupling and its influence on the elementary radiation pattern in 1D ultrasound arrays, pp. 1053–1056 in: *1999 IEEE Ultrasonics Symp. Proc.*, 1999.

111. Steinberg, B.D., The peak sidelobe of the phased array having randomly located elements, *IEEE Trans. Antennas Propagat.*, 20, 129–136, 1972.

112. Turnbull, D.H., and Foster, F.S., Beam Steering with pulsed two-dimensional transducer arrays, *IEEE Trans. Ultrason. Ferroelect. Freq. Contr.*, 38, 320–333, 1991.

113. Bruneel, C., Delannoy, B., Torguet, R., Bridoux, E., and Lasota, H., Electrical coupling effects in an ultrasonic transducer array, *Ultrasonics*, 17, 255–260, 1979.

114. Kino, G.S., and DeSilets, C.S., Design of slotted transducer arrays with matched backings, *Ultrasonic Imaging*, 1, 189–209, 1979.

115. Smith, S.W., von Ramm, O.T., and Thurstone, F.L., Angular response of piezoelectric elements in phased array ultrasound scanners, *IEEE Trans. Sonics Ultrason.*, 26, 185–191, 1979.

116. Delannoy, B., Bruneel, C., Haine, F., and Torguet, R., Anomalous behavior in the radiation pattern of piezoelectric transducers induced by parasitic Lamb wave generation, *J. Appl. Phys.*, 51, 3942–3948, 1980.

117. Larson, J.D., Non-ideal radiators in phased array transducers, pp. 673–683 in: *1981 IEEE Ultrasonic Symp. Proc.*, 1981.

118. Dias, J.F., An experimental investigation of the cross-coupling between elements of an acoustic imaging array transducer, *Ultrasonic Imaging*, 4, 44–55, 1982.

119. Dias, J.F., Construction and performance of an experimental phased array acoustic imaging transducer, *Ultrasonic Imaging*, 3, 352–368, 1982.

120. Certon, D., Felix, N., Lacaze, E., Teston, F., and Patat, F., Investigation of cross-coupling in 1–3 piezocomposite arrays, *IEEE Trans. Ultrason. Ferroelect. Freq. Contr.*, 48, 85–92, 2001.

121. t'Hoen, P.J., Aperture apodization to reduce the off-axis intensity of the pulsed-mode directivity function of linear arrays, *Ultrasonics*, 20, 231–236, 1982.

122. Harris, F.J., On the use of windows for harmonic analysis with the discrete Fourier transform, *Proc. IEEE*, 66, 51–83, 1978.

123. Daft, C.M.W., and Engeler, W.E., Windowing of wide-band ultrasound transducers, pp. 1541–1544 in: *1996 IEEE Ultrasonics Symp. Proc.*, 1996.

124. von Ramm, O.T., Smith, S.W., and Thurstone, F.L., Grey scale imaging with complex TGC and transducer arrays, pp. 266–270 in: Proc. Soc. Photo-Optical Instr. Engrs., *Application of Optical Instrumentation in Medicine*, IV, SPIE, 1975.

125. Smith, S.W., Pavy, H.G., and von Ramm, O.T., High-speed ultrasound volumetric imaging system—Part I: Transducer design and beam steering, *IEEE Trans. Ultrason. Ferroelect. Freq. Contr.*, 38, 100–108, 1991.

126. Gehlbach, S.M., and Alvarez, R.E., Digital ultrasound imaging techniques using vector sampling and raster line reconstructing, *Ultrasonic Imaging*, 3, 83–107, 1981.

127. Lockwood, G.R., Li, P-C., O'Donnell, M., and Foster, F.S., Optimizing the radiation pattern of sparse periodic linear arrays, *IEEE Trans. Ultrason. Ferroelect. Freq. Contr.*, 43, 7–14, 1996.

128. Hussain, M.A., Rigby, K.W., and Itani, L.A., Sparse two-dimensional, wideband ultrasound transducer, US Patent 5,911,692, June 1999 (filed Jan. 1998).

129. Lockwood, G.R., and Foster, F.S., Optimizing the radiation pattern of sparse periodic two-dimensional arrays, *IEEE Trans. Ultrason. Ferroelect. Freq. Contr.*, 43, 15–19, 1996.

130. Brunke, S.S., and Lockwood, G.R., Broad-bandwidth radiation patterns of sparse two-dimensional vernier arrays, *IEEE Trans. Ultrason. Ferroelect. Freq. Contr.*, 44, 1101–1109, 1997.

131. Maginness, M.G., and Walker, J.T., Induced Doppler distortions in dynamically focused array imaging systems, pp. 287–290 in: *1977 Ultrasonics Symp. Proceedings*, 1977.

132. Walker, J.T., Doppler wavefront distortion effects due to continuous dynamic array focusing, pp. 15–27 in: *Acoustical Imaging*, Vol. 8., A.F. Metherell (Ed.) (Proc. 8th Int. Symp. Acoust. Imaging, May/June, 1978), Plenum Press, New York, 1979.

133. McKeighen, R.E., Design guidelines for medical ultrasonic arrays, pp. 2–18 in: *Ultrasonic Transducer Engineering*, K.K. Shung (Ed.), Proc. SPIE Vol. 3341, Medical Imaging, 1998.

134. Foster, S.F., Larson, J.D., Mason, M.K., Shoup, T.S., Nelson, G., and Yoshida, H., Development of a 12 element annular array transducer for realtime ultrasound imaging, *Ultrasound Med. Biol.*, 15, 649–659, 1989.

135. Foster, S.F., Larson, J.D., Pittaro, R.J., Corl, P.D., Greenstein, A.P., and Lum, P.K., A digital annular array prototype scanner for realtime ultrasound imaging, *Ultrasound Med. Biol.*, 15, 661–672, 1989.

136. Kim, J.H., Song, T.K., and Park, S.B., Pipelined sampled-delay focusing in ultrasound imaging systems, *Ultrasonic Imaging*, 9, 75–91, 1987.

137. Melton, H.E., and Thurstone, F.L., Annular array design and logarithmic processing for ultrasonic imaging, *Ultrasound Med. Biol.*, 4, 1–12, 1978.

138. Dietz, D.R., Parks, S.I., and Linzer, M., Expanding-aperture annular array, *Ultrasonic Imaging*, 1, 56–75, 1979.

139. Baum, G., and Greenwood, I., Orbital lesion localization by three dimensional ultrasonography, *NY State J. Med.*, 61, 4149–4157, 1961.

140. Brown, T.G., Younger, G.W., Skrgatic, D., and Fortune, J., Multiplanar B-scanning—using the third dimension, pp. 1797–1799 in: *Ultrasound in Medicine*, Vol. 3B, D. White, and R.E. Brown (Eds.), Plenum Press, New York, 1977.

141. McDicken, W.N., Lindsay, M., and Robertson, D.A.R., Three-dimensional images using a fibre optic ultrasonic scanner, *Br. J. Radiol.*, 45, 70–71, 1972.

142. Robinson, D.E., Display of three-dimensional ultrasonic data for medical diagnosis, *J. Acoust. Soc. Am.*, 52, 673–687, 1972.

143. King, D.L., Al-Banna, S.J., and Larach, D.R., A new three-dimensional random scanner for ultrasonic/computer graphic imaging of the heart, pp. 363–372 in: *Ultrasound in Medicine*, Vol. 2, D. White, and R. Barnes (Eds.), Plenum Press, New York, 1976.

144. Brinkley, J.F., Moritz, W.E., and Baker, D.W., Ultrasonic three-dimensional imaging and volume from a series of arbitrary sector scans, *Ultrasound Med. Biol.*, 4, 317–327, 1978.

145. Brinkley, J.F., Muramatsu, S.K., McCallum, W.D., and Popp, R.L., In vitro evaluation of a an ultrasonic three-dimensional imaging and volume system, *Ultrasonic Imaging*, 4, 126–139, 1982.

146. Greenleaf, J.F., Three-dimensional imaging in ultrasound, *J. Medical Systems*, 6, 579–589, 1982.

147. Ghosh, A., Nanda, N.C., and Maurer, G., Three-dimensional reconstruction of echo-cardiographic images using the rotation method, *Ultrasound Med. Biol.*, 8, 655–661, 1982.

148. McCann, H.A., Sharp, J.C., Kinter, T.M., McEwan, C.N., Barillot, C., and Greeleaf, J.F., Multidimensional ultrasonic imaging for cardiology, *Proc. IEEE*, 76, 1063–1073, 1988.

149. Maginess, M.G., Plummer, J.D., Beaver, W.L., and Meindl, J.D., State-of-the-art in two-dimensional ultrasonic array technology, *Med. Physics*, 3, 312–318, 1976.

150. Linney, A.D., and Deng, J., Three-dimensional morphometry in ultrasound, *Proc. Inst. Mech. Eng.: Part H: J. Eng. Med.*, 213, 235–245, 1999.

151. Gilja, O.H., Hausken, T., Berstad, A., and Odegaard, S., Measurement of organ volume by ultrasonography, *Proc. Inst. Mech. Eng.: Part H: J. Eng. Med.*, 213, 247–259, 1999.

152. Fenster, A., and Downey, D.B., 3-D ultrasound imaging: a review, *IEEE Eng. Med. Biol. Mag.*, 15, 6, 41–51, 1996.

153. Downey, D.B., and Fenster, A., Three-dimensional ultrasound: a maturing technology, *Ultrasound Quarterly*, 14, 25–40, 1998.

154. Nelson, T.R., and Pretorius, D.H., Three-dimensional ultrasound imaging, *Ultrasound Med. Biol.*, 24, 1243–1270, 1998.

155. Nelson, T.R., Downey, D.B., Pretorius, D.H., and Fenster, A., *Three-Dimensional Ultrasound*, Lippincott Williams & Wilkins, Philadelphia, 1999.

156. Fenster, A., Downey, D.B., and Cardinal, H.N., Three-dimensional ultrasound imaging, *Phys. Med. Biol.*, 46, R67–R99, 2001.

157. Inerfield, M., Lockwood, G.R., and Garverick, S.L., A sigma-delta-based synthetic aperture beamformer for real-time 3-D ultrasound, *IEEE Trans. Ultrason. Ferroelect. Freq. Contr.*, 49, 243–254, 2002.

158. Rohling, R.N., Gee, A.H., and Berman, L., Automatic registration of 3-D ultrasound images, *Ultrasound Med. Biol.*, 24, 841–854, 1998.

159. Barratt, D.C., Davies, A.H., Hughes, A.D., Optimization and evaluation of an electromagnetic tracking device for high-accuracy three-dimensional ultrasound imaging, *Ultrasound Med. Biol.*, 27, 957–968, 2001.

160. Wildes, D.G., Chiao, R.Y., Daft, C.M.W., Rigby, K.W., Smith, L.S., and Thomenius, K.E., Elevation performance of 1.25D and 1.5D transducer arrays, *IEEE Trans. Ultrason. Ferroelect. Freq. Contr.*, 44, 1027–1037, 1997.

161. Daft, C.M.W., Wildes, D.G., Thomas, L.J., Smith, L.S., Lewandowski, R.S., Leue, W.M., Rigby, K.W., Chalek, C.L., and Hatfield, W.T., A 1.5D transducer for medical ultrasound, pp. 1491–1495 in: *1994 IEEE Ultrasonics Symp. Proc.*, 1994.

162. Crombie, P., *Fundamental Studies on Contrast Resolution of Ultrasound B-Mode Images*, PhD thesis, University of Toronto, 1999.

163. Guo, P., Yan, S., and Zhu, Q., Elevation beamforming performance of a 1.75D array, pp. 1113–1116 in: *2001 IEEE Ultrasonics Symp.*, 2001.

164. von Ramm, O.T., Smith, S.W., and Pavy, H.G., High-speed ultrasound volumetric imaging system—Part II: parallel processing and image display, *IEEE Trans. Ultrason. Ferroelect. Freq. Contr.*, 38, 109–115, 1991.

165. Smith, S.W., Trahey, G.E., and von Ramm, O.T., Two-dimensional arrays for medical ultrasound, *Ultrasonic Imaging*, 14, 213–233, 1992.

166. Pavy, H.G., Smith, S.W., and von Ramm, O.T., Improved real time volumetric ultrasonic imaging system, pp. 54–61 in: Proc. SPIE Vol. 1443, *Medical Imaging V: Image Physics*, R.H. Schneider (Ed.), 1991.

167. Light, E.D., Davidsen, R.E., Fiering, J.O., Hruschka, T.A., and Smith, S.W., Progress in two-dimensional imaging, *Ultrasonic Imaging*, 20, 1–15, 1998.

168. Yen, J.T., Steinberg, J.P., and Smith, S.W., Sparse 2-D array design for real time rectilinear volumetric imaging, *IEEE Trans. Ultrason. Ferroelect. Freq. Contr.*, 47, 93–110, 2000.

169. Yen, J.T., and Smith, S.W., Real-time rectilinear volumetric imaging, *IEEE Trans. Ultrason. Ferroelect. Freq. Contr.*, 49, 114–124, 2002.

170. Turnbull, D.H., and Foster, F.S., Fabrication and characterization of transducer elements in two-dimensional arrays for medical ultrasound imaging, *IEEE Trans. Ultrason. Ferroelect. Freq. Contr.*, 39, 464–475, 1992.

171. Delannoy, B., Torguet, R., Bruneel, C., Bridoux, E., Rouvaen, J.M., and LaSota, H., Acoustical image reconstruction in parallel-processing analog electronic systems, *J. Appl. Phys.*, 50, 3153–3159, 1979.

172. Shattuck, D.P., Weinshenker, M.D., Smith, S.W., and von Ramm, O.T., Explososcan: a parallel processing technique for high speed ultrasound imaging with linear phased arrays, *J. Acoust. Soc. Am.*, 75, 1273–1282, 1984.

173. Shirasaka, T., Ultrasonic imaging apparatus, US Patent No. 4,815,043, March 21, 1987 (filed July 28, 1986).

174. Snyder, R.A., Ultrasonic imaging system utilizing two or more simultaneously-active apertures, European Patent 0.335.587 A2 (filed March 22, 1989).

175. Mallart, R., and Fink, M., Improved imaging rate through simultaneous transmission of several ultrasound beams, pp. 120–130 in: *New Developments in Ultrasonic Transducers and Transducer Systems*, F.L. Lizzi (Ed.), SPIE (Int. Soc for Optical Eng.), Vol. 1773, 1992 (see also U.S. Patent 5,276,354, Jan. 4, 1994).

176. Smith, S.W., and von Ramm, O.T., Acoustic orthoscopic imaging system, US Patent 4,596,145, June 24, 1986 (filed Sept. 20, 1983).

177. Insana, M.F., and Hall, T.J., Quality management of ultrasound diagnosis, Ch. 13, pp. 161–182 in: *Advances in Ultrasound Techniques and Instrumentation (Clinics in Diagnostic Ultrasound*, Vol. 28) P.N.T. Wells (Ed.), Churchill Livingstone, New York, 1993.

178. Hand, J.W., Ultrasound hyperthermia and the prediction of heating, Ch. 8, pp. 151–176 in: *Ultrasound in Medicine*, F.A. Duck, A.C. Baker, and H.C. Starritt (Eds.), Inst. of Physics Pub., Bristol, 1998.

179. Ibbini, M.S., and Cain, C.A., A field conjugation method for direct synthesis of hyperthermia phased-array heating patterns, *IEEE Trans. Ultrason. Ferroelect. Freq. Contr.*, 36, 3–9, 1989.

180. Zel'dovich, B.Y., Pilipetsky, N.F., and Shkunov, V.V., *Principles of Phase Conjugation*, Springer-Verlag, Berlin, 1985.

181. Shkunov, V.V., and Zel'dovich, B.Y., Optical phase conjugation, *Sci. Am.*, 253, 54–59, Dec. 1985.

182. Fink, M., Time reversal of ultrasonic fields—Part I: basic principles, *IEEE Trans. Ultrason. Ferroelect. Freq. Contr.*, 39, 555–566, 1992.

183. Nikoonahad, M., and Pusateri, T.L., Ultrasonic phase conjugation, *J. Appl. Phys.*, 66, 4512–4513, 1989.

184. Ebbini, E.S., and Cain, C.A., Multiple-focus ultrasound phased array pattern synthesis: optimal driving-signal distributions for hyperthermia, *IEEE Trans. Ultrason. Ferroelect. Freq. Contr.*, 36, 540–548, 1989.

185. Karpelson, A.E., Calla, D.A., and Cobbold, R.S.C., Approximate methods for synthesis and analysis of ultrasound transducers, *IEEE Trans. Ultrason. Ferroelect. Freq. Contr.*, 42, 793–797, 1995.

8

Ultrasound Imaging Systems

Design, Properties, and Applications

This is the second of two chapters concerned with imaging systems. Its purpose is to describe a number of important matters directly related to imaging and imaging systems and to discuss some of the special ways in which clinical imaging can be performed. It begins by looking at matters concerning system design, followed by an analysis of the process of image formation, and the formation and characteristics of image speckle. Methods are then discussed for using coded excitation schemes to increase the depth to which satisfactory images can be obtained, and this is followed by a discussion of synthetic aperture schemes. Imaging using either the nonlinear properties of the propagation medium or the properties of injected contrast media are important developments. Descriptions of ultrasound tomography, elastography, and microscopy lead to the final section of this chapter: methods for imaging from within body cavities and blood vessels.

8.1 B-Mode Imaging Systems

8.1.1 Array System Design

Although several individual aspects of the design of an imaging system were considered in Chapter 7, it is perhaps helpful to consider the entire system as well. While many different variations exist, the block diagram of Fig. 8.1 is a useful starting point. The transducer T/R switch isolates the functions of

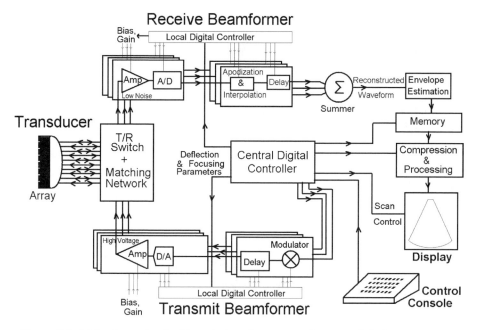

Figure 8.1 Main elements of a B-mode imaging system that uses digital beamformers for transmission and reception.

transmission and reception. For transmission beamforming, the central digital controller determines the transmitted waveforms, and these are converted into analog form by the D/A converters. Amplifiers provide the high-voltage waveforms needed to drive the individual elements. In reception, low-noise amplifiers followed by A/D converters may be used. As noted in Chapter 7, if reconstruction errors are to be avoided, the sampling frequency must be no less than $32 c_o/\lambda$, which, for a center frequency of 5 MHz, corresponds to around 200 MHz. Because the dynamic range of an A/D converter diminishes with increasing sampling frequency, such a high sampling frequency may be inconsistent with the required dynamic range. Several methods have been described for overcoming this problem [1,2]. One consists of multiplying with a local oscillator frequency so as to create sum and difference frequencies, and then, by low-pass filtering, the difference frequency portion of the spectrum can be selected. By this means the signal is converted to a lower carrier frequency, enabling a much lower sampling frequency to be used without information loss. Alternatively, by using the interpolation technique outlined in subsection 7.2.1, a lower minimum A/D sampling rate can be used, enabling an A/D converter to be used that has a much larger dynamic range. If both the preamplifier and A/D have a sufficient wide dynamic range (e.g., 96 dB $\equiv 2^{16} = 65{,}536$), time-gain compensation can be avoided, and any compression that may be needed for display or recording purposes can be performed after digitization. Summation of the delayed and apodized waveforms leads to estimating the

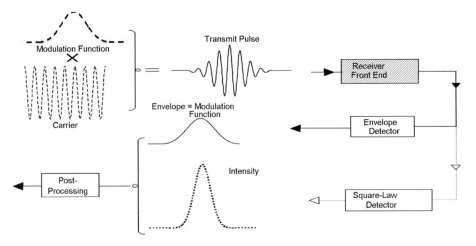

Figure 8.2 Two possible B-mode ultrasound detection schemes. For the standard envelope detector the received pressure amplitude is displayed, while for the square-law detector the intensity is displayed. The post-processing stage often involves logarithmic compression.

received signal envelope, details of which are provided in the next subsection. The final stages consist of compression, image processing, and a means for displaying and recording the images in a standard format.

8.1.2 Envelope Estimation

The envelope of the signal from a point scatterer will be the same as the incident envelope, provided there are no frequency-dependent effects. If a detector is used under these circumstances (Fig. 8.2), it should provide an estimate of the envelope that closely matches the transmitted envelope. When a square-law detector is used, the envelope will be proportional to the intensity.

Illustrated in Fig. 8.3a is a particularly straightforward method for determining the pressure envelope. If $x(t)$ is a real received signal, then its Hilbert transform [3] has a frequency spectrum identical to that of the input but whose phase components are all shifted by −90 degrees (i.e., the Hilbert transform acts as an ideal −90-degree phase shifter). As illustrated in (b), for a Gaussian received pulse, the envelope will be Gaussian and the Hilbert transformed output will be quasi-sinusoidal with a similar envelope. If the signals are in digital form, then the problem of estimating the envelope reduces to following the peak signals from the two absolute operations.

8.1.3 Imaging Theory

The point spread function (PSF) of an ultrasound imaging system represents the image response produced by a point scatterer at a particular location. The

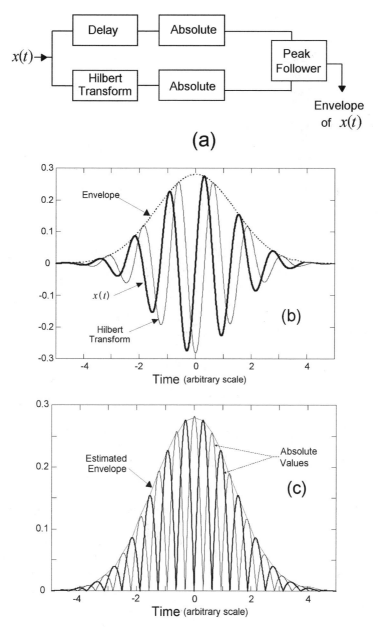

Figure 8.3 Method for estimating the envelope using the Hilbert transform. (a) Schematic of method that assumes a real input signal. (b) Gaussian received pulse, its envelope, and the Hilbert transformed input. (c) Absolute value and peak follower outputs.

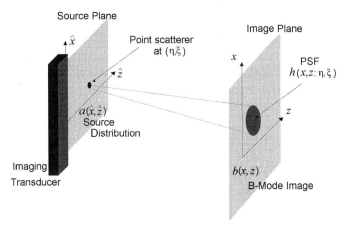

Figure 8.4 Simplified representation of a B-mode imaging system in which the source is represented by a continuous scatter distribution on a plane and the system response is represented by a 2-D point spread function (PSF).

papers by Bamber and Dickinson [4] and Fatemi and Kak [5] drew attention to the importance of this concept in describing the performance of a B-mode imaging system. Subsequently Hiller and Ermert [6] presented important extensions, particularly in relation to pulse-echo tomography, as discussed in section 8.7.2.

If the image space coordinate system is (x,y,z), then the PSF can be expressed as $h_p(x,y,z : \eta,\zeta,\xi)$, where the location of the point scatterer is (η,ζ,ξ) in the space coordinate system $(\hat{x},\hat{y},\hat{z})$. The two coordinate systems will normally be related by a magnification factor $M = x/\hat{x} = y/\hat{y} = z/\hat{z}$. Knowledge of how the PSF varies throughout the source space enables the image distribution to be predicted for a given source distribution, provided the system behaves in a *linear manner*.

A simplified representation of an imaging system is shown in Fig. 8.4, where the scattering medium is assumed to consist of a continuous 2-D distribution of scatterers represented by $a(\hat{x},\hat{z})$ and the image is given by $b(x,z)$. In practice, the transducer elevation response will cause scatterer distributions in neighboring planes to the primary source plane to influence the response. If we ignore this effect, the 2-D image can be expressed as

$$b(x,z) = \iint_{-\infty}^{\infty} a(\eta,\xi)h_p(x,z : \eta,\xi)d\eta d\xi.$$

Let us suppose that the PSF is *space invariant*. The invariance implies that the PSF depends on coordinate differences between the source and the magnified image, i.e., $h_p(x - M\eta, z - M\xi)$; consequently, the image is given by

$$b(x,z) = \iint_{-\infty}^{\infty} a(\eta,\xi)h_p(x - M\eta, z - M\xi)d\eta d\xi.$$

Changing the variables by letting $\eta' = M\eta$ and $\xi' = M\xi$, this can be expressed as a 2-D convolution:

$$b(x,z) = \frac{1}{M^2} \iint\limits_{-\infty}^{\infty} a\left(\frac{\eta'}{M}, \frac{\xi'}{M}\right) h_p\left(x - \eta', z - \xi'\right) d\eta' d\xi'.$$

which can be written in the shorthand form

(8.1)
$$b(x,z) = \frac{1}{M^2} a(\eta, \xi) \underset{x\ z}{**} h_p(x - \eta, z - \xi).$$

If we also assume that PSF is *separable* [6],

$$h_p(x - M\eta, z - M\xi) = \underset{\substack{\text{Characterizing}\\\text{Lateral Resolution}}}{\frac{h_{px}(x - M\eta)}{}} \times \underset{\substack{\text{Characterizing}\\\text{Axial Resolution}}}{\frac{h_{pz}(z - M\xi)}{}}.$$

By substituting this into (8.1) and taking the 2-D Fourier transform, the spatial frequency domain of the image for $M = 1$ is given by

(8.2)
$$\begin{aligned} B(k_x, k_z) &= A(k_x, k_z) H_{px}(k_x) H_{pz}(k_z) \\ &= A(k_x, k_z) H(k_x, k_z) \end{aligned},$$

In this equation the capital letters denote the corresponding spatial frequency (k_x, k_y) domain functions and the transfer function $H(k_x, k_z)$ is the Fourier transform of the PSF. In Fig. 8.5a the slice to be imaged is shown along with an array that generates ideal transmit/receive profiles. The spatial frequency of $a(\hat{x}, \hat{z})$ shown in (b) has frequencies in the lateral direction that exceed those that can be resolved by the transducer's lateral characteristic, and as a result only the cross-hatched portion of $A(k_x, k_z)$ is sampled. However, because the axial resolution is shown as being considerably greater, all the spatial frequency information along the k_z axis is obtained. As is evident from (c) and (d), the missing information can be obtained by rotating the transducer and repeating the B-scan: the complete set of frequency-domain data enables the image to be reconstructed by means of 2-D inverse Fourier transform.

8.2 Image Speckle

Shortly following the development of CW lasers it was discovered that shining a laser beam on a surface produced an image with a granular background appearance whose characteristic lengths bore no resemblance to the macroscopic character of the illuminated surface. It was quickly realized that because most surfaces are comparatively rough compared to the wavelength, the speckled appearance arose from interference of light scattered from various regions of the surface. The granular background appearance created by illuminating a rough surface with fairly coherent radiation is known as *speckle*, and because it reduced the resolution capabilities of the illuminating system, methods for reducing its influence were investigated. However, it was also found that the presence of speckle could be used to advantage in certain appli-

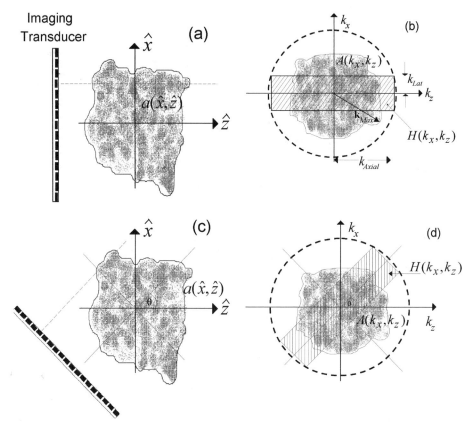

Figure 8.5 Representation of B-mode (pulse-echo) imaging in the space and spatial frequency domains. (a) Conventional scan of a region that has a backscattering function of $a(k_x, k_z)$. (b) Showing partial sampling of the spatial frequency domain $A(k_x, k_z)$. (c) Scanning at an angle θ. (d) Sampling of the spatial frequency domain at an angle θ. (Based on similar drawings in Hiller and Ermert [6].)

cations, such as providing a quantitative measure of the roughness of a surface. Imaging systems based on the use of some form of coherent illumination, including acoustic and radar systems, also exhibit speckle. Among the many papers describing the statistics of optical speckle, Goodman's [7] introduction to the topic, published in 1975, is particularly helpful.

For some time, it was known that ultrasound B-mode images of tissue contained a background that had a granular-like appearance similar to that shown in the simulated image in Fig. 8.6. In their account of the manner in which an understanding of this phenomenon developed, Abbott and Thurstone [9] indicated that it was identified as a speckle phenomenon in the mid to late 1970s. Abbott and Thurstone carefully considered some of the key differences between laser and ultrasound speckle. They pointed out that laser speckle is normally seen or detected as an intensity variation, whereas in B-mode

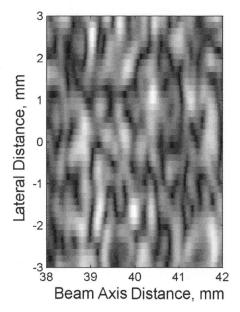

Figure 8.6 Simulation example of fully developed speckle generated in a small volume around the focal zone of a linear phased array. Simulations were performed using a scatter number density of $100/mm^3$, log compression of the image, a Gaussian pulse with a 5-MHz center frequency, and a –6-dB bandwidth of 67%. Note that in the higher-resolution axial direction, the characteristic length is considerably less than in the lateral direction. (Reproduced, with permission, from Crombie [8].)

ultrasound it is the envelope of the received pressure signal that is normally detected. Both detection schemes are illustrated in Fig. 8.2.

In a key paper in 1978, Burckhardt [10] clearly pointed out that essential ingredients for producing a speckle pattern include the presence of many small, randomly distributed scatterers, such as those due to the cellular nature of tissue, and a coherent radiation source. If each scatterer has a volume much less than the sample volume and the number within the sample volume is large, fully developed speckle will be formed. Burckhardt also presented an analytic approach and discussed potential signal-to-noise ratio (SNR) improvements that could be achieved by averaging a sequence of uncorrelated speckle images obtained by compound scanning. Although much of the initial work was focused on characterizing the speckle pattern in terms of its statistics and describing how speckle noise degraded the image contrast resolution, subsequent developments showed that, like optical speckle, its presence enables certain types of measurements to be made. For example, it can be used for assessing tissue microstructure, measuring tissue strain distribution (elastography; see section 8.8), and measuring a flow velocity field. In this final application, the movement of flowing blood causes the speckle pattern to change with time; consequently, by measuring the point-by-point displacements that occur between image frames, the 2-D flow velocity field can be mapped [11,12], as discussed further in section 8.8.

8.2.1 Speckle Analysis

Typically, a gray-scale B-mode image consists of $M \times N$ pixels, each having its magnitude represented by one byte (0 to 255). A first-order statistical analysis describes the characteristics of a given pixel. Second-order statistics are needed to describe how the gray-scale values at two different spatial locations are related. In particular, the 2-D autocovariance function will be used to characterize the patterns seen in Fig. 8.6. One of the difficulties in characterizing the statistical properties arises from the linear and nonlinear processes involved in the imaging process. For example, the effects of frequency-dependent attenuation and the use of logarithmic compression make it difficult to accurately model the statistics of speckle.

To numerically simulate tissue speckle produced by a linear array, it is fortunately not necessary to use a distribution of point scatterers having the same scatterer number density as in tissue. In the case of blood at 40% hematocrit, this would correspond to approximately $5 \times 10^6/mm^3$ scatterers, which would impose a heavy computational burden even for a relatively small test volume. In fact, it has been shown that a very much smaller number density will produce a comparable result [13], i.e., the speckle can be regarded as fully developed. For example, a Gaussian distribution of point scatterers with an average density of $100/mm^3$ may be more than sufficient to ensure that the pattern does not change with any further increase in the number density.

First-Order Statistics

The ultrasonic speckle signal arises from the effects of interference caused by microscopic scatterers from within a resolution cell as it is scanned over the region being imaged. To examine their effect we shall assume that the scatterers are randomly distributed in space and occupy a negligibly small volume. Let us consider a pulse-echo system whose transmitted waveform is approximately monochromatic, and suppose that within the sample volume there are a large number of scatterers. If the signal phasor from the n'th scatterer is denoted by[1] $a_n/\sqrt{N}$, then the complex received signal is the sum of the contributions from all N scatterers and can be written as

$$R(\mathbf{r}{:}t) = A(\mathbf{r})e^{j\omega t}.$$

As illustrated in Fig. 8.7a, the complex phasor A has real and imaginary parts given by

$$\mathrm{Re}(A) = \frac{1}{\sqrt{N}}\sum_{n=1}^{N}|a_n|\sin\phi_n \quad \text{and} \quad \mathrm{Im}(A) = \frac{1}{\sqrt{N}}\sum_{n=1}^{N}|a_n|\cos\phi_n,$$

---

1. By using the scaling factor of $1/\sqrt{N}$ the mean intensity remains finite.

Imaginary

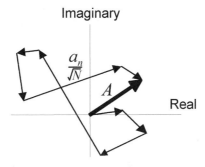

Figure 8.7 The 2-D random walk problem in which a large number of complex phasors representing the signals from a random distribution of scatterers are summed to form the phasor A.

in which ϕ_n is the phase shift of the nth component. The phase shifts account for the variations in the path lengths that arise from the positions associated with each scatterer.

Let us assume that the amplitude and phase of each scatterer are uncorrelated to one another as well as to all other scatterers, that the phases are uniformly distributed over $(-\pi,\pi)$, and that the number of scatterers is large. Using the Central Limit theorem, it can be readily shown that the real and imaginary parts of A are Gaussian random variables with the same variances and zero means. Given the above, the question as to how to determine the probability distribution function (PDF) for the phasor magnitude $|A| = \sqrt{\{\mathrm{Re}(A)\}^2 + \{\mathrm{Im}(A)\}^2}$, given the PDFs for the real and imaginary components, is part of a more general statistical transformation problem that is well documented [14,15]. By applying this transformation, the PDF of the phasor magnitude is found to be Rayleigh distributed and given by

(8.3) $$PDF(|A|) = \frac{A}{\sigma^2} e^{-A^2/(2\sigma^2)} \text{ for } A \geq 0,$$

where $\sigma^2 = \lim_{N \to \infty} \frac{1}{2N} \sum_n^N |a_n|^2$, and the mean and variance (square of the standard deviation) are given by $\overline{|A|} = \sigma\sqrt{\pi/2}$ and $\mathrm{var}(|A|) = \xi^2 = \sigma^2[2 - \pi/2]$, respectively. This result, which was obtained by Atkinson and Berry [16] in their classic analysis of the received ultrasound fluctuations created by blood, is illustrated in Fig. 8.8a. In the absence of any resolvable structures, a useful figure of merit is the ratio of the mean to the standard deviation, i.e., $\overline{|A|}/\xi = \sqrt{\pi(4-\pi)} = 1.91$ (5.6 dB), which is sometimes referred to as the SNR.

If a square-law detector is assumed, a different PDF results. For this case the 2-D image is based on the intensity $I = |A|^2 = \{\mathrm{Re}(A)\}^2 + \{\mathrm{Im}(A)\}^2$ and corresponds to that normally used optically. The PDF for the intensity can be found [15] by evaluating

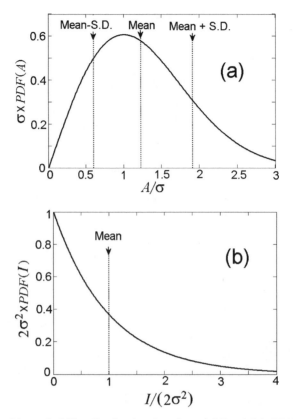

Figure 8.8 Speckle probability distribution functions. (a) Rayleigh PDF for envelope detection, showing the mean and ± one standard deviation (S.D.). (b) Exponential PDF for square law detection.

$$PDF(I) = \frac{PDF(|A|)}{|dI/dA|}.$$

With the help of (8.3) and $I = |A|^2$, the intensity PDF can be found to consist of a simple exponential given by

$$(8.4) \qquad PDF(I) = \frac{1}{2\sigma^2} e^{-I/(2\sigma^2)} \quad \text{for} \quad I \geq 0,$$

whose mean and standard deviation are both equal to $2\sigma^2$, and which is graphed in Fig. 8.8b. Moreover, the ratio of the mean to the standard deviation is unity, i.e., $SNR = 1$.

Non-Gaussian Statistics

Let us now consider the situation where the number of scatterers in the sample volume is not sufficiently large to satisfy the conditions required by the Central

Limit theorem. For this case, the real and imaginary parts of A can no longer be assumed to be Gaussian random variables, and as a result, the received signal envelope will not be Rayleigh distributed. In fact, non-Gaussian statistics are evident in many practical problems. One of the first to be investigated was that of microwave scattering by the sea surface, which led to the development of an exact solution to the finite 2-D random walk problem. For a finite number of steps, Jakeman and Pusey [17] showed that an appropriate PDF is a modified Bessel function or K-distribution given by

$$PDF(A) = \frac{2b}{\Gamma(\chi)} \left(\frac{bA}{2} \right)^{\chi} K_{\chi-1}(bA), \quad \text{for } \chi > 0,$$

where $\chi = N(1 + v)$, $b = 2\sqrt{\chi/E\{A^2\}}$, and $v > -1$ is a function that depends on the geometry and statistics. In addition, $K_{\chi-1}(.)$ is a modified Bessel function of the second order $(\chi - 1)$ and $\Gamma(.)$ is a gamma function. As the number of scatterers in the sample volume or steps in the random walk becomes large, i.e., $N \to \infty$, it can be shown that this PDF approaches a Rayleigh distribution. Moreover, Rayleigh, Rician, Poisson, and other distributions have been shown to be special cases of the generalized form of the K-distribution [18]. Because of it generality, the K-distribution has found application in ultrasound speckle analysis [19,20].

Post-Processing Statistics

The statistical analysis used above ignored the effects of any nonlinear post-processing. In B-mode systems, because of the very wide input dynamic range, limitations imposed by the image display method and an observer's ability to discriminate between gray-scale levels impose severe restrictions on the detection of weak targets. To overcome this problem, some form of nonlinear signal processing is generally used to compress a wide input signal range into a much smaller output range. Such processing, which may be in the form of a logarithmic transfer function, causes a change in the PDF. Thijssen et al. [21] were the first to examine in detail the effects of various forms of post-processing on the first- and second-order statistics of fully developed speckle. Subsequently, Kaplan and Ma [22] examined the statistics for a post-processing compression stage whose transfer function is similar to that often used in practice. Specifically, they assumed the output is given by

$$(8.5) \qquad\qquad X = D \ln(A) + G,$$

where A is the input envelope amplitude $(A > 0)$ whose statistics are given by (8.3). Also, G is a linear gain constant whose presence does not affect the output statistics, and D is another constant that is related to the dynamic range.

If X_{min} and X_{max} are the minimum and maximum values of the output corresponding to the inputs of A_{min} and A_{max}, respectively, then from (8.5)

$$D = \frac{X_{max} - X_{min}}{\ln(A_{max} - A_{min})},$$

which enables D to be estimated if the input and output ranges are known. Now the PDFs of the input and output are related by $PDF(X) = \dfrac{PDF(A)}{|dX/dA|}$, which can be evaluated with the help of (8.3) and (8.5), yielding the double exponential (Fisher-Tippet) density function given by

(8.6)
$$PDF(X) = \frac{2}{D} \exp[-\alpha - \exp(-\alpha)],$$

where $\alpha = (2/D)(\beta - X)$ and $\beta = (D/2)\ln(2\sigma^2) + G$. This enables the mean and variance to be expressed as [23, p. 930]

$$E\{X\} = D[0.5\ln 2 + \ln \sigma - \gamma/2] + G,$$

and

$$\text{var}\{X\} = D^2 \pi^2 / 24,$$

where γ is Euler's constant (≈ 0.5772).

Using a commercial linear-array scanner and two types of tissue-mimicking phantom, Kaplan and Ma [22] performed measurements to determine the pre- and post-log-compressed histograms and compared predictions to those theoretically predicted. The results shown in Fig. 8.9a indicate some differences from the Rayleigh PDF as given by (8.3). This may be due to additional nonlinear effects such as those arising from frequency-dependent attenuation. For logarithmic compression of the form given by (8.5), Fig. 8.9b shows that the PDF is in rough agreement with that theoretically predicted by (8.6). Some of the differences may be due to the differences noted in (a) being propagated to (b).

Second-Order Statistics

The 2-D autocorrelation function is a spatial domain description of the texture since it describes how the texture in one region is related to that in another. The autocorrelation function for a continuous 2-D process $f(x,z)$ whose complex conjugate is $f^*(x,z)$ is given by

$$R_{ff}(x,z) = E\{f(x,y)f^*(x,y)\} = \int\!\!\!\int_{-\infty}^{\infty} f(x'-x, z'-z)f^*(x',z')dx'dz',$$

and that for a discrete process is

$$R_{ff}(k,l) = \sum_{m=0}^{M-1} \sum_{n=0}^{N-1} f_{m,n} f_{m+k,n+l}.$$

If there is no correlation between the content of each pixel, then the autocorrelation function will be zero. The presence of correlation, such as that noted earlier in Fig. 8.6, results in a autocorrelation function whose dimensions are related to the resolution in the axial and lateral directions. Because

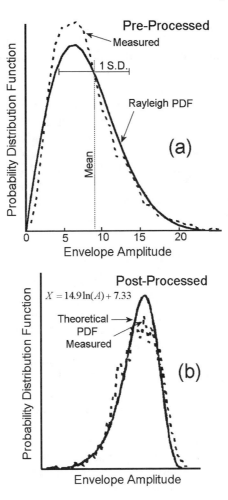

Figure 8.9 Theoretical probability distribution functions compared to the smoothed measured histograms for a tissue-mimicking phantom using a linear-array imaging system. (a) Envelope detected signal prior to post-processing. (b) With the logarithmic post-processing using the transfer function shown. (Reproduced, with permission, from Kaplan and Ma [22], *J. Acoust. Soc. Am.*, 95, 1396–1400, © 1995 Acoustical Society of America.)

an image may contain both a deterministic component and a zero-mean random component, the autocorrelation about the mean is often used, i.e.,

$$C_{ff}(k,l) = \sum_{m=0}^{M-1} \sum_{n=0}^{N-1} \left(f_{m,n} - E\{f_{m,n}\}\right)\left(f_{m+k,n+l} - E\{f_{m+k,n+l}\}\right),$$

which is the autocovariance function. Generally the autocovariance is plotted in a normalized form, and this is sometimes referred to as the correlation function.

The 2-D normalized autocovariance function for the speckle pattern illustrated in Fig. 8.6 is shown in Fig. 8.10. It will be noted that in the axial z-direction it is considerably less than in the lateral x-direction. In fact, the FWHM of the autocovariance is closely related to the resolution in the axial and lateral directions [24–27]. In the case of a circular transducer of diameter D and a transmitted Gaussian pulse with a center frequency wavelength of λ(mm) and a −6 dB bandwidth Δf(MHz), the autocovariance $FWHM_{axial} \approx 0.9/\Delta f$ and $FWHM_{lateral} \approx 0.9\lambda z/D$. As an example, consider a 5 MHz Gaussian pulse with $\Delta f = 3.35$ MHz and a transducer with an f-number $= z/D = 3$, a measure of the axial and lateral resolutions are: $FWHM_{axial} \approx 0.27$ mm, and $FWHM_{lateral} \approx 0.8$ mm. Even though the simulated image of Fig. 8.6 was obtained for a linear array, a quick assessment shows that the speckle size is in rough agreement with the above dimensions.

8.2.2 Speckle Reduction Techniques

There have been many publications describing a variety of methods for reducing the effects of speckle on B-mode images [28]. Several are based on generating a multiplicity of images whose speckle patterns are either weakly correlated or uncorrelated[2] and which are then averaged to produce a compounded image. For uncorrelated speckle images, it can be shown [10] that the ratio of the mean signal level to the standard deviation increases as $\sqrt{N}$, where N is the number of averaged images. Such methods are similar to the use of compound scanning, which, as described in Chapter 7, was originally developed for improving the image quality of hand-guided scanning systems. Subsequently, it was shown that by using an electronically steered linear array, images could be obtained at different angles [29,30], and these could then be compounded. Healey and Leeman [31] point out that the problem of speckle reduction can be usefully considered as a two-stage process in which the following questions are addressed: "(i) recognition—is the texture present in a clinical image segment the result of real (resolvable) structures or the speckle artifact?, and (ii) what would the image look like in the absence of speckle?"

Schemes for speckle reduction include:

1. Spatial movement
2. Angular movement
3. Frequency subdivision in transmit or receive
4. Post-processing methods based on filtering

The first three are compounding methods that make no use of the statistical information contained in the image itself, and these will be described more fully in the next subsection. The fourth group involves image-processing operations that can entail adaptive or nonadaptive, linear or nonlinear filtering. In the adaptive method proposed in 1986 by Bamber and Daft [32],

---

2. The changes needed to make the images reasonably well uncorrelated are of major importance and will be discussed shortly.

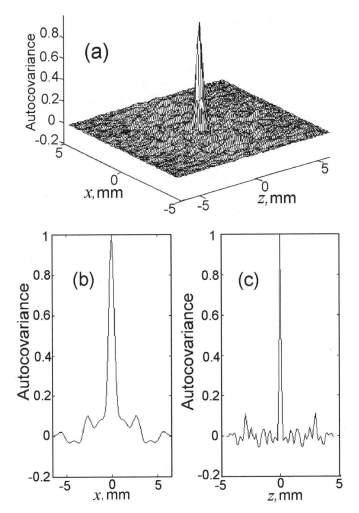

Figure 8.10 Autocovariance function of the simulated speckle image shown in Fig. 8.6. (a) 2-D form. (b) Lateral cut through $z = 0$. (c) Axial cut through $x = 0$. (Reproduced, with permission, from Crombie [8].)

use is made of the image statistics to adaptively reduce the speckle. Improvements to this method that account for the signal-processing characteristics (including log-compression) and scatterer density have also been described [20,33].

Compounding Methods

Spatial compounding can be achieved by slowly moving the transducer normal to the scan plane, enabling a sequence of images to be obtained, which can then be averaged. Because the movement between frames needed to make sure that the speckle is decorrelated is approximately the resolution in that direction, some loss in spatial resolution can be expected. Temporal resolution will also be sacrificed, depending on the number of frames to be averaged and the frame rate, but this should not be a problem if the structures are stationary or moving very slowly. Using a high-resolution scanner designed for breast imaging, this technique was first experimentally evaluated by Foster et al. [34]. The system used separate transmit and receive transducers consisting of a PVDF cone and a PZT annular array, and achieved a lateral resolution (FWHM) of 0.25 mm over a wide depth of field. Each image was produced by mechanically stepping the transducer in one direction: successive images were obtained by displacing the transducer normal to the scan plane. By averaging four image slices, separated from each other by 0.5 mm, significant improvements in the smoothness of the background were obtained, though with some loss in resolution. Bamber [28] points out that the use of filtering to perform smoothing within a single image should also be considered to be a form of spatial compounding. However, blurring of meaningful structures can result, and even when the spatial filter cutoff frequency has been properly chosen, this method has not been found to result in significant improvements.

Associated with the spatial movement technique is the angular compounding method [35–37], which is relatively simple to implement using either a linear or a phased array. Because the scatterer spacing seen from different angles differs, the speckle pattern will change, enabling image ensemble averaging to achieve a net reduction in speckle. As illustrated in Fig. 8.11a, when a phased-array aperture is displaced laterally, a fixed object will be redisplayed at a new location in the image. Because the ultrasound scan lines intersect this new region of the image at different angles, a different speckle pattern will be produced. For a linear array that is capable of being steered through different angles (see Fig. 8.11b), the images obtained for sufficiently large steering angles should also be uncorrelated.

A number of techniques based on frequency compounding have been investigated, all of which are based on the change in phase with wavelength [38–40]. For example, if the system bandwidth is sufficiently wide, then it is possible divide the received RF signal into sub-bands, each of which can be individually processed to produce an image. By compounding these images, it has been shown that speckle background can be reduced. However, the smaller bandwidth associated with each sub-band can be expected to reduce the image spatial resolution, and as a result this method, as well as other frequency compound techniques, has not shown good promise.

Correlation Coefficient

An important issue that has been addressed by several researchers concerns the transducer displacement needed to ensure that the images being compounded are statistically independent. This issue was first studied by Burckhardt [10]; it was experimentally assessed by Trahey et al. [36] and

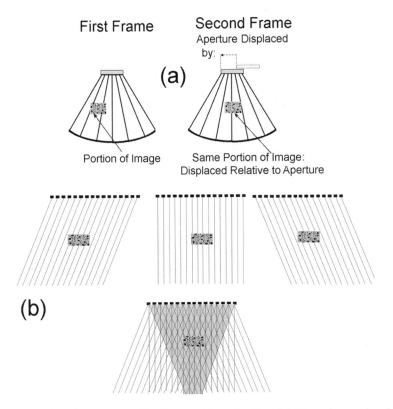

Figure 8.11 Angular compounding for speckle reduction. (a) Phased array in which the second frame is obtained after displacing the aperture. (b) With a linear array that can be steered through three angles, three sets of uncorrelated images should be obtained. The compounded image consists of a central trapezoidal region where all three images are averaged.

subsequently analyzed by Wagner et al. [27], who obtained expressions for the correlation between two images as a function of the transducer displacement. In doing so, several approximations were made, and these included (i) identical transmit and receive apertures, (ii) CW theory applies, (iii) lateral and axial point spread functions are separable, (iv) the resolution cell is in the transducer focal zone. The first step consists of obtaining an expression for the amplitude signal from a sample volume containing a distribution of point scatterers and then obtaining its intensity. The second step is to obtain an intensity expression when the transducer is displaced and angled so as to see the same scattering region. The cross-correlation between the speckle produced when the two transducer aperture locations are separated by a lateral distance b can be expressed as

$$(8.7) \qquad \rho(b) = B \left| \int |p(x)|^2 e^{j4\pi bx/(z\lambda_c)} dx \right|^2,$$

where λ_c is the wavelength corresponding to the center frequency of the pulse, z is the axial location of the sample volume, B is a normalization constant, x is the lateral coordinate, and $p(x)$ is the lateral pulse-echo response. The final quantity is simply the product of the transmit and receive directivity functions, each of which can be found by taking the spatial Fourier transform of the aperture function (see Chapter 3). Examination of (8.7) shows that it can be expressed as the square of a Fourier transform, i.e.,

$$\rho(b) = B \left\| \Im\left\{ |\mathbf{p}(x)|^2 \right\} \right|_{f=2bx/(z\lambda_c)} \right\|^2 .$$

In their investigation of the effects of multi-angle compounding, Jespersen et al. [37] used a 7.5 MHz linear array to determine the correlation between images obtained at differing angles of a speckle-generating phantom. They also determined the array transmit and receive directivity functions and, with the help of (8.7), calculated the correlation coefficient between images as a function of the beam angle. The results shown in Fig. 8.12 indicate that if a relatively small steering angle, e.g., 10 degrees, is used, the images are virtually fully decorrelated.

8.3 Resolution, Contrast, and Signal-to-Noise Ratio

The maintenance of good contrast and resolution with increasing penetration depth is of major importance in B-mode tissue imaging systems. As noted

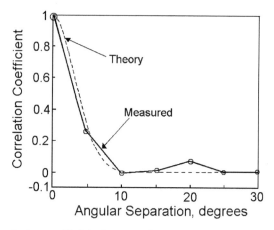

Figure 8.12 Correlation coefficient between log-compressed, envelope-detected speckle images (192 scan lines) obtained at different incident angles. Predicted and measured results were obtained using a 7.5-MHz (center frequency) linear array with a −6-dB bandwidth of ≥70%. Measurements were made on a speckle-generating phantom. Hamming windows were used for transmit and receive. (Reproduced, with permission of Dynamedia, from Jespersen et al. [37] *Ultrasonic Imaging*, 20, 81–102, © 1998 Dynamedia.)

earlier, tissue attenuation causes the backscattered signal power to diminish rapidly with increasing depth, and as a result, beyond a certain depth, there will be insufficient scattered signal with which to form a meaningful image. Limitations on the peak transmitted power that can be used arise from safety concerns and nonlinear propagation. As a result, significant difficulty can be encountered in obtaining a satisfactory image from deep regions, particularly for an obese person. Decreasing the transmission frequency provides for increased penetration, but at the same time the axial, lateral, and azimuthal resolutions are degraded. This raises the question as to the best method for increasing the imaging depth without degrading the resolution. One solution lies in devising methods for improving the SNR, such as those described in section 8.4.

8.3.1 Axial Resolution

An approximate approach for calculating the axial spatial resolution of an imaging system is to consider the transmission of a pulse consisting of several sinusoidal cycles directed towards two scatterers that are separated by Δz. As illustrated in Fig. 8.13, if the pulse duration is denoted by T, then the interval between the end of the first received pulse and the start of the second is given by $\Delta t = 2\Delta z/c_o - T$. It can be argued that it will no longer be possible to distinguish between the presence of scatterers when $\Delta t = 0$, i.e., $\Delta z = c_o T/2$, which is taken to be the axial resolution. Of course, the ability to distinguish between the two scatterers also depends on the contrast, and this depends on the SNR. As the SNR diminishes, the contrast between the noise and the signal created by the scatterers reduces to the point where the two scatterers can no longer be distinguished.

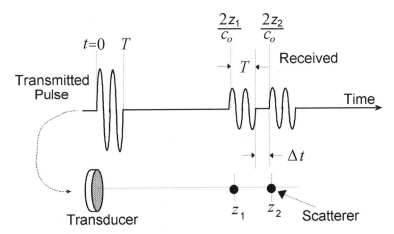

Figure 8.13 Simplified method for estimating the axial resolution for a pulse transmitted at $t = 0$ and two scatterers at locations z_1 and z_2. When the separation $\Delta t = 0$, the spatial separation of the two scatterers is given by $\Delta z = c_o T/2$, which is taken to be the axial resolution.

8.3.2 Contrast and Resolution

In judging and comparing the performance of a B-mode imaging systems designed for clinical use [41], it is has been found that specification of the resolution in the axial and lateral directions does not necessarily provide a useful measure of the performance; in fact, it can be quite misleading. In part, the problem arises from the method used to determine the resolution. In computed tomography (CT) and x-ray systems, the resolution is generally assessed by using high-contrast line pair phantoms that enable the line spread function or its Fourier transform, the modulation transfer function, to be obtained. In sonar and radar systems, the full-width at half maximum (FWHM), which is related to the classical Rayleigh criterion, is commonly used and can be measured by using two high-contrast point targets. In ultrasound systems the resolutions in the axial, lateral, and azimuthal directions generally differ and are functions of the measurement location. The contrast associated with a specific region is generally degraded through the background image speckle, and as a result an assessment of the resolution by means of high-contrast targets seems inappropriate. Moreover, if significant side lobes are present, these can contribute to the background image speckle, thereby degrading the resolution and contrast. Because the Rayleigh or FWHM assessment of the resolution depends only on the main lobe characteristics, the presence of significant side lobes can give a misleading assessment of the imaging performance [42].

The value of a B-mode clinical image for detecting abnormalities, especially those produced by low-contrast targets such as focal lesions, depends on the system contrast and resolution performance. Initial approaches to the measurement of the resolution were based on the use of phantoms containing high-contrast wire targets. However, as noted above, the results sometimes suggested that a system with an inferior FWHM could have a superior clinical performance to one with a better FWHM. Smith and Lopez [43,44] addressed this issue and pointed out the importance of properly accounting for the contrast performance. They also noted an important difference between CT and ultrasound systems. For CT systems there is a more or less fixed background noise arising from quantum mottle. Consequently, by using a higher dose, the SNR can be enhanced. However, in ultrasound the coherent speckle background increases with the incident intensity, so that provided the intrinsic system noise can be neglected, the use of a higher transmitted intensity will result in little or no improvement in performance.

To measure the performance in a realistic manner, Smith et al. [45] developed phantoms having tissue-mimicking material as a background and targets consisting of cones of varying contrast relative to the background. Using human observers, it is then possible to generate *contrast-detail* curves that enable the imaging performance of different systems to be compared [43,46]. Such a curve might be of the form illustrated in Fig. 8.14. It demarcates the boundary between the detectable and the undetectable regions, though it is somewhat observer-dependent.

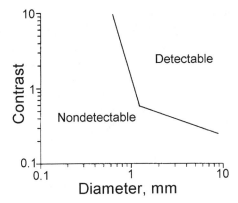

Figure 8.14 Contrast-detail graph that provides a measure of the ability to detect a circular object that has a specific contrast relative to the background. At high contrasts it is primarily the Rayleigh or FWHM resolution that governs the detectability. (Based on Hall et al. [46].)

Several proposals have been made to provide a quantitative assessment of the contrast performance, and these were based on imaging a fluid-filled spherical cyst that contained no scatterers (anechoic) embedded in a uniform medium containing scatterers. In 1983 Smith et al. [45] proposed that the contrast between the cyst and the background is given by

$$(8.8) \qquad C_1 = \frac{S_{out} - S_{in}}{\sqrt{S_{out}^2 + S_{in}^2}},$$

where S_{in} is the mean signal measured inside a region of the cyst and S_{out} is the average signal measured from the same-sized regions outside the cyst. An alternative contrast measure is that used by Patterson and Foster [47]

$$(8.9) \qquad C_2 = \frac{S_{out} - S_{in}}{S_{out}}.$$

Patterson and Foster also noted that if the variances of the signal within and outside the cyst are denoted by σ_{in}^2 and σ_{out}^2, respectively then $\sqrt{\sigma_{in}^2 + \sigma_{out}^2}\,/\,S_{out}$ is a measure of the speckle contrast fluctuations. They called the ratio of C_2 to the contrast fluctuations the "contrast-to-speckle ratio", i.e.,

$$(8.10) \qquad CSR = \frac{S_{out} - S_{in}}{\sqrt{\sigma_{in}^2 + \sigma_{out}^2}},$$

a measure that was subsequently used by several researchers for assessing imaging quality, e.g., [48].

The contrast exhibited by cysts of differing size can be used as a means for assessing the contrast resolution [43,49]. As the size of a spherical cyst is reduced, the received power will approach that of the background. For example, in the case of a *hypo*echoic cyst, the radius at which the received power is a specific number of dB's below the background can used as a quantitative measure of the performance. If a *hyper*echoic cyst is considered whose scattering strength is *above* the background by the same amount as the hypoechoic cyst was below, the radius at which the received power is a specific number of dB's *above* the background is also a measure of the performance. In general, these two radii will differ, and both may be needed for a proper assessment of the performance. The differences in image appearance of hyperechoic and hypoechoic cysts are illustrated in the simulations of Fig. 8.15 [8].

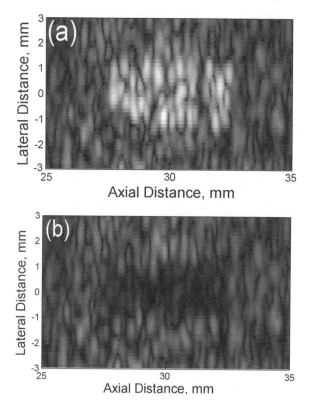

Figure 8.15 Simulations of spherical (a) hyperechoic and (b) hypoechoic cysts for a linear array with fixed transmit, receive and elevation focusing at 30 mm, and a 5-MHz center frequency pulse with a −6-dB fractional bandwidth of 67%. Logarithmic compression was used and the image was displayed using 64 gray-scale levels. The distorted outlines of the cyst positions is evident. The background (10 scatterers/mm^3) average intensity is the same for both images. The scattering strengths from within the cysts relative to the background were 4 and 1/4 for (a) and (b), respectively. (Reproduced, with permission, from Crombie [8].)

In these phased-array images, both cysts have the same fractional scattering strengths relative to the background.[3]

8.3.3 Signal-to-Noise Ratio

Noise arises from sources that include the transducer, the preamplifier, and the random nature of the background medium that gives rise to speckle. It is evident that the received signal strength due to a scatterer at a given depth will depend on the attenuation suffered by the incident and scattered signal. Consequently, the SNR is depth-dependent and can be defined by

$$(8.11) \quad SNR(z) = \frac{\text{Maximum Instantaneous Received Signal Power}}{\text{Noise Power}}.$$

If it is assumed that speckle noise can be neglected and that the noise originating from the transducer and preamplifier is white over the system bandwidth Δf, and N_n denotes the power density, then the denominator can be written as $N_n \Delta f$. If a simple sinusoidal pulse of duration T and amplitude A is considered, then the energy of the received signal can be expressed as $E = \frac{1}{2}A^2 T$. By substituting these into (8.11), we have

$$SNR(z) = \frac{A^2}{N_n \Delta f} = \frac{2E}{TN_n \Delta f}.$$

If an optimal reception filter is used, its bandwidth will be $\Delta f = 1/T$, i.e., unity *time-bandwidth* product, so that the above simplifies to

$$SNR(z) = \frac{2E}{N_n}.$$

Thus, improvements in the SNR can be achieved by reducing the noise associated with the reception process and by increasing the transmitted pulse energy. As discussed in section 6.9, the noise power is governed primarily by the properties of the transducer, the receiver preamplifier noise, matching conditions and bandwidth. Limited improvements in the SNR at the output of the preamplifier can be achieved by careful design. A more promising approach for achieving major improvements in the SNR is to increase the transmitted pulse duration by using coded transmission and/or by increasing the transmitted amplitude. Safety [51] and nonlinear propagation considerations limit the latter.

Safety Issues

In diagnostic ultrasound, safety considerations [51] impose certain limitations on the peak flux that can occur anywhere within the radiated region. For adult

---

3. When these images were displayed on a monitor, 10 independent observers stated that the hyperechoic cyst image exhibited a higher contrast relative to the background [8].

cardiac imaging, the spatial-peak pulse average[4] (I_{SPPA}) should be less than 240 W/cm^2 and the spatial peak time average[4] (I_{SPTA}) should be less than 0.73 W/cm^2. In addition, concerns about the potential harmful effects of cavitation have required that the peak negative pressure be limited. It is well known that the spatial-peak/temporal-peak negative pressure and the frequency primarily determine the potential for cavitation. In addition to this mechanical effect, the potential for tissue damage by thermal heating must be considered.

The *Mechanical Index* (*MI*) is a quantity related to the potential for damage based on mechanical effects during a diagnostic ultrasound examination. It is defined by [50]

(8.12)
$$MI = \frac{p_-(\text{MPa})}{C_{MI}\sqrt{f(\text{MHz})}},$$

where C_{MI} is 1.0 MPa/MHz$^{1/2}$ (needed to make $MI < 1$ dimensionless) and p_- is the peak value of the attenuated rarefactional pressure. Values for *MI* in diagnostic imaging generally range from 0.04 to 1.7.

The *Thermal Index* (*TI*) provides a measure of the potential for tissue damage by heating. Under model exposure conditions it is proportional to a calculated or estimated temperature rise. It is defined by [50]

(8.13)
$$TI = \frac{W_p}{W_{\text{deg}}},$$

where W_p is the attenuated output power and W_{deg} is the ultrasonic power required to raise the target tissue temperature by 1°C. For calculating or measuring the *TI*, the average ultrasonic attenuation along the beam axis is to be taken as 0.3 dB/(cm.MHz).

Under most conditions a *TI* value of 1.0 is regarded as posing negligible risk to the patient. An important report by the National Council on Radiation Protection and Measurements published in 2002 [51] indicates that under normal conditions, negligible risk to the patient requires that $MI < 0.5$ and $TI < 1$. However, higher values for *MI* may be needed to obtain adequate contrast and resolution. To provide the clinician with a means of weighing possible risks against improvements in image quality obtained by using higher transmitted power, most diagnostic systems have a real-time display of *MI*.

For linear array imaging systems that use short-duration excitation pulses, it is the peak transmitted pressure, which may be around several MPa, rather than the time-averaged flux that limits the SNR. Pressures in this range can cause significant harmonic distortion. Thus, if it is assumed that the peak transmitted pressure consistent with considerations of both safety and waveform distortion are used, the only means that remains for improving the SNR is to use a longer transmitted waveform. The question as to whether this can be

---

4. I_{SPPA} is the average flux over the time duration of the transmitted pulse. On the other hand, I_{SPTA} is a time average over the entire pulse repetition period.

done without degrading the spatial resolution will be considered in the next section.

8.4 Coded Transmission Systems

Coded excitation methods have been developed since the 1950s, initially for use in radar [52,53] to obtain improved range/resolution, and subsequently in communications systems. In these methods the duration of the transmitted waveform is substantially increased, thereby increasing the total transmitted energy, but without increasing the peak transmitted power. As illustrated in Fig. 8.16, the transmitted waveform has a coded form that could consist of a binary code or a FM chirp similar to that used by bats in locating objects. Making use of the fact that the exact form of the transmitted signal is known, correlation methods provide a means for extracting spatial scattering information from the received signal without suffering the loss of resolution associated with a long-duration transmitted pulse. The detection and decoding process involves compressing the original transmitted waveform into a signal with a much shorter duration and one that has a similar bandwidth to the transmitted signal. The resulting increase in the time-bandwidth product is a direct measure of the SNR improvement that can be realized. In the case of a radar system the improvement can be a factor of several thousand, but, as will be seen, for ultrasound systems the potential improvement is much more modest.

Some Japanese conference reports in 1970, describing the use of M-codes for Doppler flow measurements, were probably the first to recognize the potential advantages of coded excitation methods [54] in medical ultrasound. In a 1972 report Waag et al. [55] discussed the use of a coded excitation scheme for blood flow measurements that could operate in either a continuous or a burst transmission mode. Subsequently, a variety of schemes were described for NDE [56–58] applications and medical diagnostic systems [59,60]. The principles underlying these techniques were briefly discussed in subsection 6.4.2, where the use of the Barker coded transducers was described. In B-mode tissue imaging, the presence of high attenuation and nonstationary targets reduces the possible types of encoding schemes that can be used, but some still retain the potential for achieving significant SNR improvements [61]. Two different schemes that have been explored for use in diagnostic ultrasound systems will be examined in detail: the FM chirp and Golay binary codes.

8.4.1 Principles

In Fig. 8.17a the pulse-echo impulse response of a given transducer/transmission medium system has been denoted by $h(t)$. If the transducer is excited by a waveform $e_t(t)$, then the received waveform is given by the convolution

$e_r(t) = e_t(t) * h(t) = \int_{-\infty}^{\infty} e_t(t-\tau)h(\tau)d\tau$. Now the output of the cross-correlator is

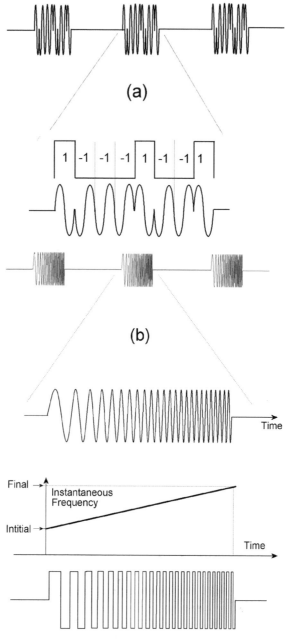

Figure 8.16 Two types of coded excitation schemes that enable the received pulse to be compressed to a fraction of the transmitted pulse length. (a) Binary encoding scheme: a single-cycle sinusoidal transmitted pulse has been assumed. (b) Linear frequency-modulated waveform (chirp), together with a square-wave pseudochirp (shown at the bottom).

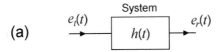

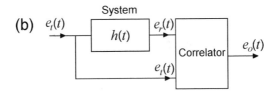

Figure 8.17 Comparison of conventional and pulse compression systems. (a) Conventional pulse-echo system in which the impulse response is that of the transducer and propagation medium. (b) Pulse compression system in which the output is the cross-correlation of the transmitted and received signal waveforms.

given by[5] $e_o(t) = \int_{-\infty}^{\infty} e_t(t + \xi) e_r(\xi) d\xi$, so that with the help of the above expression for $e_r(t)$, and noting that the autocorrelation of $e_t(t)$ is given by $R_{ee}(t) = \int_{-\infty}^{\infty} e_t(\xi + t) e_t(\xi) d\xi$, the output waveform can be expressed as

$$e_o(t) = \int_{-\infty}^{\infty} e_t(t + \xi) e_r(\xi) d\xi$$
$$= R_{ee}(t) * h(t),$$

which is the autocorrelation function of the transmitted signal convolved with the impulse response. If the autocorrelation function of the transmitted sequence is a δ-function, i.e., $R_{ee}(t) = \delta(t)$, then the impulse response is equal to the cross-correlator output, enabling the impulse response to be determined in a relatively simple manner. Continuous white noise is the best-known transmitted signal whose autocorrelation function is a δ-function, and this has been used in both radar and ultrasound NDE applications.

8.4.2 FM Chirp

Considerable effort has been made to apply the ideas developed for chirp radar for ultrasound tissue imaging. However, in ultrasound diagnostic systems, because the time-bandwidth product is around two orders of magnitude less than that for radar, the potential improvements in system performance are far less dramatic. Some significant contributions on the use of chirps for medical imaging are those of O'Donnell [62] (pseudochirp, see Fig. 8.16b)

5. See Appendix B for definitions of the cross- and autocorrelation functions.

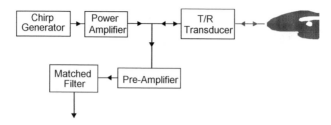

Figure 8.18 Simple pulse-echo system using an FM chirp and a matched filter.

and Rao [63]. More recently, Misaridis and Jensen [64] and Misaridis et al. [65] have used this pulse compression method to obtain enhanced SNR in deep tissue regions. One of the advantages of using the pseudochirp [66] over the CW chirp for phased-array use is that the transducer driving waveform is in a digital form.

To illustrate the use of an FM chirp, we shall consider the system shown in Fig. 8.18. If the chirp varies linearly with frequency,[6] then for a unit amplitude transmitted wave of duration T, the transmitted waveform can be expressed as

$$(8.14) \qquad e(t) = \text{rect}(t/T)\cos\left(\omega_o t + \frac{\gamma t^2}{2}\right). \qquad (a)$$

Also, the matched filter impulse response is

$$(8.14) \qquad h(t) = \text{rect}(t/T)\sqrt{\frac{2\gamma}{\pi}}\cos\left(\omega_o t - \frac{\gamma t^2}{2}\right). \qquad (b)$$

In the above equations, ω_o is the center frequency, γ specifies the rate at which the frequency changes, and the square-root factor makes the filter gain unity at $\omega = \omega_o$. In addition, it should be noted that the instantaneous frequency is given by $\omega(t) = d\varphi/dt$, where φ is the cos function argument. Consequently, by differentiating the argument of the cos function, we see that $\omega(t) = \omega_o + \gamma t$, which changes linearly with time. The filter output is the compressed waveform, as is given by the cross-correlation

$$e_o(t) = \sqrt{\frac{2\gamma}{\pi}} \int_{-T/2}^{T/2} \cos(\omega_o\tau + \gamma\,\tau^2/2)\cos\left[\omega_o(t-\tau)-\gamma(t-\tau)^2/2\right]d\tau.$$

By using the trigonometric expansion for the product of two cosine terms, it can be seen that two terms result, one of which involves a frequency of $2\omega_o t$. By ignoring this term, the matched filter output can be reduced to

---

6. There are advantages to be gained through the use of nonlinear frequency modulation [53, pp. 212–218; 67].

$$(8.15) \qquad e_o(t) = \text{rect}[t/(2T)] \sqrt{\frac{2\gamma}{\pi}} \cos(\omega_o t) \frac{\sin[\gamma t(T - |t|)/2]}{\gamma t},$$

which extends over twice the initial chirp duration, i.e., from $-T$ to $+T$.

By taking the Fourier transform of (8.14a), the transmit spectrum can be expressed as [53, pp. 136–137]

$$(8.16) \qquad S(\omega) = \sqrt{\frac{\pi}{4\gamma}} e^{-j\frac{(\omega - \omega_O)^2}{2\gamma}} [F^*(X_1) + F^*(X_2)],$$

where $X_1 = [\gamma T/2 + (\omega - \omega_o)]/\sqrt{\pi\gamma}$, $X_2 = [\gamma T/2 - (\omega - \omega_o)]/\sqrt{\pi\gamma}$ and $F^*(X)$ is the complex conjugate of the Fresnel integral as defined in Appendix C.

The above expressions can be illustrated through the example shown in Fig. 8.19a, consisting of a $10\,\mu s$ FM chirp with a center frequency of $5\,MHz$ and a bandwidth of $2.5\,MHz$. Such a waveform has a time-bandwidth product that is 25 times larger than a simple pulse-echo system. From Fig. 8.19c it can be seen that the compressed form contains *range side lobes* (sometimes referred to as *self-noise*) with amplitudes comparable to the main lobe, and these will cause difficulties in the presence of multiple scattering targets. Specifically, a weakly scattering target near a strongly scattering one will result in a main lobe that may be difficult to distinguish from the range side lobes of the strongly scattering target.

Consequently, much effort has been devoted toward devising schemes for reducing the range side lobes to levels well below $-50\,dB$. Two such schemes are generally considered. In the first, time-domain shaping of the transmitted waveform is used so that the sharp edges associated with a rectangular window are avoided. The second uses frequency-domain shaping of the received signal spectrum.

From Fig. 7.22 it will be noted that the maximum side lobe level for a signal windowed by a rectangle is $-13.2\,dB$ with respect to the main lobe, and this is the situation for the chirp shown in Fig. 8.19a. A major reduction in the range side lobes can be achieved by using a suitable window on the received output spectrum, such as the Dolph-Chebyshev window illustrated in Fig 7.23. As with other windows, its use is accompanied by some reduction of SNR[7] and broadening of the main lobe, which in turn causes a loss in axial resolution. In fact, the bandpass filter characteristics of the transducer will produce a similar effect. If the spectrum of the chirp is comparable to or wider than that of the transducer, it has been shown [64,67] that the transducer transfer function results in a major reduction in the range side lobes.

The effect of the transducer bandpass characteristics is illustrated in Fig. 8.20, where a $20\,\mu s$ rectangular transmitted chirp with a fractional bandwidth $(-6\,dB)$ of 78% has been assumed. Using a Dolph-Chebyshev window with a specified side lobe of $-90\,dB$ and neglecting the effect of the transducer (mismatched filter case), it can be seen that the near side lobes are significantly

---

7. The reduction in SNR due to the mismatch is not large [53, pp. 191–197], e.g., a few dB.

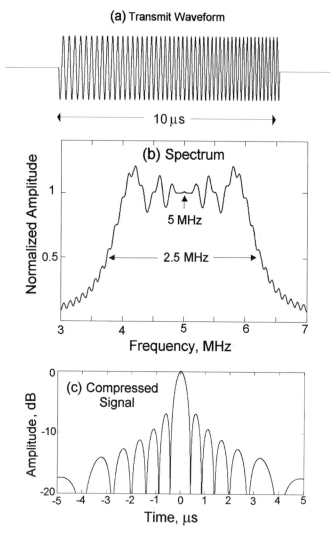

Figure 8.19 Example of a 10μs FM chirp with a time-bandwidth product of $T\Delta f =$ 25. (a) Time-domain transmitted signal calculated from (8.14a). (b) Frequency-domain representation calculated from (8.16). (c) For clarity, the envelope of the compressed signal (calculated from (8.15) without the cosine term) is plotted. It should be noted that the total signal duration is 20μs.

reduced. However, in the neighborhood of $\pm T/2$, the side lobe levels far exceed the specified value of −90 dB, and this could cause serious energy leakage from bright to dark regions of a B-mode image. The effect of including the filtering due to a 4 MHz transducer with a 65% fractional bandwidth (−6 dB) is shown in Fig. 8.20b. Even without the Dolph-Chebyshev window, the range side lobes are much less than the comparable values shown in Fig. 8.20a.

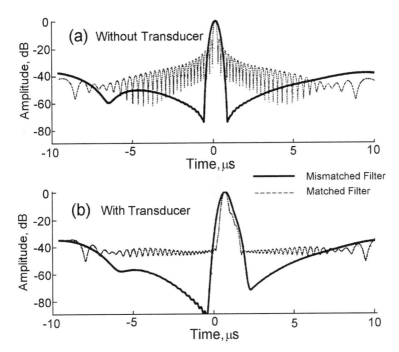

Figure 8.20 Effect of the transducer filtering effect on the compression of a 20-µs chirp generated by a square window. In (a) the compressed pulse is shown assuming no transducer filtering. The dashed line assumes a matched filter; the solid line assumes a Dolph-Chebyshev window whose side lobes have been specified to be −90 dB. In (b) the transducer filtering is present. (Reproduced, with permission, from Misaridis and Jensen [64], *1999 IEEE Ultrasonics Symp. Proc.* © 1999 IEEE.)

The high side lobes seen around ±T/2 in Fig. 8.20 are not simply a result of the frequency domain windowing but, as discussed by Kowatsch and Stocker [68], are primarily a result of the rectangular time window and are directly related to the Fresnel ripples seen in the spectrum. A major reduction can be achieved through the use of a cosine taper, i.e., a Tukey window [69], on the leading and trailing portions of the waveform. This is illustrated Fig. 8.21, where the spectra for both a rectangular and a Tukey time window are compared for a 20 µs chirp. It can be seen that the tapered waveform produces a much smoother spectrum, resulting in a substantial reduction in the far side lobes.

A major problem encountered in all coded excitation schemes arises from the effects of frequency-dependent attenuation of tissue. Problems arise from the use of TGC, which is used to partially correct for the attenuation. Specifically, the received signal from the transmitted sequence that is partially reflected from a fixed depth will not be of constant amplitude. The later parts of the transmitted sequence will be increased in amplitude, a problem that will be accentuated by longer sequence lengths. In addition, the presence of

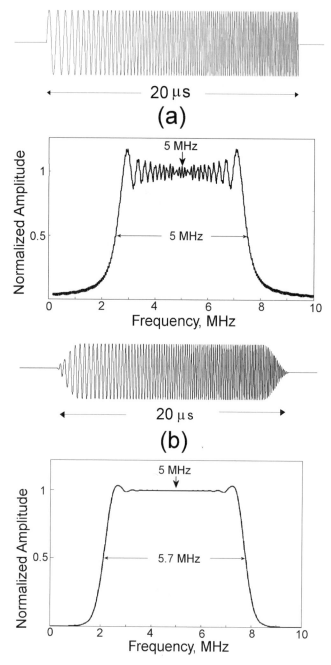

Figure 8.21 Effect of cosine (Tukey) amplitude tapering on the frequency spectrum of a 20-μs linear chirp with a center frequency of 5 MHz and a bandwidth of 5 MHz. (a) Rectangular window. (b) Cosine taper over the first and last 2.25 μs.

frequency-dependent attenuation causes the mean frequency of the returned signal to decrease with depth. As an example, consider a 5 MHz center frequency Gaussian pulse with a fractional bandwidth (–6 dB) of 60%, propagating in a medium with an attenuation of 0.7 dB/(MHz.cm). It was shown in Chapter 1 (subsection 1.8.1) that the mean frequency will be downshifted by approximately 1 MHz at a depth of 8 cm (2 MHz for two-way frequency-independent scattering from this depth). This shift and the possible depth-dependent changes in shape make it unlikely that a simple filter with sufficiently low range lobes could be realized. A depth-dependent mismatch filtering scheme has been proposed [65,70] in which a bank of filters is used, each filter being designed to operate at a certain depth.

8.4.3 Golay Code

Investigations by Golay on the design of multislit optical spectrometers [71] led to the realization that certain pairs of binary sequences have important correlation properties. If the binary sequences A and B are of equal length and if the sum of their autocorrelation functions is zero everywhere except at zero lag, the sequences are said to be a *complementary* pair. In a key paper published in 1961 by Golay [71], the properties and conditions for forming such pairs were described. Examples are {+1,+1}, {–1,+1}: {–1,–1,–1,+1}, {–1,–1,+1,–1}: {+1,–1,+1,+1,–1,+1,+1,+1}, {+1,–1,+1,+1,+1,–1,–1,–1}. The last pair of codes is shown in Fig. 8.22, together with their autocorrelation function. It can be seen that both autocorrelation functions have a peak value of 8 at zero lag and that the range side lobes are equal and opposite. As a result, the sum of the two autocorrelation functions is a triangular pulse with an amplitude of 16, a base width equal to twice the code clock period, and no range side lobes. Longer complementary sequences can be readily constructed from shorter sequences. For example, starting from a sequence with a length of 8, sequences with lengths of 16, 32, 64, and 128 can be readily constructed. Tseng and Liu [73] have generalized the ideas presented by Golay by describing the conditions for complementary sets of binary sequences to be produced, i.e., sets that can contain more than two sequences.

One of the first investigations of the possible use of Golay codes for medical imaging was that by Takeuchi [59,60] in 1979. He presented a possible design and predicted its performance. Subsequently, Lee and Furgason [74] described the operation and performance of an all-digital ultrasonic flaw detection system. The NDT imaging system described by Hayward and Gorfu [75,76] in 1988/9 used a 30-element PZT, 1.48 MHz transducer array and employed 32 bit complementary Golay codes. With this system they were able to demonstrate recognizable B-mode images of simple structures.

At least one manufacturer incorporated a form of digital coded excitation and compression and has demonstrated that this enables significant improvements in penetration depth and SNR to be achieved in clinical imaging. The improvement is illustrated in Fig. 8.23, which shows images of liver with and without the use of the encoding technology. It seems that one or more systems

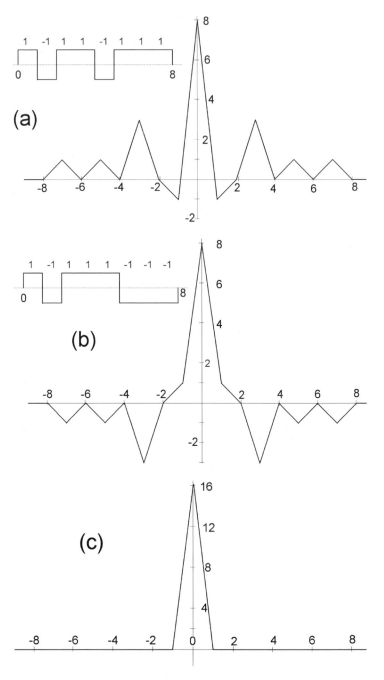

Figure 8.22 Properties of an 8-bit Golay code pair. (a) Binary code and its autocorrelation function. (b) Complementary code and its autocorrelation function. (c) Sum of the autocorrelation functions shown in (a) and (b).

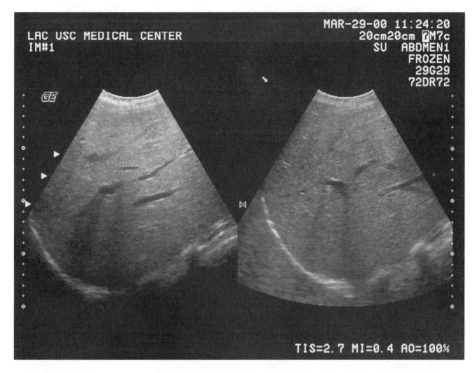

LAC USC MEDICAL CENTER
IM#1

MAR-29-00 11:24:20
20cm20cm ⁊M7c
SU   ABDMEN1
FROZEN
29G29
72DR72

GE

M

TIS=2. 7 MI=0. 4 AO=100%

Figure 8.23 Comparison of two B-mode images of liver to show the effects of coded excitation on the image quality. The right image shows that ~7MHz resolution is maintained down to a penetration depth of 20 cm. The vertical markers are separated by 1 cm and *MI* = 0.4. (From GE Medical Systems website.)

is based on the inventions disclosed in the patents[8] of Chiao and Thomas [77,78]. In these patents it is pointed out that in regions closer to the transducer, the SNR that can be achieved using conventional methods is quite adequate. At greater depths, which entail the use of larger apertures, but the same *f*-number, the code distortion due to the effects of dynamic focusing and nonlinear distortion is less. Thus, in the shallower regions the Golay code is not used, while the deeper regions benefit from the lower SNR associated with coded excitation. The need for a multiplicity of focal zones and two transmissions for Golay code compression may necessitate a reduction in frame rate. Moreover, the degrading effects of tissue movement make it necessary to ensure that the region being imaged is relatively stationary.

8.4.4 Imaging Blood Flow

Because the scattering from disaggregated blood is very weak, perhaps –30 dB below that from soft tissue, the regions of blood flow in a B-mode imaging

8. Both patents are assigned to General Electric (US).

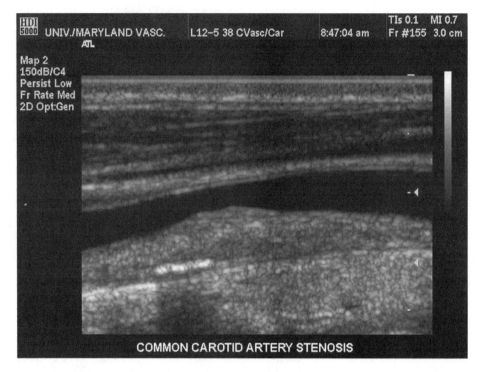

Figure 8.24 Image of a partially stenosed common carotid artery showing that the scattering from the blood flow region is very small compared to that from tissue. Also to be noted are the variations in the acoustic properties from within the heterogeneous plaque. (Reproduced from Philips/ATL ultrasonic image website.)

system will normally be displayed as a uniform black zone. This is illustrated in Fig. 8.24, which shows a section of a common carotid artery with a stenosis. To detect and display the backscattering from a blood vessel, two things must be provided. First, it is necessary to enhance the sensitivity (increase the SNR) so that the very weak backscattered signal can be measured, and second, some form of equalization filter is needed so that the backscattering from the tissue and blood are sufficiently well equalized for both to be within the main gray-scale region. Such an imaging scheme was developed by GE Medical Systems and has been described in a seven-page technology brochure [79] as well as at a conference [80]. The description given below is based on the brochure.

In the last two subsections it was shown how the SNR could be sufficiently enhanced through the use of pulse compression methods to enable satisfactory imaging of deep lying structures. These same techniques can also be used for obtaining the backscattered information from a region of blood, even though a region with far higher backscattering strength surrounds it. To ensure the signal from the blood is not masked by the range side lobe residue signal from tissue regions, the range side lobe levels must be very low.

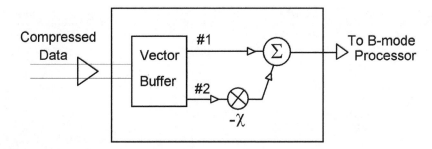

Figure 8.25 Equalization filter that enables the intensities of the moving and stationary regions to be equalized by adjusting the parameter χ. (Based on [79].)

To explain how regions of moving blood can be distinguished from regions that are fixed, it helpful to suppose that the backscattered information is acquired by two successive transmissions along the same path, even though several transmissions (in the case of Golay encoding) may be used. If there is no movement of the interrogated regions between the two transmissions, then, except for the random noise contribution, the content of the two received signals will be identical. On the other hand, if sufficient movement occurs between the two transmission times, the two received signals will differ. Thus, the weak and strong scattering portions of the A-line can be distinguished by the fact that the strong portion is stationary and the weak portion moves.

Consider the schematic shown in Fig. 8.25, in which the two transmissions are temporarily stored in the vector buffer. If the second transmission is multiplied by −1 and added to the first, then the output will consist of those regions that have moved significantly, i.e., stationary regions will be cancelled out except for a very small noise component. As $\chi \rightarrow 0$, the intensity of the moving medium will first approach that of the stationary medium and then reduce to zero. Thus, adjustment of the equalization parameter χ enables the relative intensities of the stationary and flowing regions to be changed, as illustrated in the carotid bifurcation image of Fig. 8.26.

The image intensity variations seen within the blood vessel of Fig. 8.26 can be understood with the help of Fig. 8.27. Consider the backscattered signal produced from within a small element of volume (the sample volume) that contains many red blood cells (RBCs). At low or zero flow velocities, the number and distribution of RBCs within the sample volume will not have sufficient time to change between the first and second transmissions, and consequently the number and distribution of RBCs seen in each transmission will have a high degree of correlation. As a result, the equalization filter will regard the sample volume as being closer to stationary tissue region and will reduce its intensity. As the flow velocity increases, the correlation between the two sample volumes is reduced, causing the filter to increase the image intensity for this sample volume. Because the sample volume axial length is generally less than the lateral or azimuthal dimensions, as the beam to the flow velocity vector angle diminishes, the signal intensity reaches its maximum more rapidly.

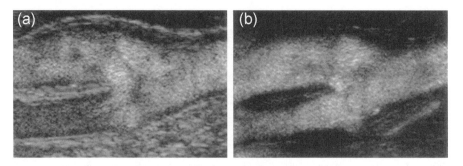

Figure 8.26 The influence of the equalization parameter χ on an image of the carotid bifurcation. In (a) the equalization filter has been adjusted so that the stationary and moving regions have similar gray-scale intensities, i.e., $\chi < 1$. For (b), $\chi = 1$, the stationary tissue background is cancelled out so that only the moving (blood) medium is displayed. (Reproduced, with permission, from GE Medical Systems [79].)

8.5 Synthetic Aperture Systems

Synthetic beamforming and focusing is the process whereby the signals recorded from individual pairs of elements are subsequently used to reconstruct the formation and focusing. It requires that the pulse-echo system obey the rules of linear superposition. The name "synthetic aperture" implies that the response of a larger array aperture is synthetically created from the response produced by smaller array elements. Thus, a basic synthetic aperture system is one that transmits from each element in turn, records the data from all possible transmit/receive combinations, and from all these recordings reconstructs an image of the scattering distribution.

Some of the first practical applications of the underlying ideas were in radar and sonar.[9] The ideas associated with synthetic beamforming and focusing for forming an ultrasound image were first explored in the 1970s [82,83], though it was not until the availability of much more powerful computational systems at reasonable cost that such techniques began to attract considerable attention [81,84–86].

To appreciate the potential value of synthetic aperture systems for generating a B-mode image, it is important to recall the method of conventional image formation. Pulses are transmitted in appropriate directions for scanning an entire area, and the received data from each pulse are collected and processed to produce an image frame. The frame rate, which is of major importance in cardiac imaging, is determined by the number of lines, the number of transmissions required for each line (depends on the number of focal zones used), and the pulse repetition frequency (depends on the imaging depth and

---

9. A useful list of references to the early developments of synthetic aperture systems is given in Karaman et al. [81].

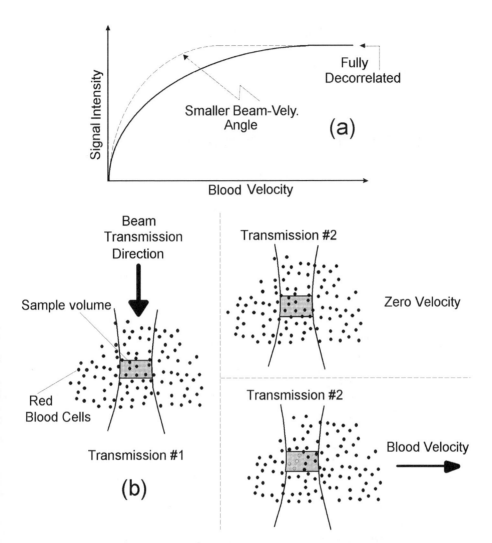

Figure 8.27 The net intensity of the signal from blood depends on its velocity. In (a) the image intensity is sketched as a function of the blood velocity. The saturation value corresponds to the situation where the backscattered signals from two successive sample volumes are uncorrelated. (b) A small sample volume is shown to illustrate that the degree of correlation between successive transmissions depends on the blood velocity. The bottom right picture shows that in the case of a higher blood velocity, new RBCs (unfilled circles) have entered the sample volume and some of the original have moved out. (Reproduced, with permission, from GE Medical Systems [79].)

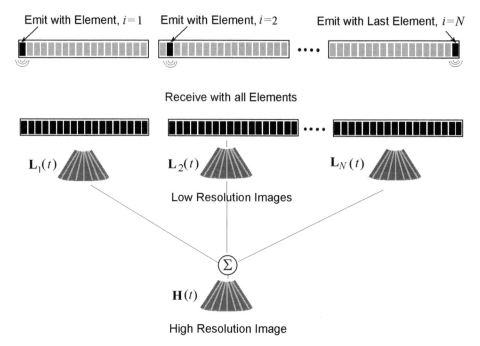

Emit with Element, $i=1$ Emit with Element, $i=2$ Emit with Last Element, $i=N$

Receive with all Elements

$\mathbf{L}_1(t)$ $\mathbf{L}_2(t)$ $\mathbf{L}_N(t)$

Low Resolution Images

Σ

$\mathbf{H}(t)$

High Resolution Image

Figure 8.28 Example of a synthetic aperture scheme in which each array element is used to emit in turn and all receive elements are used to form a rough image. From all such images a high-resolution image can be formed. (Based on a similar sketch by Nikolov and Jensen [87].)

propagation speed). Thus, for example, if the depth of the imaging area is 15 cm and the propagation speed is 1,500 m/s, each line will require 200 μs to receive the scattered data from the most distant point. If 200 lines per frame are needed to achieve adequate lateral resolution, and a single transmit focal zone is assumed, the maximum frame rate will be 25/s. As will be seen, synthetic aperture systems have the potential for high frame rates and economy in their implementation.

Various types of synthetic aperture systems can be conceived. One of the simplest is that illustrated in Fig. 8.28, in which transmission occurs from a single element at a time. If each element is sufficiently small, each emitted wavefront will be nearly spherical and will illuminate the entire region of interest. All receiving elements can be used simultaneously to sense and record the scattered signals, enabling low-resolution images to be formed. These synthesize dynamic focusing on reception, but the transmit wavefront is unfocused. When the data from all such images are summed, dynamic focusing in both transmission and reception is synthesized, yielding a high-resolution image.

Following Nikolov and Jensen [87], but assuming that all N elements are used in both transmission and reception, the high-resolution image-formation process can be conveniently expressed in matrix form. If the ith element transmits, then the lth line in the low-resolution image L_i can be expressed as

(8.17)
$$L_{il}(t) = \sum_{j=1}^{N} a_{lij}(t) r_{ij} [t - \tau_{lij}(t)].$$

In this equation, $a_{lij}(t)$ is the apodization factor for the jth receive element when transmitting from the ith element. In addition, $\tau_{lij}(t)$ is the round-trip delay from the instant of transmission from element i to the current focal point and back to receive element j. This delay is applied to the received RF signal to synthesize the effect of dynamic focusing on reception. Furthermore, $r_{ij}[t]$ denotes the signal received at element j at a time t following the transmission. Thus, a complete low-resolution image can be expressed as

(8.18)
$$\mathbf{L}_i(t) = \begin{bmatrix} L_{i1}(t_0) & L_{i2}(t_0) & \cdots & L_{iS}(t_0) \\ L_{i1}(t_1) & L_{i2}(t_1) & \cdots & L_{iS}(t_1) \\ \cdot & \cdot & \cdots & \cdot \\ \cdot & \cdot & \cdots & \cdot \\ L_{i1}(t_h) & L_{i2}(t_h) & \cdots & L_{iS}(t_h) \end{bmatrix},$$

in which the columns represent a given scan line and the rows represent the samples at a given depth corresponding to times of $t_0, t_1 \ldots t_h$. As noted by Nikolov and Jensen, because focusing is performed only on reception, such an image has a low resolution. The RF signals in each of the N images differ because a different element is used for each transmission. Now each spatial point was treated as a focal point, and as a result, summing all sub-images from the N transmit elements is equivalent to dynamic focusing on transmission, enabling a high-resolution image to be obtained. Such an image is given by

(8.19)
$$\mathbf{H}(t) = \sum_{i=1}^{N} \mathbf{L}_i(t).$$

A 1-D array having N transmit and M receive elements will require N transmissions, and the number of RF lines be stored for future processing will be $N \times M$. Each transmission will cause a diverging wavefront to be generated that passes through the entire imaging plane and which will be scattered by inhomogeneities resulting in RF signals at the receiver element locations. As discussed by Lockwood and Foster [86], a fundamental difference exists between conventional and synthetic aperture systems. In conventional imaging systems, the frame rate can be increased either by decreasing the number of scan lines, resulting in a loss of lateral resolution for the same field of view, or by decreasing the field of view. On the other hand, for a synthetic aperture system whose performance is not limited by computational speed, the frame rate can be increased by simply decreasing the number of transmit elements, i.e., by making it sparse. One example of a synthetic aperture system is the forward-viewing intravascular catheter described in section 8.10.

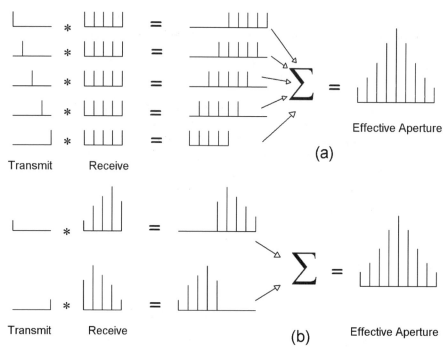

Figure 8.29 Transmit, receive, and effective apertures for a 5-element array. (a) Dense (fully populated) system. (b) A sparse system in which just two transmission elements are used and the five-element receive aperture has a triangular weighting. (Based on a similar drawing in Lockwood and Foster [86].)

A simple example [86] of a synthetic aperture beamforming system is illustrated in Fig. 8.29. The system shown in (a) is a synthetic *transmitting* aperture that uses five transmit/receive elements: each transmit element is fired in turn and the signals received by the five-element aperture are stored. It can be seen that the effective aperture is obtained by summing all the convolutions of the individual transmit elements with the receive aperture. For the sparse arrangement illustrated in (b), which uses the two end elements for transmission, it can be seen that by appropriately weighting the receive aperture, an identical effective aperture can be obtained. This aperture is also identical to that obtained with a five-element aperture conventional imaging system.

An important advantage of a synthetic aperture system is the ability to achieve dynamic focusing both on transmission[10] and reception. As discussed earlier, transmission requires the use of delays that cannot be changed once the elements have been excited, and hence a fixed focal point with a limited

10. A retrospective filtering technique that deconvolves a defocused transmit pattern, given a dynamically focused received image, has been described by Freeman et al. [89]. While this method reduces the effects of a fixed transmission focus, it does so in a retrospective manner and is quite different from the synthetic aperture method.

depth of focus. To improve the overall image quality, multiple transmissions with different focal zones are needed, causing a loss in frame speed. On the other hand, dynamic focusing on both transmission and reception can be achieved in a synthetic aperture system without sacrificing frame speed. A second advantage arises from the need for just a single transmitter and receiver for each firing, thereby simplifying the transmit/receive circuitry. This is particularly significant in designing a catheter-tip intravascular imaging probe (see section 8.10). Here, the size constraints severely limit the number of elements, the number of connecting wires, and the volume occupied by the integrated circuits used for preprocessing [88]. The design for a mechanically scanned sparse synthetic aperture 1-D array for real-time 3-D imaging has been proposed by Lockwood et al. [90]. By incorporating a $\Delta\Sigma$ modulator (see subsection 7.2.1) into this system, Inerfeld et al. [91] estimate that it should be possible to obtain frame rates of up to 1,700/s.

A major potential difficulty with synthetic aperture systems concerns a loss in SNR. By following one of the schemes outlined in Fig. 8.29, it is evident that unless the transmitted power is increased, there will be major loss in SNR associated with transmission from a single element. O'Donnell et al. [88] have pointed out that for an N-element array in which single elements are used for transmission and reception, the electronic noise causes the SNR to be reduced by approximately a factor of $10\log(2N)$. Although the power can be increased, limits are imposed by the onset of nonlinear effects and the mechanical index (MI). Several means have been proposed for overcoming this problem. One involves the use of arrays of defocused transmit elements [81]. Because the delays to each element are chosen so that the focal point is on the opposite side of the transducer array from the image, the power can be increased without exceeding regulatory limits. A second method uses a synthetic transmit aperture composed of a number of elements [78,92]. By using a Hadamard[11] matrix for spatial encoding of the transmission process and its inverse for decoding the received data, the information needed for reconstructing the image information can be obtained.

8.6 Linear and Nonlinear Imaging

Two types of harmonic imaging can be distinguished: one is based on the introduction of a contrast agent, the other on nonlinear wave propagation properties in tissue. Both require the use of fairly high excitation powers. Ultrasound contrast agents approved for clinical use are biocompatible media that can be organ- or tumor-specific and are designed to achieve contrast enhancement in a number of ways. Their nonlinear scattering properties provide a means for generating harmonics that mark their presence and enhance the contrast in the regions where they reside. The resulting imaging process is sometimes called *contrast media harmonic imaging*. On the other hand, for sufficiently

---

11. The elements of a Hadamard matrix are either +1 or −1.

high incident pressure fields, the nonlinear properties of the transmission medium become apparent, causing higher harmonics to be generated that, because of the increased frequency and compact region where they are generated, can enhance the image quality. This second form of imaging is generally called *tissue harmonic imaging*.

8.6.1 Contrast Media Imaging

The use of contrast agents is valuable in a wide range of clinical situations where unenhanced images are limited in quality. Moreover, because of their special properties, they offer the opportunity for obtaining structural or functional information that may be difficult to obtain by alternative noninvasive techniques [93].

Gramiak and Shah [94,95] in 1968 were the first to show that bubbles created by the rapid injection of either indocyanine green (used for measuring cardiac output) or saline were capable of greatly enhancing the contrast in ultrasound M-mode recordings. Some 20 years later, extensive efforts were made [96,97] to develop encapsulated microbubble contrast agents that could be intravenously injected. Such agents must be sufficiently small to pass through the capillary bed of the lungs and have a sufficiently long half-life to enable them to appear in the systemic circulation following intravenous injection.

Two primary approaches have been used to achieve a sufficiently long microbubble half-life: the first was to use a shell that limits the transport of gas from within the shell, the second was to use gas with a high molecular weight with reduced diffusivity and solubility. Contrast agents typically consist of gas-filled microbubbles encapsulated in a biodegradable shell with mean diameters in the range from 2 to 6 µm. Encapsulated microbubbles have a very large impedance difference compared to tissue, and consequently they act as highly efficient scatterers and can thereby create greatly increased contrast in the regions where they lodge or flow. However, when the ratio of blood to tissue volume is small, the contrast enhancement that can be achieved with fundamental B-mode imaging can be rather disappointing [98]. For example, the volume ratio for the myocardium is ~10%, enabling only a few dB's of enhancement to be obtained at the contrast agent concentrations used clinically.[12] Moreover, when the incident intensity is increased to obtain improved contrast, bubble destruction can occur, causing the scattered signal enhancement to be of a temporary nature [99]. Thus, the behavior of contrast agents is complex and depends on the nature of the suspending medium, the acoustic pressure, and the characteristics of the shell [100–102]. The relation between the mechanical index and its effects on the bubble response is approximately represented in Fig. 8.30. It is also important to recognize that microbubbles have a resonant frequency and consequently can be expected to have a very strong response when this coincides with the pulse center frequency. More-

---

12. In such situations harmonic B-mode imaging, which makes use of the nonlinear characteristics of the contrast agent (see subsection 8.6.1), has important advantages.

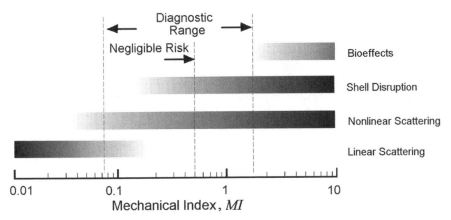

Figure 8.30 The approximate acoustic response of contrast agents for ultrasound imaging as a function of the mechanical index, which is defined by (8.12). At a center frequency of 4.0 MHz, an *MI* of 1.0 corresponds to a peak negative pressure of 2 MPa. Bioeffects have been observed above the *MI* range used diagnostically. (Reproduced with permission from David Hope Simpson [103].)

over, because the expansion and contraction of a microbubble in an applied pressure field are unequal, they can behave in a highly nonlinear manner, generating harmonics, subharmonics, and ultraharmonics.

Bubble Theory

To describe the behavior of a contrast agent bubble in an incident pressure field, such as that produced by a B-mode imaging system, the influence of the shell is sometimes ignored so that the enclosed medium behaves like a free gas bubble in a fluid. Even so, the behavior of a bubble in an incident pressure field is complex. The incident pressure wave causes the bubble to expand and contract, resulting in flow of the surrounding fluid whose viscosity and compressibility influence the behavior. Moreover, the changing pressure in the bubble, along with its changing surface area, causes diffusion of gas into or out of the surrounding fluid, and this can result in a net growth in the bubble size over several cycles, a phenomenon known as *rectified diffusion*. Proper accounting for these and other effects is difficult.

If the effects of gas diffusion can be ignored, then the Rayleigh-Plesset equation provides a reasonably accurate description of the dynamics. For a bubble whose initial radius is R_o subjected to a pressure field $p(t)$, the instantaneous radius $R(t)$ is given by [104, pp. 302–306]

$$
\rho_o R \frac{\partial^2 R}{\partial t^2} + \frac{3\rho_o}{2}\left(\frac{\partial R}{\partial t}\right)^2 = \left(p_o + \frac{2\sigma}{R_o} - p_v\right)\left(\frac{R_o}{R}\right)^{3\varsigma} - p(t) - \frac{4\mu}{R}\frac{\partial R}{\partial t}
$$
$$
(8.20) \qquad\qquad\qquad\qquad - \left(p_o + \frac{2\sigma}{R_o} - p_v\right),
$$

where ζ is the polytropic exponent varying between 1.0 for the isothermal case and γ (ratio of specific heats) for the adiabatic case, σ is the liquid-vapor surface tension, ρ_o is the fluid density, p_o is the hydrostatic pressure in the liquid, p_v is the vapor pressure within the bubble, and μ is the shear viscosity.

For small sinusoidal excitation amplitudes, i.e., $p(t) = P_o\cos(\omega t)$, and negligible vapor pressure and viscosity, the microbubble angular resonant frequency can be found from (8.20) as [104, p. 306]

(8.21)
$$\omega_o = \frac{1}{R_o}\sqrt{\frac{3\zeta}{\rho_o}\left(p_o + \frac{2\sigma}{R_o}\right) - \frac{2\sigma}{R_o}} \; .$$

As can be seen from Fig. 8.31, the resonant frequency increases rapidly with decreasing radius. With increasing excitation amplitude, nonlinear effects become significant: in particular, the resonant frequency diminishes and the bubble boundary generates harmonics.

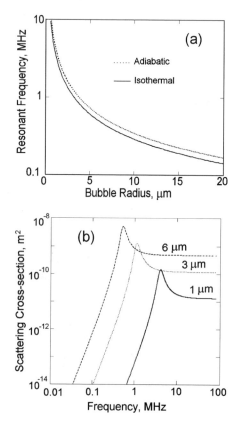

Figure 8.31 Microbubble characteristics. (a) Resonant frequency as calculated from (8.21) for a bubble in water at atmospheric pressure. (b) Scattering cross-section calculated using (8.22) for three ideal bubbles of differing radii and a damping constant of $b = 0.1$.

Anderson and Hampton [105] give the approximate small signal scattering cross-section as

$$(8.22) \qquad \sigma_s = \frac{4\pi R_o^2}{\left(\omega_o^2/\omega^2 - 1\right)^2 + \left(\omega_o^4/\omega^4\right)b^2} \approx \frac{4\pi R_o^2}{\left(\omega_o^2/\omega^2 - 1\right)^2 + \left(\omega_o^4/\omega^4\right)k^2 R_o^2},$$

where b is a damping constant and the second form is for a bubble with no damping. Fig. 8.31b shows that close to resonance the scattering cross-section increases well beyond the bubble cross-sectional area and for $\omega \gg \omega_o$ reaches a value that is close to four times higher.

As the bubble oscillates under the influence of the incident pressure field, it emits radiation [106]. The effect of increasing incident pressure is illustrated in Fig. 8.32, where the incident pressure field is taken to be a pulse similar to that used in a B-mode imaging system [107]. As shown in (a), the −6 dB bandwidth is roughly 40% of the 3 MHz center frequency. In (b) two columns are shown: the percentage change in radius with time and the pressure produced by the oscillating bubble at a distance of 40 mm from the bubble. In fact, the radius waveform enables the radial velocity of the bubble radius (identical to the particle velocity) to be determined, and this enables the pressure to be predicted. The center frequency of 3 MHz is greater than the resonant frequency of a 3.0 μm bubble (1.3 MHz), considerably less than that for a 0.6-μm bubble (9.1 MHz), and close to that for a 1.5 μm bubble (2.9 MHz). For low-level excitation (i and ii), both the percentage radius change and the radiated pressure waveforms for the 0.3 μm and 3.0 μm bubbles are very similar to the transmitted waveform. On the other hand, for the resonant bubble size, the waveform shows considerable ring-down (see iii). When the incident peak pressure is increased to 100 kPa (see iv), radial oscillations become highly nonlinear, and the radiated pressure predicted at 40 mm from the bubble indicates that an appreciable portion of the energy is radiated at harmonic frequencies.

A number of papers have described the radiated spectrum from a bubble for various excitation pressures. For example, using the Rayleigh-Plesset equation, Lauterborn [108], Eatock et al. [109], and de Jong et al. [110] have numerically predicted the spectrum produced for CW and pulse excitation. An example[13] is illustrated in Fig. 8.33a, which shows the spectrum radiated by a 1.5-μm-radius bubble when the amplitude is increased from 5 kPa to 100 kPa. Although the fundamental remains essentially the same, the second harmonic amplitude increases to within 12 dB of the fundamental.

The presence of a surface layer that surrounds the bubble can have a very significant effect on the behavior, depending on its thickness and elastic properties. Based on the assumption that the layer is an incompressible solid elastic material whose properties include viscous damping, Church [100] has derived an equation that describes the dynamic behavior. It is of the same form as the

---

13. I am grateful to Chien Ting Chin for providing the data that enabled the plots to be made and wish to acknowledge the help his PhD thesis provided in preparing this subsection.

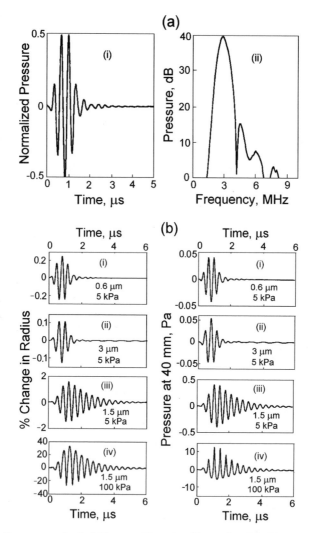

Figure 8.32 Response of a bubble to a Gaussian-like pulse. (a) Characteristics of the transmitted pulse assumed for the simulations. (b) Fractional change in radius and pressure waveform produced at 40 mm by bubbles of differing radii. (Reprinted by permission of Elsevier from Chin and Burns [107], *Ultrasound Med. Biol.*, 26, 1293–1300, © 2000 World Federation of Ultrasound in Medicine and Biology.)

Rayleigh-Plesset equation, as given by (8.20), but it includes terms that are governed by the properties of the encapsulating layer thickness, density, rigidity, and viscosity. As illustrated in Fig. 8.34, the scattering cross-sections are highly dependent on the presence of a shell and changes in viscous damping. For a cloud of bubbles, Church also examined the frequency dependence of the speed of sound, attenuation, and total scattering cross-section.

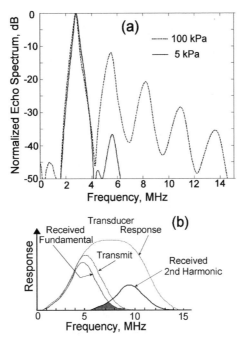

Figure 8.33 Contrast media harmonic imaging. (a) Harmonic generation by a bubble with an initial radius of 1.5 μm excited by the pulse shown in Fig. 8.32a for small (5 kPa) and large (100 kPa) excitations. The two plots correspond to the two waveforms (iii) and (iv) shown on the RHS of Fig. 8.32b. Both spectra have been normalized to the peak fundamental component, which are almost identical.[13] (b) Sketch showing the overall transducer frequency response, the transmitted spectrum, and the received fundamental and second harmonic components. The shaded portion indicates the overlap.

Harmonic Imaging

The ideas associated with the development of contrast media harmonic imaging can be traced back to the proposals of Tucker and Welsby [111]. Work first reported by others in 1968 showed that gas bubbles generated during decompression of deep-sea divers could be detected by Doppler ultrasound. That same year, Tucker and Welsby suggested that the detectability of small bubbles should be significantly enhanced by looking at the second harmonic emission of bubbles excited at close to their resonant frequency. Some 13 years later, Miller [112] described the advantages of second harmonic emission measurements for counting resonant bubbles. Subsequent to this, Schrope et al. [113,114] demonstrated theoretically as well as through in vitro and in vivo measurements the advantages of using the second harmonic produced by an excited contrast agent for pulse wave flow estimation in small vessels. At approximately the same time (1992), Burns et al. [115] presented the first in vitro demonstration of contrast agent harmonic imaging using a modified

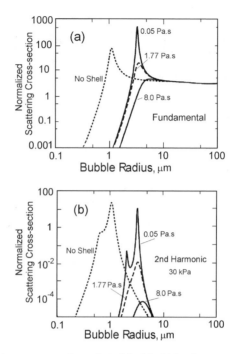

Figure 8.34 Scattering cross-section of air-filled bubbles in water at a driving frequency of 3.5 MHz. It was assumed that the shell had a thickness of 15 nm, a rigidity modulus of 88.8 MPa, and the viscosity values indicated. Computed cross-section variations with the bubble radii for (a) the fundamental and (b) second harmonic (30-kPa driving pressure). The maximum cross-sectional area of the bubble was used for normalization. (Reproduced, with permission, from Church [100], *J. Acoust. Soc. Am.*, 97, 1510–1521, © 1995 Acoustical Society of America.)

imaging system that transmitted at a center frequency of 4 MHz and received at frequencies of around 8 MHz. Subsequent clinical use [96] with improved contrast agents demonstrated the advantages and limitations.

Depending on their fabrication and ingredients, microbubble contrast agent lifetimes can range from seconds to many minutes. With fundamental imaging, the range of times over which the image can be formed is quite limited, as indicated in Fig. 8.35. But with harmonic imaging, the decreased tissue clutter signal enables the detection threshold to be greatly reduced, allowing far longer image-formation times [116].

For a transmit spectrum of the form sketched in Fig. 8.33b and sufficient intensity, scattering from regions containing the contrast medium will cause the received signal to contain both the fundamental and a second harmonic component. For wideband excitation, the broad distribution of bubble sizes will cause a fairly wide harmonic spectrum, especially for peak amplitudes corresponding to those typically used in diagnostic imaging, e.g., 1 MPa. However, because shell disruption occurs with increasing acoustic pressure [99,102],

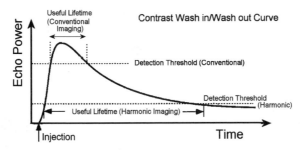

Figure 8.35 Effects of the contrast agent lifetime on conventional and harmonic contrast imaging. The agent is assumed to be injected as a bolus. (Reproduced, with kind permission of Springer Science and Business Media, from Powers et al. [116], Chapter 8 in *Advances in Echo Imaging Using Contrast Echo Enhancement*, © 1997 Kluwer Academic Publishers.)

improvements in the second harmonic response by increasing the transmit pulse intensity may be limited.

The presence of the second harmonic component is the signature that in principle enables the presence of the contrast medium to be distinguished from tissue scattering, the latter being at the fundamental frequency. The effect of using harmonic imaging on the contrast is illustrated schematically in Fig. 8.36, where darker regions correspond to less scattering and light regions to strong scattering. Assuming that the contrast medium is present only in the blood vessel, the second harmonic image (c) will show little or no scattering from the tissue and very strong scattering from the blood vessel.

The transducer must have a considerably greater bandwidth for harmonic imaging. Filtering of the RF signal is generally used to extract the harmonic component whose spectrum may overlap the fundamental, as shown in Fig. 8.33b. Issues concerning the design of matched filters to optimize the contrast agent to tissue response have been discussed by Simpson et al. [117]. Moreover, Powers et al. [116] have provided an excellent discussion of the issues concerning the system design. Reducing the transmitted bandwidth diminishes the overlap but also causes a loss in axial resolution. At higher transmitted intensities, scattering of the tissue-generated harmonics may partially mask the harmonic signal produced by contrast bubbles. One method proposed for reducing its effects is based on transmitting a signal at the second harmonic frequency in the absence of a contrast agent and then using the received signal to cancel out the received second harmonic tissue signal that is produced when the contrast agent is present [118]. An alternative approach, as described below, is to use subharmonic imaging.

Subharmonic Imaging

When encapsulated gas bubbles are excited at higher pressures, in addition to the harmonics $(2f, 4f\ldots)$, subharmonics $(f/2)$ and ultraharmonics $(3f/2, 5f/2$

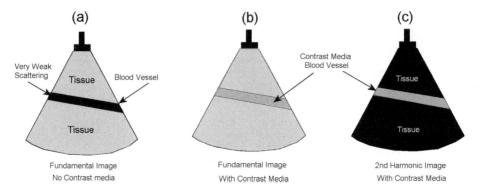

Figure 8.36 Contrast media harmonic imaging. (a) Standard B-mode image. (b) B-mode image using fundamental scattering signal from tissue and from contrast agent in blood vessel. (c) Second harmonic image showing strong contrast: the blood vessel produces a strong scattering signal, the tissue a much smaller one.

...) can be produced [104,119]. Investigations [120] of the subharmonic generation properties of certain contrast agents approved for clinical use, e.g., Optison, have shown that for bubbles with a resonant frequency of f_o, the threshold for generating subharmonics is minimized when the excitation frequency is at $2f_o$, i.e., the subharmonic is at f_o. Moreover, it is found that the subharmonic component undergoes a fairly rapid increase in the intermediate incident pressure range, i.e., 0.5–1 MPa, as compared to lower and higher pressures. Given the right excitation conditions, it has been reported that certain types of contrast agents can generate more subharmonic power than that generated at the second harmonic frequency.

Because subharmonics do not appear to be generated by nonlinear propagation in tissue, for imaging applications, subharmonic scattering should avoid the reduced blood-to-tissue contrast that can occur in harmonic imaging. This idea appears to have been first reported by Shi et al. [121] in 1997 and subsequently implemented [122,123]. Some potential advantages and disadvantages of this contrast imaging mode have been considered by Shankar et al. [124]. They point out that although the resolution may be less than that achieved with harmonic imaging, it should be no more so than with conventional imaging at a frequency of $2f_o$. Moreover, because the subharmonic signal suffers less attenuation than either the fundamental or the second harmonic, the imaging depth should be improved.

Perfusion Measurement and Imaging

A noted earlier, the shells of microbubble contrast agents can be disrupted when the incident pressure pulse (or a succession of pulses) has sufficient intensity and duration. For certain agents, a catastrophic disruption of the shell occurs, causing the gas inside to be very rapidly ejected. The sudden localized pressure change produces a wideband acoustic signal that can be readily detected. This stimulated acoustic emission mode [125,126] offers opportunities for blood perfusion[14] imaging and measurements.

Measurement of the flow into an organ is a challenging task, especially if the flow is pulsatile. A very important application is for myocardial blood flow imaging, whose objective is to determine the adequacy or otherwise of flow to certain regions. A widely used method for myocardial stress testing requires the intravenous injection of a short-lived radioactive isotope (e.g., Tc99m with a half-life of 6.03 hours, emitting gamma-2 rays with a mean energy of 140.5 eV). A tomographic detection technique SPECT (single photon emission computed topography) can be used to obtain the perfusion image pattern in fairly thin (~5 mm) myocardial slices. The disadvantage of using radioactive isotopes and the expense of complex nuclear imaging equipment makes the use of contrast-based ultrasound methods a rather attractive possibility. In 1998 Wei et al. [127] described and demonstrated a scheme that used high *MI* ultrasound for sudden microbubble destruction and B-mode harmonic imaging for subsequent microbubble concentration measurements. Harmonic power contrast flow imaging (see subsection 10.10.4) was subsequently used for the purpose of detecting coronary artery stenosis by measuring the transient changes associated with bubble destruction in the myocardium [128].

Suppose that the concentration of microbubbles in an organ is allowed to reach a steady state during a steady intravenous infusion. If the concentration is suddenly reduced to zero by performing a high *MI* scan over the region of interest (see Fig. 8.37), the perfusion will cause the contrast agent concentration to eventually return to its earlier state. It is reasonable to expect that the normalized microbubble image intensity can be characterized by $A[1 - \exp(-t/\tau)]$, where τ is a time constant. Wei et al. [127] showed experimentally that A/τ and $1/\tau$ are proportional to the perfusion rate. Thus, by performing low *MI* imaging scans, subtracting the background, integrating each scan to determine the average backscattered intensity, and fitting the results to an exponential, τ can be estimated. However, to find the actual perfusion rate from this requires additional information concerning the imaging slice thickness and the relation between the intensity and the microbubble concentration.

Multipulse Transmission Methods

Several methods have been proposed and used to overcome the limitations on the contrast and resolution imposed by the spectral overlap seen in Fig. 8.33b. In the *pulse inversion* detection scheme [129–131] illustrated in Fig. 8.38a, two transmission pulses are used, the second being an inverted copy of the first. If we suppose that the first transmitted pressure pulse is denoted by $p_1(t)$, then the second will be $p_2(t) = -p_1(t - T)$, where T is the pulse interval. Let us suppose that both pulses are scattered by a bubble at a fixed depth z, corresponding to a transit time of $\tau = 2z/c_o$, so that the echoes can be denoted

---

14. The blood perfusion of a volume of tissue is defined as the volume of blood per unit time that flows through the microvessels.

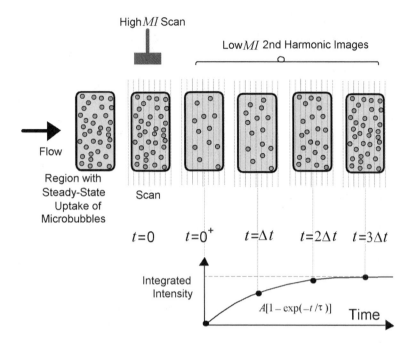

Figure 8.37 Sketch illustrating the principle used to determine the relative volumetric perfusion of blood into a tissue region. Following the start of a continuous contrast agent injection, this region (represented by the rectangle) is allowed to reach a steady-state microbubble concentration. A high MI frame is then used to fragment the bubbles and subsequent low MI images are used to plot the change in the intensity (integrated over each area) with time. The concentration of microbubbles, following their extinction, can approximately be represented by an exponential. After subtracting the background from each image and then by fitting an exponential to the integrated intensity curve, the characteristic time-constant τ and the saturation intensity A can be determined.

by $p_{1e}(t - \tau)$, $p_{2e}(t - T - \tau)$. To gain a physical understanding of the process, we shall assume that the returned echo can be written as a power series expansion of the incident pulse pressure, i.e.,

$$p_{1e}(t - \tau) = \sum_{n=1}^{\infty} a_n p_1^n(t - \tau) \text{ and } p_{2e}(t - T - \tau) = \sum_{n=1}^{\infty} a_n p_2^n(t - T - \tau),$$

where the a_n's depend on the scattering properties of the bubble (for a linear scattering process $a_n = 0$ when $n > 1$). If we form the sum of the received pressures (time-shifted by T), then, because the odd terms cancel out,

$$p_{1e}(t - \tau) + p_{2e}(t - \tau) = 2 \sum_{n=1}^{\infty} a_{2n} p_1^{2n}(t - \tau) ,$$

and for the difference, the even terms cancel, i.e.,

$$p_{1e}(t-\tau) - p_{2e}(t-\tau) = 2\sum_{n=1}^{\infty} a_{2n-1}p_1^{2n-1}(t-\tau) .$$

As an example, we take $a_1 = 1$, $a_2 = 0.4$, $a_3 = 0.1$, $a_4 = 0.05$, $a_n = 0$ for $n > 4$, and assume a Gaussian transmit pulse. Although several simplifying approximations have been made, it will be noted from Fig. 8.38a that the fundamental component has been eliminated from the sum. However, movement of the contrast medium between transmissions will degrade the result.

Jiang et al. [132] have considered an alternative approach, the scaling or *power modulation* method, and have compared its performance to the inversion technique. As illustrated in Fig. 8.38b, the two waveforms are identical except that the second pulse is a scaled version of the first. Consequently, if the scaling factor is denoted by k, the echo from the second pulse can be written as

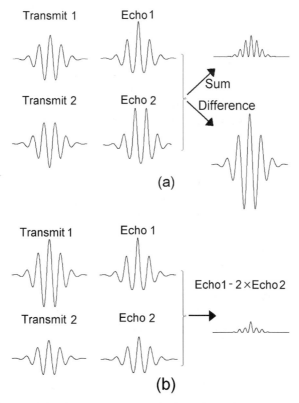

Figure 8.38 Methods for improving harmonic detection using two transmissions of a Gaussian pulse. Note that the bubble echoes have not been accurately calculated. (a) Pulse inversion technique [129–131]. (b) Scaling scheme [132] in which a scaling factor (k) of 2 has been assumed.

$$p_{2e}(t - T - \tau) = \sum_{n=1}^{\infty} a_n \frac{p_1^n(t - T - \tau)}{k^n}.$$

Taking the product of the second echo with k and then subtracting this from the first echo, we obtain

$$p_{1e}(t - \tau) - kp_{2e}(t - \tau) = \sum_{n=2}^{\infty} \frac{a_n p_1^n(t - \tau)}{k^{n-1}},$$

which is independent of a_1, though it does depends on $a_2, a_3, \ldots$ Because of the reduced size of the second signal, it is reasonable to expect that the SNR of the scaling method will be inferior to the inversion technique, as noted by Jiang et al.

8.6.2 Tissue Harmonic Imaging

The idea of using the nonlinearity of a medium to generate harmonics of the incident field can be traced back to the work of Kompfner and Lemons [133] in 1976. They described a transmission scanning acoustic microscope with a fundamental frequency of around 400 MHz that was capable of generating second harmonic images at 800 MHz. Using a ~5 μm thick specimen of a mouse larynx, they obtained transmission images demonstrating that second harmonic images had improved resolution. They noted that these harmonic images were generated in the region of the beam focus and differed somewhat from linear transmission images that they also made at 800 MHz. Shortly thereafter, Muir [134] described an underwater harmonic imaging system that used an approach very similar to that of subsequent diagnostic systems. The sonar system illustrated in Fig. 8.39a used a $100 \times 10 \, cm^2$ transducer operating at a fundamental frequency of 100 kHz, emitting 200 μs CW pulses at a pulse power of 1.3 kW. The bandpass filters enabled images to be constructed from the fundamental up to the fifth harmonic. For targets between 50 and 200 m from the source, the images of a floating barge shown in (b) clearly demonstrate improved angular resolution. Specifically, the measured beam profile showed improvement in the −6 dB resolution from 0.8 to 0.5 degrees in going from the fundamental to the second harmonic.

Proposals for using tissue harmonic imaging to improve the quality of ultrasound diagnostic systems were first described at a 1995 conference by Ward et al. [135], fuller details being presented early in 1997 [136]. At the same time, Christopher [137], who may have been unaware of Muir's earlier sonar paper and the conference presentation of Ward et al., also presented proposals, though no images were shown until his subsequent paper [143]. In late 1997 Averkiou et al. [138] presented the first in vivo harmonic images. Since then, a number of papers [139–141] have studied the clinical advantages on a qualitative basis and found significant advantages in terms of penetration, increased contrast resolution, improved side lobe suppression, and overall image quality. In addition, computational studies of image formation including simulated tissue images based on the KZK equation using a simple focused disk transducer have been presented by Li and Zagzebski [145]. They also

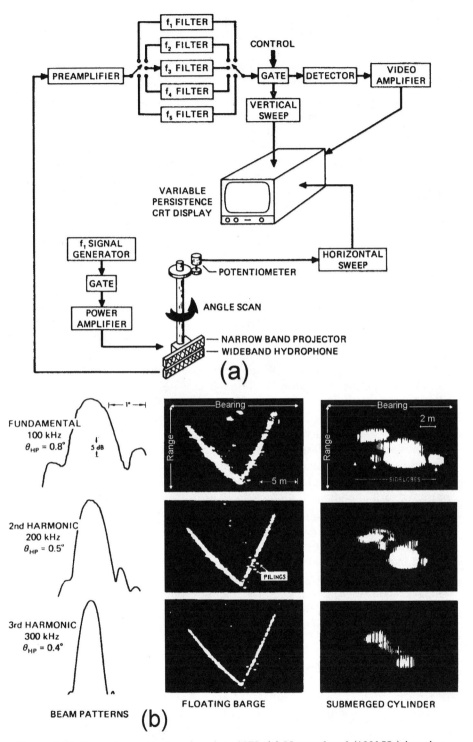

Figure 8.39 Sonar harmonic imaging circa 1979. (a) Narrowband (100 kHz) imaging system for generating images up to the fifth harmonic. (b) Underwater image of a floating barge and a submerged cylinder using the fundamental, second, and third harmonics. The pilings are about 15 cm in diameter. Also shown are the measured beam patterns. (Reproduced, with kind permission of Springer Science and Business Media, from Muir [134], Vol. 9 of *Acoustical Imaging*, Plenum Press, © 1980 Kluwer Academic Publishers.)

demonstrated small improvements to the image quality by using the pulse inversion (two-pulse) technique [130,131] discussed earlier in this section.

An important issue to consider is whether a harmonic imaging system can offer improved performance over a conventional system that operates at twice the fundamental frequency of the harmonic system. For the harmonic system, the harmonic amplitudes become greatest in the regions of high intensity, i.e., close to the focal point. Because of the frequency-dependent attenuation, a conventional system operating at twice the fundamental frequency of the harmonic system, i.e., $2f_0$, would require increased transmitted pulse energy to achieve the same scattered signal strength. But because the second harmonic is typically 10 dB below the fundamental, there may be little or no net gain in efficacy. Further issues concern the resolution and side lobe levels. As noted in Chapter 4 (Fig. 4.11), the side lobes in the lateral response of the harmonics fall off more rapidly than the fundamental, and as a result it can be expected that image haze due to side lobes should be reduced. On the other hand, the lateral resolution may be somewhat worse than that of a conventional $2f_0$ system. To help answer some of these questions, the lateral and elevation responses of a 64-element phased array, when excited at 2 and 4 MHz, are compared in Fig. 8.40. It can be seen that for 4 MHz excitation at low amplitudes, the fundamental response has a narrower main lobe but much higher side lobes.

Maps of the azimuthal and elevational fields for CW excitation of a 64-element phased array are shown in Fig. 8.41 [142]. The calculations were performed using an operator splitting approach (see subsection 4.10.1) that used incremental steps of diffraction, attenuation, and nonlinear propagation. An angular spectrum algorithm was used to calculate the effects of diffraction and attenuation, and a frequency-domain solution to Burgers' equation was used for nonlinear propagation. The calculations assumed a focal distance of 10 cm in the azimuthal plane and no focusing lens in the elevation plane. Some features that have previously been mentioned in Chapter 4 should be noted. For example, in (a) and (c) it can be seen that the peak response occurs at a location somewhat prior to the azimuthal focus. In addition, it can be seen that the second harmonic contains substantially lower side lobes.

The effect of lower side lobes is evident in the clinical images shown in Fig. 8.42. Also contributing to the improvement may be the reduced effects of distortion caused by inhomogeneities in the surface layer [137,144] and reduced reverberation effects [144].

8.7 Ultrasound Computed Tomography

In x-ray computed tomography[15] (CT) as originally developed,[16] an image of the attenuation coefficient distribution in a slice was reconstructed from a

---

15. The word "tomography" is in part derived from the Greek word *tomos*, meaning slice or section.

16. The development of x-ray CT originated with the work of Cormack published in 1963 and 1964 and the work of Hounsfield, who independently developed the first practical CT system for medical use in 1972. Cormack and Hounsfield were jointly awarded the 1979 Nobel Prize in Medicine.

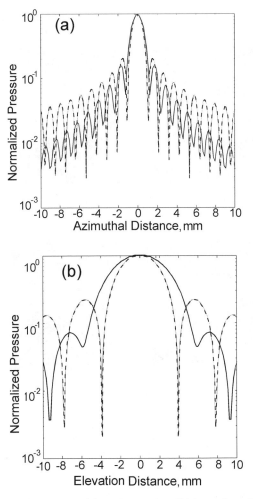

Figure 8.40 Computed azimuthal (a) and elevation (b) lateral profiles of a CW excited 64-element phased array with no elevation lens in a tissue-like medium. Solid lines are the nonlinear second harmonic profiles when excited at 2 MHz with a source pressure amplitude of 347 kPa. Dashed curves are the profiles in the absence of any nonlinear propagation when excited at 4.0 MHz. Note that the harmonic profiles have a wider main lobe than that for the higher-frequency source, but much lower side lobes. For both excitation frequencies the azimuthal focusing was at $z = 10$ cm and the 64-element had the following dimensions: $H = 10$ mm, $W = 375$ μm, inter-element gap = 93.8 μm. The tissue was assumed to be characterized by $c_o = 1550$ m/s, $\rho_o = 1050$ kg/m^3, $n = 1.1$, $\beta = 5$, and $\alpha_o = 3$ dB/(cm × MHz$^{1.1}$). (Reproduced, with permission, from Zemp et al. [142], *J. Acoust. Soc. Am.*, 113, 139–152, © 2003 Acoustical Society of America.)

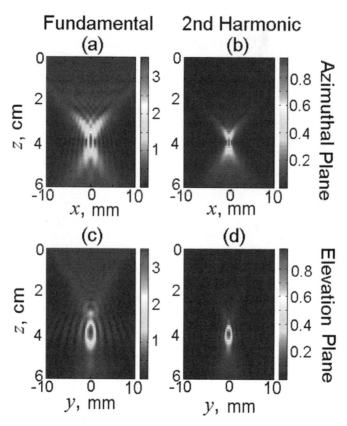

Figure 8.41 Computed transmit profiles for nonlinear propagation in a liver-like medium from a linear phased array excited with a 2-MHz CW signal. Fundamental and second harmonic profiles in: (a), (b) azimuthal plane and (c), (d) elevation plane. The array had 64 elements, each with a height of 20 mm, width of $\lambda/2$, and spacing of $\lambda/4$, giving a total length ≈ 3.7 cm. Focusing in both the azimuthal and elevation directions was at a depth of 4 cm. The properties of the medium are the same as those listed Fig. 8.40. The scale gives the pressure in MPa. The source velocity amplitude was 0.23 m/s (source pressure amplitude $\approx$ 347 kPa). See also color insert. (Reproduced, with permission, from Zemp et al. [142], *J. Acoust. Soc. Am.*, 113, 139–152, © 2003 Acoustical Society of America.)

sequence of transmission measurements. With the enormous success enjoyed by x-ray CT, it was perhaps natural to suggest that it could be used in other medical imaging modalities, including ultrasound. In particular, it was suggested that images of the distribution of the absorption coefficient or the propagation speed distribution throughout the region being examined could be obtained. However, it was soon realized that the use of ultrasound posed certain problems that were not present with x-rays. First, refraction causes the

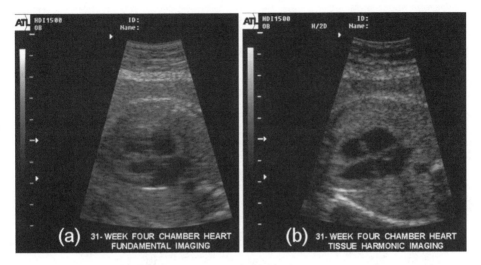

Figure 8.42 Comparison of (a) fundamental and (b) harmonic images of the fetal heart at 31 weeks, showing the four chambers. (Reproduced from Philips Medical Systems website.)

paths of the incident radiation to differ from straight lines. Second, because every object point should be insonated over a wide range of angles to achieve error-free reconstruction, the presence of highly reflecting regions such as bone would cause serious difficulties.

The objective of ultrasound CT is to enable one or more of the intrinsic properties of the medium to be reconstructed from a sequence of experimental measurements. It is an inverse problem of considerable difficulty that seeks to discover the distribution that gives rise to the measurements. In x-ray CT, because of the very small associated wavelengths, the effects of diffraction can be ignored, so that the laws of geometric optics govern the ray paths.[17] In ultrasound CT the wavelengths are no longer small compared to the structures, and as a result diffraction should be accounted for. However, finding an inverse solution is a challenging task, and in most approaches the laws of geometric optics are generally assumed.

8.7.1 Transmission Tomography

The first work concerning the practical development of ultrasound CT was that reported in 1973 by Greenleaf et al. [148], in which they described a

17. Starting from Euler's equation and the continuity equation, which describe the acoustic field in an inhomogeneous medium, Greenleaf [146] has shown that if $\lambda \to 0$ and the density is constant, these equations reduce to the Eikonal (from Greek: εικῶνν = image) equation. As discussed in Born and Wolf [147, pp. 109–113], this is the basic equation of geometric optics.

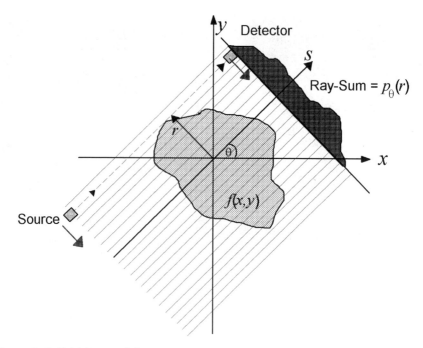

Figure 8.43 Initial part of the process for determining the 2-D property of an object from projections by first performing a sequence of measurements along parallel beam paths to find the ray-sum for a fixed θ.

method for reconstructing the 2-D ultrasound absorption coefficient distribution from a large sequence of projection transmission measurements made at different incident angles. Subsequently, the same group described [149] how the speed distribution could be reconstructed through time-of-flight measurements. Glover and Sharp [150–151] have described development of a system that was used for preliminary clinical tests of the speed distribution and have reported on the results obtained for breast imaging.

As shown in Fig. 8.43, a rectangular coordinate system is assumed to be fixed in the region being measured, and the function $f(x,y)$ specifies the quantity being imaged. For example, $f(x,y)$ could describe how the ultrasound attenuation or the propagation speed is distributed. If the beam path is assumed to be a straight line, then the coordinates r, s, and θ can be used to denote the location, the distance along it, and the angle it makes with respect to the x-axis. Measurement of a property of the beam, such as the amplitude, transit time, or intensity, along each of the paths shown enables a 1-D function to be constructed from the samples. This ray-sum or projection will be denoted by $p_\theta(r)$, in which the subscript indicates that the measurements were made with the beam direction inclined at an angle θ. In fact, $p_\theta(r)$ is the Radon [152, 154, p. 517] transform of $f(x,y)$. It is the line integral of f along the path s, i.e.,

$$\mathcal{R}\{f(x,y)\} = p_\theta(r) = \int_{r,\theta} f(x,y)\,ds \,,$$

where $\mathcal{R}$ is the 2-D Radon transform operator. This equation can be expressed as

$$\mathcal{R}\{f(x,y)\} = \iint_{-\infty}^{\infty} f(x,y)\delta(s - x\cos\theta - y\sin\theta)\,dxdy \,,$$

in which $\delta(.)$ is the Dirac δ-function.

To relate $f(x,y)$ to the attenuation coefficient distribution, we note that

$$I(r) = I_0 e^{-2\int \alpha(x,y)ds} \,,$$

and that $f(x,y) \equiv \alpha(x,y)$. It therefore follows that the ray-sum is related to the normalized transmitted beam intensity by

$$p_\theta(r) = -\frac{1}{2}\ln[I(r)/I_0].$$

If the function $f(x,y)$ is continuous, then an infinite number of projections would be needed to perform an exact reconstruction of the function. In practice, a finite number of equally spaced projections are used over the range from $\theta = 0$ to π. A variety of reconstruction methods have been developed for determining the 2-D distribution function from projection measurements [152,153, 154 Chapter 15]. One of these is based on a fundamental relationship between the Radon transform and the 2-D Fourier transform, which was recognized and illuminated by Bracewell [155, 154 Chapter 14] in relation to the problem of obtaining a map of the microwave emission from the sun's disk. In his classic 1956 paper,[18] Bracewell developed what is now widely referred to as the (2-D) projection-slice theorem, which is used in a variety of fields as the basis for reconstructing a distribution function from projection measurements. In one form it states that the 1-D Fourier transform of the ray-sum at a given angle θ is equal to the 2-D Fourier transform of $f(x,y)$ along a line in the spatial frequency plane that makes the same angle, i.e.,

$$\Im_{1D}\{p_\theta(r)\} = [\Im_{2D}\{f(x,y)\}]_\theta \,.$$

Thus, as illustrated in Fig. 8.44, by taking the Fourier transform of the ray-sum obtained at an angle θ, the set of values on the line that makes an angle of θ with the k_x axis is obtained. By making measurements over 180 degrees the Fourier plane can be fully defined, enabling $f(x,y)$ to be reconstructed from a 2-D inverse Fourier transform:

$$f(x,y) = \Im_{2D}^{-1}[\Im_{1D}\{p(r,\theta)\}].$$

18. Bracewell was not aware of Radon's 1917 paper, whose translated title is "On the determination of certain functions from their integrals along certain manifolds" (a translated copy appears as Appendix A in [156]).

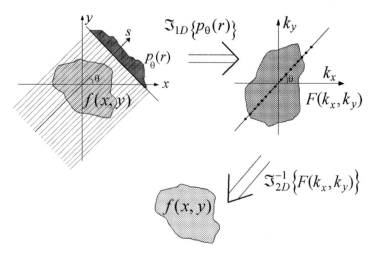

Figure 8.44 The steps involved in reconstructing the function $f(x,y)$ from sets of projections by using the projection-slice theorem. Note that interpolation is needed prior to taking the inverse Fourier transform to determine the spatial frequencies on a rectangular basis.

This final step assumes that the nonrectangular points obtained on the Fourier plane have been interpolated to enable the values to be specified on a rectangular coordinate system.

8.7.2 Pulse-Echo Tomography

Although the primary focus of ultrasound CT has been in transmission measurements, it should be noted that Norton [156–158] proposed methods for tomographic reconstruction from pulse-echo backscattering measurements. As illustrated in Fig. 8.45, he assumed a 2-D distribution of scatterers whose distribution function was to be determined from a sequence of measurements and an appropriate reconstruction technique. The transmit/receive (T/R) transducer element is assumed to launch a cylindrical wave consisting of a short pulse. If the propagation speed is constant throughout the object space, then the backscattered signal at any given time will consist of the contributions from all scatterers that lie on a circle whose radius corresponds to this propagation time. As the wavefront expands, information from the entire object space is generated. By assuming weak scattering and a negligible attenuation, the received signal consists of the line integral of the scattering function over each circle. When the T/R element is located at an angle ϕ on the circle of radius a that encompasses the region, the integral over the circle of radius $R(t)$ shown in (b) can be written as

$$p_\phi(r) = \oint_\phi f(x,y)ds,$$

which can be expressed as

$$p_\phi(R{:}t) = \int\limits_0^\infty \int\limits_0^{2\pi} rf(r,\theta)\delta\left[\sqrt{r^2 + a^2 - 2ar\cos(\theta - \phi)} - R(t)\right]drd\theta.$$

By repeating the measurements over a suitably chosen aperture, Norton showed that sufficient information could be acquired to enable the reconstruction to be performed. Specifically, for the circular aperture geometry shown in Fig. 8.45, Norton [157] found that the above equation can be exactly inverted and that numerical evaluation requires measurements of $p_\phi(R{:}t)$ for a range of ϕ from 0 to 2π. Norton [156] also examined the alternative case in which an omnidirectional T/R element was translated linearly along the boundary of a half-plane containing the 2-D object.

An alternative pulse-echo CT method described by Hiller and Ermert [159] is illustrated in Fig. 8.46. It is based on transmitting a narrow, pencil-like beam. With the object orientated at an angle ϕ, A-mode traces are recorded from a sequence of locations sufficiently closely spaced so that the entire object region is scanned, as could be achieved by using a linear array. Such a set of recordings contains the information that is normally used for displaying a B-mode image. However, in this case integration (averaging) is performed at a constant depth to form the pseudo-projection shown. This bears some similarity to the ray-sum described earlier, but instead of integrating $f(x,y)$ along the beam, it is now performed in a perpendicular direction. This process is repeated for small increments of ϕ over a range from 0 to π. From this set of pseudo-projections $f(x,y)$ can be reconstructed by using, for example, a filtered backprojection algorithm. The additional pulse-echo information gathered by varying ϕ is similar to that obtained in B-mode imaging by using compound scanning. Experimental results using test objects and excised organs were reported by Maderlechner et al. [160].

8.8 Ultrasound Elastography

Palpation is a valuable and traditional qualitative method that is widely used by physicians for detecting abnormalities and enables some of the physical properties of a region to be described. It is also widely used for self-examination of the breast. By applying pressure to a region it is possible from a combination of "feel" and experience to determine the presence of any abnormal structures that might indicate the presence of a tumor. In essence, palpation is a means of assessing the elastic behavior, though its qualitative nature and the inability to access many regions limit its use. For many years ultrasound has been seen as a potential tool to provide such an access, and beginning in the mid-1980s, the possibility of generating 2-D images of the elastic properties was actively explored. Sarvazyan et al. [162] have pointed out that the development of methods for producing elastic images would provide the physician with a "virtual finger," enabling internal regions of the body to be quantitatively assessed. Of particular importance in these developments was

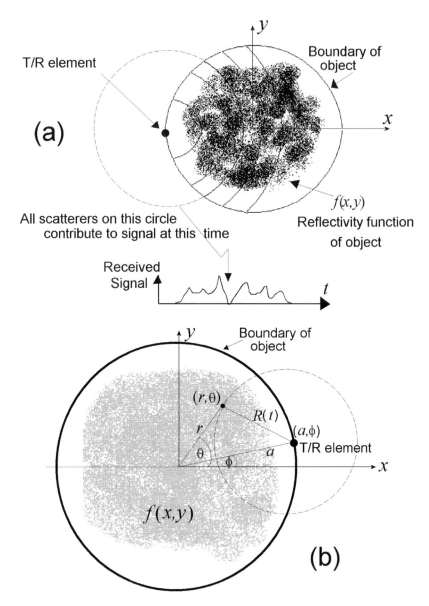

Figure 8.45 Principles of reflection tomography as described by Norton for a 2-D object. A T/R transducer is moved to a sequence of points on the boundary of a circle encompassing the object. The T/R transducer is assumed to transmit a cylindrical wave consisting of a brief pulse. (a) At any given instant of time, the received signal consists of the contributions from all scatterers that lie on a circle whose center is at the T/R element. (b) Assumed geometry in which the T/R element is located at (a,ϕ) and a scatterer is at (r,θ).

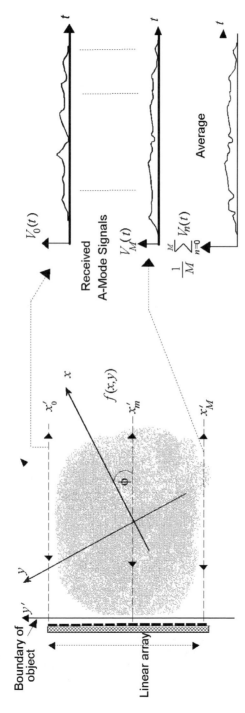

Figure 8.46 A method for using a linear array for acquiring pulse-echo data for CT reconstruction of the function $f(x,y)$.

the earlier work of Wilson and Robinson [163] and Dickenson and Hill [164]. Wilson and Robinson proposed methods of determining the strain and velocity distribution along an A-line caused by aortic pulsations and demonstrated their application for in vivo measurements in the liver. Dickenson and Hill proposed a method for estimating tissue displacement based on cross-correlating successive A-scans. Two reviews[19] [165,168] published in 1996 and one [169] in 1999 provide a good summary of the background leading to these developments and outline the measurement techniques, some of which are discussed below.

Elastography was the name used by Ophir et al. [166] to describe ultrasound methods for visualizing the elastic properties of a medium. Subsequently, when it was realized that several other imaging techniques can also be used (e.g., magnetic resonance [170–173]), it was suggested [165] that elastography is appropriate for all such visualization techniques, and that the more specific name of *sonoelastography* [167] could be used for ultrasound methods.

To obtain a strain image, it is necessary that the region under examination be subjected to a stress and that the resulting strain be measured. Generally speaking, soft tissue is an anisotropic medium that possesses hysteresis, making it very difficult to characterize its behavior from a measurement of the strain distribution. In soft tissue sonoelastography, isotropy and elastic behavior are usually assumed; moreover, because the stress may be non-uniformly distributed and the measured strain may be a single component, not necessarily in the direction of the stress, it may be difficult to deduce the elastic constants. Stress in soft tissue can be generated internally by the periodic expansion and contraction of vessels that normally occur in pulsatile flow. The vessel movement produces a periodic stress in the surrounding tissue regions. Unfortunately, the magnitude and direction of such stresses are not readily determined, making it difficult to estimate the spatial distribution of the elastic properties from a measurement of the strain distribution. A stress can also be generated externally, and this could consist of a quasi-static, a periodic, or transient force. Bercoff et al. [174] have investigated the use of a transient force, produced by a simple electromagnetic vibrator, for breast tumor detection. The system used a two cycle, 60 Hz sinusoid pulse in conjunction with a very high frame rate imaging system (6000 Hz) to obtain a shear modulus map of the medium [175,176].

An alternative method for producing low-frequency vibrations is that based on the radiation force produced by an intense focused ultrasound beam.[20] An equation relating the instantaneous vector force to the acoustic intensity

19. An important source of information is the special issue of *Phys. Med. Biol.* (Vol. 45, June 2000) entitled "Tissue Motion and Elasticity Imaging," guest edited by M.F. Insana and J.C. Bamber. It includes papers involving both ultrasound and magnetic resonance imaging.

20. The effect of viscous losses on the propagation of shear, longitudinal, and coupling waves in soft viscoelastic tissue has been described by Bercoff et al. (*IEEE Trans. Ultrason. Ferroelect. Freq. Contr.*, 51, 1523–1536, 2004). They obtained the Green's function solution to the linearized Navier-Stokes equation. As noted at the beginning of Chapter 2, this problem was previously addressed by Poisson and Stokes.

vector $\mathbf{I}(\mathbf{r}{:}t)$ and to the amplitude attenuation coefficient α of the medium is commonly taken to be given by

$$\mathbf{F}(\mathbf{r}{:}t) = \frac{2\alpha\mathbf{I}(\mathbf{r}{:}t)}{c_o}.$$

Its use for generating low-frequency shear waves was probably first described by Andreev et al. [161]. Subsequently, Sarazyan et al. [162] discussed its application for medical diagnosis. They used a focused ultrasonic source of several MHz that was amplitude-modulated at a frequency in the kHz range, enabling low-frequency shear waves to be generated in the focal zone. Their presence was detected by using either magnetic resonance imaging or a laser-based optical detection method. In the somewhat different scheme discussed by Nightingale et al. [177], several long CW transmissions, e.g., four $28\,\mu s$ pulses in $0.7\,ms$, from a linear array were used to produce a transient radiation force in the focal zone. Using correlation-based tracking they measured in vivo tissue displacements of around $10\,\mu m$. Using a high frame rate B-mode imaging system, Bercoff et al. [178] obtained images of shear wave propagation from the focal zone where the radiation force was created. By using very high frame rate imaging, they also demonstrated shear wave generation by a supersonic source that created quasi-plane shear wavefronts propagating in opposite directions.

An alternative method for generating a localized radiation force is that described by Fatimi and Greenleaf [179,180]. It uses two fairly intense high-frequency ultrasound sources whose frequencies differ by a small amount. In the zone where the two beams overlap, a time-varying radiation force is produced at the difference frequency. The use of this technique was theoretically and experimentally investigated by Konofagou and Hynynen [181] using sources of around $2.27\,MHz$, with difference frequencies in the range of 200 to $800\,Hz$.

The use of ultrasound for measuring the displacement field produced by either an internal or external force requires the presence of scattering structures, such as those due to the cellular nature of tissue that are also responsible for B-mode speckle. It is the changes in the backscattered signal arising from the movement that makes it possible to determine the spatial distribution of displacement. In the case of blood flow, the force is internal and produces a pressure gradient that causes the speckle pattern to change with time. As noted earlier (section 8.2), changes in the location of a particular speckle pattern between successive frames can be used as the basis for estimating the local 2-D velocity field. As illustrated in Fig. 8.47, the displacement of a small area of the speckle pattern can be found by searching in the succeeding B-mode frame for the position of a maximum in the cross-correlation. Repeating this for the entire B-mode area enables the 2-D displacement field to be imaged, enabling the 2-D flow velocity field to be estimated. The basic idea underlying this approach for measuring the soft tissue velocity distribution was reported in 1982 by Dickenson and Hill [164] and by Robinson et al. [184]. It

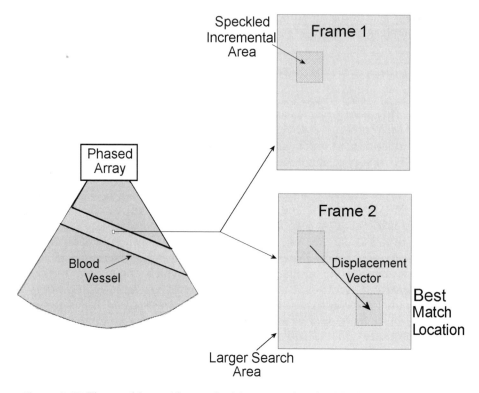

Figure 8.47 The speckle tracking method for measuring the 2-D flow velocity vector in a blood vessel. Two image frames are acquired. A small kernel region is selected, and the best match of this within a larger search region of the second frame enables the displacement vector to be estimated. From this and the time between frames, the velocity vector can be calculated. By repeating this cross-correlation process throughout the vessel, a map of the 2-D velocity profile can be obtained.

was subsequently developed for 1-D and 2-D blood flow velocity mapping [11,12,182,183] as well as for determining tissue displacement [185,188,189], such as for mapping localized movement of the myocardium [186].

By extending these ideas to much higher frequencies, the elastic properties on a microscopic scale can be imaged. Cohn et al. [190–192] have described an elasticity microscope operating in the neighborhood of 50 MHz that enables strain images to be achieved with resolutions of less than 100 μm.

8.8.1 Correlation Methods

A technique based on the using of a quasi-static force and time-domain correlation was developed by Ophir et al. [166]. Fig. 8.48 shows a cross-section of tissue with a force plate on the upper surface. Not shown is a simple pulsed transducer placed at the center of the force plate. In the absence of any force

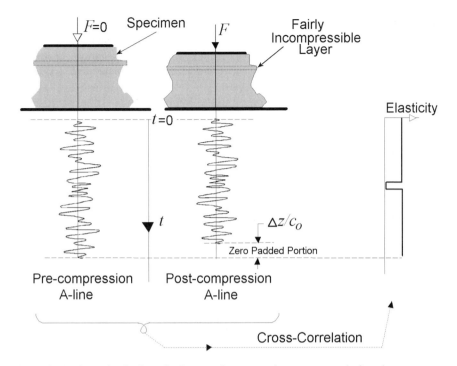

Figure 8.48 A method of producing an elastogram by cross-correlating the pre- and post-compression A-scan lines [166]. For simplicity, a specimen with a fairly incompressible layer is illustrated. It is assumed that a simple pulsed transducer element is embedded in the center (at the arrowhead) of the force plate, and that it produces an ideal pencil-like beam.

other than that needed to make good acoustic contact to the specimen, an A-scan is recorded and digitized; then, following the application of a force, a second A-scan is digitized. Because of the reduction in the path length, the signal duration will be reduced by $2\Delta z/c_o$, where Δz is the reduction in path length. To equalize the number of digital samples of the two A-scan lines, either zero padding or a stretching process can be used on the post-compression signal. The two pairs of lines are then divided into overlapping time segments, and corresponding segments are compared by cross-correlation methods to determine the change in the time of arrival due to the compression. If the time shift for the i'th segment is Δt_i, then the strain in the axial for this segment is given by

$$(8.23) \qquad\qquad s_i = \frac{\Delta t_{i+1} - \Delta t_i}{2\Delta z / c_o}.$$

By repeating the above process for all segments and then duplicating for different lateral transducer positions, a 2-D image of the axial strain can be obtained. Better ways exist for determining the time shift than simply cross-correlating portions of the two (real) RF signals. For example, as discussed by Ledoux et al. [189], performing a cross-correlation of the analytic form of the RF signals improves the accuracy with which the time shift can be estimated. The analytic[21] form of a signal in fact consists of two signals: the first is the original real signal and the second consists of a −90-degree phase-shifted copy of the real RF signal, which can be obtained by means of a Hilbert transform. The results of this method are illustrated in Fig. 8.49, where two analytic signals are shown that could correspond to portions of the pre- and post-compression RF signals from the same location. Calculation of the magnitude of the spatial correlation function accounts for both the real and imaginary parts and results in an improved estimation of the delay.

In practice, problems arise in accurately estimating the strain, and these can be attributed to the presence of a gradient operation in (8.23). Alternative estimation methods have been developed [194] that make use the power

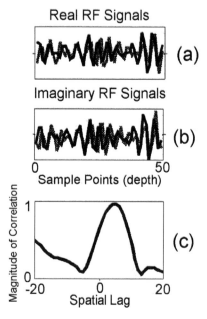

Figure 8.49 Cross-correlation of an analytic signal consisting of real (a) and imaginary (b) parts. Two RF lines are shown that could correspond to the pre- and post-compression signals. (c) The magnitude of the cross-correlation has a well-defined peak, enabling a better estimation of the delay to be made. (Reprinted by permission of Elsevier from Ledoux et al. [189], *Ultrasound Med. Biol.*, 24, 1383–1396, © 1998 World Federation of Ultrasound in Medicine and Biology.)

21. The analytic signal associated with a real signal $x(t) = a(t) \cos[\phi(t)]$, in which $a(t)$ is the instantaneous amplitude, and $\phi(t)$ is the instantaneous phase, can be written as $z(t) = a(t) \exp[j\phi(t)]$. Note that $\text{Re}[z(t)] = a(t) \cos[\phi(t)] = x(t)$ and that $\text{Im}[z(t)] = a(t) \sin[\phi(t)]$. For a careful discussion of the issues surrounding the properties and definitions, see [193].

spectrum, and these, because they make no use of the phase, are incoherent. In essence, power spectrum methods are based on the scaling property of the Fourier transform, whereby compression in the time domain corresponds to expansion in the frequency domain and vice versa. It can be shown that some of these methods are able to estimate the strain in a direct manner without requiring a gradient operation and hence are more immune to the effects of noise. For example, by estimating the power spectrum from a region in the pre- and post-compressed state, it has been shown that a cross-correlation between the two estimates is sensitive to small shifts in the spectra and therefore to the estimation of small strains [195].

From the sketch of Fig. 8.48 it can be seen that compression of the tissue in the axial direction will also cause a lateral strain in off-axis locations unless the tissue is clamped laterally. For in vivo application this would not be practical. A measure of the coupling between the axial and lateral strains is Poisson's ratio (subsection 1.2.2): a value of zero means no coupling and a value of 0.5 implies perfect coupling. Soft tissue is generally considered to be nearly incompressible, with a Poisson's ratio very close to 0.5. Consequently, to estimate the axial strain in response to axial force, it is necessary to correct for the lateral deformation. A procedure for doing this has been described by Konofagou and Ophir [196], who also demonstrated imaging of the lateral displacement (lateral elastogram) in tissue.

In vivo examples of breast B-mode images and elastograms are illustrated in Fig. 8.50 [197]. It should be noted that the apparent transverse diameter of the benign tumor is less than that of the B-mode image, whereas for the malignant tumor the opposite is true. A possible explanation is that the benign tumor is weakly coupled to the surrounding tissue, whereas for the malignant tumor the opposite is true, making the surrounding tissue less compliant and thereby expanding the apparent size.

8.8.2 Pulsed Velocity Estimation Methods

The use of pulsed wave velocity estimation schemes (see Fig. 8.51) for sonoelastography have been described by Yamakoshi et al. [198] and Learner et al. [167,199,200]. The idea of measuring the characteristics of a low-frequency wave as it propagates through tissue has been explored for many years. When a low-frequency periodic force is applied to a tissue specimen, the scatterers present will be displaced in a periodic manner. As described in Chapter 10, the scatterer velocity can be estimated from the change in reception time of the scatterer signature between successive transmissions. If the ultrasound PRF is synchronized to the vibration frequency, the velocity spectrum will consist of symmetric array of discrete harmonic components, each separated from its neighbor by the vibration frequency. As will be shown, the spectral components enable the displacement amplitude to be estimated, enabling an image to be produced that represents the disturbance created by the propagation of the low-frequency wave. It can be expected that any localized nonuniformity in the propagation medium should be evident in such an image.

Sonogram   **Elastogram**

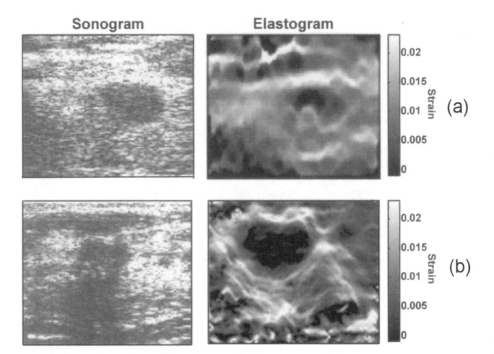

Figure 8.50 In-vivo B-mode and elastogram images. (a) Benign breast tumor (fibroadenoma) and (b) malignant breast tumor (invasive ductal carcinoma). The strain used was approximately 0.01. Note that the darker regions correspond to stiffer regions where there is less strain. In (a) the patient was sitting and the direction of compression was parallel to the body. For (b) the patient was supine and the compression was applied perpendicular to the body. (Reproduced, with permission, from Konofagou et al. [197], *IEEE Trans. Ultrason. Ferroelect. Freq. Contr.*, 48, Frontispiece, © 1997 IEEE.)

The analysis can be simplified by assuming that the vibration angular frequency is ω_L and that the ultrasound beam is aligned with the tissue movement directions so that the insonation angle is zero. Also, the transmitted pulse will be treated as a narrowband signal whose angular center frequency is ω_c. If the tissue displacement at a particular location for a given instant of time is denoted by $\xi(t) = \xi_o \sin(\omega_L t + \phi)$, then its velocity is given by $v(t) = \xi_o \omega_L \cos(\omega_L t + \phi)$. The instantaneous angular center frequency of the slow-time received signal can be obtained by substituting the latter into (10.2) and adding an offset frequency of ω_o, yielding

$$\omega_{PW}(t) = \frac{2\omega_c \zeta_o \omega_L \cos(\omega_L t + \phi)}{c_o} + \omega_o$$

where, to ensure that ω_{PW} is always positive, $\omega_o > 2\omega_c \xi_o \omega_L / c_o$.

Now the normalized slow wave received signal can be written as $X(t) = \sin[\theta(t)]$, where the phase angle is given by

Pulse Wave Velocity Measurement

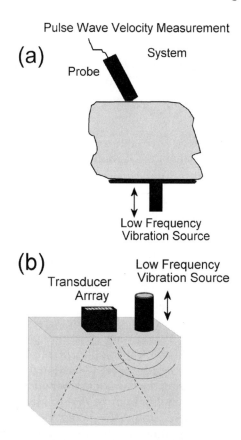

Figure 8.51 Measurement of tissue elastic properties using a low-frequency vibration source. (a) Simplified scheme using a single-element transducer with a pulsed velocity estimation method. (b) Elasticity imaging system using a phased array.

$$\theta(t) = \int_{-\infty}^{t} \omega_{PW}(t)dt = M_f \sin(\omega_L t + \phi) + \omega_o + \varphi,$$

where $M_f = 2\omega_c \xi_o / c_o$ and φ is a constant. Consequently, the slow wave signal can be written as

(8.24) $$X(t) = \sin[\omega_o t + M_f \sin(\omega_L t + \phi) + \varphi].$$

This is identical in form to that of a frequency-modulated wave with a modulation index of M_f. To obtain the spectrum, first expand (8.24) by using the expression for the sum of two angles, namely $\sin(\alpha + \beta) = \sin\alpha\cos\beta + \cos\alpha\sin\beta$. Then the following Bessel function expansions

$$\cos(\alpha \sin \beta) = J_0(\alpha) + 2\sum_{m=1}^{\infty} J_{2m}(\alpha)\cos(2m\beta)$$

(8.25)

$$\sin(\alpha \sin \beta) = 2\sum_{m=0}^{\infty} J_{2m+1}(\alpha)\sin[(2m+1)\beta],$$

can be used. These enable (8.24) to be rewritten as

$$X(t) = \sin(\omega_o t + \varphi)\left\{ J_0(M_f) + 2\sum_{m=1}^{\infty} J_{2m}(M_f)\cos[2m(\omega_L t + \phi)] \right\}$$
$$+ \cos(\omega_o t + \varphi)\left\{ 2\sum_{m=1}^{\infty} J_{2m-1}(M_f)\sin[(2m-1)(\omega_L t + \phi)] \right\}.$$

Using $2\sin\alpha\cos\beta = \sin(\alpha + \beta) + \sin(\alpha - \beta)$, the above equation can be rearranged in a form that enables the frequency components to be obtained as

$$\begin{aligned}
X(t) = {} & J_0(M_f)\sin(\omega_o t + \varphi) \\
& + J_1(M_f)\{\sin[(\omega_o + \omega_L)t + \varphi + \phi] - \sin[(\omega_o - \omega_L)t + \varphi - \phi]\} \\
& + J_2(M_f)\{\sin[(\omega_o + 2\omega_L)t + \varphi + 2\phi] + \sin[(\omega_o - 2\omega_L)t + \varphi - 2\phi]\} \\
& + J_3(M_f)\{\sin[(\omega_o + 3\omega_L)t + \varphi + 3\phi] - \sin[(\omega_o - 3\omega_L)t + \varphi - 3\phi]\} \\
& + \ldots
\end{aligned}$$

(8.26)

This demonstrates the presence of harmonic components whose amplitudes depend on the modulation index through the Bessel functions and whose frequencies differ from the offset frequency by a multiple of the vibration frequency. The manner in which spectral component amplitudes change for two displacement amplitudes $\{\xi_o = c_o M_f/(2\omega_c)\}$ is illustrated in Fig. 8.52. The modulation index can be found from the harmonic component amplitudes, thereby enabling the displacement amplitude to be determined. This process can be repeated throughout the observation slice plane, yielding a 2-D map representing the displacement amplitude of the low-frequency disturbance in the propagation medium.

8.8.3 Shear Wave Propagation in Tissue

The question as to the manner in which low-frequency vibrations propagate in tissue has been studied for many years [201,202]. When a low-frequency (10–500 Hz) periodic uniaxial stress is applied to tissue, in the manner illustrated in Fig. 8.51, the energy propagates primarily as transverse (shear) waves with a speed of propagation several orders of magnitude less than compressional waves. In fact, the wavelength of a compressional wave may be several hundred times less than the dimensions of an organ examined, whereas for a low-frequency transverse wave it may be of similar magnitude. With increasing frequency the shear wave suffers increasing attenuation, and eventually the energy it contributes becomes small in comparison to the compressional wave.

In B-mode imaging it is the changes in acoustic properties, primarily the bulk modulus, that determine the image. However, such changes are relatively small compared to the shear modulus, whose values may change by many orders of magnitude, depending on the tissue. A comparison of the bulk and

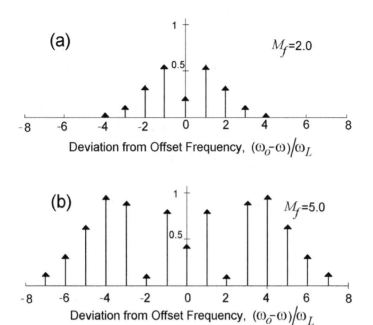

Figure 8.52 Frequency spectra from a pulse wave system due to scattering from a sinusoidally displaced region by a low-frequency vibration source. A narrowband transmitted signal was assumed. The spectra for two modulation indices are shown. Assuming a transmitted frequency of 4 MHz, the displacement amplitude (ξ_o) in water would be 0.06 mm for (a) and 0.15 mm for (b).

shear moduli properties, as summarized from the literature, is shown in Fig. 8.53. This suggests that by imaging one or more characteristics of shear wave propagation, improved sensitivity to localized changes in elastic properties could be achieved [162].

Because of the rapidly increasing attenuation with frequency, it is not possible to use high-frequency shear waves, which suggests that the spatial resolution might be rather limited. However, the presence of even a relatively small non-uniformity in elasticity could create an appreciably larger disturbance to the shear wave propagation: much like dropping a small pebble into a pond and observing the resulting surface wave disturbance.

For waves propagating in a viscous medium of density ρ_o whose shear modulus is denoted by μ_ℓ and shear viscosity by μ, the propagation speed and attenuation can be obtained by starting with the linearized Navier-Stokes equation for an isotropic solid as given by (1.66). By splitting this into irrotational and incompressible components, the elastic equations for longitudinal and transverse waves were obtained as (1.68). For plane harmonic transverse waves, it can be readily shown from (1.68b) that the propagation speed and attenuation are given by [201]:

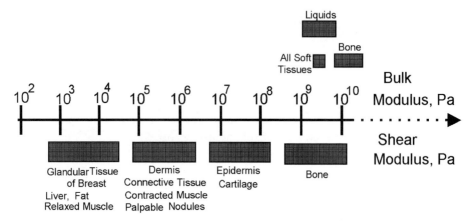

Figure 8.53 Summary and comparison of the shear (μ_ℓ) and bulk moduli ($1/\kappa$) of hard and soft tissue. The lower half shows the shear modulus and the upper shows the bulk modulus ($N/m^2 \equiv Pa$). (Reprinted by permission of Elsevier from Sarvazyan et al. [162], *Ultrasound Med. Biol.*, 24, 1419–1436, © 1998 World Federation of Ultrasound in Medicine and Biology.)

$$c_T = \sqrt{\frac{2(\mu_\ell^2 + \omega^2\mu^2)}{\rho_o(\mu_\ell + \sqrt{\mu_\ell^2 + \omega^2\mu^2})}}$$

(8.27)

$$\alpha_T = \sqrt{\frac{\rho_o\omega^2(\sqrt{\mu_\ell^2 + \omega^2\mu^2} - \mu_\ell)}{2(\mu_\ell^2 + \omega^2\mu^2)}}.$$

In the limit as $\omega \to 0$, or if the shear modulus dominates over the viscous losses ($\mu_\ell \gg \omega\mu$), then $c_T \to \sqrt{\mu_\ell/\rho_o}$, which is the result given in Chapter 1. Examining (8.27), it can be seen that the speed is strongly influenced by the angular frequency, and this is illustrated in Fig. 8.54 for soft tissue. Also shown are the wavelength and attenuation as a function of frequency. For the assumed parameters, the wavelength at 200 Hz is 2.8 cm and attenuation is about $2\,cm^{-1}$ ($\sim$17 dB/cm).

The corresponding equations for compressional waves can be obtained from (1.68a) as

$$1/c_L = \sqrt{\rho_o}\, R_e\{B\}$$

(8.28)

$$a_L = -\omega\sqrt{\rho_o}\, Im\{B\},$$

where $B = 1/\sqrt{(\lambda_\ell + 2\mu_\ell) + j\omega\left(\mu_B + \frac{4}{3}\mu\right)}$, in which λ_ℓ is the first Lamé constant and μ_B is the bulk viscosity. Assuming that $(\lambda_\ell + 2\mu_\ell) \gg \omega\left(\frac{4}{3}\mu + \mu_B\right)$, (8.28) simplifies to

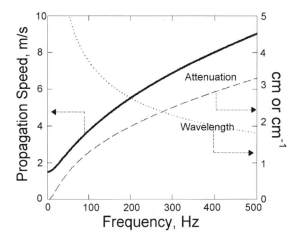

Figure 8.54 Propagation characteristics of low-frequency shear waves in a tissue-like medium ($\rho_o = 1100\,\mathrm{kg/m^3}$, $\mu_\ell = 2500\,\mathrm{Pa}$, $\mu = 15\,\mathrm{Pa.s}$). Note that the LH scale for the speed is in m/s, while for the wavelength and attenuation the RH scale is in cm and $\mathrm{cm^{-1}}$. Note that the strong dispersion is associated with the high shear attenuation.

(8.29)
$$c_L \approx \sqrt{(\lambda_\ell + 2\mu_\ell)/\rho_o}$$

$$\alpha_L \approx \omega^2\left(\mu_B + \frac{4}{3}\mu\right)/\left(2\rho_o c_L^3\right)$$

The first approximate equation for the speed was previously obtained as (1.70), while the second equation is identical to the classic Stokes formula for the attenuation of a viscous liquid, which was derived as (3.113).

Equation (8.27) suggests that the viscoelastic properties of soft tissue can be determined by measuring the phase speed and attenuation using low-frequency CW excitation. Catheline et al. [203] point out that three sources of error can arise in attempting to do so on a confined specimen. The first arises from the interference of waves reflected from boundaries, the second from diffraction effects associated with the use of a finite-size source, and the third from the effects of interference between the axial components of shear and compressional waves. To overcome these problems they used an impulse technique in which the characteristics of the propagating shear and compressional waves were measured prior to any boundary effects becoming important.

8.9 Ultrasound Microscopy and Biomicroscopy

8.9.1 Background

The invention of the optical microscope opened a window that enabled the optical properties of matter to be visually perceived at a microscopic level, and this led to many important discoveries in biology and medicine. The subsequent invention of other imaging modalities, such as the electron microscope, the scanning electron microscope, and the atomic force microscope, provided additional important new tools for research. These modalities generated the image contrast through microvariations in the medium properties or topography, sometimes revealing important new features. Likewise, one of the aims in using ultrasound radiation as a means for generating image contrast at the microscopic level was to provide a detailed view of the acoustic properties.

Ultrasound *biomicroscopy*[22] [204] is generally associated with the imaging of living tissue (see subsection 8.9.3). It is a more recently developed field than acoustic microscopy, and its resolution is generally limited by a compromise between the depth of penetration and the frequency-dependent attenuation. Rapid expansion of this field has been made possible through improved methods of fabricating high-frequency transducers [e.g., 205,206] and the development of piezoelectric materials with enhanced characteristics (see subsection 6.1.2). Initially, high-frequency imaging was performed using single-element mechanically scanned transducers [207]. More recently, considerable effort has been made to develop arrays [208–210] that can provide the flexibility needed to enable tissue acoustic microstructure to be imaged at frame rates sufficient to resolve rapid dynamic changes.

One method that avoids the difficulties associated with fabricating high-frequency arrays has been described by Tutwiler et al. [211]. It uses an array with much wider elements, e.g., 2λ, displaced in sub-wavelength steps by a piezoelectric actuator. After each step the data needed for synthetic image reconstruction were acquired. To demonstrate feasibility, they used a 12-element 50 MHz phased array with an inter-element spacing of 105 μm and an actuator that performed 14 steps of 7.5 μm ($14 \times 7.5 = 105$). Each step was equivalent to moving the array by a distance of $\lambda/4$. By this means they were ale to demonstrate a lateral resolution performance (~22 μm) equivalent to that of a 64-element array operating at the same center frequency.

The idea of using ultrasound for imaging at the microscopic level appears to have originated with the work of Sokolov [212,213] in the former USSR. In a short paper published in 1949[23] that described a possible means to achieve this, he appears to be the first to use the term "ultrasound microscope" and pointed out that at a frequency of 3 GHz the wavelength would be similar to optical wavelengths, yielding a similar resolution. It was some 10 years later that the first practical steps were taken towards its realization. Dunn and Fry [214] used a very fine thermocouple wire junction (~13 μm) placed immediately adjacent to the specimen to measure the absorption of ultrasound by the specimen when irradiated with ultrasound pulses at a center frequency of 12 MHz. By slowly moving the specimen they were able to demonstrate that

22. As pointed out by Foster et al. [204], *optical biomicroscopy* is well-established term used to describe an optical means for visualizing living tissue, and hence it is logical to use the term *ultrasound biomicroscopy* to describe the same using ultrasound.

23. A number of papers have suggested that Sokolov developed the basic ideas in the 1930s and have quoted various patents and publications to support this.

a graph could be produced that represented the local absorption characteristics.

In the early 1970s, two different approaches to ultrasound microscopy were developed [221]. Korpel and Kessler [215,216] developed a scheme that made use of a scanning laser beam to detect the local acoustic field transmitted through the specimen. The resulting scanning laser acoustic microscope (SLAM), which used excitation in the 100 to 500 MHz range, could provide simultaneous acoustic and optical images at standard TV frame rates [216,217]. The group under Quate, used a different approach in which an ultrasound beam was mechanical scanned over the specimen to form C-mode images. The transmission and reflection acoustic microscopes [218–220] initially developed by this group operated in the sub-GHz range. Subsequent research showed that systems of this type were capable of operating at frequencies of over 15 GHz, though under cryogenic conditions.

8.9.2 Scanning Acoustic Microscope

The earliest form of scanning acoustic microscope developed by Quate's group was a CW transmission system with separate transmission and receiving lenses. However, the very small focal zone places considerable demands in ensuring that the two lenses are maintained confocal. Moreover, the very high attenuation required that the specimen be extremely thin. Reflection mode acoustic microscopy has the advantage that the same lens is used for both transmission and reflection that is, by definition, a confocal arrangement. In addition, specimen thickness is no longer an issue. The first reflection scanning acoustic microscope operated using CW excitation at 600 MHz and was able to resolve details of around 2 μm. Pulsed excitation is generally preferred since it enables interface reflection artifacts to be more readily separated.

In the system illustrated in Fig. 8.55, single crystal sapphire (Al_2O_3) is used to form a hemispherical lens whose radius of curvature for a 1 GHz design may be around 40 μm. At high frequencies sapphire has a very low attenuation (0.2–0.5 dB/cm at 1 GHz), and the speed of sound (11,000 m/s) is about 7.3 times that of water. As a result, the refraction at the sapphire/water interface of the spherical cavity causes the ultrasound beam to focus close to the center of curvature (~1.3 times the radius of curvature) in a nearly ideal manner.

The properties of the fluid used to couple the lens to the specimen are of major importance. In a pulsed system, a single $\lambda/4$ matching layer will not eliminate all reflections from the sapphire/fluid interface. Hence, it is necessary to separate the specimen from the sapphire by a sufficient thickness of fluid to enable the signal from the specimen to be separated in time from that produced by the interface. For most fluids, the attenuation increases as the square of the frequency, which limits the maximum frequency that can be used for a given lens radius. According to the Rayleigh resolution criterion, the lateral resolution is given by (3.57)], i.e.,

$$(8.30) \qquad R_L = 1.22\lambda \frac{\text{Focal Length}}{\text{Aperture}} = 1.22\lambda \times \textit{f-number}.$$

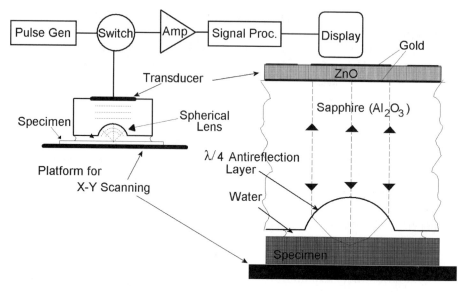

Figure 8.55 Simplified representation of a reflection scanning acoustic microscope. An enlarged view of the sapphire lens, transducer, and sample is also shown. A vacuum-deposited layer of zinc oxide is often used as the piezoelectric medium.

Also, the depth of field is expressed by (3.58),

$$(8.31) \qquad Z_F(3\text{dB}) = 7.2\lambda \times (f\text{-}number)^2 .$$

For a water-coupled system, the smallest *f-number* that can be achieved is around 0.65 (1.3/2) yielding the lateral resolutions listed in Table 8.1. Also shown in this table are the attenuation coefficients of water at 20°C over a range of frequencies. Cryogenic acoustic microscopy [222] exploits the properties of certain gases in a liquid state. For example, liquid helium has a much lower speed of sound than water (~230 m/s), and consequently the wavelength is approximately one sixth of those listed. Furthermore, the attenuation below 1°K rapidly decreases, dropping to about 0.04 dB/mm at 0.1°K for 1 GHz. These properties made it possible to achieve resolutions well beyond that possible with an optical microscope [223].

8.9.3 Scanning Biomicroscopy

The group led by Foster at the University of Toronto recognized the importance of developing a form of acoustic microscopy that would enable living cellular matter to be imaged and pointed out that such an instrument could enable normal cellular growth to be studied as a function of time. Moreover, the penetration of ultrasound enables visualization of subsurface planes that

Table 8.1. Resolution and Attenuation for Acoustic Microscopy

Frequency, MHz	λ, in H_2O	Lateral Resolution			Attenuation of H_2O at 20°C
		f/0.65	f/1.0	f/3.0	
10	150 µm	120 µm	180 µm	550 µm	0.022 dB/mm
30	50 µm	40 µm	61 µm	183 µm	0.2 dB/mm
100	15 µm	1.2 µm	18 µm	55.0 µm	2.2 dB/mm
300	5 µm	4.0 µm	6.1 µm	18.3 µm	0.02 dB/µm
1000	1.5 µm	1.2 µm	1.8 µm	5.50 µm	0.22 dB/µm
3000	0.5 µm	0.4 µm	0.61 µm	1.83 µm	2 dB/µm

are inaccessible to optical methods. One of the first instruments they developed is the 100 MHz backscatter microscope [224] illustrated in Fig. 8.28. It contained a cylindrically symmetric focused PVDF transducer with a 3.0-mm aperture and a focal length of 4.0 mm so that the f-number was 1.33. The measured slice thickness was around 30 µm, with a lateral resolution (FWHM) of 17.5 µm. It was mechanically scanned on the x–y plane to obtain a C-scan image at a given depth: each scan consisted of 256 × 256 pixels and took about 10 minutes to acquire. Additional subsurface planes were obtained by changing the transducer/specimen distance. The system performance was illustrated by obtaining images of several subsurface planes through a tumor spheroid.[24]

A problem with the above system was the length of time (10 minutes) required for each scan. By changing from C- to B-mode Sherar et al. [225] reported that the performance was dramatically improved, since this required mechanical scanning in just one direction. They used a PVDF focused transducer similar to that illustrated in Fig. 8.56, though with a smaller aperture corresponding to an f-number of 2.0. From (8.30) and (8.31) this results in a greater depth of field (0.43 mm), though with some loss in axial resolution (35 µm). With this system and an image size of 512 × 512 pixels, they were able to achieve five frames per second.

The success of the above methods stimulated high-frequency B-mode imaging work in a several clinical areas, specifically ophthalmology, dermatology, and intravascular ultrasound. It also stimulated investigations into the use of frequencies in the 100 to 200 MHz range [226]. The depth to which satisfactory images can be obtained depends on the frequency-dependent attenuation, the backscattering coefficient, and the depth of field. For soft tissue, the approximate frequency dependence of the attenuation and backscattering coefficient are illustrated in Fig. 8.57.

---

24. A spheroid is a aggregate of living cells that is grown in vitro; it has been used to model the effects of tumor growth [224].

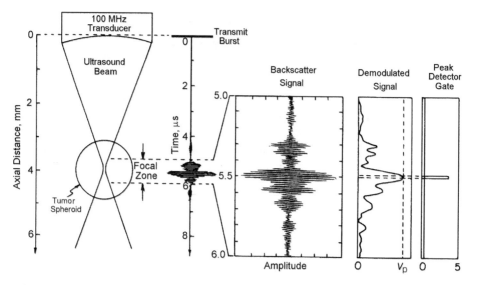

Figure 8.56 Principles of an ultrasound backscatter microscope designed for obtaining C-scan images of living tissue by mechanical *x-y* scanning. To obtain the peak backscattered signal corresponding to the focal plane, the received signal was sampled by a gate. C-scan images from various planes were obtained by changing the transducer/tumor separation. (Reprinted, with permission of Macmillan Magazines Ltd., from Sherar et al. [224], *Nature*, 330, 493–495, © 1987 Macmillan Magazines Limited.)

8.9.4 Biomicroscopy of the Eye

In ophthalmology, the group directed by Foster [227–229] developed a high-frequency imaging system that made use of an oscillating lever to achieve real-time imaging. The first commercial system[25] based on their prototype is illustrated in Fig. 8.58. The increase in attenuation with frequency limits the depth to which structures can be satisfactorily imaged, though this is partially offset by the increase in the backscattering coefficient. To obtain satisfactory images of the globe and orbit, frequencies in the range of 10 to 20 MHz are generally used, but for the anterior structures much higher frequencies are possible.

For frequencies much above 20 MHz, the attenuation and limited depth of field restricts the imaging and measurement capability to the anterior segment of the eye. Nonetheless, the cornea is the most significant refractive element of the eye and is the site of surgical intervention for correcting refractive problems. In addition, the trabecular network at the junction (the angle) of the iris and sclera is the site for aqueous fluid drainage, and abnormalities in this region can be a cause of glaucoma. A high-frequency image of the anterior portion of the eye obtained with a wideband 50 MHz system is presented in

---

25. Paradigm Medical Industries, Salt Lake City, UT.

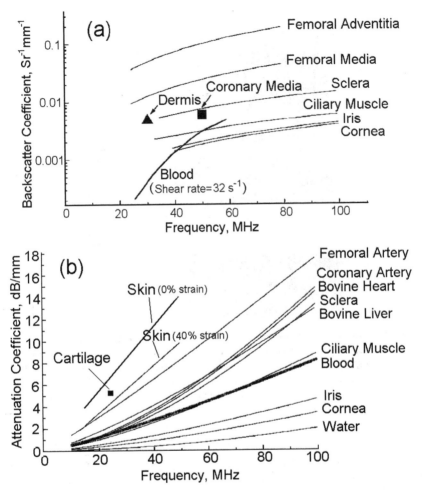

Figure 8.57 Approximate (a) backscattering and (b) attenuation properties of soft tissue at higher frequencies. All measurements were made 37°C except the bovine tissues, skin, and dermis, all of which were made at 22 to 24°C. (See [204] for sources of the original data. Reprinted by permission of Elsevier from Foster et al. [204], *Ultrasound Med. Biol.*, 26, 1–27, © 2000 World Federation of Ultrasound in Medicine and Biology.)

Fig. 8.59, together with an anatomic map. A normal cornea is approximately 12 mm in diameter, with a central region thickness of about 0.5 mm. In vitro imaging of the cornea at 200 MHz has also been demonstrated, enabling its various layers to be clearly visualized [226].

Lateral images of the entire anterior portion of the eye are shown in Fig. 8.60 under light and dark conditions. These were obtained with a system designed to automatically perform a B-scan scan over nearly the entire lateral dimension of the cornea using a transducer with a nominal frequency of

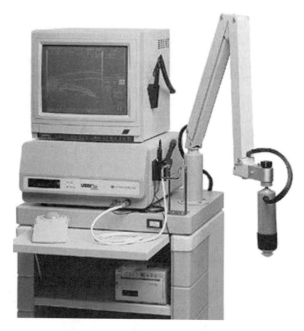

Figure 8.58 Commercial version [25] of a B-mode eye scanning system. An articulated arm supports the probe housing. The probe makes acoustic contact to the eye through a coupling fluid such a physiologic saline. This version can be used with a low-frequency probe (10 MHz, 13 or 18 frames/s) for examination of the globe and orbit, and with a high-frequency probe (50 MHz, 8 frames/s) for examination of the anterior segment of the eye.

50 MHz. The scanning motion was in the form of an arc that closely matched the cornea, thereby maintaining normal incidence and a constant range relative to the cornea. By scanning at various meridians and using appropriate signal-processing software, 2-D color-encoded maps were produced showing the thickness variations of the cornea and its various sublayers [230]. This information could be particularly useful for planning and evaluation of corneal excimer laser-assisted refractive surgery [231].

8.9.5 Biomicroscopy of Skin

A second field of application for high-frequency imaging that could be clinically important is in dermatology. Some of the first applications were to measure the thickness of the skin both in a normal and an abnormal condition [232]. Subsequently, imaging methods were developed and applied by Dines et al. [233] using 25 and 50 MHz transducers, though the 50-MHz transducer gave inferior images to the 25 MHz transducer due to a long ringdown time. Serup [234] has provided a useful review of many of these early developments. During the 1990s a number of groups described the development of

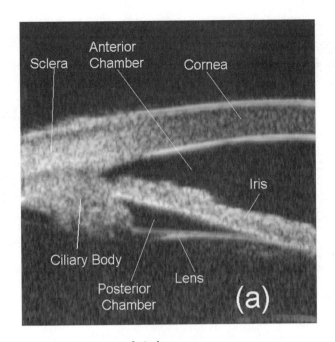

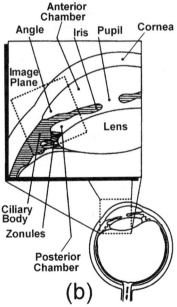

Figure 8.59 Ultrasound biomicroscope imaging of the anterior portions of the eye. (a) Image of approximately $4 \times 4\,\text{mm}^2$ made at 50 MHz: only a small section of the lens boundary is visible. (b) Schematic identifying the various structures. (Reproduced, with permission, from Foster et al. [229], *IEEE Trans. Ultrason. Ferroelect. Freq. Contr.*, 40, 608–617, © 1993 IEEE.)

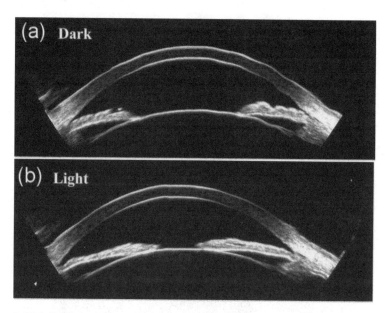

Figure 8.60 Ultrasound arc-scans of the anterior portion of a normal eye showing the effects of pupil adaptation to (a) the absence and (b) the presence of light. Images were obtained with a 50 MHz Artemis system (Ultralink LLC, St. Petersburg, FL). (Reproduced, with permission, from Ultralink LLC.)

systems with center frequencies up to 200 MHz that were used for dermatologic imaging [226,235–238].

8.10 Endoluminal and Intravascular Imaging

With the development of miniature transducers, imaging became possible from within various body cavities and vascular lumina. *Intravascular* ultrasound imaging is the term usually used to describe the technique that enables a vessel to be imaged from the inside and that can provide a high-resolution picture of the vessel wall and the tissue that immediately surrounds it. Strictly speaking, *endoluminal* ultrasound is a more general term referring to all nonpercutaneous methods, but it is often used to describe all nonvascular applications.

The beginnings of endoluminal and intravascular imaging [239] can be traced to the early work reported by Wild and Reid [240] in 1955. They constructed a rigid probe with a piezoelectric transducer mounted at one end that projected a beam at right angles to the probe axis. By means of an electric motor and worm gear, the transducer could be simultaneously rotated and slowly withdrawn, enabling a sequence of radial 360 degree B-mode images to be recorded. The system was used on a volunteer by inserting the probe into the rectum and recording on film the sequence of B-mode images of the wall of the bowel. Probes sufficiently small for use in intravascular imaging were first developed during the 1960s by Cieszynski [241], Omoto et al. [242,243], and Wells [244]. Commercial versions of several mechanically scanned systems became commercially available toward the end of the 1980s. More modern versions of these side-viewing probes use either rotation of the transducer or rotation of a 45-degree mirror with the transducer fixed. In addition, they may be equipped with a motorized transport to slowly withdraw the catheter from the vessel, enabling images to be obtained from successive locations within the vessel. The long mechanical coupling cable (drive cable) that passes through the catheter lumen can cause nonuniform rotation when the vessel is long and tortuous, resulting in image distortion [245].

8.10.1 Side-Viewing Transducers

In the early 1970s the group led by Bom [246] developed the cylindrically organized phased array transducer illustrated in Fig. 8.61, in which 8 of the 32 elements were used to form each B-mode line. This scheme avoided the need for mechanical rotation of either the transducer or a reflecting mirror. However, the image quality was relatively poor, due in part to the high side lobes and a long ringdown time that prevented imaging close to the catheter surface.

The technical challenges associated with designing and manufacturing a cylindrical phased array sufficiently small to be incorporated into an intravascular catheter for coronary arterial examinations are considerable. O'Donnell et al. [88,248] adopted a synthetic aperture approach (see section 8.5) using transmission and reception from a single pair of elements at a time. With this scheme, the signal processing to be performed in close proximity to the PZT elements is simplified and, most importantly, the number of wires required to be threaded down the catheter lumen is greatly reduced, e.g., six. Schulze-Clewing et al. [247] have provided details of a practical form of this catheter-tip design, and a sketch is presented in Fig. 8.62. In this design, five custom IC chips were needed to multiplex the array into a single channel at a time. The chips incorporated the preamplifiers, driving amplifiers, and all the circuits needed for selecting a single transducer for transmission and one for reception [249]. Of the 64 elements, a group of 14 can be used as an active aperture. For such a group, it can be shown [88] that the number of non-redundant transmit/receive firing combinations needed to synthetically reconstruct a single beam line is 105. If the group of 14 is incremented around the 64-element array, one element at a time, a total of $14 \times 64 \times 105 = 94,080$ firings would be required to provide all the data needed for reconstructing a complete frame.

A coronary intravascular image obtained with an early version of this phased array is illustrated in Fig. 8.63. In this image a central black region corresponds to the region occupied by the catheter. A ring arising from scattering/reverberation by the outer acoustically transparent sheath of the catheter surrounds it. Between about 3 and 5 o'clock can be seen a very strongly scattering region, which likely consists of calcified plaque, and this creates a strong

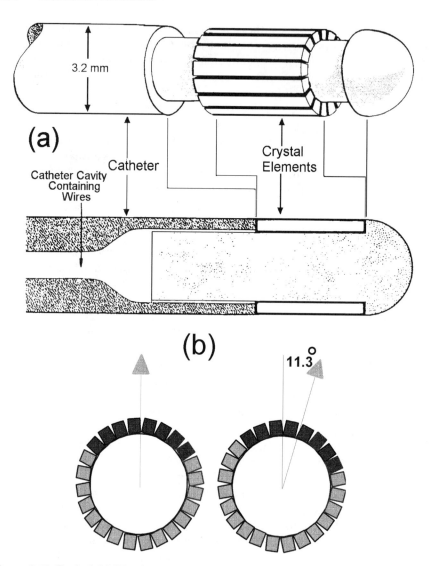

Figure 8.61 Early 5.6-MHz phased-array endoluminal imaging catheter with an outer diameter of 3.2 mm (9F) and consisting of 32 crystal elements. (a) Sketch of phased array. (Reprinted by permission of Elsevier from Bom et al. [246], © 1972.) (b) Cross-sectional view showing some elements and illustrating the scanning scheme in which successive groups of eight elements were used for each angular increment of 360/32 = 11.25 degrees.

shadow. Between 10 and 1 o'clock can be seen a crescent-shaped area that probably consists of soft plaque.

With increasing frequency, improved radial and lateral resolution can be expected. For example, at 40 MHz the radial resolution for a single-element transducer can be expected to be less than 100 μm, and the lateral resolution,

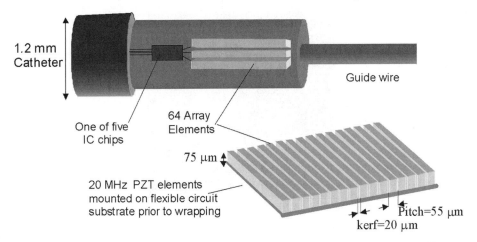

1.2 mm Catheter

Guide wire

One of five
IC chips

64 Array
Elements

75 μm

20 MHz PZT elements
mounted on flexible circuit
substrate prior to wrapping

Pitch=55 μm
kerf=20 μm

Figure 8.62 Sketch of a synthetic aperture intravascular imaging catheter according to the design of Schulze-Clewing et al. [247]. The PZT slab is mounted on a preprinted flex-circuit prior to dicing. The ICs needed for element driving, amplification, and selection are also mounted on the flex circuit.

which decreases with radial distance and depends on the number of imaging lines, would be substantially less. However, with increasing frequency, the scattering from blood surrounding the probe increases more rapidly relative to that from other media (see Fig. 8.57a). As a result it becomes increasingly difficult to distinguish between the two, thereby diminishing the accuracy with which the ratio of the areas of the plaque to lumen can be estimated. One method to help restore the contrast is to make use of the fact that the speckle produced by moving blood will be time-dependent, making it possible to devise filter schemes for reducing its effect [250,251]. Observation of the time-dependent region of the image can help delineate the lumen boundary, as can the use of contrast agents. An example of the contrast improvement made possible by using a filter is illustrated in Fig. 8.64 [252]. These images, which show mild atherosclerosis, were obtained using a single-element 40 MHz transducer rotated at 1,800 rpm, which corresponds to 30 frames/s. They display what appears to be a fairly uniform thickness of soft plaque that can be more readily distinguished from the region containing blood when filtering is used. The medium (weak scattering, ring-like region) surrounded by the more strongly scattering adventitia also appears to be more clearly delineated.

8.10.2 Three-Dimensional Imaging

The ability to slowly withdraw the catheter probe and record successive images enables longitudinal and cylindrical visualization of an entire vessel segment to be made. As noted in Chapter 7, 3-D reconstruction from freehand 2-D images obtained with a 1-D array normally requires a 3-D position

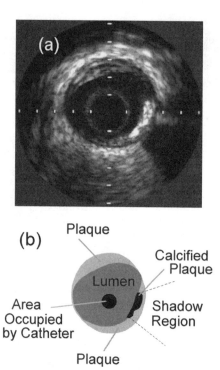

Figure 8.63 Single-frame coronary intravascular image using a 20-MHz synthetic phased-array imaging system at 30 frames/s and a catheter with a diameter of 1.2 mm (3.5F). (a) Image with tick mark separation of 1 mm. (Reproduced with permission from O'Donnell et al. [88], *IEEE Trans. Ultrason. Ferroelect. Freq. Contr.*, 44, 714–721, © 1997 IEEE.) (b) Sketch indicating the likely characteristics of various regions.

measurement system. However, if it is assumed that the catheter moves in a straight line, the only information needed for a simple 3-D reconstruction is the catheter displacement. Software has been designed and clinically used to provide a variety of other 3-D image display formats and also to automate the determination of plaque and lumen volumes as a function of the axial location [253,254].

Three-Dimensional imaging at a given location in a vessel can also be performed using the forward viewing, 2-D synthetic aperture array that is described in the next subsection. An alternative approach developed by a group at Duke University is designed for intracardiac imaging [255,256] and makes use of a full 2-D transducer array mounted in a 3.8 mm (12F) or a 2.8 mm (9F) catheter. The 5-MHz array consisting of 13 × 11 PZT elements spaced by 200 μm with a 25 μm kerf is mounted on a flexible polyamide substrate. Subsequently, the same group described [257] a 7 MHz catheter-mounted PZT array fabricated on a silicon substrate.

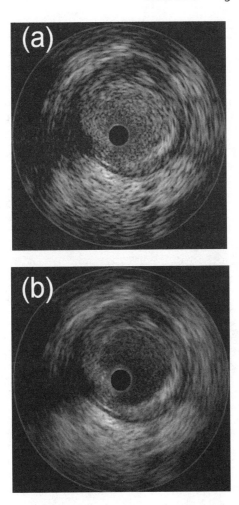

Figure 8.64 Examples of 40-MHz coronary intravascular images in a 0.87-mm-diameter (2.6F) catheter. (a) Without filtering algorithm. (b) Same image but using a filter algorithm to reduce the contrast produced by the moving blood. (Reproduced with permission from Hibi et al. [252], *Circulation*, 102, 1657–1663, © 2000 American Heart Association.)

A major challenge associated with a more conventional method of beam-forming is the need for a large number of active channels required for simultaneously transmitting data along the inside of the catheter. As briefly discussed in subsection 6.8.2, ribbon cables provide a partial solution to this problem. For example, Smith et al. [256] have reported that up to 143 channels can be activated in a 3.8-mm catheter. As illustrated in Fig. 8.65a, two array mounting designs have been considered: a side-viewing array and a beveled, the latter providing a mixture of side and forward imaging. The

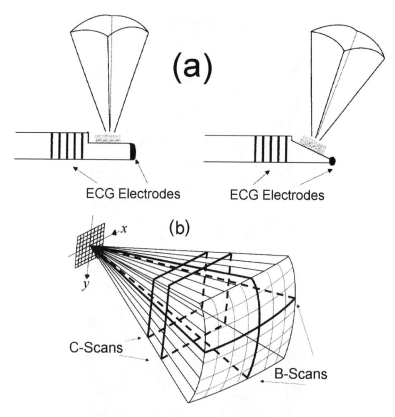

Figure 8.65 Catheter-based echocardiography 2-D array intracardiac imaging system. (a) Side and beveled mounting at the catheter tip along with ring electrodes for collecting electrocardiography signals and for delivering RF ablation energy. (b) Pyramidal scan volume from which various 2-D images can be displayed. (Reprinted by permission of Elsevier from Light et al. [255], *Ultrasound Med. Biol.*, 27, 1177–1183, © 2001 World Federation of Ultrasound in Medicine and Biology.)

pyramidal imaging volume provided by the array enables both B- and C-mode displays to be obtained.

8.10.3 Forward-Viewing Transducers

By 1990 it was appreciated that the inability to view ahead was a significant limitation of side-viewing intravascular imaging systems. Specifically, the side-viewing transducer must traverse the lesion by several millimeters to obtain an image. In the case of severe partial blockages of a vessel, there is a danger that the tip could restrict the flow; this, for a coronary artery, would increase the risk of myocardial ischemia. The ability to assess a severe lesion without having to cross it could help decide on the most appropriate interventional therapeutic approach and to measure its effects.

In 1991 a design [258] based on the use of a single-element transducer that could be rotated to achieve conventional side imaging (Fig. 8.66a, top) was proposed. By withdrawing the drive cable, the beam was reflected by a conical mirror and formed a conical image in the forward direction (Fig. 8.66a, bottom). About the same time, Busse and Dietz [259] described the results of simulations and scaled up experimental investigations of a sparse 2-D array of elements mounted on a disk at the tip of a catheter. This avoided the need for mechanical actuators, offered the possibility of real-time 3-D imaging, and represented an important initial step toward a more practical solution to the design problems.

An alternative design [260] is illustrated in Fig. 8.66b. In this, a mechanism was used for converting a single rotation of the drive cable into a 90-degree rocking movement of the crystal mount, thereby enabling sector scan to be produced. Subsequently, Liang and Hu [261] described a forward-viewing catheter (1.7 mm, 5F) that used a fixed transducer and a rotating mirror that redirects the beam into an arc. However, both of these, along with a more recent design [261,262], lacked side-view imaging, a feature considered important for clinical use.

To perform both side and forward imaging in the same catheter, the scheme illustrated in Fig. 8.67 was proposed by O'Donnell et al. [88] and subsequently described in more detail [263,264]. It contains two synthetic aperture transducer arrays. For side viewing, a 64-element 20 MHz array, similar to that illustrated in Fig. 8.62, was proposed. For forward viewing it was proposed that the array consist of 64 radially oriented elements equally spaced around an annular ring with inner and outer diameters of 1.1 and 1.3 mm, respectively, and with a resonant frequency of 10.4 MHz. The lower frequency was to provide increased depth of penetration and to avoid interference with the side-viewing array.

The question as to how the radially oriented elements of this array could provide forward viewing over a range of angles with adequate resolution is vital to the success of this proposal. Norton [84] studied the problem of synthesizing a full disk aperture by means of a large number of arbitrarily small elements equally spaced around an annular ring. He showed that by suitably weighting all the received signals obtained from all possible transmit/receive pairs of elements, it was possible to obtain a point spread function (PSF) equal to that of a full disk whose diameter was twice the annulus diameter.

For elements of non-zero size, it is helpful to first consider the effective receive aperture function that was defined in subsection 7.2.10. Although this is a CW approach, it does give a fair idea as to the pulse-echo characteristics. For 2-D apertures whose transmit and receive apertures are expressed in polar coordinates, i.e., $S_T(r,\theta)$ and $S_\Re(r,\theta)$, the effective aperture is given by

$$S_E(r,\theta) = S_T(r,\theta) ** S_\Re(r,\theta),$$

where the origin is at the center of the aperture.

If the two apertures are identical and are of the form shown in Fig. 8.67b, then the effective aperture will be the 2-D convolution of the array aperture with itself, i.e.,

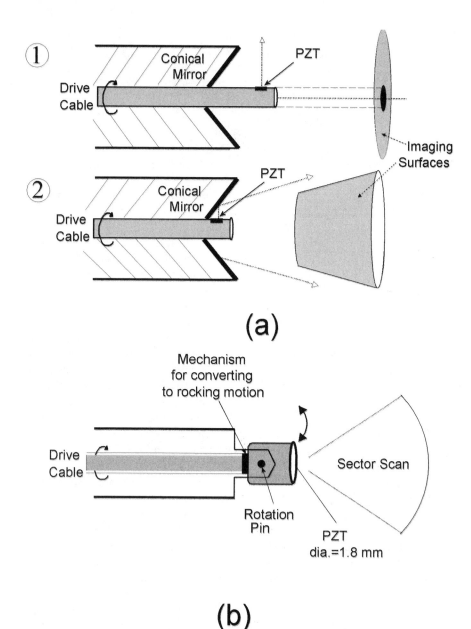

Figure 8.66 Some early designs of a forward-viewing intravascular catheter (a) ①
Side-view imaging: the central rod is displaced forward so that the beam misses the
edge of the conical mirror. ② Forward viewing: the central rod is withdrawn so that a
conical mirror producing an image that is formed from the surface of a cone reflects
the beam. (Based on Lee and Benkser [258].) (b) Rotation of the drive cable causes
the transducer to be rocked through 90 degrees, enabling a sector scan to be
produced.

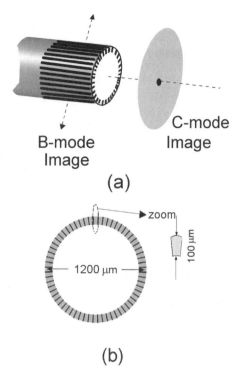

Figure 8.67 Side- and forward-imaging intravascular catheter. (a) Showing two 64-element arrays. (b) Forward-imaging synthetic aperture 64-element array. (Reproduced with permission from Wang et al. [263], pp. 1573–1576 in: *2001 IEEE Ultrasonics Symp.*, © 2001 IEEE.)

$$(8.32) \qquad S_E(r,\theta) = \left[\sum_{n=0}^{N-1} S_n \right] ** \left[\sum_{m=0}^{N-1} S_m \right],$$

where S, with the appropriate subscript, denotes the aperture function of an individual element of the N-element array [266]. Two examples are shown in Fig. 8.68. In (a) a full transmit aperture is convoluted with receive aperture elements at 0 and 90 degrees. In (b) a full transmit aperture is convoluted with receive elements at 180 and 270 degrees. Also indicated in this case are the contributions of 0 and 90 degrees, had they been present. From these examples it can be seen that the center region is common to all transmit elements and that a full self-convolution would be expected to result in an effective aperture whose amplitude is fairly intense at the center. This is evident in Fig. 8.69, which also demonstrates that the effective receive aperture diameter is twice that of the annular ring. The non-uniform amplitude of the response can be expected to give rise to strong side lobes that would seriously degrade the imaging performance. By using various non-uniform receiver-weighting

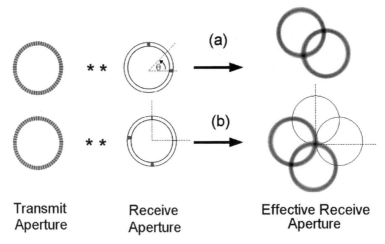

Transmit
Aperture

Receive
Aperture

Effective Receive
Aperture

Figure 8.68 Effective receive aperture for a full transmit array and two receive elements (a) at 0 and 90 degrees, and (b) at 180 and 270 degrees. (c) Central cross-section of the effective aperture for full transmit and receive apertures. (Modified version reproduced, with permission, from Wang et al. [263], pp. 1573–1576 in: *2001 IEEE Ultrasonics Symp.*, © 2001 IEEE.)

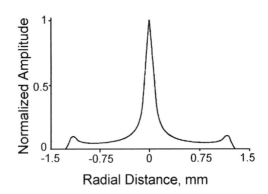

Figure 8.69 Effective receive aperture response for the annular array of Fig. 8.67b. Because of near-cylindrical symmetry, this graph represents the entire result of the 2-D convolution as expressed by (8.32). (Reproduced, with permission from Dynamedia, from Crowe et al. [266], *Ultrasonic Imaging*, 23, 19–38, © 2001 Dynamedia.)

functions, it has been shown that the response [263,266] can be improved, though with some loss in SNR.

Full coverage of the effective receive aperture using the 64-element ring array described earlier requires $64 \times 33 = 2{,}112$ single transmit/receive pair firings. For an intravascular catheter, using a single transmit/receive pair at a time, the length of time required for this number of transmissions would result

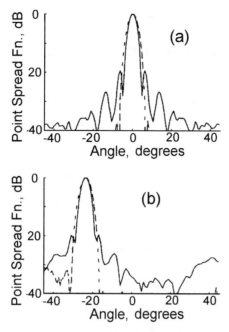

Figure 8.70 Point spread function for a 64-element annular ring for (a) no steering and (b) steering of 23.6 degrees. The PSF (solid lines) are for 210 firings; the dashed lines are for all 2112 firing combinations. (Reproduced, with permission, from Wang et al. [263], pp. 1573–1576 in: *2001 IEEE Ultrasonics Symp.*, © 2001 IEEE.)

in serious motion artifacts. Wang et al. [263] have proposed a sparse scheme that uses only 210 firings to form a complete image, though with some additional (to the apodization method) loss in SNR. They computed the PSF for a 10-MHz system with no steering and steering of 23.6 degrees, and the results are shown in Fig. 8.70. Wang and O'Donnell [265] have also explored the use of compounding (see subsection 8.2.2) to reduce the effects of speckle noise, with encouraging results.

8.10.4 Flow Measurement

A method of measuring the blood flow within a vessel using a side-viewing transducer is that proposed by Li et al. [267,268]. It makes use of the relation between the flow velocity and decorrelation. Specifically, the received RF signal from successive transmissions through a moving scattering medium decorrelates more rapidly as the velocity increases in the direction normal to the beam. Thus, if the relation between the correlation coefficient and the displacement is known, measurement of the correlation coefficient between successive A-mode transmissions should enable the velocity to be calculated.

The above method was subsequently used with a side-viewing imaging array catheter [269]. Suppose that such a catheter is positioned coaxially in a

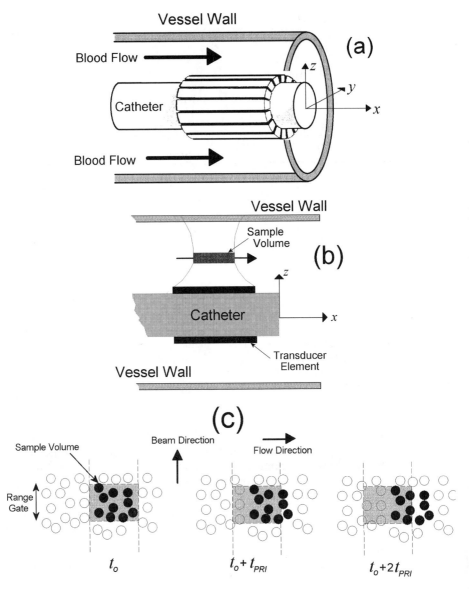

Figure 8.71 Method for measuring blood flow using decorrelation of the RF signal from an intravascular catheter array. (a) Intravascular side-viewing catheter array. (b) Sample volume generated by excitation of several adjacent elements. (c) Decorrelation of an ensemble of scatterers as they pass through the sample volume.

vessel, as illustrated in Fig. 8.71a. If a small number of adjacent elements are joined together, e.g., 4 out of 64, and these are used for A-mode transmissions and receptions, then the range-gated sample volume could be as illustrated in (b). Suppose that the RBC scatterer locations in relation to the sample volume for an A-mode transmission at a time t_o are those shown in (c). If the scatterers are moving in the transverse direction, then, for a subsequent transmission at $t_o + t_{PRI}$, the number of original scatterers in the sample volume will be less, and even less for transmission at $t_o + 2t_{PRI}$. A new scatterer ensemble would have replaced the one that was displaced from the sample volume. Consequently, successive A-mode RF signals become decorrelated.

It is reasonable to expect the correlation coefficient to decrease nearly linearly with increasing velocity and with increasing t_{PRI} (see subsection 10.4.2 for further details). These relationships provide a potential means of measuring the volumetric flow rate [268,270]. Specifically, a transducer calibration is performed of the correlation coefficient versus displacement of an ensemble of scatterers. This enables the slope to be determined as a function of z. Then, the RF signals from successive transmissions are measured and correlated to determine the correlation versus time relation as a function of z. For a given z, the ratio of the measured time slope (s^{-1}) to the calibration displacement slope (m^{-1}) can be shown to be equal to the blood velocity (m/s). By performing the same process for each group of transducer elements around the catheter, the velocity distribution between the catheter and the vessel wall can be found. By using the B-mode images to determine the spacing between the vessel and the catheter, the volumetric flow can then be determined.

In Fig. 8.71, it was assumed that flow was along the vessel axis and that the catheter was coaxial with the vessel. In practice, the blood velocity may have an appreciable component in the beam direction, and this will cause decorrelation. Other effects, such as the presence of noise in the RF signal or a velocity distribution within the sample volume, can also contribute to errors in flow velocity estimation [267].

References

1. Powers, J.E., Phillips, D.J., Brandestini, M.A., and Sigelmann, R.A., Ultrasound phased array delay lines based on quadrature sampling techniques, *IEEE Trans. Sonics Ultrason.*, 27, 287–294, 1980.
2. Thomenius, K.E., Evolution of ultrasound beamformers, pp. 1615–1622 in: *1996 IEEE Ultrasonics Symp. Proc.*, 1996.
3. Bracewell, R.N., *The Fourier Transform and its Applications*, 3rd Ed., McGraw-Hill, New York, 2000.
4. Bamber, J.C., and Dickinson, R.J., Ultrasonic B-scanning: a computer simulation, *Phys. Med. Biol.*, 25, 463–479, 1980.
5. Fatemi, M., and Kak, A.C., Ultrasonic B-scan imaging: theory of image formation and a technique for restoration, *Ultrasonic Imaging*, 2, 1–47, 1980.

6. Hiller, D., and Ermert, H., System analysis of ultrasound reflection mode computerized tomography, *IEEE Trans. Sonics Ultrasonics*, 31, 240–250, 1984.

7. Goodman, J.W., Statistical properties of laser speckle patterns, Ch. 2, pp. 9–75 in: *Laser Speckle and Related Phenomena*, J.C. Dainty (Ed.), 2nd Ed., Springer-Verlag, Berlin, 1984.

8. Crombie, P., *Fundamental Studies on Contrast Resolution of Ultrasound B-Mode Images*, PhD thesis, University of Toronto, 1999.

9. Abbot, J.G., and Thurstone, F.L., Acoustic speckle: theory and experimental analysis, *Ultrasonic Imaging*, 1, 303–324, 1979.

10. Burckhardt, C.B., Speckle in ultrasound B-mode scans, *IEEE Trans. Sonics Ultrasonics*, 25, 1–6, 1978.

11. Trahey, G.E., Allison, J.W., and von Ramm, O.T., Angle independent ultrasonic detection of blood flow, *IEEE Trans. Biomed. Eng.*, 34, 965–967, 1987.

12. Trahey, G.E., Hubbard, S.M., and von Ramm, O.T., Angle independent ultrasonic blood flow detection by frame-to-frame correlation of B-mode images, *Ultrasonics.*, 26, 271–276, 1988.

13. Oosterveld, B.J., Thijssen, J.M., and Verhoef, W.A., Texture of B-mode echograms: 3-D simulations and experiments of the effects of diffraction and scatterer density, *Ultrasonic Imaging*, 7, 142–160, 1985.

14. Goodman, J.W., *Statistical Optics* (Chapter 2), Wiley, New York, 1985.

15. Papoulis, A., and Pillai, S.U., *Probability, Random Variables and Stochastic Processes*, 4th Ed., McGraw-Hill, New York, 2002.

16. Atkinson, P., and Berry, M. V., Random noise in ultrasonic echoes diffracted by blood, *J. Phys. A. Math. Nucl. Gen.*, 7, 1293–1302, 1974.

17. Jakeman, E., and Pusey, P.N., A model for non-Rayleigh sea echo, *IEEE Trans. Antennas Propagation*, 24, 806–814, 1976.

18. Jakeman, E., and Tough, R.J.A., Non-Gaussian models for the statistics of scattered waves, *Advances in Physics*, 37, 471–529, 1988.

19. Weng, L., Reid, J.M., Shankar, P.M., and Soetanto, K., Ultrasound speckle analysis based on the K distribution, *J. Acoust. Soc. Am.*, 89, 2992–2995, 1991.

20. Dutt, V., and Greenleaf, J.F., Adaptive speckle reduction filter for log-compressed B-scan images, *IEEE Trans. Med. Imaging*, 15, 802–813, 1996.

21. Thijssen, J.M., Oosterveld, B.J., and Wagner, R.F., Grey level transforms and lesion detectability in echographic images, *Ultrasonic Imaging*, 10, 171–195, 1988.

22. Kaplan, D., and Ma, Q., On the statistical characteristics of log-compressed Rayleigh signals: theoretical formulation and experimental results, *J. Acoust. Soc. Am.*, 95, 1396–1400, 1995.

23. Abramowitz, M., and Stegun, I.A. (Eds.), *Handbook of Mathematical Functions*, Dover, New York, 1965.

24. Dickinson, R.J., A computer model for speckle in ultrasound images: theory and Application, pp. 115–129, in: *Acoustical Imaging*, Vol. 10, P. Alias, and A.F. Metherell (Eds.), Plenum Press, New York, 1982.

25. Smith S.W., Sandrik, J.M., Wagner, R.F., and von Ramm, O.T., Measurement and analysis of speckle in ultrasound B-scans, pp. 195–211, in: *Acoustical Imaging*, Vol. 10, P. Alias, and A.F. Metherell (Eds.), Plenum Press, New York, 1982.

26. Wagner, R.F., Smith S.W., Sandrik, J.M., and Lopez, H., Statistics of speckle in ultrasound B-scans, *IEEE Trans. Sonics Ultrasonics*, 30, 156–163, 1983.

27. Wagner, R.F., Insana, M.F., and Smith, S.W., Fundamental correlation lengths of coherent speckle in medical ultrasonic images, *IEEE Trans. Ultrason. Ferroelect. Freq. Contr.*, 35, 34–44, 1988.

28. Bamber, J.C., Speckle reduction, Chapter 5, pp. 55–67, in: *Advances in Ultrasound Techniques and Instrumentation (Clinics in Diagnostic Ultrasound*, Vol. 28) P.N.T. Wells (Ed.), Churchill Livingstone, New York, 1993.

29. Carpenter, D.A., Dadd, M.J., and Kossoff, G., A multimode real time scanner, *Ultrasound Med. Biol.*, 6, 279–284, 1980.

30. Berson, M., Roncin, A., and Pourcelot, L., Compound scanning with an electrically steered beam, *Ultrasonic Imaging*, 3, 303–308, 1981.

31. Healey, A.J., and Leeman, S., Speckle definitions, pp. 259–269, in: *Acoustical Imaging*, Vol. 21, J.P. Jones (Ed.), Plenum Press, New York, 1995.

32. Bamber, J.C., and Daft, C., Adaptive filtering for reduction of speckle in ultrasonic pulse-echo images, *Ultrasonics*, 24, 41–44, 1986.

33. Crawford, D.C., Bell, D.S., and Bamber, J.C., Compensation for the signal processing characteristics of ultrasound B-mode scanners in adaptive speckle reduction, *Ultrasound Med. Biol.*, 19, 469–485, 1993.

34. Foster, F.S., Patterson, M.S., Arditi, M., and Hunt, J.W., The conical scanner: a two transducer ultrasound scatter imaging technique, *Ultrasonic Imaging*, 3, 62–82, 1981.

35. Shattuck, D.P., and von Ramm, O.T., Compound scanning with a phased array, *Ultrasonic Imaging*, 4, 93–107, 1982.

36. Trahey, G.E., Smith, S.W., and von Ramm, O.T., Speckle pattern correlation with lateral aperture translation: experimental results and implications for spatial compounding, *IEEE Trans. Ultrason. Ferroelect. Freq. Contr.*, 33, 257–264, 1986.

37. Jespersen, S.K., Wilhjelm, J.E., and Sillesen, H., Multi-angle compound imaging, *Ultrasonic Imaging*, 20, 81–102, 1998.

38. Magnin, P.A., von Ramm, O.T., and Thurstone, F.L., Frequency compounding for speckle contrast reduction in phased array images, *Ultrasonic Imaging*, 4, 267–281, 1982.

39. Trahey, G.E., Allison, J.W., Smith, S.W., and von Ramm, O.T., A quantitative approach to speckle reduction via frequency compounding, *Ultrasonic Imaging*, 8, 151–164, 1986.

40. Galloway, R.L., McDermott, B.A., and Thurstone, F.L., A frequency diversity process for speckle reduction in real-time ultrasonic images, *IEEE Trans. Ultrason. Ferroelect. Freq. Contr.*, 35, 45–49, 1988.

41. Sharp, P.F., Display and perception of ultrasound images, Ch. 1, pp. 1–18, in: *Advances in Ultrasound Techniques and Instrumentation (Clinics in Diagnostic Ultrasound)* Vol. 28, P.N.T. Wells (Ed.), Churchill Livingstone, New York, 1993.

42. Vilkomerson, D., Greenleaf, J., and Dutt, V., Towards a metric for medical ultrasonic imaging, pp. 1405–1410, in: *1995. IEEE Ultrasonics Symp. Proc.*, 1995.

43. Smith, S.W., and Lopez, H., A contrast-detail analysis of diagnostic ultrasound imaging, *Med. Phys.*, 9, 4–12, 1982.

44. Smith, S.W., Wagner, R.F., Sandrik, J.M., and Lopez, H., Low contrast detectibility and contrast/detail analysis in medical ultrasound, *IEEE Trans. Sonics Ultrason.*, 30, 164–173, 1983.

45. Smith, S.W., Lopez, H., and Bodine, W.J., Frequency independent ultrasound contrast-detail analysis, *Ultrasound Med. Biol.*, 11, 467–477, 1985.

46. Hall, T.J., Insana, M.F., Cook, L.T., et al., Ultrasound contrast-detail analysis: a preliminary study in human observer performance of image degradation due to lossy compression, *Med. Phys.*, 20, 117–127, 1993.

47. Patterson M.S., Foster F.S., The improvement and quantitative assessment of B-mode images produced by an annular array/cone hybrid, *Ultrasonic Imaging*, 5, 195–213, 1983.

48. Stetson, P.F., Sommer, F.G., Macovski, A., Lesion contrast enhancement in medical ultrasound imaging, *IEEE Trans. Medical Imag.*, 16, 416–425. 1997.

49. Johnson, R., Contrast response analysis for medical ultrasound imaging, *IEEE Trans. Ultrason. Ferroelect. Freq. Contr.*, 44, 805–809, 1997.

50. Abbott, J.G., Rationale and derivation of MI and TI, a review, *Ultrasound Med. Biol.*, 25, 431–441, 1999.

51. National Council on Radiation Protection, *Exposure Criteria for Medical Diagnostic Ultrasound: II. Critera Based on all Known Mechanisms*, Report No. 140, 2002.

52. Klauder, J.R., Price, H.C., Darlington, S., and Albersheim, W.J., Theory and design of chirp radars, *Bell Syst. Tech. J.* 39, 745–808, July 1960.

53. Cook, C.E., and Bernfeld, M., *Radar Signals: An Introduction to Theory and Application*, Academic Press, New York, 1967 (republished: Artech House Inc., Boston, 1993).

54. Ohtsuki, S., and Okujima, M., Ultrasonic Doppler velocity meter by M-sequence modultaion method [in Japanese], *J. Acoust. Soc. Japan*, 29, 347–355, 1973. See the conference presentation listings of 1970, as referenced in [59].

55. Waag, R.C., Myklebust, J.B., Rhoads, W.L., and Gramiak, R., Instrumentation for noninvasive cardiac chamber flow rate measurement, pp. 74–77, in: *1972 IEEE Ultrasonics Symp. Proc.*, 1972.

56. Newhouse, V.L., Furgason, E.S., Bilgutay, N.M., and Cooper, G.R., Random signal flaw detection, pp. 711–715 in: *1974 IEEE Ultrasonics Symp. Proc.*, 1974.

57. Bendick, P.J., and Newhouse, V.L., Ultrasonic random-signal flow measurement system, *J. Acoust. Soc. Am.*, 56, 860–865, 1974.

58. Newhouse, V.L., Cathignol, D., and Chapelon, J.Y., Introdution to ultrasonic pseudo-random code systems, Ch. 5, pp. 215–226, in: *Progress in Medical Imaging*, V.L. Newhouse (Ed.), Springer-Verlag, New York, 1988.

59. Takeuchi, Y., An investigation of a spread energy method for medical ultrasound systems. Part one: theory and investigation, *Ultrasonics*, 17, 175–182, 1979.

60. Takeuchi, Y., An investigation of a spread energy method for medical ultrasound systems. Part two: proposed system and possible problems, *Ultrasonics*, 17, 219–224, 1979.

61. Benkhelifa, M.A., Gindre, M., Le Huerou, J-Y., and Urbach, W., Echography using correlation techniques: choice of coding signal, *IEEE Trans. Ultrason. Ferroelect. Freq. Contr.*, 41, 579–587, 1994.

62. O'Donnell, M., Coded excitation system for improving the penetration of real-time phased-array imaging systems, *IEEE Trans. Ultrason. Ferroelect. Freq. Contr.*, 39, 341–351, 1992.

63. Rao, N.A.H.K., Investigation of a pulse compression technique for medical ultrasound: a simulation study, *Med. Biolog. Eng. Comput.*, 32, 181–188, 1994.

64. Misaridis, T.X., and Jensen, J.A., An effective coded excitation scheme based on a predistorted FM signal and an optimized digital filter, pp. 1589–1593 in: *1999 IEEE Ultrasonics Symp. Proc.*, 1999.

65. Misaridis, T.X., Pedersen, M.H., and Jensen, J.A., Clinical use and evaluation of coded excitation in B-mode images, pp. 1689–1693. in: *2000 IEEE Ultrasonics Symp. Proc.*, 2000. See also: Pedersen, M.H., Misaridis, T.X., and Jensen, J.A., Clinical evaluation of chirp-coded excitation in medical ultrasound, *Ultrasound Med. Biol.*, 29, 895–905, 2003.

66. Pollakowski, M., and Ermert, H., Chirp signal matching and signal power optimization in pulse-echo mode ultrasonic nondestructive testing, *IEEE Trans. Ultrason. Ferroelect. Freq. Contr.*, 41, 655–659, 1994.

67. Pollakowski, M., Ermert, H., Bernus, L. von., and Schmeidl, T., The optimum bandwidth of chirp signals in ultrasonic applications, *Ultrasonics*, 31, 417–420, 1993.

68. Kowatsch, M., and Stocker, H.R., Effect of Fresnel ripples on sidelobe suppression in low time-bandwidth product linear FM pulse compression, *IEEE Proc.*, 129, Part F, 41–44, 1982.

69. Harris, F.J., On the use of windows for harmonic analysis with the discrete Fourier transform, *Proc. IEEE.*, 66, 51–83, 1978.

70. Brenner, A.R., Eck, K., Wilhelm, W., and Noll, T.G., Medical ultrasound imaging using pulse compression and depth-dependent mismatched-filtering, pp. 35–40. in: *Acoustical Imaging*, Vol. 23, S. Lees, and L.A. Ferrari (Eds.), Plenum Press, New York, 1997.

71. Golay, M.J.E., Static multislit spectrometry and its application to the panoramic display of infrared spectra, *J. Opt. Soc. Am.*, 41, 468–472, 1951.

72. Golay, M.J.E., Complementary series, *IRE Trans. Inf. Theory*, IT-9, 82–87, 1961.

73. Tseng, C.-C, and Liu, C.L., Complementary sets of sequences, *IEEE Trans. Inf. Theory*, 18, 644–652, 1972.

74. Lee, B.B., and Furgason, E.S., High-speed digital Golay code flaw detection system, *Ultrasonics*, 21, 153–161, 1983.

75. Hayward, G., and Gorfu, Y., A digital hardware correlation system for fast ultrasonic data acquisition in peak power limited applications, *IEEE Trans. Ultrason. Ferroelect. Freq. Contr.*, 35, 800–808, 1988.

76. Hayward, G., and Gorfu, Y., Low power ultrasonic imaging using digital correlation, *Ultrasonics*, 27, 288–296, 1989.

77. Chiao, R.Y., and Thomas, L.J, Method and apparatus for ultrasonic beamforming using Golay-coded excitation, US patent 5,984,869, Nov. 1999 (filed April 1998).

78. Chiao, R.Y., and Thomas, L.J, Method and apparatus for ultrasonic synthetic transmit aperture imaging using orthogonal complementary codes, US patent 6,048,315, April 2000 (filed Sept. 1998).

79. Ultrasound technology update: B-flow. A new way of visualizing blood flow, GE Medical Systems Brochure, 1999.

80. Chiao, R.Y., Mo, L.Y., Hall, A.L., Bashford, G.R., Muzilla, D.J., Owen, C.A., Washburn, M., Miller, S.C., and Thomenius, K.E., B-mode blood flow imaging, Abstract #710, American Institute of Ultrasound in Medicine (AIUM), 44th Annual Convention, April 2–5, 2000.

81. Karaman, M., Li, P-C., and O'Donnell, M., Synthetic aperture imaging systems for small scale systems, *IEEE Trans. Ultrason. Ferroelect. Freq. Contr.*, 42, 429–442, 1995.

82. Burckhardt, C.B., Grandchamp, P.-A., and Hoffmann, H., An experimental 2 MHz synthetic aperture sonar system intended for medical use, *IEEE Trans. Sonics Ultrason.*, 21, 1–6, 1974.

83. Corl, P.D., and Kino, G.S., A real-time synthetic-aperture imaging system, pp. 341–355, in: *Acoustical Imaging*, Vol. 9, K.Y. Wang (Ed.), Plenum Press, New York, 1979.

84. Norton, S.J., Annular array imaging with full-aperture resolution, *J. Acoust. Soc. Am.*, 92, 3202–3206, 1992.

85. Cooley, C.R., Robinson, B.S., Synthetic focus imaging using partial data sets, pp. 1539–1542, in: *1994 IEEE Ultrasonics Symp. Proc.*, 1994.

86. Lockwood, G.R., and Foster, F.S., Design of sparse array imaging systems, pp. 1237–1243, in: *1995 IEEE Ultrasonics Symp. Proc.*, 1995.

87. Nikolov, S.I., and Jensen, J.J., Comparison between different encoding schemes for synthetic aperture imaging, pp. 1–12, in: *Ultrasonic Imaging and Signal Processing*, M.F. Insana, and W.F. Walker (Eds.), Proc. SPIE Vol. 4687, Medical Imaging, 2002.

88. O'Donnell, M., Eberle, M.J., Stephens, D.N., Litzza, J.L., San Vincente, K., and Shapo, B.M., Synthetic phased arrays for intraluminal imaging of coronary arteries, *IEEE Trans. Ultrason. Ferroelect. Freq. Contr.*, 44, 714–721, 1997.

89. Freeman, S., Li, P-C., and O'Donnell, M., Retrospective dynamic transmit focusing, *Ultrasonic Imaging*, 17, 173–196, 1995.

90. Lockwood, G.R., Talman, J.R., and Brunke, S.S., Real time 3-D ultrasound imaging using sparse synthetic aperture beamforming, *IEEE Trans. Ultrason. Ferroelect. Freq. Contr.*, 45, 980–988, 1998.

91. Inerfield, M., Lockwood, G.R., and Garverick, S.L., A sigma-delta-based synthetic aperture beamformer for real-time 3-D ultrasound, *IEEE Trans. Ultrason. Ferroelect. Freq. Contr.*, 49, 243–254, 2002.

92. Chiao, R.Y., Thomas, L.J., and Silverstein, S.D., Sparse array imaging with spatially-encoded transmits, pp. 1679–1682, in: *1997 IEEE Ultrasonics Symp. Proc.*, 1997.

93. Cosgrove, D.O., Why do we need contrast agents for ultrasound? *Clin. Radiol.*, 51 (suppl. 1), 1–4, 1996.

94. Gramiak, R., and Shah, P.M., Echocardiography of the aortic root, *Invest. Radiol.*, 3, 356–366, 1968.

95. Gramiak, R., The beginnings of ultrasound contrast, Ch. 1, pp. 1–7, in: *Ultrasound Contrast Agents*, B.B. Goldberg, (Ed.), Martin Dunitz, London, 1997. See also: Shah, P.M., Contrast echocardiography: a historical perspective, Chapter 1, pp. 3–9, in: *Advances in Echo Imaging Using Contrast Echo Enhancement*, N.C. Nanda, R. Schlief, and B.B. Goldberg (Eds.), 2nd Ed., Kluwer Academic Pub., Boston, 1997.

96. Goldberg, B.B., Liu, J-B., and Forsberg, F., Ultrasound contrast agents: a review, *Ultrasound Med. Biol.*, 20, 319–333, 1994.

97. Hoff, L., *Acoustic Characterization of Contrast Agents for Medical Ultrasound Imaging*, Kluwer Academic Publishers, Boston, 2001.

98. Frinking, P.J.A., Bouakaz, A., Kirkhorn, J., TenCate, F.J., and deJong, N., Ultrasound contrast imaging: currennt and new potential methods, *Ultrasound Med. Biol.*, 26, 965–975, 2000.

99. Shi, W.T., Forsberg, F., Tornes, A., Ostensen, J., and Goldberg, B.B., Destruction of contrast microbubbles and the association with inertial cavitation, *Ultrasound Med. Biol.*, 26, 1009–1019, 2000.

100. Church, C.C., The effects of an elastic solid surface layer on the radial pulsations of gas bubbles, *J. Acoust. Soc. Am.*, 97, 1510–1521, 1995.

101. Frinking, P.J.A., and de Jong, N., Acoustic modeling of shell-encapsulated gas bubbles, *Ultrasound Med. Biol.*, 24, 523–533, 1998.

102. Sboros, V., Moran, C.M., Pye, S.D., and McDicken, W.N., Contrast agent stability: a continuous B-Mode imaging approach, *Ultrasound Med. Biol.*, 27, 1367–1377, 2001.

103. Simpson, D.H., *Detecting and Imaging Microbubble Contrast Agents with Ultrasound*, PhD thesis, University of Toronto, 2000.

104. Leighton, T.G., *The Acoustic Bubble*, Academic Press, London, 1994.

105. Anderson, A.L., and Hampton, L.D., Acoustics of gas-bearing sediments. I. Background, *J. Acoust. Soc. Am.*, 67, 1865–1889, 1980.

106. de Jong, N., Physics of microbubble scattering, Chapter 3, pp. 39–64, in: *Advances in Echo Imaging Using Contrast Echo Enhancement*, N.C. Nanda, R. Schlief, and B.B. Goldberg (Eds.), 2nd Ed., Kluwer Academic Pub., Boston, 1997.

107. Chin, C.C., and Burns, P.N., Predicting the acoustic response of a microbubble population for contrast imaging in medical ultrasound, *Ultrasound Med. Biol.*, 26, 1293–1300, 2000.

108. Lauterborn, W., Numerical investigation of nonlinear oscillations of gas bubbles in liquids, *J. Acoust. Soc. Am.*, 59, 283–293, 1976.

109. Eatock, B.C., Nishi, R.Y., and Johnston, G.W., Numerical studies of the spectrum of low-intensity ultrasound scattered by bubbles, *J. Acoust. Soc. Am.*, 77, 1692–1701, 1985.

110. de Jong, N., Cornet, R., and Lancee, C.T., Higher harmonics of vibrating gas-filled microspheres. Part one: simulations, *Ultrasonics*, 32, 447–453, 1994.

111. Tucker, D.G., and Welsby, V.G., Ultrasonic monitoring of decompression, *Lancet*, 1, 1253, 1968.

112. Miller, D.L., Ultrasonic detection of resonant cavitation bubbles in a flow tube by their second-harmonic emissions, *Ultrasonics*, 19, 217–224, 1981.

113. Schrope, B., Newhouse, V.L., and Uhlendorf, V., Simulated capillary blood flow measurement using a nonlinear ultrasonic contrast agent, *Ultrasonic Imaging.*, 14, 134–158, 1992.

114. Schrope, B., and Newhouse, V.L., Second harmonic ultrasonic blood perfusion measurement, *Ultrasound Med. Biol.*, 19, 567–579, 1993.

115. Burns, P.N., Powers, J.E., and Fritzsch, T., Harmonic imaging: a new imaging and Doppler method for contrast enhanced ultrasound, *Radiology*, 185 (suppl.), 142 (Abstr.), 1992. See also the excellent review: Burns, P.N., Harmonic imaging with ultrasound contrast agents, *Clin. Radiol.*, 51 (suppl. 1), 50–55, 1996.

116. Powers, J.E., Burns, P.N., and Souquet, J., Imaging instrumentation for ultrasound contrast agents, Chapter 8, pp. 139–170, in: *Advances in Echo Imaging Using Contrast Echo Enhancement*, N.C. Nanda, R. Schlief, and B.B. Goldberg (Eds.), 2nd Ed., Kluwer Academic Pub., Boston, 1997.

117. Simpson, D.H., Burns, P.N., and Averkiou, A., Techniques for perfusion imaging with microbubble contrast agents, *IEEE Trans. Ultrason. Ferroelect. Freq. Contr.*, 48, 1483–1494, 2001.

118. Krishnan, S., Hamilton, J.D., and O'Donnell, M., Suppression of propagating second harmonic in non-linear imaging, pp. 1567–1579, in: *1997 IEEE Ultrasonics Symp. Proc.*, 1997.

119. Neppiras, E.A., Subharmonic and other low-frequency emission from bubbles in sound-irradiated liquids, *J. Acoust. Soc. Am.*, 46, 587–601, 1968.

120. Shi, W.T., and Forsberg, F.B., Ultrasonic characterization of the nonlinear properties of contrast microbubbles, *Ultrasound Med. Biol.*, 26, 93–104, 2000.

121. Shi, W.T., Forsberg, F.B., and Goldberg, B., Subharmonic imaging with gas-filled microbubbles [Abstract], *J. Acoust. Soc. Am.*, 101, 3139, 1997.

122. Shi, W.T., Forsberg, F., Hall, A.L., Chiao, R.Y., Liu, J.B., Miller, S., Thomenius, K.E., Wheatley, M.A., and Goldberg, B.B., Subharmonic imaging with microbubble contrast agents: initial results, *Ultrasonic Imaging*, 21, 79–94, 1999.

123. Forsberg, F., Shi, W.T., Chiao, R.Y., Hall, A.L., Lucas, S.D., and Goldberg, B.B., Implementation of subharmonic imaging, pp. 1673–1676, in: *1999 IEEE Ultrasonics Symp. Proc.*, 1999.

124. Shankar, P.M., Krishna, P.D., and Newhouse, V.L., Advantages of subharmonic over second harmonic backscatter for contrast-to-tissue echo enhancement, *Ultrasound Med. Biol.*, 24, 395–399, 1998.

125. Uhlendorf, V., and Hoffmann, C., Nonlinear acoustical response of coated microbubbles in diagnostic ultrasound, pp. 2559–1562, in: *1994 IEEE Ultrasonics Symp. Proc.*, 1994.

126. Hauff, P., Fritzsch, T., Reinhardt, M., Weitschies, W., Luders, F., Uhlendorf, V., and Heldmann D., Delineation of experimental liver tumors in rabbits by a new ultrasound contrast agent and stimulated acoustic emission, *Invest. Radiol.*, 32, 94–99, 1997.

127. Wei, K., Jayaweera, A.R., Firoozan, S., Linka, A., Skyba, D.M., and Kaul, S., Quantification of myocardial blood flow with ultrasound induced destruction of microbubbles administered as a constant venous infusion, *Circulation*, 97, 473–483, 1998.

128. Villanueva, F.S., Gertz, E.W., Csikari, M., Pulido, G., Fisher, D., and Sklenar, J., Detection of coronary artery stenosis with power Doppler imaging, *Circulation*, 103, 2624–2630, 2001.

129. Chapman, C.S., and Lazenby, J.C., Ultrasound imaging system employing phase inversion subtraction to enhance the image, US Patent 5,632,277, May 1997 (filed June 1996).

130. Hwang, J-J, and Simpson, D.H., Two pulse technique for ultrasonic harmonic imaging, US patent 5,951,478, Sept. 1999 (filed Dec. 1997).

131. Simpson, D.H., Chin, C.T., and Burns, P.N., Pulse inversion Doppler: a new method for detecting nonlinear echoes from microbubble contrast agents, *IEEE Trans. Ultrason. Ferroelect. Freq. Contr.*, 46, 372–382, 1999.

132. Jiang, P., Mao, Z., and Lazenby, J.C., A new tissue harmonic imaging scheme with better fundamental frequency cancellation and higher signal-to-noise ratio, pp. 1589–1594, in: *1998 IEEE Ultrasonics Symp. Proc.*, 1998.

133. Kompfner, R., and Lemons, R.A., Nonlinear acoustic microscope, *Appl. Phys. Lett.*, 28, 295–297, 1976.

134. Muir, T.G., Nonlinear effects in acoustic imaging, pp. 93–109, in Vol. 9: *Acoustical Imaging*, K.Y. Wang (Ed.), Plenum Press, New York, 1980. (Proc. 9th Int. Symp. Acoust. Imaging, Dec. 1979).

135. Ward, B., Baker, A.C., and Humphrey, V.F., Non-linear propagation applied to the improvement of lateral resolution in medical ultrasound scanners, pp. 965–968, in: *Proc. 1995 World Congress on Ultrasonics*, J. Herbertz (Ed.), Berlin, 1995.

136. Ward, B., Baker, A.C., and Humphrey, V.F., Nonlinear propagation applied to the improvement of resolution in diagnostic medical imaging, *J. Acoust. Soc. Am.*, 101, 143–154, 1997.

137. Christopher, T., Finite amplitude distortion-based inhomogeneous pulse echo imaging, *IEEE Trans. Ultrason. Ferroelect. Freq. Contr.*, 44, 125–139, 1997.

138. Averkiou, M., Roundhill, D.N., and Powers, J.E., A new imaging technique based on the nonlinear properties of tissues, pp. 1561–1566, in: *1997 IEEE Ultrasonics Symp. Proc.*, 1997.

139. Shapiro, R.S., Wagreich, J., Parsons, R.B., Stancato-Pasik, A., Yeh, H.C., and Lao, R., Tissue harmonic imaging sonography: evaluation of image quality compared with conventional sonography, *Am. J. Roentgenol.*, 171, 1203–1206, 1998.

140. Thomas, J.D., Rubin, D.N., Tissue harmonic imaging: why does it work? *J. Am. Soc. Echocardiogr*, 11, 803–808, 1998.

141. Tranquast, F., Grenier, N., Eder, V., and Purcelot, L., Clinical use of ultrasound tissue harmonic imaging, *Ultrasound Med. Biol.*, 25, 889–894, 1999.

142. Zemp, R.J., Tavakkoli, J, and Cobbold, R.S.C., Modeling of nonlinear ultrasound propagation in tissue from array transducers, *J. Acoust. Soc. Am.*, 113, 139–152, 2003.

143. Christopher, T., Experimental investigation of finite amplitude distortion-based, second harmonic pulse echo ultrasonic imaging, *IEEE Trans. Ultrason. Ferroelect. Freq. Contr.*, 45, 158–162, 1998.

144. Humphrey, V.F., Nonlinear propagation in ultrasonic fields: measurements, modelling and harmonic imaging, *Ultrasonics*, 38, 267–272, 2000.
145. Li, Y., and Zagzebski, J.A., Computer model for harmonic ultrasound imaging, *IEEE Trans. Ultrason. Ferroelect. Freq. Contr.* 47, 1000–1013, 2000.
146. Greenleaf, J.F., Computerized tomography with ultrasound, *Proc. IEEE*, 71, 330–337, 1983.
147. Born, M., and Wolf, E., *Principles of Optics*, 6th ed., Pergamon Press, Oxford, 1980.
148. Greenleaf, J.F., Johnson, S.A., Lee, S.L., Herman, G.T., and Wood, E.H., and Algebraic reconstruction of spatial distributions of acoustic absorption within tissue from their two-dimensional acoustic projections, pp. 591–603, in: *Acoustic Holography*, Vol. 5, P.S. Green (Ed.), Plenum Press, New York, 1974. (Proceedings of the 5th Int. Symp., on Acoustic Holography, July 1973).
149. Greenleaf, J.F., Johnson, S.A., Samayoa, W.F., and Duck, F.A., Algebraic reconstruction of spatial distributions of acoustic velocities in tissue from their time-of-flight profiles, pp. 71–90, in: *Acoustic Holography*, Vol. 6, N. Booth (Ed.), Plenum Press, New York, 1976. (Proceedings of the 6th Int. Symp., on Acoustic Holography, Feb. 1975).
150. Glover, G.H., and Sharp, J.C., Reconstruction of ultrasound propagation speed distributions in soft tissue: time-of-flight tomography, *IEEE Trans. Sonics Ultrasonics.*, 24, 229–234, 1977.
151. Glover, G.H., Computerized time-of-flight ultrasonic tomography for breast examination, *Ultrasound Med. Biol.*, 3, 117–127, 1977.
152. Deans, S.R., *The Radon Transform and Some of its Applications*, Wiley, New York, 1983.
153. Kak, A. C., and Slaney, M., *Principles of Computerized Tomographic Imaging*, IEEE Press, New York, 1988.
154. Bracewell, R.N., *Two-Dimensional Imaging*, Prentice Hall, Englewood Cliffs, NJ, 1995.
155. Bracewell, R.N., Strip integration in radio astronomy, *Aust. J. Phys.*, 9, 198–217, 1956.
156. Norton, S.J., Reconstruction of a reflectivity field from line integrals over circular paths, *J. Acoust. Soc. Am.*, 67, 853–863, 1980.
157. Norton, S.J., Reconstruction of a two-dimensional reflecting medium over a circular domain: exact solution, *J. Acoust. Soc. Am.*, 67, 1266–1273, 1980.
158. Norton, S.J., and Linzer, M., Ultrasonic reflectivity tomography: reconstruction with circular transducer arrays, *Ultrasonic Imaging*, 1, 154–184, 1979.
159. Hiller, D., and Ermert, H., Tomographic reconstruction of B-scan images, pp. 347–364, in: *Acoustic Imaging*, Vol. 10, P. Alias, and A.F. Metherell (Eds.), Plenum Press, New York, 1982.
160. Maderlechner, G., Hundt, E., Kronmuller, E., and Trautenberg, E., Experimental results of computerized ultrasound echo tomography, pp. 415–425, in: *Acoustic Imaging*, Vol. 10, P. Alias, and A.F. Metherell (Eds.), Plenum Press, New York, 1982.
161. Andreev, V.G., Dmitriev, V.N., Rudenko, O.V., and Sarvazyan, A.P., Remote generation of shear wave in soft tissue by pulsed radiation pressure [abstract], *J. Acoust. Soc. Am.*, 102, 3155, 1997.
162. Sarvazyan, A.P., Rudenko, O.V., Swanson, S.D., Fowlkes, J.B., and Emelianov, S.Y., Shear wave elasticity imaging: a new ultrasonic technology of medical diagnostics, *Ultrasound Med. Biol.*, 24, 1419–1436, 1998.
163. Wilson, L.S., and Robinson, D.E., Ultrasonic measurement of small displacements and deformation of tissue, *Ultrasonic Imaging*, 4, 71–82, 1982.

164. Dickinson, R.J., and Hill, C.R., Measurement of soft tissue motion using correlation between A-scans, *Ultrasound Med. Biol.*, 8, 263–271, 1982.
165. Gao, L., Parker, K.J., Lerner, R.M., and Levison, S.F., Imaging of the elastic properties of tissue, a review, *Ultrasound Med. Biol.*, 22, 959–977, 1996.
166. Ophir, J., Cespedes, I., Ponnekanti, H., Yazdi, Y., and Li, X., Elastography: a quantitatative method for imaging the elasticity of biological tissues, *Ultrasonic Imaging*, 13, 111–134, 1991.
167. Lerner, R.M., Parker, K.J., Holen, J., Gramiak, R., and Waag, R.C., Sono-elasticity: medical elasticity images derived from ultrasound signals in mechanically vibrated targets, pp. 317–327, in: *Acoustical Imaging*, Vol. 16, L.W. Kessler (Ed.), Plenum Press, New York, 1988.
168. Ophir, J., Cespedes, I., Garra, B., Ponnekanti, H., Huang, Y., and Maklad, N., Elastography: ultrasonic imaging of tissue strain and elastic modulus in vivo, *Eur. J. Ultrasound.*, 3, 49–70, 1996.
169. Ophir, J., Alam, K.A., Garra, B., Kallel, F., Konofagou, E.E., Krouskop, T.A., and Varghese, T., Elastography: ultrasonic estimation and imaging of the elastic properties of tissues, *Proc. Inst. Mech. Eng.: Part H: J. Eng. Med.*, 213, 203–233, 1999.
170. Muthupillai, R., Lomas, D.J., Rossman, P.J., Greenleaf, J.F., Manduca, A., and Ehman, R.L., Magnetic resonance elastography by direct visualization of propagating acoustic strain waves, *Science*, 269, 1854–1857, 1995.
171. Fowlkes, J.B., Emelianov, S.Y., Pipe, J.P., Skovorada, S.R., Carson, P.L., Adler, R.S., and Sarvazyan, A.P., Magnetic resonance imaging techniques for detection of elasticity variation, *Med. Phys.*, 22, 1771–1778, 1995.
172. Lewa, C.J., and de Certaines, J.D., MR imaging of viscoelastic properties, *J. Magn. Res. Imag.*, 5, 242–244, 1995.
173. Plewes, D.B., Betty, I., Urchuk, S.N., and Soutar, I., Visualizing tissue compliance with MR imaging, *J. Magn. Res. Imag.*, 5, 733–738, 1995.
174. Bercoff, J., Chaffai, S., Tanter, M., Sandrin, L., Catheline, S., Fink, M., Gennisson, J. L., and Meunier, M., *In vivo* breast tumor detection using transient elastography, *Ultrasound Med. Biol.*, 29, 1387–1396, 2003.
175. Sandrin, L., Tanter, M., Catheline, S., and Fink, M., Shear modulus imaging using 2D transient elastography, *IEEE Trans. Ultrason. Ferroelect. Freq. Contr.*, 49, 426–435, 2002.
176. Sandrin, L., Tanter, M., Gennisson, J.L., Catheline, S., and Fink, M., Shear elasticity probe for soft tissues with 1D transient elastography, *IEEE Trans. Ultrason. Ferroelect. Freq. Contr.*, 49, 436–446, 2002.
177. Nightingale, K., Soo, M.S., Nightingale, R., and Trahey, G., Acoustic radiation force impulse imaging: in vivo demonstration of clinical feasibility, *Ultrasound Med. Biol.*, 28, 227–235, 2002.
178. Bercoff, J., Tanter, and Fink, M., Supersonic shear imaging: a new technique for soft tissue elasticity mapping, *IEEE Trans. Ultrason. Ferroelect. Freq. Contr.*, 51, 396–409, 2004.
179. Fatimi, M., and Greenleaf, J.F., Ultrasound-stimulated vibro-acoustic spectrography, *Science*, 280, 82–85, 1998.
180. Fatimi, M., and Greenleaf, J.F., Application of radiation force in noncontact measurement of the elastic parameters, *Ultrasonic Imaging*, 21, 147–154, 1999.
181. Konofagou, E. E., and Hynynen, K., Localized harmonic motion imaging: theory, simulations and experiments, *Ultrasound Med. Biol.*, 29, 1405–1413, 2003.

182. Bohs, L.N., Geiman, B.J., Anderson, M.E., Breit, S.M., and Trahey, G.E., Ensemble tracking for 2D vector velocity measurement: experimental and initial clinical results, *IEEE Trans. Ultrason. Ferroelect. Freq. Contr.*, 45, 912–924, 1998.

183. Bohs, L.N., Geiman, B.J., Anderson, M.E., Gebhart, S.C., and Trahey, G.E., Speckle tracking for multi-dimensional flow estimation. *Ultrasonics*, 38, 369–375, 2000.

184. Robinson, D.E., Chen, F., and Wilson, L.S., Measurement of velocity of propagation from ultrasonic pulse-echo data, *Ultrasound Med. Biol.*, 8, 413–420, 1982.

185. Bertrand, M., Meuniere, J., Doucet, M., and Ferland, G., Ultrasonic biomechanical strain gauge, based on speckle tracking, pp. 859–863, in: *1989 IEEE Ultrasonics Symp. Proc.*, 1989.

186. Meuniere, J., Bertrand, M., Mailloux, G.E., and Petitclerc, R., Local myocardial deformation computed from speckle motion, pp. 133–136, in: *1988 IEEE Computers in Cardiology*, 1988.

187. O'Donnell, M., Skovoroda, A.R., Shapo, B.M., and Emelianov, S.Y., Internal displacement and strain imaging using ultrasonic speckle tracking, *IEEE Trans. Ultrason. Ferroelect. Freq. Contr.*, 41, 314–325, 1994.

188. Lubinski, M.A., Emelianov, S.Y., and O'Donnell, M., Speckle tracking methods for ultrasonic elasticity imaging using short-time correlation, *IEEE Trans. Ultrason. Ferroelect. Freq. Contr.*, 46, 82–96, 1999.

189. Ledoux, L.A.F., Willigers, J.M., Brands, P.J., and Hoeks, A.P.G., Experimental verification of the correlation behavior of analytic ultrasound radiofrequency signals received from moving structures, *Ultrasound Med. Biol.*, 24, 1383–1396, 1998.

190. Cohn, N.A., Emelianov, S.Y., Lubinski, M.A., and O'Donnell, M., An elasticity microscope. Part I: methods, *IEEE Trans. Ultrason. Ferroelect. Freq. Contr.*, 44, 1304–1319, 1997.

191. Cohn, N.A., Emelianov, S.Y., and O'Donnell, M., An elasticity microscope. Part II: experimental results, *IEEE Trans. Ultrason. Ferroelect. Freq. Contr.*, 44, 1320–1331, 1997.

192. Cohn, N.A., Kim, B.S., Erkamp, R.Q., Mooney, D.J., Emelianov, S.Y., Skovoroda, A.R., and O'Donnell, M., High-resolution elasticity imaging for tissue engineering, *IEEE Trans. Ultrason. Ferroelect. Freq. Contr.*, 47, 956–966, 2000.

193. Picinbono, B., On instantaneous amplitude and phase of signals, *IEEE Trans. Sig. Processing*, 45, 552–560, 1997.

194. Konofagou, E.E., Varghese, T., Ophir, J., and Alam, S.K., Power spectral strain estimators in elastography, *Ultrasound Med. Biol.*, 25, 1115–1129, 1999.

195. Varghese, T., Konofagou, E.E., Ophir, J., Alam, S.K., and Bilgen, M., Direct strain estimation in elastography using spectral cross-correlation, *Ultrasound Med. Biol.*, 26, 1525–1537, 2000.

196. Konofagou, E., and Ophir, J., A new elasographic method for estimation and imaging of latreral displacements, lateral strains, corrected axial strains and Poisson's ratios in tissue, *Ultrasound Med. Biol.*, 24, 1183–1199, 2000.

197. Konofagou, E., Garra, B., and Ophir, J., *IEEE Trans. Ultrason. Ferroelect. Freq. Contr.*, 48, Frontispiece (No. 3), May 2001.

198. Yamakoshi, J., Sato, and Sato, T., Ultrasonic imaging of internal vibration of soft tissue under forced vibration, *IEEE Trans. Ultrason. Ferroelect. Freq. Contr.*, 37, 45–53, 1990.

199. Lerner, R.M., Huang, S.R., and Parker, K.J., Tissue response to mechanical vibrations for "sonoelasticity imaging," *Ultrasound Med. Biol.*, 16, 231–239, 1990.

200. Parker, K.J., Huang, S.R., Musulin, R.A., and Lerner, R.M., "Sonoelasticity" images derived from ultrasound signals in mechanically vibrated tissues, *Ultrasound Med. Biol.*, 16, 241–246, 1990.

201. Oestreicher, H.L., Field and impedance of an oscillating sphere in a viscoelastic medium with an application to biophysics, *J. Acoust. Soc. Am.*, 23, 707–714, 1951.

202. von Gierke, H.E., Oestreicher, H.L., Franke, E.K., Parrack, H.O., and von Wittern, W.W., Physics of vibration in living tissue, *J. Appl. Physiol.*, 4, 886–900, 1952.

203. Catheline, S., Wu, F., and Fink, M., A solution to diffraction biases in sonoelasticity: the acoustic impulse technique, *J. Acoust. Soc. Am.*, 105, 2941–2950, 1999.

204. Foster, F.S., Pavlin, C.J., Harasiewicz, K.A., Christopher, D.A., and Turnbull, D.H., Advances in ultrasound biomicroscopy, *Ultrasound Med. Biol.*, 26, 1–27, 2000.

205. Foster, F.S., Ryan, L.K., and Turnbull, D.H., Characterization of lead zirconate titanate (PZT) ceramics for use in miniature high frequency (30–80 MHz) transducers, *IEEE Trans. Ultrason. Ferroelect. Freq. Contr.*, 38, 446–453, 1991.

206. Zipparo, M.J., Shung, K.K., and Shrout, T.R., Piezoceramics for high frequency (20–100 MHz) single element imaging transducers, *IEEE Trans. Ultrason. Ferroelect. Freq. Contr.*, 44, 1038–1048, 1997.

207. Lethiecq, M., Berson, M., Feuillard, G., and Patat, F., Principles and applications of high-frequency medical imaging, Chapter 2, pp. 39–102, in: *Advances in Acoustic Microscopy*, Vol. 2, A. Briggs and W. Arnold (Eds.), Plenum Press, 1996.

208. Ritter, T.A., Shrout, T.R., and Shung, K.K., Development of high frequency medical ultrasound arrays, pp. 1127–1133, in: *2001 IEEE Ultrasonics Symp.*, 2001.

209. Ritter, T.A., Shrout, T.R., Tutwiler, R., and Shung, K.K., A 30-MHz piezocomposite ultrasound array for medical imaging applications, *IEEE Trans. Ultrason. Ferroelect. Freq. Contr.*, 49, 217–230, 2002.

210. Morton, C.E., and Lockwood, G.R., Design of a 40 MHz annular array, pp. 1135–1138, in: *2001 IEEE Ultrasonics Symp.*, 2001.

211. Tutwiler, R.L., Stitt, J.P., Ritter, T.A., Shung, K.K., Hackenberger, W.S., Jiang, X.N., and Rehrig, P.W., Precision mechanically scanned HF ultrasound arrays, pp. 873–876, in: *2003 IEEE Ultrasonics Symp.*, 2003.

212. Sokolov, S.Ya., The ultra-acoustic microscope, *Zh. Tekh. Fiz.*, 19, 271–273, 1949.

213. Sokolov, S.Ya., The ultrasonic microscope [in Russian], *Dokl. Akad. Nauk. SSSR*, 64, 333–335, 1949. See also: *Selected Papers on Scanning Acoustic Microscopy*, B.T. Khuri-Yakub and C.F. Quate (Eds.), SPIE Press, 1992.

214. Dunn, F., and Fry, W.J., Ultrasonic absorption microscope, *J. Acoust. Soc. Am.*, 31, 632–633, 1959.

215. Korpel, A., Kessler, L.W., and Palermo, P.R., Acoustic microscope operating at 100 MHz, *Nature*, 232, 110–111, 1971.

216. Kessler, L.W., Korpel, A., and Palermo, P.R., Simultaneous acoustic and optical microscopy of biological specimens, *Nature*, 239, 111–112, 1972.

217. Kessler, L.W., and Yuhas, D.E., Acoustic microscopy, 1979, *Proc. IEEE*, 67, 526–536, 1979.

218. Lemons, R.A., and Quate, C.F., A scanning acoustic microscope, pp. 18–21, in: *Ultrasonics Symp. Proc.*, 1973.

219. Lemons, R.A., and Quate, C.F., Acoustic microscope, scanning version, *Appl. Phys. Lett.*, 24, 163–165, 1974.

220. Quate, C.F., Atalar, A., and Wickramasinghe, H.K., Acoustical microscopy with mechanical scanning, a review, *Proc. IEEE*, 67, 1092–1114, 1979.

221. Briggs, A., *Acoustic Microscopy*, Oxford University Press, Oxford, 1992.

222. Foster, J.S., and Rugar, D., Low-temperature acoustic microscopy, *IEEE Trans. Sonics Ultrason.*, 32, 139–151, 1985.

223. Muha, M.S., Moulthrop, A.A., Kozlowski, G.C., and Hadimioglu, B., Acoustic microscoy at 15.3 GHz in pressurized superfluid helium, *Appl. Phys. Lett.*, 56, 1019–1021, 1990.

224. Sherar, M.D., Noss, M.B., and Foster, F.S., Ultrasound scatter microscopy images the internal structure of living tumour spheroids, *Nature*, 330, 493–495, 1987.

225. Sherar, M.D., Starkoski, B.G., Taylor, W.B., and Foster, F.S., A 100 MHz B-scan backscatter microscope, *Ultrasonic Imaging*, 11, 95–105, 1989.

226. Knapik, D.A., Starkoski, B., Pavlin, C.J., and Foster, F.S., A 100–200 MHz ultrasound biomicroscope, *IEEE Trans. Ultrason. Ferroelect. Freq. Contr.*, 47, 1540–1549, 2000.

227. Pavlin, C.J., Sherar, M.D., and Foster, F.S., Subsurface ultrasound microscopic imaging of the intact eye, *Ophthalmology*, 97, 244–250, 1990.

228. Pavlin, C.J., and Foster, F.S., *Ultrasound Biomicroscopy of the Eye*, Springer-Verlag, New York, 1994.

229. Foster, F.S., Pavlin, C.J., Lockwood, G.R., Ryan, L.K., Harasiewicz, K.A., Berube, L., and Rauth, A.M., Principles and applications of backscatter microscopy, *IEEE Trans. Ultrason. Ferroelect. Freq. Contr.*, 40, 608–617, 1993.

230. Silverman, R.H., Reinstein, D.Z., Lizzi, F.L., and Coleman, D.J., Ultrasound signal processing for characterization and enhanced biometry of the cornea, pp. 346–355, in: *Ultrasonic Imaging and Signal Processing*, M.F. Insana, and K.K. Shung (Eds.), Proc. SPIE vol. 4325, Medical Imaging, 2001.

231. Reinstein, D.Z., Silverman, R.H., Raevsky, T., Simoni, G.J., Lloyd, H.O., Najafi, D.J., Rondeau, M.J., and Coleman, D.J., Arc-scanning very high-frequency digital ultrasound for 3D pachymetric mapping of the corneal epithelium and stroma in laser in situ keratomileusis, *J. Refract. Surg.*, 16, 414–430, 2000.

232. Alexander, R., and Miller, D.L., Determining skin thickness with pulsed ultrasound, *J. Invest. Dermatol.*, 72, 17–19, 1979.

233. Dines, K.A., Sheets, P.W., Brink, J.A., Hanke, C.W., Condra, K.A., Clendenon, J.L., Goss, S.A., Smith, D.J., and Franklin, T.D., High frequency ultrasonic imaging of skin: experimental results, *Ultrasonic Imaging*, 6, 408–434, 1984.

234. Serup, J., Ten years' experience with high-frequency ultrasound examination of the skin: development and refinement of technique and equipment, pp. 41–54, in: P. Altmeyer, S. El Gammal, and K. Hoffmann (Eds.), *Ultrasound in Dermatology*, Springer Verlag, Berlin, 1992.

235. Passmann, C., and Ermert, H., A 100-MHz ultrasound imaging system for dermatologic and ophthalmologic diagnostics, *IEEE Trans. Ultrason. Ferroelect. Freq. Contr.*, 43, 545–552, 1996.

236. Turnbull, D.H., Starkoski, B.G., Harasiewicz, K.A., Semple, J.L., From, L., Gupta, A.K., Sauder, D.N., and Foster, F.S., A 40–100 MHz B-scan ultrasound backscatter microscope for skin imaging, *Ultrasound Med. Biol.*, 21, 79–89, 1995.

237. Yokosawa, K., Shinomura, R., Sano, S., Ito, Y., Ishikawa, S., and Sato, Y., 120 MHz ultrasound probe for tissue imaging, *Ultrasonic Imag.*, 18, 231–239, 1996.

238. Kaspar, K., Vogt, M., Ermert, H., Altmeyer, P., and El Gammal, S., 100-MHz-Sonographie zur Dar-stellung des Stratum corneum an der Palmarhaut nach Anwendung verschiedener Externa, *Ultraschall in Med.*, 20, 110–114, 1999.

239. Roelandt, J.R.T.C., and Bom, N., The history of intravascular ultrasound, pp. 11–15, Chapter 2, in: *Intravascular Ultrasound*, R. Erbel, J.R.T.C. Roelandt, J. Ge, and G. Gorge (Eds.), Martin Dunitz, London, 1998.

240. Wild, J.J., and Reid, J.M., Progress in the techniques of soft tissue examination by 15MC pulsed ultrasound, pp. 30–48, in: *Ultrasound in Biology and Medicine*, E. Kelly (Ed.), (Proc. of 1955 Symp. at Allerton Park, Illinois), Am. Inst. Biological Sciences, Washington, 1957.

241. Cieszynski, M., Intracardiac method for investigation of structure of the heart with the aid of ultrasonics, *Archiwum Immunologi i Terapii Doswiadezalnej*, 8, 551–557, 1960.

242. Omoto, R., Tsunemoto, M., Hirose, M., Muroi, T., Hori, M., Saigusa, M., Kimoto, S., and Uchida, R., Ultrasonic tomography of the heart with ultrasonic intravenous probe, pp. 296–297, in: *Digest of papers, 6th Int. Conf. Med. Biolog. Eng.*, Tokyo, 1965.

243. Omoto, R., Ultrasonic tomography of the heart: an intracardiac scan method, *Ultrasonics*, 5, 80–83, 1967.

244. Wells, P.N.T., Developments in medical ultrasonics, *World Medical Electronics*, 4, 272–277, 1966.

245. ten Hoff, H., Korbijn, A., Smit, T.H., Kinkhamer, J.F.F., and Bom, N., Imaging artifacts in mechanically driven ultrasound catheters, *Int. J. Cardiac Imaging*, 4, 195–199, 1989.

246. Bom, N., Lancee, C.T., and van Egmond, F.C., An ultrasonic intracardiac scanner, *Ultrasonics*, 10, 72–76, 1972.

247. Schulze-Clewing, J., Eberle, M.J., and Stephens, D.N., Miniaturized circular array, pp. 1253–1254, in: *2000 IEEE Ultrasonics Symp.*, 2000.

248. O'Donnell, M., Eberle, M.J., Stephens, D.N., Litzza, J.L., Shapo, B.M., Crowe, J.R., Choi, C.D., Chen, J.J., Muller, D.M.W., Kovach, J.A., Lederman, R.L., Ziegenbein, R.C., Wu, C.C., SanVincente, K., and Bleam, D., Catheter arrays: can intravascular ultrasound make a difference in managing coronary artery disease? pp. 1447–1456, in: *1997 IEEE Ultrasonics Symp.*, 1997.

249. Black, W.C., and Stephens, D.N., CMOS chip for invasive ultrasound imaging, *IEEE J. Solid State Circuits*, 29, 1381–1387, 1994.

250. Gronningsaeter, A., Angelsen, B.A.J., Heimdal, A., and Torp, H.G., Vessel wall detection and blood noise reduction in intravascular ultrasound imaging, *IEEE Trans. Ultrason. Ferroelect. Freq. Contr.*, 43, 359–369, 1996.

251. Evans, A.N., and Nixon, M.S., Biased motion-adaptive temporal filtering for speckle reduction in echocardiography, *IEEE Trans Med. Imaging.*, 15, 39–50, 1996.

252. Hibi, K., Takagi, A., Zhang, X., Teo, T-J., Bonneau, H.N., Yock, P.G., and Fitzgerald, P.J., Feasibility of a novel blood noise reduction algorithm to enhance reproducibility of ultra-high-frequency intravascular ultrasound images, *Circulation*, 102, 1657–1663, 2000.

253. Birgelen, C. von, Mallus, M.T., and Serruys, P.W., Three-dimensional intravascular ultrasound reconstruction and quantification: a valuable approach for clinical decision-making, Chapter 10, pp. 177–203, in: *Intravascular Ultrasound Imaging in Coronary Artery Disease*, R.J. Siegel (Ed.), Marcel Dekker, New York, 1998.

254. Birgelen, C. von, de Feyter, P.J., and Roelandt, J.R.T.C., Three-dimensional reconstruction of intracoronary ultrasound, pp. 51–60, Chapter 6, in: *Intravascular Ultrasound*, R. Erbel, J.R.T.C. Roelandt, J. Ge, and G. Gorge (Eds.), Martin Dunitz, London, 1998.

255. Light, E.D., Idriss, S.F., Wolf, P.D., and Smith, S.W., Real-time three-dimensional intracardaic echocardiography, *Ultrasound Med. Biol.*, 27, 1177–1183, 2001.

256. Smith, S.W., Light, E.D., Idriss, S.F., Lee, W., Dixon-Tullch, E., and Wolf, P.D., Real-time three dimensional intracardiac echo for guidance of cardiac ablation, pp. 1307–1310, in: *2001 IEEE Ultrasonics Symp.*, 2001.

257. Lee, W., and Smith, S.W., Intracardiac catheter 2-D arrays on a silicon substrate, *IEEE Trans. Ultrason. Ferroelect. Freq. Contr.*, 49, 415–425, 2002.

258. Lee, C.K., and Benkeser, P.J., Investigation of a forward-looking IVUS imaging transducer, pp. 691–694, in: *1991 IEEE Ultrasonics Symp.*, 1991.

259. Busse, L.J., and Dietz, D.R., Sparse circular array methods, performance and application to intravascular imaging, pp. 641–644, in: *1991 IEEE Ultrasonics Symp.*, 1991.

260. Evans, J.L., Ng, K-H, Vonesh, M.J., Kramer, B.L., Meyers, S.N., Mills, T.A., Kane, B.J., Aldrich, W.N., Jang, Y-T., Yock, P.G., Rold, M.D., Roth, S.I., and McPherson, D.D., Arterial imaging with a new forward-looking intravascular ultrasound catheter, I: initial studies, *Circulation*, 89, 712–717, 1994.

261. Liang, D.H., and Hu, B.S., Forward-looking catheters, *Seminars Intervent. Cardiol.*, 2, 75–81, 1997.

262. Gatzoulis, L., Watson, R.J., Jordan, L.B., Pye, S.D., Anderson, T., Uren, N., Salter, D.M., Fox, K.A.A., and McDicken, W.N., Three-dimensional forward-viewing intravascular ultrasound imaging in human arteries in vitro, *Ultrasound Med. Biol.*, 27, 969–982, 2001.

263. Wang, Y., Stephens, D.N., and O'Donnell, M., A forward-viewing ring-annular array for intravascular imaging, pp. 1573–1576, in: *2001 IEEE Ultrasonics Symp.*, 2001.

264. Wang, Y., Stephens, D.N., and O'Donnell, M., Optimizing the beam pattern of a forward-viewing ring-annular ultrasound array for intravascular imaging, *IEEE Trans. Ultrason. Ferroelect. Freq. Contr.*, 49, 1652–1664, 2002.

265. Wang, Y., and O'Donnell, M., Compounding for a forward viewing ring-annular ultrasound array system, *Ultrasonic Imaging*, 23, 147–160, 2001.

266. Crowe, J.R., Hamilton, J.D., Stephens, D.N., Wang, Y., and O'Donnell, M., Modified weighting method for forward-looking ring-annular arrays, *Ultrasonic Imaging*, 23, 19–38, 2001.

267. Li, W., Lancee, C.T., Cespedes, E.I., van der Steen, A.F.W., and Bom, N., Decorrelation of intravascular echo signals: potentials for blood velocity estimation, *J. Acoust. Soc. Am.*, 102, 3785–3794, 1997.

268. Li, W., Lancee, C.T., van der Steen, A.F.W., Cespedes, E.I., and Bom, N., Blood flow imaging and volume flow quantitation with intravascular ultrasound, *Ultrasound Med. Biol.*, 24, 203–214, 1998.

269. van der Steen, A.F.W., Cespedes, E.I., Carlier, S.G., Mastik, F., Lupotti, F., Borsboom, J.M.G., Li, W., Serruys, P.W., and Bom, N., Flow estimation using an intravascular imaging catheter, *Ultrasonics*, 38, 363–368, 2000.

270. Lancee, C.T., Cespedes, E.I., and van der Steen, A.F.W., Decorrelation characteristics of transverse blood flow along an intravascular array catheter, *IEEE Trans. Ultrason. Ferroelect. Freq. Contr.*, 47, 1582–1592, 2000.

9

Principles of Doppler Ultrasound

9.1 Historical Background

In a paper given in 1842 before the Royal Bohemian Society of Learning, Christian Doppler (1803–1853) [1] proposed that when a wave source is moving with respect to an observer, the frequency perceived by the observer will differ from that transmitted by an amount proportional to the relative velocity and the transmitted frequency. A full account of this work was published in the society's proceedings in the following year [2]. Three years later a young Dutch scientist confirmed the application of this theory to acoustic waves. As recounted by Jonkman [3], Buys-Ballot (1817–1890) arranged for a locomotive to transport brass horn players through a station where musicians recorded the change in pitch. Within the experimental errors, the results corresponded well with the predictions made by Doppler's theory.

The first recorded observations concerning the Doppler effect at ultrasonic frequencies appear to be those made just prior to the end of World War I. This work, conducted in the United States off Key West in the Gulf of Mexico, established ultrasonic transmission over a 3 km path and showed that a pronounced change in the received frequency was caused by a moving target. It may not have been appreciated by those conducting the experiments that measurement of the frequency shift could provide a means for measuring the velocity component of the target in the beam direction. At about the same time, Chilowski and Langevin [4], working in France, filed a U.S. patent relating to ship and submarine motion measurement methods that clearly described the underlying principles. Filed at the U.S. Patent office in May 1917, the patent contains the following statement: "The relative motion of the obstacle and the observation post may be determined by applying Doppler's method, that is to say, by observing the change in frequency due to the movement." In Chilowski's subsequent patent [5] filed in 1924, specific methods are described for measuring the speed of a vessel by beams projecting from the bottom of the vessel onto the underlying sea bed, measuring the backscattered frequency, and using a heterodyne method for determining the frequency shift.

Lynnworth [6], in a review of ultrasonic flow measurement methods, lists eight categories of principles and methods, and this includes transit-time, Doppler, correlation [7], and deflection techniques. Of these, the transit-time and Doppler methods have been most widely used for biomedical flow estimation. In the transit-time method, which makes no use of the Doppler effect, the difference in transit time or phase between acoustic waves propagated upstream and downstream enables the fluid velocity to be determined. Although the first practical *noninvasive* transit-time method for fluid flow measurement was described by Kamus et al. [10] in 1954, it should be noted that the method is based on an idea that was disclosed many years earlier. For example, in 1928 Rutten [8] described a means based on transducers that were mounted within the flow field. Even earlier (1921), Kunze [9] described a transit-time technique for measuring air velocity. Subsequent developments, along with the availability of improved electronic techniques, resulted in their widespread use for industrial flow measurements [6] as well as for blood flow estimation.

Satomura et al. [11], working at Osaka University, first described in-vivo Doppler signal measurements. Their results[1], as presented in 1956, provided convincing evidence that the signals were created by moving tissue structures. They pointed out the potential of the method in the diagnosis of cardiovascular abnormalities [13]. Using a 3 MHz continuous wave ultrasound source and system (Fig. 9.1), they observed and recorded Doppler-shifted ultrasonic return echoes from moving structures in the heart. The externally placed transducer consisted of an annular structure with separate transmit and receive elements.

In subsequent experiments, first described in 1958, Satomura reported the presence of Doppler-shifted ultrasound signals from blood vessels [15–17]. In fact, he and Kaneko performed a frequency analysis of these signals and showed that quite broad ranges of frequencies were present, ranging up to several kilohertz. With the 5 MHz system illustrated in Fig. 9.2, they measured Doppler signals from a number of vessels and showed that the Doppler frequency was related to the blood velocity. Satomura and Kaneko correctly anticipated that the technique would be of clinical value in assessing arteriosclerosis. However, they were mistaken in suggesting that the observed Doppler-shifted signals arose primarily from reflections of the incident ultra-

---

1. Dr. Kaneko, a research colleague of Dr. Satomura, has written an authoritative account of the early stages in the development of the Doppler flowmeter [12].

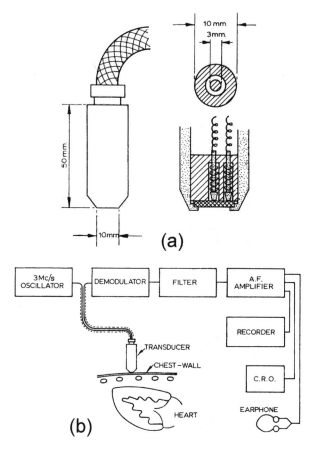

Figure 9.1 Transducer (a) and schematic (b) of system used by Satomura to show how movement of the cardiac structures could be detected by the ultrasonic Doppler effect. (Reproduced, with permission of the International Federation for Medical & Biological Engineering, from Satomura et al. [14], © 1961 IFMBE.)

sound from regions of turbulent flow in the vessel. It was not until the early 1960s that the origin of the observed Doppler signals from within blood vessels was correctly identified. In 1962 Kato and his colleagues [18] offered conclusive evidence that the primary cause, at least for the low-hematocrit blood used in their experiments, was due to red blood cell (RBC) scattering. Subsequently, Reid et al. [19,20] demonstrated the same was true for normal-hematocrit blood and also showed that the backscattered power was proportional to the fourth power of the frequency, in agreement with the predicted behavior of Rayleigh scatterers.

Like the design used by Satomura, early CW Doppler ultrasound systems had separate transmit and receive transducer elements and did not have directional sensing capabilities. Consequently, if the velocity in a vessel reversed during part of the cardiac cycle, as it does in certain vessels, the reverse veloc-

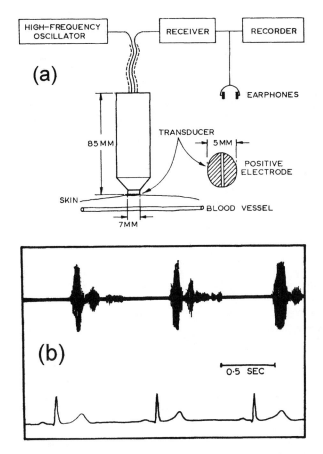

Figure 9.2 Doppler blood flow velocity measurement system as first described by Satomura. (a) System. (b) Recording from the radial artery along with the ECG waveform. (Reproduced, with permission of the International Federation for Medical & Biological Engineering, from Satomura et al. [14], © 1961 IFMBE.)

ity signal would appear incorrectly as a forward flow signal. The importance of developing methods for extracting the flow direction was quickly recognized. Kato and Izumi [21] in Japan were the first (1966) to describe a method based on the use of the heterodyne technique. Subsequently (1967), McLeod [22], working at Cornell University, described a Doppler system that used phase-quadrature demodulation for extracting the forward and reverse flow velocity components.

9.2 Ultrasonic Transit-Time and Phase-Delay Methods

Transit-time and phase-delay methods are based on the change in the apparent speed of propagation caused by motion of the propagation medium with

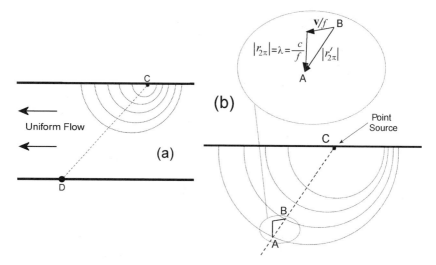

Figure 9.3 Snapshot showing the idealized CW wavefronts produced by a point source in a medium with a uniform flow velocity. (a) Effect of flow on the wavefronts from a stationary source at C. A stationary observer at D would find that the wavefront separation increases with flow velocity. (b) Analysis of the wavefront crest separation as seen by a stationary observer.

respect to the source and receiver.[2] These methods, unlike Doppler methods, do not require the presence of moving scatterers: they rely on the change in propagation caused by the moving medium. In the case of pulse transmission, it is the upstream/downstream transit-time difference that enables the fluid flow to be determined. On the other hand, for a CW source, it is the change in phase of the received signal due to propagation in the two directions that provides the flow information. In fact, the first practical flowmeter, as described by Kamus et al. [10], used this technique.

Franklin et al. [23,24], whose publications concerning transit-time and phase-delay measurement methods started in 1959, pioneered the development of pulsed transit-time ultrasonic techniques for animal blood flow studies. About the same time, Herrick and Anderson [25], using a CW phase-delay method, reported the measurement of blood flow in animals using the phase-delay method. Also proposed by Franklin [26] was the use of frequency modulation as a means of avoiding the need to switch between the pairs of elements.

The effect of uniform flow on the wavefronts is illustrated in Fig. 9.3a, where the pressure wave created by the point source can be expressed as

2. Because flow velocity measurements are a major application of both ultrasonic Doppler and transit-time flow velocity measurement techniques, it seems appropriate to discuss them in this chapter, even though, as previously noted, the Doppler effect is not involved in transit-time methods.

$$p(\mathbf{r};t) = \frac{A}{r} e^{j(\omega t - \mathbf{k} \cdot \mathbf{r})},$$

and the wavenumber vector $\mathbf{k}$ is taken to be normal to the wavefront in the propagation direction. A downstream observer at the point D will see crests that are further apart, while the opposite will be true for an upstream observer. Next, an expression will be obtained that relates the upstream–downstream phase difference over a path length L to the flow velocity.

If the medium is stationary, the crests will be separated by $r_{2\pi} = \lambda = c/f$. However, for a medium flowing with a uniform velocity $\mathbf{v}$, adjacent crests will be separated by a distance that generally differs from λ. As illustrated in Fig. 9.3b, the crest separations are now given by

$$\mathbf{r}'_{2\pi} = \mathbf{r}_{2\pi} + \mathbf{v}/f = \mathbf{r}_{2\pi} + \mathbf{v}\lambda/c.$$

By evaluating the modulus squared and noting that $r_{2\pi} = \lambda$, we obtain

$$\lambda^2 = v^2 \lambda^2/c^2 + (\mathbf{r}'_{2\pi})^2 - 2\mathbf{v} \cdot \mathbf{r}'_{2\pi} \lambda/c.$$

Noting that $\mathbf{v} \cdot \mathbf{r}'_{2\pi} = vr'_{2\pi}\cos\theta$, where θ is the angle between $\mathbf{r}'_{2\pi}$ and $\mathbf{v}$, the crest separation can be expressed as

$$|\mathbf{r}_{2\pi}|_\theta = \lambda \left(\varepsilon_M \cos\theta + \sqrt{1 - \varepsilon_M^2 \sin^2\theta} \right),$$

where $\varepsilon_M = v/c$ is the Mach number. If the transmission is in the opposite direction, then

$$|\mathbf{r}_{2\pi}|_{\pi-\theta} = \lambda \left(\varepsilon_M \cos(\pi-\theta) + \sqrt{1 - \varepsilon_M^2 \sin^2(\pi-\theta)} \right)$$
$$= -\lambda \left[\varepsilon_M \cos\theta - \sqrt{1 - \varepsilon_M^2 \sin^2\theta} \right].$$

It therefore follows that the upstream–downstream phase difference over a path length L is given by

(9.1)
$$\Delta\varphi = \frac{2\pi L \{ r_{2\pi}|_\theta - r_{2\pi}|_{\pi-\theta} \}}{\lambda^2} = \frac{4\pi v}{c_o} \frac{L}{\lambda} \cos\theta.$$

Thus, the change in phase is directly proportional to the velocity component in the measurement direction.

To account for a non-uniform flow velocity profile over the measurement path, we assume the transmission of an acoustic pulse and that the upstream–downstream transit-time difference is determined using the transducer arrangement shown in Fig. 9.4a. Over an incremental distance ds, the travel time for a pulse is given by $dt = ds/(c_o \pm v\cos\theta)$, so that the total transit time is given by

$$t = \int_C^D \frac{1}{c_o (1 + \varepsilon_M \cos\theta)} ds \approx \int_C^D \frac{1}{c_o} (1 - \varepsilon_M \cos\theta) ds,$$

for $\varepsilon_M \ll 1$. Consequently, the upstream–downstream transit-time difference is

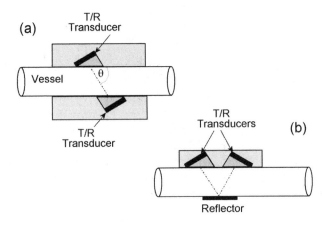

Figure 9.4 Transit-time transducer schemes for volume flow estimation. (a) Direct transmission. (b) Reflector scheme.

(9.2)
$$\Delta t \approx \frac{2}{c_o^2} \int_C^D v \cos\theta \, ds.$$

For example, consider the case of a parabolic velocity profile in a circular pipe of radius R, i.e., $v = v_{\max}[1 - (r/R)^2]$. It can readily be shown that for the same average flow velocity, the non-uniform flow will cause a 33% overestimation of the volume flow rate as compared to that estimated for uniform flow. Because of the dependency on the flow profile, calibration corrections may be needed to improve the accuracy. In the presence of pulsatile flow, because the velocity profile generally changes over the flow cycle, calibration corrections become difficult.

An extensive range of transit-time ultrasonic flowmeters and transducers exist for use in production monitoring and measurements. For the measurement and monitoring of blood flow in animals, a variety of clamp–on transducers are available for vessels with diameters ranging down to about a millimeter; they generally have one of the transducer arrangements shown in Fig. 9.4.

9.3 Doppler Equation for Moving Scatterers

The formula that characterizes the frequency change due to ultrasound scattering by a particle that moves with the local flow field can be derived in two steps. The first consists of obtaining the Doppler frequency shift seen by an observer located on the moving particle. The second consists of obtaining the frequency shift seen by an observer on a fixed (laboratory) frame of reference due to emission by the scatterer moving with the fluid. By combining both results, the overall Doppler shift can be calculated.

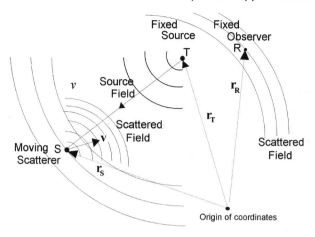

Figure 9.5 Deriving the Doppler equation due to a scatterer S that moves with the fluid velocity v, a fixed transmitter at T, and a fixed observer at R (the receiver).

To simplify the analysis, the flow field will be assumed constant throughout the region of interest. As illustrated in Fig. 9.5, a transmitter T located at $\mathbf{r}_T$ emits a monochromatic wave into a flowing medium. A scatterer S, located at $\mathbf{r}_S$ at a time t, is assumed to be moving with a constant velocity $\mathbf{v}$ when measured in a fixed laboratory coordinate system. The frequency seen by an observer located on the moving scatterer can be found by noting that the two coordinate systems are related by a *Galilean* transform. As shown below, frequency is not a Galilean invariant, and therefore the observed frequency depends on the velocity.

Consider the Galilean transform from an unprimed to a primed Cartesian coordinate system moving with a constant velocity $\mathbf{v}$. Such a transform can be expressed by

(9.3)
$$\begin{bmatrix} t \\ x \\ y \\ z \end{bmatrix} = \begin{bmatrix} 1 & 0 & 0 & 0 \\ -v_x & 1 & 0 & 0 \\ -v_y & 0 & 1 & 0 \\ -v_z & 0 & 0 & 1 \end{bmatrix} \begin{bmatrix} t' \\ x' \\ y' \\ z' \end{bmatrix},$$

where v_x, v_y, and v_z are the components of the fluid velocity measured with respect to the fixed (unprimed) system. We will first apply this transformation to the gradient function $\phi \equiv \phi(x, y, z : t)$, i.e.,

$$\nabla\phi = \tilde{\mathbf{x}}\frac{\partial\phi}{\partial x} + \tilde{\mathbf{y}}\frac{\partial\phi}{\partial y} + \tilde{\mathbf{z}}\frac{\partial\phi}{\partial z},$$

where the curly overscore denotes a unit vector. Now the x-component can be expressed as

$$\frac{\partial\phi}{\partial x} = \frac{\partial\phi}{\partial x'}\frac{\partial x'}{\partial x} + \frac{\partial\phi}{\partial t'}\frac{\partial t'}{\partial x},$$

with similar expressions for $\partial\phi/\partial y$ and $\partial\phi/\partial z$. Using (9.3), these reduce to

$$\frac{\partial\phi}{\partial x} = \frac{\partial\phi}{\partial x'}, \quad \frac{\partial\phi}{\partial y} = \frac{\partial\phi}{\partial y'}, \quad \frac{\partial\phi}{\partial z} = \frac{\partial\phi}{\partial z'},$$

and consequently the gradient is a Galilean invariant, i.e., $\nabla\phi = \nabla'\phi$.

We now identify $\phi(\mathbf{r}':t')$ as the phase function as seen in the moving coordinate system and use the chain rule to express its partial derivative with respect to t' as

$$\frac{\partial\phi}{\partial t'} = \frac{\partial\phi}{\partial t}\frac{\partial t}{\partial t'} + \frac{\partial\phi}{\partial x'}\frac{\partial x'}{\partial t'} + \frac{\partial\phi}{\partial y'}\frac{\partial y'}{\partial t'} + \frac{\partial\phi}{\partial z'}\frac{\partial z'}{\partial t'}.$$

Using the transformation given by (9.3) and the Galilean invariance of the gradient, this equation simplifies to

$$\frac{\partial\phi(\mathbf{r}_S':t')}{\partial t'} = \frac{\partial\phi(\mathbf{r}_S:t)}{\partial t} + \mathbf{v}\cdot\nabla\phi(\mathbf{r}_S:t).$$

Now, the angular frequency of a harmonic function can be defined as the derivative of the phase, i.e., $\omega = \partial\phi/\partial t$. Thus, the transmitted angular frequency seen by a stationary observer in the laboratory coordinate system can be written as $\omega_0 = \partial\phi(\mathbf{r}_s:t)/\partial t$ and that seen by the observer on the moving scatterer is $\omega' = \partial\phi(\mathbf{r}_s':t')/\partial t'$. In addition, because the wavenumber vector is given by $\mathbf{k}_T = -\nabla\phi(\mathbf{r}_s:t) = (\omega_0/c_0)\mathbf{k}_T/|\mathbf{k}_T|$, the above equation simplifies to

(9.4) $$\omega' = \omega_0 - \mathbf{v}\cdot\mathbf{k}_T. \tag{a}$$

The second step in the derivation is to consider the scatterer as a radiation source that has an angular frequency of ω' in the primed frame of reference and that moves with the local flow field. We wish to determine the angular frequency ω'' that would be measured by an observer whose position is fixed at $\mathbf{r}_R$ in the laboratory frame of reference. This also involves a Galilean transformation and results in

(9.4) $$\omega' = \omega'' - \mathbf{v}\cdot\mathbf{k}_R, \tag{b}$$

where, as indicated in Fig. 9.6a, $\mathbf{k}_R = (\omega''/c_o)\mathbf{k}_R/|\mathbf{k}_R|$ is the vector whose direction is from the scatterer to the receiver. Subtracting (9.4a) from (b) enables the Doppler angular frequency shift to be expressed as

$$\omega_D = \omega'' - \omega_0 = \mathbf{v}\cdot(\mathbf{k}_R - \mathbf{k}_T) = \frac{1}{c_o}\mathbf{v}\cdot\left(\omega''\frac{\mathbf{k}_R}{k_R} - \omega_0\frac{\mathbf{k}_T}{k_T}\right)$$

or as

(9.5) $$\omega_D = -\frac{v\omega_0}{c_o}\left(\frac{\omega''}{\omega_0}\cos\theta_R + \cos\theta_T\right).$$

Both of the angles in this equation are shown in Fig. 9.6a and are given by

$\cos\theta_R = -\dfrac{\mathbf{v}\cdot\mathbf{k}_R}{vk_R}$ and $\cos\theta_T = -\dfrac{\mathbf{v}\cdot\mathbf{k}_T}{vk_T}$. For small Mach numbers ($v/c_o \ll 1$), (9.5) simplifies to

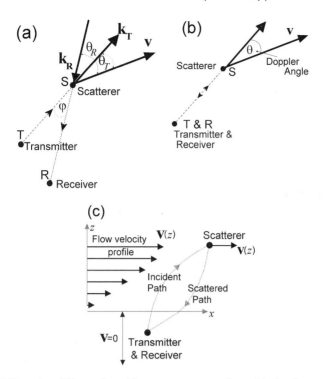

Figure 9.6 Doppler shift produced by a scatterer moving with the flow velocity **v**. In (a), the directions of the wave vectors are indicated. A simplified sketch is shown in (b) for the case where the transmitter and receiver are at the same location. (c) The incident and scattered beams paths can no longer be assumed to be straight lines when the scatterer is transported at high speed by flowing medium. The change in transport speed results in refraction, causing the incident and scattered beams to differ.

$$\omega_D \approx \frac{v}{c_o}\omega_0\left(\frac{\mathbf{v}\cdot\mathbf{k}_R}{vk_R} - \frac{\mathbf{v}\cdot\mathbf{k}_T}{vk_T}\right) = -\frac{v}{c_o}\omega_0\left(\cos\theta_R - \cos\theta_T\right).$$

When the transmitter and receiver lie on the same straight line joining them to the scatterer (Fig. 9.6b), the well-known Doppler formula for the change in frequency produced by a moving scatterer results, namely

(9.6)
$$\boxed{f_D = f_R - f_T = -\frac{2v}{c_o}f_0\cos\theta}\,,$$
(a)

in which the negative sign indicates that the received frequency is less than the transmitted frequency when flow is away from the source. The angle θ is generally referred to as the Doppler angle. Suppose that the transmitter and receiving crystals are mounted in the same probe holder at an angle φ to one another. If the angle made by the bisector between the transmitting and receiving transducers and the velocity vector is now defined as θ, it can be readily shown that

(9.6)

$$\boxed{f_D = -\frac{2v}{c_o}f_0\cos\theta\cos(\varphi/2)}.$$

(b)

9.3.1 Refractive Effects

In the presence of a non-uniform flow velocity profile with velocities approaching c_o, the incident and scattered ray paths can be quite different from the geometric paths. The change in the speed of propagation relative to the laboratory coordinate system causes refractive bending of the beam in the manner illustrated in Fig. 9.6c. Depending on the flow profile, the incident and scattered angles can differ substantially.

To illustrate this effect, we shall assume a linear change on flow velocity with depth. For an ultrasound beam incident at an angle of θ_i at (x_o, z_o) on a region whose flow velocity is in the x-direction and increases linearly with depth (z), Ziomek [27, Chapter 5] has shown that the path of the ultrasound ray can be determined from

$$z = z_o + \frac{c_o}{b}\left\{\frac{\sin[\theta_r(z)]}{\sin\theta_i} - 1\right\}, \text{ and } \cos[\theta_r(z)] = \cos\theta_i - b\frac{\sin\theta_i}{c_o}(x - x_o),$$

where $\theta_r(z)$ is the angle of refraction at a depth z and b is the slope given by $b = [c(z) - c_o]/(z - z_0)$ By eliminating θ_r from these two equations, the coordinates of the beam can be obtained, enabling the path to be calculated. This is illustrated in Fig. 9.7 for a fluid whose velocity in the lateral direction is assumed to change linearly with depth. Such conditions are not realistic in practice. Moreover, for physiologic flow conditions, because the peak flow velocities are less than 0.1% of c_o, worst-case angle corrections for the incident or scattered beam are well below one degree.

9.4 Continuous-Wave Doppler Systems

As noted previously, early versions of CW Doppler systems were insensitive to the flow direction. Consequently, when both forward and reverse flow components are present in a vessel, as occurs in some arteries, the flow velocity profile can be misinterpreted. Subsequent development of a variety of demodulation methods enabled the forward and reverse flow signals to be separated. One such technique, using phase-quadrature demodulation, will be described shortly.

Over the 10-year period from the mid 1970s, CW Doppler systems were widely used for the assessment of vascular disease and provided a relatively simple means by which the normality or otherwise of the flow could be determined in a noninvasive manner. Unlike pulsed measurement systems, CW systems have limited depth discrimination; therefore, when the sensitive (sample) volume intersects more than one vessel, the required Doppler signal can be seriously corrupted. As will be shown, pulsed systems do not make use

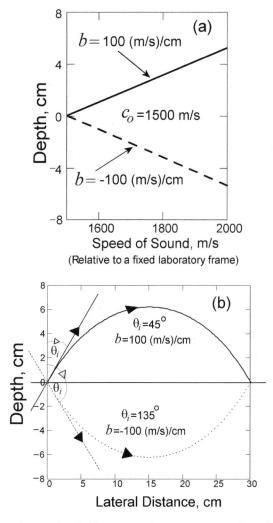

Figure 9.7 Effect of a moving fluid on acoustic wave propagation when the fluid speed varies linearly with depth. It is assumed that at a depth of $z = z_o$ the speed of sound $c(z_o) = c_o = 1500 \, \text{m/s}$. (a) Sound speed depth profile $c(z)$, i.e., speed relative to a fixed laboratory frame as a function of depth). (b) The beam path in the depth-lateral plane for incident angles of 45 and 135 degrees.

of the Doppler effect (see section 10.1). Nonetheless, because the approximate equations relating the velocity and frequency shift are identical for both types of system, a description and analysis of CW systems provides a good foundation for understanding pulsed systems. Subsequently, these will be referred to as *pulsed wave* (velocity estimation) systems, in accordance with the terminology used by Jensen [35].

For typical clinical peak flow velocities (e.g., 100 cm/s) and transmission frequencies (3–10 MHz), the Doppler frequencies are in the audio frequency range. For example, if the peak flow velocity ranges from 4 to 70 cm/s for a 7 MHz system, and the Doppler angle is 60 degrees, then, from (9.6), the peak Doppler frequency would be in the range from 190 Hz to 3.3 kHz. Because of this, the Doppler signal is generally converted to an audio output, enabling the time variations of the Doppler frequency to be assessed. In Chapter 8 it was noted that the backscattered signal from non-aggregating whole blood is typically several orders of magnitude smaller than that from tissue; as a result, obtaining a Doppler signal that has a good SNR is normally of considerable importance. Generally, CW systems, with their very narrow bandwidth and relatively large insonated blood volume, can achieve a better SNR than for pulsed wave systems.

9.4.1 Probe Design

The design and performance of CW Doppler probes has been reported and discussed in several papers [28–30]. Although it is possible to use the same element for both transmission and reception [33], most CW systems use probes with separate elements, thereby enhancing the SNR and avoiding the problem of cancelling out the large transmit signal at the receiver input. Of major importance in vascular assessment is the size and shape of the sample volume. For CW systems this is determined by the transducer geometry. The D-shaped transducer design illustrated in Fig. 9.8a consists of two transducers mounted a small angle to one another. Roughly speaking, the Doppler sample volume can be expected to correspond to the region of geometric overlap. Measurement and calculation of this volume is of considerable practical importance, and a variety of methods have been used. One scheme is to use a small vibrating target immersed in water that can be scanned through the transmit–receive field [30–32]. The nature of the sample volume shape will be discussed in Chapter 10 (subsection 10.3.4) when discussing pulsed wave flow measurement systems.

9.4.2 Extracting the Doppler Signal

To extract the forward and reverse components of the Doppler signal, a variety of methods are feasible. In the early stages of development three demodulation techniques prevailed: single-sideband, heterodyne, and phase-quadrature demodulation. The basic principles, along with design details, are given in the books by Atkinson and Woodcock [34], Jensen [35], and Evans and McDicken [36]. The phase-quadrature demodulation method, one of the most widely used techniques for both CW and pulsed wave systems, will be briefly described.

The phase-quadrature method illustrated in Fig. 9.9 provides in-phase and quadrature output signals that enable the flow velocity components to be readily extracted. It consists of two multipliers that generate sum and difference frequencies and two bandpass filters.

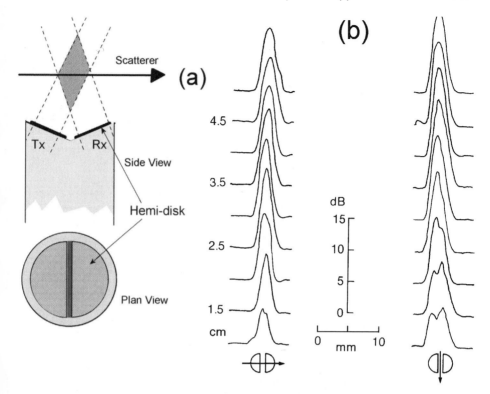

Figure 9.8 Example of an 8-MHz CW Doppler probe showing the two-way spatial response characteristics. (a) Transducer with separate transmit and receive hemi-disks elements, mounted at an angle to one another. (b) The measured (two-way) response in two lateral directions at various axial distances as obtained using a small vibrating target in water. (Reproduced, with permission, from Douville et al. [30], *J. Clin. Ultrasound*, 11, 83–90, © 1983 Wiley. This material is used by permission of John Wiley & Sons, Inc.)

A simple approach for understanding this method is to assume that the received signal consists of three frequency components: a forward ($2A_f$, ω_f, ϕ_f), a reverse ($2A_r$, ω_r, ϕ_r), and a carrier component ($2A_o$, ω_o, ϕ_o), where the amplitudes, angular frequencies, and phases are denoted by $2A$, ω, and ϕ, respectively. Thus, the received signal can be written as:

$$R(t) = 2A_o\cos(\omega_o t + \phi_o) + 2A_f\cos[(\omega_o + \omega_f)t + \phi_f] + 2A_r\cos[(\omega_o - \omega_r)t + \phi_r],$$

which, when multiplied by $\cos(\omega_o t)$ and $\sin(\omega_o t)$, enables the in-phase (I) and quadrature (Q) signals to be expressed as

$$I(t) = A_o\cos[(2\omega_o t + \phi_o) + \cos\phi_o] + A_f\{\cos(\omega_f t + \phi_f) + \cos([2\omega_o + \omega_f]t + \phi_f)\}$$
$$+ A_r\{\cos(\omega_r t - \phi_r) + \cos([2\omega_o - \omega_r]t + \phi_r)\},$$

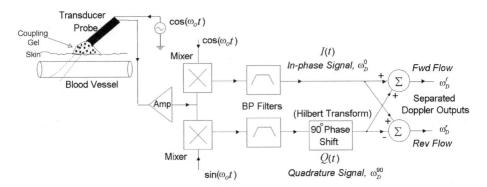

Figure 9.9 Example of an analog CW Doppler system for flow velocity estimation using a phase-quadrature demodulator. The flow separator is based on performing an analog Hilbert transform, enabling the forward and reverse flow components to be extracted.

and

$$Q(t) = A_o[\sin(2\omega_o t + \phi_o) - \sin\phi_o] - A_f\{\sin(\omega_f t + \phi_f) + \sin([2\omega_o + \omega_f]t + \phi_f)\}$$
$$+ A_r\{\sin(\omega_r t - \phi_r) + \sin([2\omega_o - \omega_r]t + \phi_r)\}.$$

If a bandpass filter is used to reject the DC and high-frequency components, these equations reduce to

$$I(t) = A_f\cos(\omega_f t + \phi_f) + A_r\cos(\omega_r t - \phi_r) \tag{a}$$

(9.7)
$$Q(t) = -A_f\sin(\omega_f t + \phi_f) + A_r\sin(\omega_r t - \phi_r)$$
$$= A_f\cos\left(\omega_f t + \phi_f + \frac{\pi}{2}\right) + A_r\cos\left(\omega_r t - \phi_r - \frac{\pi}{2}\right). \tag{b}$$

Comparison of these two equations shows that there is a 90 degree phase difference between the two signals. If flow is away from the Doppler probe, then the in-phase signal leads the quadrature signal by 90 degrees.

Because of the pulsatile nature of arterial flow and the elastic nature of vessel walls, substantial vessel wall movement (e.g., 5%) occurs over the cardiac cycle. The associated velocity creates a strong low-frequency clutter component in the Doppler spectrum, and this typically has frequency components extending to around 200 Hz. If a bandpass filter is used to eliminate this and the high-frequency sum components of the mixer, the low-frequency cutoff is generally set within the range 100 to 200 Hz. However, this also removes the Doppler signal arising from slow-moving RBCs in the immediate vicinity of the vessel wall. To minimize noise, the high-frequency cutoff should be set to around the maximum Doppler frequency anticipated, e.g., 10 kHz.

A wide variety of methods have been proposed and used for extracting the forward and reverse Doppler frequency signals from the I and Q components. A particularly straightforward method is that illustrated in Fig. 9.9. It uses a

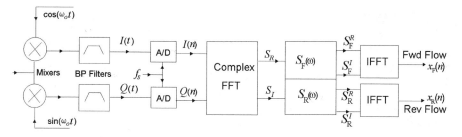

Figure 9.10 Method for extracting the spectra and forward and reverse flow signals. The subscripts or superscripts R and I refer to the real and imaginary parts, respectively, and the subscripts R and F (not italicized) refer to the forward and reverse flow components, respectively. (Based on a similar drawing by Aydin et al. [38].)

Hilbert transform (the equivalent to a filter that performs a 90 degree phase shift over the frequency band of the Doppler signal), followed by addition and subtraction. For the I and Q signals given by (9.7), it can be seen that this process extracts the forward and reverse signal components, i.e.,

$$V_f = I(t) + Q(t) = 2A_f \cos(\omega_f t + \phi_f)$$
$$V_r = I(t) - Q(t) = 2A_r \cos(\omega_r t - \phi_r).$$

For the analog systems initially used, achieving a 90 degree phase shift with sufficient accuracy over the entire Doppler signal bandwidth (e.g., 10 Hz to 15 kHz), was particularly challenging. Digital methods provide a more accurate and convenient means for performing the Hilbert transform, enabling the time-domain form of the velocity signals to be extracted, as has been described by Aydin and Evans [37,38]. Their scheme is illustrated in Fig. 9.10. It uses a complex FFT to extract the real and imaginary parts of the spectrum, filters to obtain the in-phase and quadrature components of the forward and reverse flow spectra, and finally an inverse FFT (IFFT) to obtain the time-domain signals.

9.5 Continuous-Wave Doppler Spectrum Related to Velocity Profile

Spectral analysis of the Doppler signal can provide information concerning the underlying hemodynamics. The potential clinical importance of this relation was first appreciated in the 1960s by the group working with Kaneko [12,39] in Japan. They developed several on- and off-line frequency analysis schemes that were used in the early clinical studies [40].

As described in Chapter 5, the CW backscattered signal from stationary blood arises from the interference effects produced by scattering from a very large number of RBCs. Moreover, it was noted that the signal is a zero-mean Gaussian random process that can be completely specified by its autocorrelation function. If a range of RBC velocities are present in the sample volume, a corresponding spectrum of frequencies will be present in the Doppler signal, and this will vary in a periodic manner over the cardiac cycle. Of considerable importance in the noninvasive assessment of arterial disease is the relation between the Doppler spectrum and the flow velocity profile. In principle, with the pulsed method it is possible to use a sufficiently small sample volume so that the flow velocity at a given location can be sampled and measured over a cardiac cycle. However, in CW Doppler the sample volume tends to be large and may completely envelop the entire cross-section of a vessel. Moreover, attenuation can cause the sensitivity to vary with depth. These added complications can make it more difficult to properly interpret the spectrum in terms of the flow velocity profile.

9.5.1 Steady Flow Spectra

The relation between the flow velocity profile and the Doppler power spectrum can be derived in a simple manner by ignoring the stochastic aspects of the problem and making a number of additional simplifying assumptions. Roevros [41] used this approach in studying the Doppler spectrum produced by a suspension of scatterers flowing in a cylindrical tube. The predicted spectrum corresponds to that determined from a very long time-domain record under steady flow conditions. His derivation also assumed fully developed laminar flow in a cylindrical tube of inner radius R, and a flow velocity profile given by

$$(9.8) \qquad v(r) = v_{max}\left[1 - (r/R)^n\right],$$

where n characterizes the flow velocity profile and v_{max} is the flow velocity at the center. As illustrated in Fig. 9.11, Poiseuille (parabolic) flow conditions

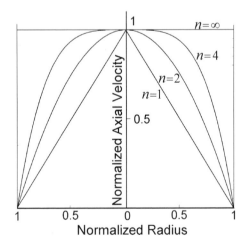

Figure 9.11 Examples of flow velocity profiles in a circular tube according to (9.8).

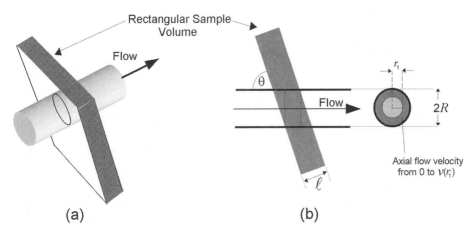

Figure 9.12 Geometry used for calculating the CW Doppler power spectrum due to flow in a circular tube, assuming a rectangular slab sample volume.

correspond to $n = 2$, while $n = \infty$ corresponds to a flat profile. Roevros also assumed that the ultrasound sample volume intersected the vessel at an angle θ and that the intersection region consisted of the volume whose length in the flow direction is given by $\ell/\sin\theta$ (Fig. 9.12). The scattered signal was assumed to arise from randomly distributed point scatterers within the intersection volume. For a constant sensitivity in the intersection volume, the total received signal intensity could therefore be taken as the sum of the intensities from each individual scatterer, thereby making it unnecessary to consider interference effects. In addition, by ignoring the effects of attenuation and spectral broadening, his analysis predicted the correct ensemble averaged form of the power spectrum.

The first effort to account for the stochastic nature of the backscattered signal from blood and to relate the Doppler spectrum to the velocity profile appears to be that presented by Fahrbach in 1969/70 [42]. In fact, this work precedes the often-quoted 1971 report by Brody [43] and the paper by Roevros [41] in 1974 that also addressed these issues. Brody assumed that the RBCs could be modeled as independent point scatterers and derived an expression for the autocovariance function. By taking its Fourier transform, an expression was then obtained for the power spectrum. A more general approach based on the analysis given by Bascom and Cobbold [44] is presented below.

We shall assume that the scatterers have a non-zero size and their spatial distribution is as described in Chapter 5. From the definition of the backscattering coefficient σ_{BSC} {see (5.59)}, the backscattered power from an elemental volume dV of scatterers is given by

(9.9) $$dP = \sigma_{BSC}\Omega dV,$$

where Ω is the solid angle suspended at the receiving transducer by dV. Such a volume element can be taken to encompass all scatterers having a velocity range from v to $v + dv$, provided its dimensions are small compared to its distance from the receiving transducer. If the velocity profile is monotonic and axiymmetric, this velocity range will correspond to an incremental radial distance range from r to $r + dr$. With the help of Fig. 9.12b, the elemental volume can therefore be expressed as

$$(9.10) \qquad dV = \frac{\ell}{\sin\theta} 2\pi r dr.$$

According to (5.71), the backscattering coefficient is given by $\sigma_{BSC} = \sigma_b HW(H)/V_s$, where σ_b is the scattering cross-section, H is the hematocrit, the scatterer volume is denoted by V_s, and the packing factor W, is a function of the hematocrit. By substituting this expression and (9.10) into (9.9), the backscattered power is given by

$$(9.11) \qquad dP = \frac{\sigma_b HW(H)}{V_s} \Omega 2\pi \frac{\ell}{\sin\theta} r dr.$$

In velocity space, the Doppler power spectrum $\Phi(v)$ can be defined by

$$dP(v) = \Phi(v)dv = \Phi(v)\frac{dv}{dr}dr,$$

which, when substituted into (9.11), enables the Doppler spectrum to be expressed as

$$\Phi(v) = \frac{\sigma_b HW(H)}{V_s} \frac{\Omega 2\pi\ell}{\sin\theta} r \left(\frac{dv}{dr}\right)^{-1}.$$

When the differential coefficient of (9.8) is substituted into this equation, we obtain

$$\Phi(v) = \frac{\sigma_b HW(H)}{V_s} \frac{\Omega 2\pi\ell}{\sin\theta} \frac{R^2}{n v_{max}} \left(1 - \frac{v}{v_{max}}\right)^{\frac{2-n}{n}}.$$

This can be expressed in Doppler frequency space by using the Doppler equation given by (9.6), yielding

$$(9.12) \qquad \Phi(f_D) = \frac{\sigma_b HW(H)}{V_s} \frac{\Omega 2\pi\ell}{\sin\theta} \frac{R^2}{n f_D^{max}} \left(1 - \frac{f_D}{f_D^{mas}}\right)^{\frac{2-n}{n}},$$

where $f_D^{max} = 2(v_{max}/c_o)f_o\cos\theta$ is the maximum Doppler shift and $\Phi(f_D)df_D$ is the total backscattered power in the frequency range from f_D to $f_D + df_D$. This equation is similar to that derived by Roevros [41], except that it now accounts for the scatterer size.

For parabolic flow ($n = 2$), (9.12) predicts a constant power density spectrum from zero frequency up to a maximum corresponding to the spectra generated by scatterers at the center of the vessel that move with the peak velocity. This case, together with the other flow profiles of Fig. 9.11, are illus-

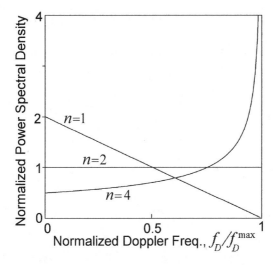

Figure 9.13 Relation of the flow velocity profile to the CW Doppler spectrum. For parabolic flow ($n = 2$), the spectrum is flat extending up to a frequency determined by the maximum flow velocity. For a flat velocity profile ($n = \infty$), the profile is a δ-function at $f_D/f_D^{max} = 1$.

trated in Fig. 9.13. In practice, the sample volume is unlikely to be well modeled by a rectangular slab, and other assumptions such as a circular beam [45] and a Gaussian weighted beam [46] have been numerically and analytically examined.

Based on certain simplifying assumptions, Brody [43], Arts and Roevros [47], and Nakayama and Furuharta [48] have shown that the mean Doppler shift is proportional to the mean scatterer velocity and is independent of the velocity profile. Specifically, if the transmit/receive sensitivity is uniform over the insonated volume and spectral broadening effects (see section 9.7) can be neglected, the mean velocity estimate can be expressed in terms of the complex power spectral density as

$$(9.13) \qquad \hat{\bar{v}} = \frac{c_o}{2 f_o \cos\theta} \int_{-\infty}^{\infty} f_D \Phi(f_D) df_D \bigg/ \int_{-\infty}^{\infty} \Phi(f_D) df_D,$$

which is independent of $v(r)$. Now, for a cylinder with an inner radius of R, the instantaneous volume flow rate (e.g., ml/sec) is given by $\hat{Q} = \pi R^2 \hat{\bar{v}}$. This relation and (9.13) have frequently been used as the basis for determining the volume flow rate in blood vessels.[3]

9.5.2 Characteristics of Pulsatile Blood Flow in Arteries

For pulsatile flow, the Doppler spectrum will change over the cardiac cycle, with the maximum flow velocity occurring close to peak systole. As an

---

3. See subsection 10.11.2 for further details of CW Doppler techniques based on this approach.

Table 9.1. Values Used for Calculating the Velocity Profiles in Fig. 9.14

Artery	Diameter (mm)	Kinematic Viscosity (cS)	Mean Flow (ml/s)	Peak Flow (ml/s)	α_0	Period (sec)
Common carotid	7.31	3.60	7.4	28	5.22	0.85
Common femoral	9.0	3.60	5.8	35	6.42	0.85

Data obtained from Shehada et al. [49].

example, we shall consider blood flow in the common carotid and femoral arteries of man. Based on the unscaled waveforms given by Evans and McDicken [36, p. 13] for a normal volunteer and the data given in Shehada et al. [49], volumetric flow waveforms are shown in Fig. 9.14 along with computed velocity profiles over a flow cycle. The basis of these calculations is the method described by Evans [50] that makes use of equations derived by Womersley [51] for the velocity profile produced by a sinusoidal flow waveform in a rigid tube. These equations assume that the flow is fully developed so that the profile does not depend on the axial distance; the flow is laminar; the fluid is incompressible; and the fluid viscosity is independent of the shear rate. The overall velocity profile can be determined by first Fourier analyzing the flow waveform. The flow profile associated with each component can then be determined and finally, by summation, the overall profile can be found. Further details of this process are given below.

For fully developed pulsatile laminar flow through a tube of radius R, the velocity profile can be expressed in terms of the radial coordinate r. If the volumetric flow $Q(t)$ is periodic with a fundamental angular frequency ω_0, the flow can be expressed as a complex Fourier series:

$$(9.14) \qquad Q(t) = Q_0 + \sum_{m=1}^{\infty} Q_m e^{j(m\omega_0 t - \phi_m)},$$

where Q_m and ϕ_m denote the amplitude and phase of the mth harmonic, respectively, and Q_0 is the steady flow component. Following the procedure given by Evans [50], the following form for the instantaneous velocity profile can then be obtained from (9.14) in combination with the Womersley equations:

$$v(r{:}t) = \frac{1}{\pi R^2} \operatorname{Re}\left\{ 2Q_0\left[1 - (r/R)^2\right] + \sum_{m=1}^{\infty} Q_m\left(\frac{\tau_m J_0(\tau_m) - \tau_m J_0(r_N \tau_m)}{\tau_m J_0(\tau_m) - 2 J_1(\tau_m)}\right) e^{j(m\omega_0 t - \phi_m)} \right\},$$
(9.15)

where $\tau_m = \alpha_m i^{3/2}$, in which $\alpha_m = R\sqrt{m\omega_o \, \rho/\mu}$ is the Womersley number for the m'th harmonic, μ is the shear viscosity, and ρ is the fluid density. Examination of this equation shows that in the absence of any pulsatile components the velocity profile is parabolic, with a maximum value equal to $2Q_0/(\pi R^2)$, as expected.

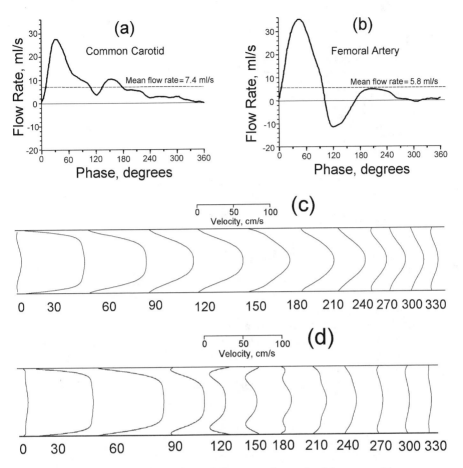

Figure 9.14 Examples of the estimated flow waveforms for (a) a normal human common carotid artery and (b) a normal femoral artery. The corresponding flow velocity profiles shown in (c) and (d) were calculated using (9.15) together with the data in Table 9.1.

9.5.3 Characteristics of the Doppler Signal and its Power Spectrum

Two 10-ms segments of a CW Doppler signal measured at peak diastole and late diastole from a common carotid artery are shown in Fig. 9.15. Both segments were Fourier transformed, and the resulting power spectra are shown in (b) and (d). Although the Doppler signal is non-stationary, the 10 ms interval in late diastole is likely sufficiently short so that the signal can be considered quasi–stationary over this period. Around peak systole, the flow profile changes much more rapidly, and an analysis window of around 5 ms would be preferable. Examination of systolic spectrum indicates that most of the power is concentrated at higher frequencies. According to the results of Fig. 9.13, this

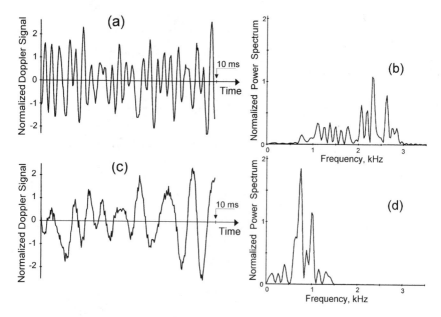

Figure 9.15 Measured time-domain segments of 10-ms duration from a normal common carotid artery, together with Doppler signals and their spectra. (a) Close to the systolic peak. (c) Close to late diastole. In (b) and (d) are shown the spectra of the two time-domain signals of (a) and (c), respectively. (Reprinted by permission of Elsevier from Cobbold et al. [52], Ch. 5, in *Cardiovascular Applications of Doppler Ultrasonography*, Churchill Livingstone, © 1989 Longman Group, UK, Limited.).

suggests that the velocity profile is closer to being flat rather than parabolic, which is in agreement with the theoretical profile shown in Fig. 9.14c for the phase angle of 30 degrees. Some noise is present, and this is particularly evident at frequencies where the Doppler signal power is negligible.

A traditional method of displaying the time-varying spectra is to use a gray scale for the spectral power or amplitude, as illustrated in Fig. 9.16. This picture for a normal human internal carotid artery clearly indicates the absence of lower-frequency components in the region of the systolic peak. Apart from the effects of the high-frequency filter (~300 Hz), in the diastolic region the spectrum looks much flatter, corresponding to a velocity profile that is closer to parabolic. At peak systole, the power is primarily confined to frequencies between f_D^{max} and f_D^{min}. Instead of gray scale, color encoding can also be used to display the amplitude, and by using tracking algorithms, the variations of f_D^{max} and f_D^{min} can be displayed. Moreover, all of this information can be shown as a running display that is continuously updated.

An alternative display format is the pseudo-3D graphs shown in Fig. 9.17. In (a), the absence of low-frequency components in the neighborhood of the

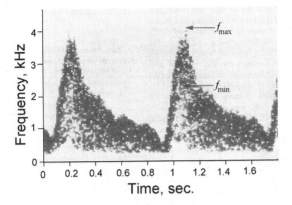

Figure 9.16 Gray-scale display of the amplitude spectrum from a normal human internal carotid artery. Each spectrum was calculated for a 10-ms segment and displayed in gray scale. (Reprinted by permission of Elsevier, from Kassam et al. [53], *Ultrasound Med. Biol.*, 11, 425–433, 1985, © 1995 World Federation of Ultrasound in Medicine and Biology.)

systolic peak should be noted. For (b), much higher frequencies are seen throughout the flow cycle, particularly in the neighborhood of peak systole. This indicates the presence of a stenosis that would cause the flow to be confined to a smaller cross-section area, possibly resulting in the formation of a jet and accompanied by flow separation. Such methods of analyzing and displaying the Doppler signals are sometimes referred to as *spectral Doppler*. This is in contrast to methods that analyze and display the mean flow as a 2-D color map, which will be referred to as *pulsed wave flow imaging* (see section 10.7).

To help interpret the Doppler spectra obtained from insonating normal and diseased vessels, a flow model can be very helpful [54]. Such a model can be either physical or mathematical. Computational fluid dynamic models have the advantage that changes in geometry and flow conditions can be readily made, often enabling predictions to be made that would be difficult to test experimentally. Because such a model enables the velocity vector throughout the vessel to be predicted at each instant of time, the Doppler spectrum for a given sample volume shape can be estimated. Such models do make a number of assumptions that are not required for a physical model. A physical model extensively studied is that illustrated at the top of Fig. 9.18. It consists of an acrylic tube with an inside diameter of 4.6 mm and a 70% asymmetric area stenosis in the entrance region. It is designed to approximately simulate the conditions seen in a partially blocked vessel, without causing a significant reduction in the mean volumetric flow. This model has been used to study the changes in spectra obtained with insonation location [44, 55, 56] using either steady or pulsatile flow and either CW or pulsed wave [57] measurement systems.

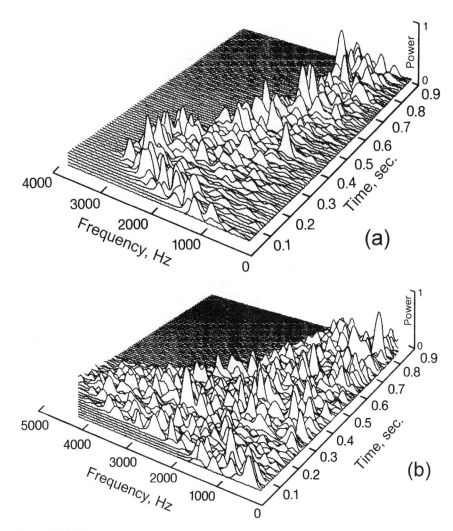

Figure 9.17 3-Dspectral displays of CW Doppler spectra from human carotid arteries. (a) Normal and (b) abnormal Doppler spectra. For (b), the much higher-frequency components correspond to higher flow velocities and indicate the presence of a moderately severe stenosis. (Reprinted by permission of Elsevier from Cobbold et al. [52], Chapter 5, in *Cardiovascular Applications of Doppler Ultrasonography*, Churchill Livingstone, © 1989 Longman Group, UK, Limited.)

The fluid displacement profile sketches shown in Fig. 9.18 were based on measurements of the displacement profiles obtained with a nearly identical model using a photochromic dye visualization technique [58]. For both CW Doppler and pulsed wave measurements, a fluid consisting of a suspension of outdated human RBCs suspended in saline (to prevent aggregation) was used. A CW probe was directed downstream at an angle of 50 degrees to the axis of the tube, whose inner diameter was 4.6 mm. For the photochromic measurements, the test section had an inner diameter of 5.1 mm and the fluid consisted of kerosene with small amount of dye. A pulsed laser beam was used to activate the dye. By photographing the trace shortly after the pulse, the velocity profile was measured, and this was repeated at various axial locations. To ensure similar flow conditions in the two sets of experiments (the fluids had different kinematic viscosities), the same Reynolds number ($R_E = 2R\bar{v}\rho/\mu$) was used for both. For pulsatile flow, both the Reynolds number and Wormersly parameter were matched for the two sets of experiments.

Using a parabolic inlet velocity profile at a Reynolds number of 545, four regions distal to the stenosis can be identified, and these are associated with Doppler spectra that have distinctly different characteristics [55]. As can be seen from the middle portion of Fig. 9.18, prior to the stenosis the spectrum is quite flat, corresponding to the parabolic inlet flow. In the first region (I) the high jet velocity gives rise to a high Doppler frequency. In addition, the retrograde flow in the separation zone causes a reverse Doppler spectrum. As the probe is moved further downstream (II), the maximum Doppler frequency is reduced, the spectrum becomes peaked at the low-frequency end, and the reverse spectral power is diminished. Further downstream (III), the Doppler spectrum becomes peaked toward the high-frequency end and the maximum frequency is further reduced as a result of the complete dissipation of the jet flow. The spectrum is similar to that expected from a velocity profile that is relatively flat, such as that arising from steady turbulent flow in a circular tube. As the insonation point is moved even further downstream (IV), the flow field begins to re-laminarize, and at $20D$ the Doppler spectrum is essentially flat, indicating a return to parabolic flow.

The total backscattered power at seven locations is shown at the bottom of Fig. 9.18. In the laminar flow regions, apart from the reduction in the throat of the stenosis, the power remains reasonably constant. However, in the turbulent zone, a significant increase in the backscattered power occurs. As briefly discussed in Chapter 5 (see Fig. 5.24), turbulence can be expected to cause an increase in the local variance of RBC number density, thereby increasing the backscattering coefficient. Measurements made with 4% hematocrit blood showed no significant change in backscattered power in the turbulent zone, which is in agreement with the discussion in subsection 5.9.4.

9.6 Properties of the Doppler Signal

9.6.1 Statistical Properties

In considering the statistical properties of the Doppler signal, we shall assume that the sample volume contains N identical scatterers, each of which has a scattering cross-section of σ_b. The backscattered RF signal from the ith scatterer moving with a velocity $\mathbf{v}_i$ can be written as

$$x_i(t) = A\sqrt{\sigma_b}\cos\left[(\omega_o - \omega_D^i)t + \phi_i\right],$$

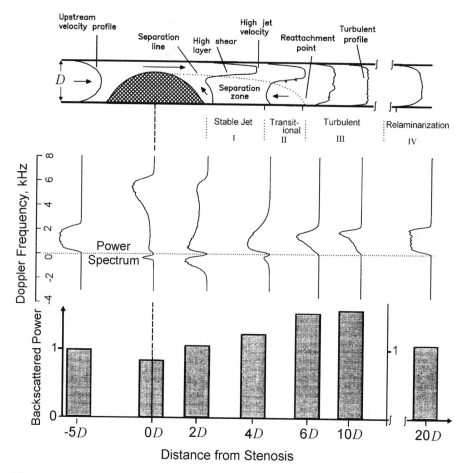

Figure 9.18 Changes seen in the Doppler spectrum and total backscattered power for a 5 MHz CW system as the insonation site was moved relative to a 70% (by area) stenosis. The experimental results were obtained under steady flow conditions at a Reynolds number of 545 using a 40% suspension of human RBCs in saline. The Doppler probe axis was at 50 degrees to the tube axis. Note that the power reaches a maximum in the turbulent region. (Reproduced, with permission, from Bascom and Cobbold [44], *IEEE Trans. Biomed. Eng.*, 43, 562–571, © 1996 IEEE, and reprinted by permission of Elsevier from Bascom et al. [55], *Ultrasound Med. Biol.*, 19, 197–210, © 1993 World Federation of Ultrasound in Medicine and Biology.)

where A is a constant and where the Doppler equation, namely (9.6), expresses ω_D^i in terms of $\mathbf{v}_i$, i.e.,

$$(9.16) \qquad \omega_D^i = 2(\omega_o/c_o)v_i \cos\theta = 2\mathbf{k}\cdot\mathbf{v}_i.$$

Using this to eliminate ω_D^i from the previous equation yields

$$x_i(t) = A\sqrt{\sigma_b}\cos\big[(\omega_o + 2\mathbf{k}\cdot\mathbf{v}_i)t + \phi_i\big].$$

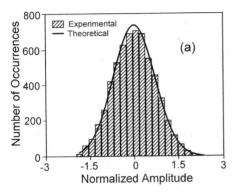
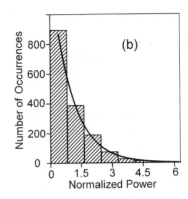

Figure 9.19 Statistical properties of the Doppler signal. (a) Measured CW Doppler amplitude distribution in the time domain for steady flow of a 42% hematocrit suspension of RBCs. A Gaussian distribution is shown for comparison. (b) Power distribution at 1.5 kHz measured over 1,500 successive 10-ms time intervals, providing evidence that the power at a specific frequency is chi-squared distributed with two degrees of freedom. (Reprinted by permission of Elsevier from Bascom et al. [55], *Ultrasound Med. Biol.*, 19, 197-210, © 1993 World Federation of Ultrasound in Medicine and Biology.)

When all such components are summed over the N identical scatterers within the sample volume and the resulting signal is demodulated and low-pass filtered, the Doppler signal is obtained as

$$x(t) = A\sqrt{\sigma_b} \sum_{i=1}^{N} \cos\left[(2\mathbf{k}\cdot\mathbf{v}_i)t + \phi_i\right].$$

In this equation $\mathbf{v}_i$ is a function of $\mathbf{r}_i$, which, like ϕ_i, is a random variable. Because $x(t)$ is formed from the sum of a large number of independent contributions, it tends toward a Gaussian random process that has a zero mean; consequently, it can be completely specified by its autocorrelation function [59].

Experimental evidence that the Doppler signal in the time domain is Gaussian distributed has been presented by Bascom et al. [55]. Using the model illustrated in Fig. 9.18 with a 42% hematocrit suspension of RBCs, a 1.0 s duration demodulated Doppler signal was recorded and digitized from a region where laminar flow was expected to be present. As can be seen in Fig. 9.19a, the sampled amplitude has a distribution that is close to Gaussian. Measurements at other locations, using short-duration windows, also indicated that throughout the flow model the signal was Gaussian. A second aspect concerns the statistics of the power spectrum: specifically, the characteristics of the power distribution at a specific frequency. For a Gaussian-distributed time series it can be shown [60, pp. 466–468] that the power distribution at a specific frequency should be chi-squared distributed with two degrees of freedom.[4]

4. An exponential distribution is the same as the special case of a chi-squared distribution with 2 degrees of freedom.

Experimental results obtained in a laminar flow region are shown in Fig. 9.19b, and these show close agreement with the predicted distribution. However, in the turbulent zone, Bascom et al. [55] reported that the hypothesis of a chi-squared distribution should be rejected.

9.6.2 Doppler Simulation Models

A Doppler signal model [61,62] can be based on a voxel approach for describing the scattering by blood; as will be seen, this results in a form that is particularly convenient for simulation purposes. In Chapter 5, it was pointed out that if the sample volume is divided into elements of volume that are small compared to a wavelength, then each voxel will contain differing numbers of RBCs, depending on the statistics. The backscattered pressure waveform was shown to arise from the effects of these variations throughout the sample volume. We first recall (5.66), which was derived for the backscattered RF pressure waveform created by a given stationary realization of RBCs within the sample volume. This equation can be readily adapted to account for the effects of flow and demodulation through the following steps. First, the crystallographic term can be ignored. Second, to obtain the Doppler demodulated signal we replace ω by ω_D', as expressed by (9.16). Third, we divide the total range of velocities within the sample volume into M velocity bins and use the index i to denote one of these bins. The number of voxels in the ith bin whose velocities are $\mathbf{v}_i$ will be denoted[5] by m_i.

From (5.66), making use of the above substitutions and notational changes, the demodulated time-domain Doppler signal can be expressed as

$$(9.17) \qquad x(t) = A\sqrt{\sigma_b} \sum_{i=1}^{M} \sum_{j=1}^{m_i} n_{i,j}(t - t_{i,j}) \cos(2t\mathbf{k} \cdot \mathbf{v}_i + \phi_{i,j}),$$

where $n_{i,j}(t-t_{i,j})$ denotes the deviation of the number of RBCs in the jth voxel of the ith bin from the mean value at a time $(t - t_{i,j})$, where $t_{i,j}$ is the time taken for the scattered wave to travel back to the transducer. Also, $\phi_{i,j}$ is the corresponding voxel phase that can reasonably be assumed to be uniformly distributed over $(-\pi, \pi)$.

By proceeding in a manner similar to that enabling (5.60) to be transformed into (5.62), it can be shown [61] that (9.17) can be transformed to

$$(9.18) \qquad x(t) = A\sqrt{\sigma_b} \sum_{i=1}^{M} a_i(t) \cos(2t\mathbf{k} \cdot \mathbf{v}_i + \psi_i),$$

where the phase ψ_i is uniformly distributed over $(-\pi, \pi)$ and $a_i(t) = \sqrt{\sum_{j=1}^{m_i} n_{i,j}^2(t - t_{i,j})}$ is a Rayleigh distributed random variable. If each bin has an

---

5. The sum of the m-values over all velocity bins will equal the number of voxels in the sample volume, i.e., $\sum_{i=1}^{M} m_i = N_x$.

incremental frequency range of Δf, then the Doppler signal power of the ith bin is given by

$$\Delta P_i(f_D^i, t) = \Phi(f_D^i, t)\Delta f_D^i.$$

But from (9.18), the power of the ith component is $\Delta P_i(t) = \sigma_b a_i^2(t)/2$. Consequently, (9.18) can be written as

$$x(t) = \sum_{i=1}^{M} \sqrt{2\Delta f_D^i \Phi(f_D^i, t)\chi_i} \cos(2t\mathbf{k}\cdot\mathbf{v}_i + \psi_i), \tag{9.19}$$

where χ_i is a chi-squared random variable with two degrees of freedom and a mean value of unity. The advantage of this model is that it enables the Doppler signal to be simulated for any assumed spectral shape. As shown by Mo and Cobbold, (9.19) enables realistic Doppler signals to be simulated for both steady [63] and pulsatile flow [64] conditions. For example, in the case of steady parabolic flow, it may be reasonable to specify a flat spectrum extending from a wall cutoff frequency of f_D^{min} up to f_D^{max}. Then, with $M = (f_D^{max} - f_D^{min})/\Delta f_D^i$ and a constant value of $\Phi(f_D^i, t)$ over this frequency range, (9.18) can be used to generate the Doppler signal. On the other hand, if the flow is pulsatile, the variation of the Doppler spectrum must be specified over a complete flow cycle. However, the model does not simulate the effects of the low-frequency clutter signal created by vessel wall movement. As noted earlier, these movements create signal components with spectra that are typically below 200 Hz, though with amplitudes many times stronger than that from blood.

An alternative simulation approach is to assume that the backscattered signal is created by a random distribution of small identical particles transported in fully developed pulsatile flow. The velocity profile equation given by (9.15) can be used to determine the velocity distribution within the insonated volume. This, together with an appropriate scattering model, enables the backscattered signal and its non-stationary spectrum to be predicted. Bastos et al. [65] used this simulation method to examine the influence of acceleration and other parameters on the spectra obtained with a pulsed wave measurement system. Subsequently, in studying methods for removing the clutter component, Zhang et al. [66] extended this simulation approach by including a low-frequency component that simulated the effect of vessel wall movement. For various clutter-to-blood ratios, they showed that a wavelet approach could be used to advantage for separating the clutter signal with minimum loss of the true flow signal.

9.7 Doppler Spectral Broadening

An ideal Doppler velocity determining system when measuring a single scatterer moving with a constant velocity should have a power spectrum with a δ-function response at the Doppler frequency. Spectral broadening refers to an increase of the spectral bandwidth; as will be described, several potential sources can be identified. Spectral broadening is also important in optics, particularly in association with Doppler laser flow measurements, in weather radar (wind shear information can be derived from the Doppler broadening), as well as in Doppler ultrasound.

In Doppler radar, it is well established that ambiguity (uncertainty) exists in simultaneously measuring the range and speed of an object. This is also true for Doppler ultrasound measurements. To illustrate this, we shall consider the accuracy that can be achieved using long- (pseudo-CW) and short-pulse radar transmissions for determining the range and speed of an object. Long-pulse radar is a narrowband process, and the accuracy with which the Doppler shift can be measured is limited by the SNR and the transit time of the object through the beam. However, considerable uncertainty will exist as to the target range. Short-pulse transmissions enable the range to be determined much more accurately, but the wider bandwidth and the resulting higher noise increase the ambiguity in determining the Doppler frequency. It can be shown that for an optimal matched filter reception system, the product of the range and speed measurement errors is determined by the SNR and the time-bandwidth product of the measurement system. For such a system, the ambiguity function introduced by Woodward [67] provides a useful means of optimizing the system so that it best meets the desired performance. Similar limitations and optimization tasks are present in Doppler ultrasound. First, it is helpful to look at the ambiguity arising from spectral broadening.

Green [68] seems to have been the first to identify and analyze several distinct causes of spectral broadening in Doppler ultrasound flowmeters. This work was extended by Brody [43], who included both the transit-time and geometric effects as distinct causes of broadening (see also [69] and [70]). As indicated in Table 9.2, the many possible causes of Doppler spectral broadening can best be discussed by categorizing them according to whether they are intrinsic or extrinsic to the transduction and analysis processes. Intrinsic refers to those processes that are an inherent part of the measurement and analysis methods. Extrinsic processes are those associated with the nature of the velocity field. Using the pulsatile-flow Doppler signal simulation model described in the last subsection, Bastos et al. [65] have examined the influence of several of these processes on the overall spectral broadening.

The contribution of Brownian motion to the overall broadening has been shown to be very small [68], and consequently it will be ignored in the ensuing

Table 9.2. Causes of Doppler Spectral Broadening

Intrinsic	Extrinsic
†Transit-time	Spatial velocity distribution
†Geometric	Vector velocity direction
Brownian motion	Turbulence
*Spectral analysis window	*Acceleration

†* Not independent sources: see discussion.

discussion of intrinsic and extrinsic processes. Although our focus is on CW Doppler spectral broadening, it should be noted that many of the sources of spectral broadening in pulsed wave systems are identical.

9.7.1 Intrinsic Broadening

Transit-time broadening can be understood by considering the Doppler signal produced by the movement of a scatter through a sample volume. For simplicity, we shall assume that within the sample volume the phase iso-contours are planes. As sketched in Fig. 9.20a, the Doppler waveform from a single scatterer is gated by the movement into and out of the sample volume, resulting in a spectral spread about the center frequency, i.e., broadening arises from windowing a constant frequency waveform.

On the other hand, Fig. 9.20b shows that as the scatterer moves through the sample volume, it suspends a range of angles to various spatial locations on the transducer surface. At each location, the scatterer will see elemental sources on the transducer surface at different angles; thereby producing a spectrum of Doppler frequencies, and this spectrum changes as the scatterer traverses the sample volume. This spectrum will be further broadened on reception because every point on the receiving transducer aperture also subtends a range of angles. Thus, ambiguities in the vector directions on both transmission and reception are present, and both must be accounted for to determine the overall spectral shape. When the same transducer is used for both transmission and reception, Bascom et al. [45] pointed out that by using the principle of reciprocity the received amplitude spectrum can be expressed as the autocorrelation of the complex spectrum seen by the scatterer, i.e., by

$$(9.20) \qquad \mathcal{A}_R(\omega_D) = \frac{1}{2\omega_{BW}} \int\limits_{-\omega_{BW}}^{\omega_{BW}} \mathcal{A}_T(\omega_D')\mathcal{A}_T^*(\omega_D' - \omega_D)d\omega_D', \qquad (a)$$

where ω_{BW} is the angular frequency bandwidth and the complex conjugate of the spectrum seen by the scatterer is denoted by $\mathcal{A}_T^*(\omega_D)$. An alternative form for (9.20a) is that subsequently obtained by Censor et al. [71], in which the received spectrum is expressed in the form of a self-convolution given by

$$(9.20) \qquad \mathcal{A}_R(\omega_D) \propto \mathcal{A}_T(\omega_D) * \mathcal{A}_T(\omega_D), \qquad (b)$$

which they called the Doppler spectrum convolution theorem. In fact, this and (9.20a) can be shown to be equivalent.

The spectrum seen by the scatterer as it traverses the beam can be obtained by treating the transducer as a distribution of incremental sources and the spectrum as a distribution of incremental frequency bins. By summing the complex signal amplitudes that contribute to each frequency bin, the complex amplitude spectrum $\mathcal{A}_T(\omega_D)$ can be obtained. Then, by evaluating (9.20), the received Doppler amplitude spectrum can be calculated. Details of a method that uses this approach have been reported for calculating the CW Doppler

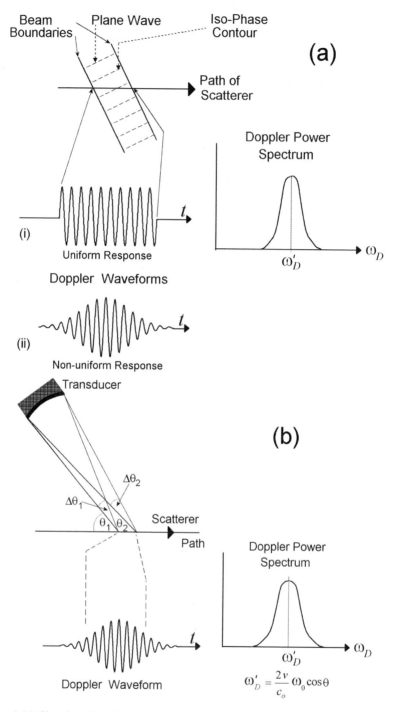

Figure 9.20 Sketches showing how spectral broadening can arise from the movement of a constant velocity scatterer through the sample volume. (a) Broadening due to the transit time of a scatterer through the sample volume. The time waveform is shown for (i) a constant response over the beam width and (ii) a Gaussian-like response. (b) Broadening due to a range of angles that the particle suspends to different points on the transducer surface. All points on the transducer surface act as both transmitters and receivers: both frequency and amplitude modulation occur.

spectrum for transducers with square and circular geometries and when these insonate various flow velocity profiles [45].

A somewhat different approach originally discussed by Fish [72] was subsequently implemented by Ata and Fish [73]. It requires that the complex pressure $p(\mathbf{r})$ of the transmitted field be determined at incremental points along the scatterer trajectory. If it is assumed that the same transducer is used for both transmission and reception, then the principle of reciprocity can also be used to calculate the received signal from the signal seen by the moving scatterer. Specifically, if the scatterer position is denoted by $\mathbf{r}$, the backscattered signal will be proportional to $p^2(\mathbf{r})e^{j\omega_o t}$. Because the scatterer is moving, its position $\mathbf{r}$ will be a function of time, and since the demodulation process eliminates the carrier frequency ω_o, the analytic Doppler signal over the entire trajectory will be proportional to $p^2(\mathbf{r})$. Because the spectrum is simply the Fourier transform, i.e., $\mathcal{A}_R(\omega_D) = \Im\{p(t)p(t)\}$, by using the convolution product theorem as given in Appendix B, this is seen to be proportional to $\mathcal{A}_T(\omega_D)$ * $\mathcal{A}_T(\omega_D)$, which is the same as that given by (9.20).

As an example of the above method, Fig. 9.21 shows both the waveform and the spectrum of a single scatterer as it moves with a constant velocity (10 cm/s) on a path at 45 degrees to the axis of a simple piston transducer. The two sets of results correspond to a path that intersects the transducer axis at half the last maximum (a^2/λ) and one that intersects the last maximum. In the first case it will be noted that because the scatterer passes through an axial region close to the last minimum, the Doppler signal amplitude is greatly reduced for a substantial time, and this is partially responsible for the complex nature of the spectrum. A much smoother spectrum results when the scatterer path passes through the last maximum.

Spectral broadening in laser Doppler flowmeters is directly related to broadening in Doppler ultrasound. Edwards et al. [74] presented a detailed analytical study of spectral broadening in laser Doppler flowmeters. They showed that transit-time (referred to as Doppler radar ambiguity) broadening and geometric (referred to as wave vector ambiguity) broadening are equivalent to one another in the focal region. In other words, calculation of transit-time broadening also accounted for geometric broadening, and vice versa. As part of continuing studies on Doppler ultrasound broadening, Newhouse et al. [75] stated "that geometrical broadening and transit time broadening are one and the same effect under the conditions that hold for Doppler ultrasound measurement." In discussing this statement, Jones [76] used a simple example to illustrate why this equivalence is not necessarily true.

Consider the sketch of Fig. 9.22, in which a scatterer is moving with a constant velocity through the CW field produced by a point source. It can be seen that as the scatterer starts to approach the source, the amplitude increases and the Doppler frequency reduces, as expressed by the Doppler equation {see (9.6a)}. On passing by the source, the instantaneous frequency then starts to increase in a negative direction and the amplitude starts to diminish, approaching zero as the distance approaches infinity: at this point, the Doppler frequency approaches $-2vf_o/c_o$. Consequently, the Doppler signal is modulated

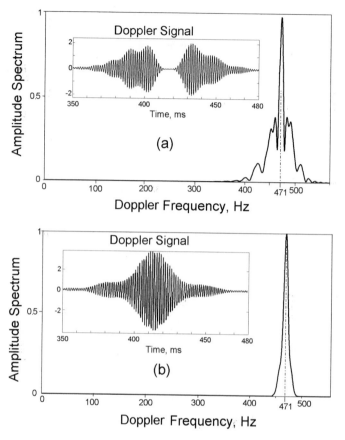

Figure 9.21 Calculated CW Doppler waveform and its amplitude spectrum produced by a point scatterer moving with a velocity of 10 cm/s at 45 degrees to the axis of a 5 mm radius piston transducer excited at 5 MHz. For a straight-line path through the axis at (a) 0.5 of the last maximum and (b) the last maximum. In the absence of spectral broadening, the spectrum would be a δ-function at 741 Hz. The results were obtained by using (3.22) with $f_r(z, R) = 1$ for calculating the normalized pressure.

in both amplitude and frequency. It should be noted that the assumption of a point source/detector means that just a single angle is subtended at any given scatterer location. This should be contrasted to the situation shown in Fig. 9.20b, where a range of angles exists at each scatterer location, causing a spectrum of Doppler frequencies, and this spectrum changes as the scatterer moves through the sample volume.

For a point source and detector, the demodulated backscattered signal can be written as $A(t)e^{j2f[\mathbf{k}(t)\cdot\mathbf{v}]}$, in which both the magnitude and direction of $\mathbf{k}$ are functions of $\mathbf{r}$ and therefore of time. Jones [76] pointed out that the amplitude modulation term $A(t)$ leads to what one might intuitively regard as transit-

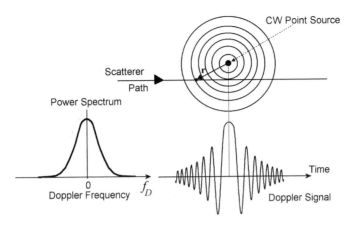

Figure 9.22 Sketch showing the time-domain Doppler signal and its spectrum produced by a scatterer moving with a constant velocity in the field produced by a CW point source that also acts as a receiver. Note that both the amplitude and frequency are functions of r, and therefore of time. (Based on a similar sketch by Jones [76].)

time spectral broadening. On the other hand, the exponent contains the term $v\cos[\theta(\mathbf{r})]$, which describes a change in Doppler frequency with the scatterer position. However, this term, which can be considered to account for the effect of geometric broadening, is not equivalent to $A(t)$. As noted by Jones, the theoretical proof given by Edwards et al. [74] assumed a constant angle between $\mathbf{k}$ and $\mathbf{v}$ within the sample volume, i.e., the wavefronts are planes. While this may be a reasonable approximation in the focal region, it is unlikely to be the case elsewhere. Fig. 9.23a provides an intuitive picture of how changes in the direction of $\mathbf{k}$ over the scatterer trajectory can affect the Doppler waveform.

Ata and Fish [73] examined the planarity assumption using a computational model that calculates $p(\mathbf{r})$ over the path as described earlier in this section. They calculated the CW Doppler spectrum produced by a small scatterer as it traversed the field produced by apodized and unapodized plane and focused disk transducers. They assumed that it moved with a constant velocity at 45 degrees to the beam axis and intercepted the axis at either the focal point or halfway from it. Comparison of the spectral shapes with and without frequency modulation showed that when the particle passed through the focus, the effect of the planar assumption was relatively good (<16%). However, at half the focal distance, much larger errors (up to 234%) were found. Part of the confusion over the statement concerning the equivalence of transit-time and geometric broadening arises from the failure to provide a clear definition of geometric spectral broadening. If it is defined in terms of the angles subtended to all points on the transducer surface from the scatterer, as depicted in Fig. 9.20b, then transit-time broadening is not equal to geometric broadening; rather, it is a subset of it [76].

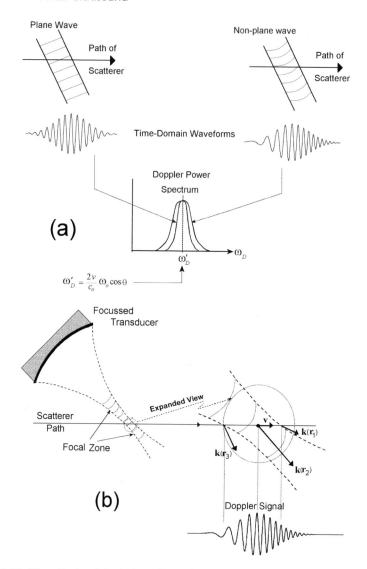

Figure 9.23 The effects of deviations from plane-wave conditions on the Doppler signal and spectrum. (a) Simplified sketch for plane wave and non-plane wave conditions. Note that for non-planar conditions, the frequency increases as the scatterer moves through the sample volume. (Modified version, reproduced, with permission, from Ata and Fish [73].) (b) More realistic sketch showing the change in the wave vector direction and magnitude as the scatterer moves through the focal zone. (Based on a similar sketch by Fish [72].)

Another contribution to intrinsic spectral broadening arises from the method of spectral analysis and the choice of signal sample window. For measurements on human arteries, it is generally assumed that the signal is quasi-stationary over a duration of around 5 ms. This suggests that by dividing the signal into overlapping 10-ms segments every 5 ms and performing an FFT on each segment, a reasonably accurate representation of the true spectral variation can be obtained. However, the windowing process is a cause of spectral broadening, and this becomes more severe as the duration is reduced.

9.7.2 Extrinsic Broadening

Extrinsic broadening refers to effects extrinsic to the Doppler system. The simplest case, corresponding to the first form of broadening listed in Table 9.2, arises when the scatterers within the insonated volume have a range of velocities but their vectors all point in the same direction. For example, in the case of a small vessel, the range of velocities will range from zero to a maximum and give rise to the spectra described in section 9.5.

A second form of extrinsic broadening arises from a distribution of velocity directions within the insonated volume. This can arise from the flow boundary causing a change in the flow direction or the inclusion of a separation line. In a turbulent region, there will be a range in velocity vector directions. In addition, because a turbulent region can be expected to have an increased variance of the voxel scatterer number density (see subsection 5.9.4), resulting in increased backscattering, the spectrum may be broadened.

In pulsatile flow, changes in the mean velocity will occur within the window used for spectral analysis, giving rise to spectral broadening. Acceleration broadening (also called non-stationary broadening) has been studied by several groups using theoretical analysis [77,78], Doppler signal simulation methods [65], and experimental measurements [79]. In their simulation study using a common femoral artery waveform, Bastos et al. [65] showed that for windows of very short duration, e.g., 2 ms, broadening will be dominated by the nature of the window rather than by the effects of acceleration. However, for longer windows, the effects of acceleration become important and need to be accounted for in predicting the overall spectral broadening.

9.7.3 Maximum Velocity Estimation Errors

Pulsed wave ultrasound measurements of the peak systolic velocity are widely used for determining the severity of a stenosis in a variety of vessels. Typically, a phased-array transducer is used to position a small sample volume in a central region of the vessel. The method is used as a clinical screening tool to determine which patients need an angiogram prior to surgery; in some institutions, peak velocity measurement is the only preoperative diagnostic technique used prior to carotid endarterectomy and reoperative surgery on bypass grafts. However, studies using phased-array transducers have shown the presence of significant errors in peak velocity estimations; these can range from −4% up to 47% [80], leading to serious misdiagnoses. Several potential sources of error have been suggested [81]: those associated with the ultrasound system itself; those associated with the technologist, including the examination technique; and those arising from the geometry of the vessel, such as its tortuosity. Spectral broadening is a primary cause of errors in the ultrasound system itself. Spreading out the frequency distribution causes the measured peak frequency to be higher than the value corresponding to the true peak velocity.

Several methods for error correction have been proposed and evaluated depending on the assumed origin of the spectral broadening. Correction techniques for intrinsic spectral broadening have been proposed by several groups [82–86]. In addition, a correction method to account for the effects of acceleration and window broadening has been proposed by Wang and Fish [87].

In the method proposed and experimentally verified by Tortoli et al. [83], it is assumed that the beam-to-flow angle is relatively large, so that the scatterers cross the waist of the ultrasound beam, and the influence of the sample volume axial dimensions is unimportant. If it can be assumed that the Doppler spectrum is close to symmetric about the value given by the Doppler equation, then the maximum frequency and the Doppler bandwidth B_D are related to the velocity of a streamline by

$$f_D^{\max} = \frac{2v}{c_o} f_o \cos\theta + \frac{1}{2} B_D.$$

For a focused transducer with cylindrical symmetry, Censor et al. [71] have shown that the bandwidth is proportional to the scatterer velocity component normal to the ultrasound beam direction ($v\sin\theta$) and inversely proportional to the *f-number*. Specifically, they found the Doppler bandwidth associated with a streamline of velocity v is given by

$$B_D = \frac{2f_o}{c_o} \frac{\mathcal{D}}{F} v \sin\theta,$$

where $\mathcal{D}$ is the transducer aperture and F is the focal length. Although this relation was derived for a focused transducer with cylindrical symmetry, Newhouse and Reid [88] state that the above proportionality relations can be extended to focused rectangular apertures [89]. By combining the above two equations, it can be seen that the observed maximum frequency is related to the true velocity by

(9.21)
$$f_D^{\max} = \frac{2f_o v}{c_o} \left[\cos\theta + \frac{1}{2} \frac{\mathcal{D}}{F} \sin\theta \right].$$

Using a pulsed wave ultrasound system with a focused piston transducer, Tortoli et al. [83] reported experimental results over a range of beam-to-flow angles. By using (9.21) to predict the scatterer velocity in the beam direction from the measured maximum velocity, they showed that the accuracy was significantly improved over a range of angles from 70 to 90 degrees.

References

1. White, D.N., Johann Christian Doppler and his effect, a brief history, *Ultrasound Med. Biol.*, 8, 583–591, 1982.

2. Doppler, C., Uber das farbige Licht der Doppelsterne und einiger anderer Gestirne des Himmels (On the coloured light of double stars and certain other stars of the heavens), *Abh. Konigl. Bohm. Ges. Wiss.*, 2, 465–482, 1843.

3. Jonkman, E.J., Doppler research in the nineteenth century, *Ultrasound Med. Biol.*, 6, 1–5, 1980.

4. Chilowski, C., and Langevin, P., Production of submarine signals and the location of submarine objects, US patent 1,471,547 Oct. 1923 (filed May 1917).

5. Chilowski, C., Method and means for the observation and measurement of the speed of a vesel by directed beams of ultra-audible waves, US patent 1,864,638, June 1932 (filed Dec. 1924).

6. Lynnworth, L.A., Ultrasonic flowmeters, Chapter 5, pp. 407–525 in: *Physical Acoustics*, Vol. 14, W.P. Mason, and R.N. Thurston (Eds.), Academic Press, New York, 1979.

7. Beck, M.S., and Plaskowski, A., *Cross Correlation Flowmeters: Their Design and Application,* IOP Press, Bristol, UK, 1987.

8. Rutten, O., Verfahren und Vorrichtung zum Messen von stromenden Flussigkeits: Gas-oder Dampfmengen [Method and means for measuring fluid, gas or steam volume flow], German Patent No. 520,484, Feb. 1931 (applied for Sept. 1928).

9. Kunze, W., Uber eine Methode Geschwindigkeiten auf akustischem Wege zu messen [On an acoustic method of measuring air velocities], *Physikalische Zeitscr.*, 21, 437–443, 1920.

10. Kamus, H.P., Hedrloh, A.L., and Pardue, D.R., The acoustic flowmeter using electroric switching, *Trans. IRE Prof. Group on Ultrasonics Engineering*, 1, 49–62, 1954.

11. Satomura, S., Matsubara, S., and Yoshioka, M., A new method of mechanical vibration measurement and its application, *Memoirs Inst. Scient. Indust. Res. Osaka Univ.*, 13, 125–133, 1956.

12. Kaneko, Z., First steps in the development of the Doppler flowmeter, *Ultrasound Med. Biol.*, 12, 187–195, 1986.

13. Satomura, S., Astracts of papers #231–234 presented at a meeting and reported in: *Jpn. Circ. J.*, 20, 227–228, 1956. See also: Satomura, S., Ultrasonic Doppler method for the inspection of cardiac functions, *J. Acoust. Soc. Am.*, 29, 1181–1185, 1957.

14. Satomura, S., Nimura, Y., and Yoshida, T., Ultrasonic Doppler cardiograph, *Proc. 3rd Int. Conf. on Medical Electronics*, pp. 249–253, 1960.

15. Satomura, S., Tamura, A., and Kido, Y., Study of blood flow in vessels by ultrasonics. (Abstr. of meeting: *Acoust. Soc. Jpn.*, 1958, 81–82, Oct., 1958.

16. Satomura, S., Study of the flow patterns in peripheral arteries by ultrasonics [in Japanese], *J. Acoust. Soc. Jpn.*, 15, 151–158, 1959.

17. Satomura, S., and Kaneko, Z., Ultrasonic blood rheograph, *Proc. 3rd Int. Conf. on Medical Electronics*, pp. 254–258, 1960.

18. Kato, K., Kido, Y., Motomiya, M., Kaneko, Z., and Kotani, H., On the mechanism of generation of detected sound in ultrasonic flowmeter, *Memoirs Inst. Scient. Indust. Res., Osaka Univ.*, 19, 51–57, 1962.

19. Reid, J.M., Sigelmann, R.A., Nasser, M.C., and Baker, D.W., The scattering of ultrasound by human blood, Paper 10–7 in: *Proc. 8th Int. Conf. Med. Biolog. Eng.*, Chicago, 1969.

20. Sigelmann, R.A., and Reid, J.M., Analysis and measurement of ultrasound backscattering from an ensemble of scatterers excited by sine-wave bursts, *J. Acoust. Soc. Am.*, 53, 1351–1355, 1973.

21. Kato, K., and Izumi, T., A new ultrasonic flowmeter that can detect flow direction, *Jpn. Med. Ultrasonics*, 5, 28–30, 1966.

22. McLeod, F.D., A directional Doppler flowmeter, p. 213 in: *Digest. 7th Int. Conf. Med. Biolog. Eng.*, Stockholm, 1967.

23. Franklin, D.L., Baker, D.W., Ellis, R.M., and Rushmer, R.F., A pulsed ultrasonic flowmeter, *IRE Trans. Bio-Med. Electronics*, 6, 204–206, 1959.

24. Franklin, D.L., Baker, D.W., and Rushmer, R.F., Pulsed ultrasonic transit time flowmeter, *IRE Trans. Bio-Med. Electronics*, 9, 44–49, 1962.

25. Herrick, J.F., and Anderson, J.A., Circulatory system: methods; ultrasonic flowmeter, pp. 181–184 in: *Medical Physics*, Vol. 3, O. Glasser (Ed.), Year Book Pub., Chicago, 1960.

26. Franklin, D., Frequency modulated ultrasound technique for measurement of fluid velocity, US Patent 3,568,661, March 1971 (filed Oct. 2, 1968).

27. Ziomek, L.J., *Fundamentals of Acoustic Field Theory and Space-Time Signal Processing*, CRC Press, Boca Raton, FL, 1995.

28. Wells, P.N.T., Ultrasonic Doppler probes, Chapter 9, pp. 125–131 in: *Cardiovascular Applications of Ultrasound*, R.S. Reneman (Ed.), North-Holland Pub., Amsterdam, 1974.

29. Evans, D.H., and Parton, I., The directional characteristics of some ultrasonic Doppler blood-flow probes, *Ultrasound Med. Biol.*, 7, 51–62, 1981.

30. Douville, Y., Arenson, J.W., Johnston, K.W., Cobbold, R.S.C., and Kassam, M., Critical evaluation of continuous-wave Doppler probes for carotid studies, *J. Clin. Ultrasound*, 11, 83–90, 1983.

31. Hoeks, A.G.P., Ruissen, C.J., Hick, P., and Reneman, R.S., Methods to evaluate the sample volume of pulsed Doppler systems, *Ultrasound Med. Biol.*, 10, 427–434, 1984.

32. Hoskins, P.R., and Ramnarine, K.V., Doppler test devices, Appendix 2, pp. 382–404 in [36].

33. Reid, J.M., Davis, D.L., Ricketts, H.J., and Spencer, M.P., A new Doppler flowmeter system and its operation with catheter mounted transducers, Chapter 14, pp. 183–192 in: *Cardiovascular Applications of Ultrasound*, R.S. Reneman (Ed.), North-Holland Pub., Amsterdam, 1974.

34. Atkinson, P., and Woodcock, J.P., *Doppler Ultrasound and its Use in Clinical Measurement*, Academic Press, London, 1982.

35. Jensen, J.A., *Estimation of Blood Velocities Using Ultrasound*, Cambridge Univ. Press, Cambridge, 1996.

36. Evans, D.H., and McDicken, W.N., *Doppler Ultrasound: Physics, Instrumentation and Signal Processing*, 2nd Ed., Wiley, New York, 2000.

37. Aydin, N., and Evans, D.H., Implementation of directional Doppler techniques using a digital signal processor, *Med. Biolog. Eng. Comput.*, 32, S157–164, 1994.

38. Aydin, N., Fan., L., and Evans, D.H., Quadrature to directional format conversion of Doppler signals using digital methods, *Physiol. Meas.*, 15, 181–199, 1994.

39. Kaneko, Z., Shiraishi, J., Omizo, H., Kato, K., Motomiya, M., Izumi, T., and Okumura, T., An analyzing method of ultrasonic blood-rheograph with sonograph, pp. 286–287 in: *Digest of 5th Int. Conf. Med. Electron. Biolog. Eng.*, Tokyo, 1965.

40. Kaneko, Z., Shiraishi, J., and Omizo, H., Analysis of ultrasonic blood rheogram by a band pass filter, *Angiology*, 19, 10–24, 1968.

41. Roevros, J.M.J.G., Analog processing of C.W. Doppler flowmeter signals to determine average frequency shift momentaneously without the use of a wave analyzer, Chapter 4, pp. 43–54 in: *Cardiovascular Applications of Ultrasound*, R.S. Reneman (Ed.), North-Holland Pub., Amsterdam, 1974.

42. Fahrbach, K., Ein beitrag zur blutgeschwindigkeitsmessung unter anwendungdes Dopplereffektes [A major contribution to blood speed measurement using the Doppler effect], *Elektromedizin*, 14, 233–246, 1969 and 15, 26–36, 1970.

43. Brody, W.R., Theoretical analysis of the ultrasonic flowmeter, PhD thesis, Dept. Elect. Eng., Stanford University, 1971 (Technical report # 4958-1). See also: Brody, M.R., and Meindl, Theoretical analysis of the CW ultrasonic flowmeter, *IEEE Trans. Biomed. Eng.*, 21, 183–192, 1974.

44. Bascom, P.A.J., and Cobbold, R.S.C., Origin of the Doppler ultrasound spectrum from blood, *IEEE Trans. Biomed. Eng.*, 43, 562–571, 1996.

45. Bascom, P.A.J., Cobbold, R.S.C., and Roelfs, B.H.M., Influence of spectral broadening on continuous wave Doppler ultrasound spectra: a geometric approach, *Ultrasound Med. Biol.*, 12, 387–395, 1986.

46. Bascom, P.A.J., and Cobbold, R.S.C., Effects of transducer beam geometry and flow velocity profile on the Doppler power spectrum: a theoretical study, *Ultrasound Med. Biol.*, 16, 279–295, 1989.

47. Arts, M.G.J., and Roevros, J.M.J.G., On the instantaneous measurement of blood flow by ultrasonic means, *Med. Biolog. Eng.*, 10, 23–34, 1972.

48. Nakayama, K., and Furuharta, H., Necessary requirements for blood flowmetering by ultrasonic Doppler method, *Electron. Comm. Jpn.*, 57-C, 85–92, 1974.

49. Shehada, R.E.N., Cobbold, R.S.C., Johnston, K.W., and Aarnink, R., Three-dimensional display of calculated velocity profiles for physiological flow waveforms, *J. Vasc. Surg.*, 17, 656–660, 1993.

50. Evans, D.H., Some aspects of the relationship between instantaneous volumetric blood flow and continuous wave Doppler ultrasound recording—III. The calculation of Doppler power spectra from mean velocity waveforms, and the results of processing these spectra with maximum, mean, and RMS frequency processors, *Ultrasound Med. Biol.*, 18, 617–623, 1982.

51. Womersley, J.R., Method for the calculation of the velocity, rate of flow and viscous drag in arteries when the pressure gradient is known, *J. Physiol.*, 127, 553–563, 1955.

52. Cobbold, R.S.C., Mo, L.Y.L., and Johnston, K.W., Methods for processing, displaying and recording Doppler signals, Chapter 5, pp. 43–70 in: *Cardiovascular Applications of Doppler Ultrasonography*, A.N. Nicolaides, and A.M. Salmasi (Eds.), Churchill Livingstone, Edinburgh, 1989.

53. Kassam, M., Johnston, K.W., and Cobbold, R.S.C., Quantitative estimation of spectral broadening for the diagnosis of carotid arterial disease: method and in-vitro results, *Ultrasound Med. Biol.*, 11, 425–433, 1985.

54. Routh, H.F., Law, Y.F., Mo, L.Y.L., Ojha, M., Vaitkus, P.J., Cobbold, R.S.C., Johnston, K.W., and Bascom, P.A.J., Role of models in understanding and interpreting clinical Doppler ultrasound, *Medical Progress through Technology*, 15, 155–169, 1989.

55. Bascom, P.A.J., Cobbold, R.S.C., Routh, H.F., and Johnston, K.W., On the Doppler signal from a steady flow asymmetrical stenosis model: effects of turbulence, *Ultrasound Med. Biol.*, 19, 197–210, 1993.

56. Bascom, P.A.J., Johnston, K.W., Cobbold, R.S.C., and Ojha, M., Relation of the flow field distal to a moderate stenosis to the Doppler power, *Ultrasound Med. Biol.*, 23, 25–39, 1997.

57. Bascom, P.A.J., Johnston, K.W., Cobbold, R.S.C., and Ojha, M., Defining the limitations of measurements from Doppler spectral recordings, *J. Vasc. Surg.*, 24, 34–45, 1996.

58. Ojha, M., Hummel, R.L., Cobbold, R.S.C., and Johnston, K.W., Development and evaluation of a high resolution photochromic dye method for pulsatile flow studies, *J. Physics, E., Sci. Instrum.*, 21, 998–1004, 1988.

59. Mo, L.Y-L., and Cobbold, R.S.C., A stochastic model of the backscattered Doppler ultrasound from blood, *IEEE Trans. Biomed. Eng.*, 33, 20–27, 1986.

60. Priestley, M.B., *Spectral Analysis and Time Series*, Vol. 1, Academic Press, New York, 1981.

61. Mo, L.Y-L., and Cobbold, R.S.C., A unified approach to modelling the backscattered Doppler ultrasound from blood, *IEEE Trans. Biomed. Eng.*, 39, 450–461, 1992.

62. Mo, L.Y-L., and Cobbold, R.S.C., Theoretical models of ultrasonic scattering in blood, Chapter 5, pp. 125–170 in: *Ultrasonic Scattering in Biological Tissues*, K.K. Shung and G.A. Thieme (Eds.), CRC Press, Boca Raton, FL, 1993.

63. Mo, L.Y-L, and Cobbold, R.S.C., "Speckle" in C.W. ultrasound spectra: a simulation study, *IEEE Trans. Ultrason. Ferroelec. Freq. Contr.*, 33, 747–753, 1986.

64. Mo, L.Y-L., and Cobbold, R.S.C., A non-stationary signal simulation model for continuous wave and pulsed Doppler ultrasound, *IEEE Trans. Ultrason. Ferroelec. Freq. Contr.*, 36, 522–530, 1989.

65. Bastos, C.A.C., Fish, P.J., and Vaz, F., Spectrum of Doppler ultrasound signals from nonstationary blood flow, *IEEE Trans. Ultrason. Ferroelec. Freq. Contr.*, 46, 1201–1217, 1999.

66. Zhang, Y., Cardoso, J.C., Wang, Y., Fish, P.J., Bastos, C.A.C., and Wang, W., Time-scale removal of "wall thump" in Doppler ultrasound signals: a simulation study, *IEEE Trans. Ultrason. Ferroelec. Freq. Contr.*, 51, 1187–1192, 2004.

67. Woodward, P.M., *Probability and Information Theory, with Applications to Radar*, Pergamon Press, London, 1953.

68. Green, P.S., Spectral broadening of acoustic reverberation in Doppler-shift fluid flowmmeters, *J. Acoust. Soc. Am.*, 36, 1383–1390, 1964.

69. Newhouse, V.L., Bendick, P.J., and Varner, L.W. Analysis of transit-time effects in Doppler flow measurement, *IEEE Trans. Biomed. Eng.*, 23, 381–387, 1976.

70. Griffith, J.M., Brody, W.R., and Goodman, L., Resolution performance of Doppler ultrasound flowmeters, *J. Acoust. Soc. Am.*, 60, 607–610, 1976.

71. Censor, D., Newhouse, V.L., Vontz, T., and Ortega, H.V., Theory of ultrasound Doppler-spectra velocimetry for arbitrary beam and flow configurations, *IEEE Trans. Biomed. Eng.*, 35, 740–751, 1988.

72. Fish, P.J., Doppler methods, Chapter 11, pp. 338–376 in: *Physical Principles of Medical Ultrasonics*, Hill, C.R. (Ed.), Ellis Horwood (Wiley), Chichester, UK, 1986.

73. Ata, O.W., and Fish, P.J., Effect of deviation from plane wave conditions on the Doppler spectrum from an ultrasonic blood flow detector, *Ultrasonics*, 29, 395–403, 1991.

74. Edwards, R.V., Angus, J.C., French, M.J., and Dunning, J.W., Spectral analysis of the signal from laser Doppler flowmeter: time-independent systems, *J. Appl. Phys.*, 42, 837–850, 1971.

75. Newhouse, V.L., Furgason, E.S., Johnson, G.F., and Wolf, D.A., The dependence of ultrasound Doppler bandwidth on beam geometry, *IEEE Trans. Sonics Ultrason.*, 27, 50–59, 1980.

76. Jones, S.A., Fundamental sources of error and spectral broadening in Doppler ultrasound signals, *Critical Reviews in Biomed. Eng.*, 21, 399–483, 1993.

77. Kikkawa, S., Yamaguchi, T., Tanishita, K., and Sugawara, M., Spectral broadening in ultrasonic Doppler flowmeters due to unsteady flow, *IEEE Trans. Biomed. Eng.*, 34, 388–391, 1987.

78. Fish, P.J., Nonstationarity broadening in pulsed Doppler spectrum measurements, *Ultrasound Med. Biol.*, 17, 147–155, 1991.

79. Cloutier, G., Shung, K.K., and Durand, L.G., Experimental evaluation of intrinsic and nonstationary ultrasonic Doppler spectral broadining in steady and pulsatile flow loop models, *IEEE Trans. Ultrason. Ferroelec. Freq. Contr.*, 40, 786–795, 1999.

80. Hoskins, P.R., Accuracy of maximum velocity estimates made using Doppler ultrasound systems, *Br. J. Radiol.*, 69, 172–177, 1996.

81. Steinman, A.H., Errors in phased array pulse-wave ultrasound velocity estimation systems. PhD Thesis, University of Toronto, 2004.

82. Tortoli, P., Guidi, G., Guidi, F., and Atzeni, C. A review of experimental transverse Doppler studies. *IEEE Trans. Ultrason. Ferroelec. Freq. Contr.*, 41, 84–49, 1994.

83. Tortoli, P., Guidi, G., and Newhouse, V.L., Improved blood velocity estimation using the maximum Doppler frequency. *Ultrasound Med. Biol.*, 21, 527–532, 1995.

84. Winkler, A.J., and Wu, J., Correction of intrinsic spectral broadening errors in Doppler peak velocity measurements made with phased sector and linear array transducers, *Ultrasound Med. Biol.*, 21, 1029–1035, 1995.

85. Routh, H.F., Ultrasonic Doppler measurement of blood flow velocities by array transducers, US Patent 5,606,972, Mar. 4, 1997 (filed Aug. 10, 1995).

86. Mo, L.Y.L., and Otterson, S.D., Method and apparatus for estimation and display of spectral broadening error margin for Doppler time-velocity waveforms, US Patent 6,176,143, Jan. 23, 2001 (filed Dec. 1, 1997).

87. Wang, Y., and Fish, P.J., Correction for nonstationarity and window broadening in Doppler spectrum estimation, *IEEE Signal Processing Lett.*, 4, 18–21, 1997.

88. Newhouse, V.L., and Reid, J., Invariance of the Doppler bandwidth with flow displacement in the illuminating field. *J. Acoust. Soc. Am.*, 90, 2595–2601, 1991.

89. Newhouse, V.L., Faure, P., Cathignol, D., and Chapelon, J-Y., The transverse Doppler spectrum for focused transducers with rectangular apertures. *J. Acoust. Soc. Am.*, 95, 2091–2098, 1994.

10

Pulsed Methods for Flow Velocity Estimation and Imaging

The question as to whether pulsed Doppler makes use of the Doppler effect has been considered on several occasions. To address this question in a satisfactory manner requires that we first agree on a definition of the effect that bears Doppler's name.

Christian Doppler studied the optical spectrum emitted by stars and proposed a theory that described the change in wavelength (frequency) of each component of the received spectrum caused by the relative movement of the source and observer. It is clear from the discussion in Chapter 9 that when a CW acoustic source is used and there is relative motion between the source and target, the apparent change in frequency should be referred to as the Doppler effect.

Unlike the line optical spectrum from a star, the spectrum of a single brief acoustic pulse is continuous. Thus, when such a pulse is transmitted from a moving source, each incremental spectral component would be subject to a frequency change proportional to its frequency, causing a small change in the received spectral shape from that transmitted. In principle, then, by measuring the change in spectrum of the received pulse, it should be possible to estimate the target velocity from the information provided by transmitting a single pulse. Here again, the basis of this technique for estimating the velocity is the Doppler effect. An alternative but equivalent way of examining the classic Doppler effect on a pulse is to consider the transmission of a square ultrasound pulse and a scatterer moving with a velocity of v in the beam direction. In the absence of any attenuation and frequency-dependent scattering, it is shown in section 10.3 that the received pulse duration would be changed by a factor of $(c_o + v)/(c_o - v)$. This factor is exactly the same as that calculated from a frequency-domain analysis using the classic Doppler formula to determine the change to each frequency component and then performing an inverse transform to determine the received pulse duration. However, as discussed below, if the transmission medium has frequency-dependent attenuation and/or the target has frequency-dependent scattering, and if these properties are not precisely known, velocity estimation would be very difficult, if not impossible. Thus, unlike the line spectra produced by stars, whose components can be clearly identified on reception, the spectrum of a single pulse is continuous, thereby preventing identification of the changes that occur to a specific component on reception.

It is therefore apparent that a possible definition of the Doppler effect would include any phenomenon for which a change occurs in the spectral content due to a relative motion of the source and target and from which the relative velocity can be estimated. Such a definition is restricted in its scope and does not include methods based on measuring the change in position of a target at two or more instants of time. This definition is the one adopted in this book. A much broader definition could have been chosen, such as that used by Gill [3, p. vii]. He defines the Doppler effect as "the change in apparent time interval between two events, which arises from the motion of an observer, together with the finite velocity of transmission of information about the events." Such a definition makes no distinction between a process in which successive pulse-echo measurements are made to determine the change in position of a target (such as that used in M-mode ultrasound) and measurements based on the frequency change caused by relative motion of the source and target. Nonetheless, it should be pointed out that prior to the development of pulsed "Doppler" ultrasound, radar techniques had been developed and widely used for estimating the velocity from changes to the received signal between successive transmissions. At least one book [4] refers to this as *pulsed doppler* radar, with no capitalization of Doppler's name.

10.1 Introduction

If a single transmit pulse is used and the transmission medium has frequency-dependent attenuation, the shape of the spectrum will be changed. In fact, as discussed in Chapter 1 (subsection 1.8.1), a transmitted pulse will be down-shifted in frequency—an effect that could easily mask the Doppler effect. As an example, consider a Gaussian modulated 5-MHz sinusoidal transmitted pulse with a −6-dB fractional bandwidth of 5%. Moreover, we will assume an attenuation factor of $\alpha_o = 0.7$ dB/(cm × MHz) (i.e., one that is directly proportional to the frequency). The analytical expression as given by (1.126) gives the change in peak frequency as 9 kHz at a 1-cm depth. For a typical blood flow measurement, such a change is considerably greater than the Doppler shift. Second, as discussed in Chapter 5, scattering is a frequency-dependent process, and for a scatterer whose dimensions are small compared to the wavelength, the backscattered pressure increases as the square of the frequency, causing the peak frequency of the returned echo to be upshifted. Thus, for a transmitted pulse with a relatively broad bandwidth, the backscattered spectrum from a moving target can be significantly changed. Newhouse et al. [1] provided the first detailed discussion and showed that both effects on the spectrum could be accounted for by a linear filter. Subsequently, the combination of both effects was examined by Round and Bates [2], who derived an analytical expression for the pulse-echo response in the case of a Gaussian transmit pulse and a power law frequency dependence of the attenuation and scattering. In the absence of knowledge concerning the spatial and frequency dependence of both effects, the task of extracting the scatterer velocity from a single pulse appears to be intractable.

How, then, do pulsed "Doppler" ultrasound systems work? As will be seen, they require a minimum of two transmit pulses and, based on our decision to use the narrow definition of the Doppler effect, they make no use of the Doppler effect. However, the Doppler effect is present in the form of a small artifact that has a negligible influence on the accuracy with which the velocity can be estimated. The velocity component in the beam direction can be estimated from changes to the received signal caused by movement of the target in the interval between two transmit pulses. Such changes include a change in phase and/or a change in delay. Based on our choice of a narrow definition of the Doppler effect, it seems inappropriate to use Doppler's name for characterizing the operation of pulsed-wave flow systems. Furthermore, use of the name can cause confusion and lead to a misunderstanding of the basic operating principle of such systems.

An important step toward a proper understanding of pulsed wave systems was the 1983 paper by Newhouse and Amir [5] in which they correctly described many of the key properties. In 1986 Bonnefous and Pesque [8] pointed out that pulsed "Doppler" systems do not measure the Doppler frequency shift; rather, they measure the target displacement. Thomas and Leeman in their 1991 conference paper [9] also addressed this issue. In a section entitled "Pulsed Doppler Flowmeters—The Missing Doppler Effect," a theoretical basis was developed. Subsequently, they created a more complete picture [6,7] that formed the basis of the theory of pulsed Doppler measurements presented in the book by Jensen [10]. The simplified theory given in section 10.3 is partially based on their work.

A useful means of illustrating the differences between velocity estimation based on the changes that occur between successive received signals and that based on the classical Doppler effect is illustrated in Fig. 10.1. In this, the scatterer displacement waveform is assumed periodic with a frequency of exactly half the PRF and the medium is assumed to contain no frequency-dependent scattering and attenuation effects. In (a), the transmit pulse arrives at the scatterer when its velocity is zero, so that the received pulse will have exactly the same shape as that transmitted, i.e., no Doppler-shift change. In (b) the transmit pulse arrives when the scatterer displacement is zero but the velocity is

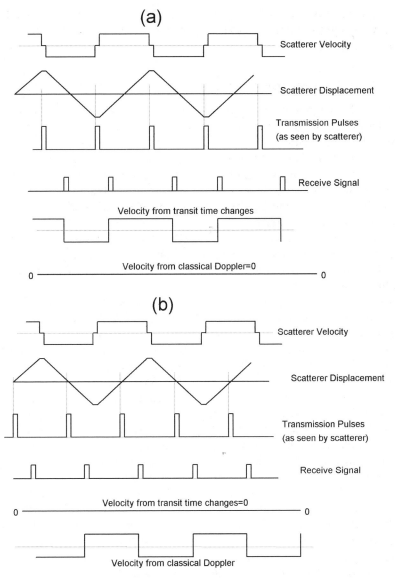

Figure 10.1 The differences between velocity estimation based on the change in scatterer location and that from the classical Doppler effect. (a) The velocity estimated from the change in transit time correctly reproduces the velocity waveform. However, because the received signal is identical to that transmitted, no Doppler shift occurs and the Doppler velocity is zero. (b) Here, the transmitted pulses arrive when the scatterer displacement is zero. No transit time changes occur, yielding a velocity of zero. However, each received pulse will be slightly distorted due to the classical Doppler effect, enabling the velocity to be extracted. (Based on the example presented by Thomas and Leeman [9].)

non-zero. For this case, the classic Doppler effect will cause the received pulse to have a slightly different spectrum, which in principle enables the velocity to be extracted.

10.1.1 Historical Background

Much of the initial work on the development of pulsed "Doppler" systems centered around four groups in the late 1960s: one in England, one in France, and two in the United States. It seems that a common motivation was to overcome some of the limitations of CW systems, such as the need for two transducers and the absence of any depth discrimination. It could be argued that the work by Peronneau in France had precedence in that he filed a patent application in April 1967 describing a pulsed system [11]. It used a single transducer and generated a relatively long pulse to encompass the entire blood vessel, while rejecting signals from other vessels in the beam path. Although the patent does not seem to suggest that a much shorter gate could enable the flow velocity profile to be measured, the ability of such a system to measure the velocity profiles was experimentally demonstrated two years later [12] and is well described in subsequent papers [13] by the same group. Also in 1967, Baker and Watkins [14] at the University of Washington (Seattle) described a range-gated pulsed system that was under development and that used separate transmit and receive transducer elements. Details of the method, together with measured velocity profiles both in vitro and in vivo, were subsequently described [15,16]. A second group in the United States also reported on the development of a pulsed system [17], though details were limited to a one-page conference digest. The final report, also in 1969, was that by Wells [18], who provided a full description of a pulsed system that used a single transducer element. The system was designed to explore the potential of pulsed velocity measurements, and its application was illustrated for measuring the velocity of cardiovascular structures but not for blood flow.

An important development was that of combining B-mode imaging with pulse velocity measurements in the same system. Initially developed in the 1970s by the group at the University of Washington, they are generally referred to as *duplex scanners* [19,20]. By incorporating B-mode imaging, the sample volume placement and the beam-to-vessel angle could be determined, enabling the velocity to be estimated. It was found that with the addition of spectral flow analysis, such systems were especially valuable for the diagnosis of vascular disease. Although separate transducers for imaging and velocity measurements were initially used, recent systems use the array elements to perform both imaging and velocity estimation roles.

These early reports and many subsequent papers appear to base their discussions and explanations on the classic Doppler effect, which was subsequently shown to be an artifact in pulsed wave systems. Specifically, it was assumed that the change in phase of the received signal between successive transmissions resulted from Doppler frequency changes. It seems likely that contributing to this misunderstanding is the fact that under the same approx-

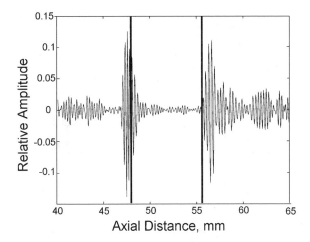

Figure 10.2 Received signal obtained from a single line-of-sight transmission through liver. Vertical lines mark the approximate location of a portal vein. (Reproduced, with permission of Cambridge University Press, from Jensen [10], *Estimation of Blood Velocities using Ultrasound.* ©1996 Cambridge University Press.)

imation, namely $v_z \ll c_o$, the equation relating the velocity to the frequency for pulsed wave systems is identical to the CW Doppler equation.[1] Nonetheless, this early work did provide a vital stimulus for research on the development of pulsed velocity measurement systems, leading eventually to color flow imaging.

One of the difficulties associated with blood velocity measurements is the relatively weak scattering produced by red blood cells (RBCs) in comparison with the surrounding structures. This is illustrated in Fig. 10.2, where an in vivo portion of the received RF signal from liver is shown [10]. It can be seen that within the portal vein, whose boundaries are marked by vertical lines, the signal is much smaller than the surrounding tissue, especially from the vessel wall–blood boundary. Typically, the signal from blood may be 20 to 60 dB less and have an SNR in the range 0 to 20 dB. Associated with pulsatile arterial blood flow is the radial movement of the vessel wall, which may be about 5% of the vessel radius, depending on its elastic constants and the pressure change over a cardiac cycle. Because of the strong vessel wall signal and its associated velocity, separating out the signal caused by blood moving close to the vessel wall can be a particularly challenging task.

---

1. It appears that Atkinson and Woodcock in their 1982 book [21, pp. 32–36], were the first to point this out. However, in describing "Pulse-Doppler" systems they speak of the Doppler-shifted components.

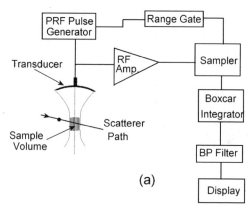

(a)

Sample Volume≡ SV
SV lateral dimension=2.0 mm
Scatterer velocity=33 cm/s
Scatterer path through SV=2.3 mm
Scatterer enters SV at 1.5 cm from transducer
Angle to beam axis = 60°
Center Frequency, 5.0 MHz,
Pulse Duration, approx =1μs (5 cycles)
PRF=5 kHz
Assumed c_o=1500 m/s

(b)

Figure 10.3 Simplified pulsed-wave system for determining the velocity component in the beam direction of a scatterer. (a) A concave transducer is shown with a sample volume whose dimensions are given in (b). Passage of the scatterer through the SV at an angle of 60 degrees is shown. The center frequency is an integer multiple of the PRF. Direct sampling of the RF signal is assumed to be coherent, and the resulting samples go to a boxcar integrator. A bandpass filter removes the abrupt changes as well as the pseudo-stationary clutter component.

10.2 Physical Principles of Pulsed Systems

Before providing a theoretical explanation, it is helpful to consider a simplified model of a pulsed system that ignores attenuation and frequency-dependent scattering. This will be used to develop a physical picture of the process by which a single scatterer generates a signal whose frequency after sampling and reconstruction is proportional to its velocity. For this purpose, consider the block diagram of Fig. 10.3, where a simple concave transducer produces the sample volume indicated. A single scatterer is shown moving through this volume with a constant velocity in the direction away from the transducer. We shall assume that the response is constant within the sample volume and drops to zero at its boundaries. Consequently, a scatterer anywhere within this volume creates a similar response. Let us assume that the transmitter produces

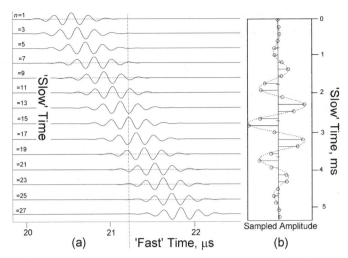

Figure 10.4 Waveforms corresponding to the simplified pulsed velocity measurement system shown in Fig. 10.3(a) for the parameter values of Fig. 10.3(b). (a) Portions of the backscattered RF signals due to transmission of a Gaussian pulse. The first signal corresponds to a moving point target as it enters the sample volume at 1.5 cm from the transducer. Each waveform (only alternate pulses are shown) corresponds to a PRI of 200 μs ($f_{PRF} = 5.0$ kHz). Movement of the scatterer through the sample volume causes its distance from the transducer to increase for each transmission. The RF received signal is sampled at the same instant of time (vertical dashed line) following transmission. (b) Sampled amplitudes sampled once each PRI at the times indicated by the dashed line in (a). With sufficient samples, the entire shape of the transmitted pulse can be reconstructed though the reconstructed time axis is now scaled by a factor of $2v \cos \theta / c_o$ and is sometimes referred to as "slow" time. The particle velocity component in the beam direction is related to the center frequency of this waveform by (10.2).

a simple Gaussian modulated pulse with a center frequency of 5 MHz. In the absence of frequency-dependent effects, the received signal will also consist of a Gaussian pulse with the same shape but with a delay that increases with each PRI. We shall assume that sampling is performed on the RF received signal in a coherent manner, i.e., the sampling frequency is synchronized to the center frequency and PRF.

Suppose that the scatterer moves sufficiently slowly so that a large number of received signals are obtained over the transit time of the scatterer through the sample volume, such as those shown in Fig. 10.4a. As can be seen, these start when the scatterer enters the sample volume ($n = 1$) and finishes when it leaves ($n = 28$). If each received signal is sampled with exactly the same delay from transmission, then, as shown in subsection 10.3.1, the sampled signal will be a sampled replica of the transmitted signal but with a time scale that is greater by a factor of approximately $c_o/(2v \cos \theta)$. Thus, if the waveform is represented by $G(t)$ and there are N transmissions, the sampled signal can be expressed as the convolution

$$G\left\{\frac{c_o(t-\tau)}{2v\cos\theta}\right\} * \sum_{n=1}^{N}\delta(t-nt_{PRI}),$$

where τ is the time of flight to and from the scatterer.

The terms "slow" and "fast" are used to refer to the time scale for the received waveform and the sampled waveform, respectively. The spectrum will be identical to the transmitted spectrum but scaled down in frequency by $2v\cos\theta/c_o$. Consequently, the fractional bandwidth will be the identical to that of the transmitted pulse. Fig. 10.4b shows the sampled received pulse together with the reconstructed signal when the scatterer is moving away from the transducer, as in Fig. 10.3. Had it been moving in the opposite direction, the reconstructed signal would be a time-reversed, time-stretched replica of the incident pulse. All of the above properties were predicted in the paper by New-house and Amir [5].

If the scatterer velocity is denoted by v and t_{PRI} denotes the pulse repetition interval, then the distance moved in the beam axis direction between successive transmissions is given by $\Delta z = (v\cos\theta)t_{PRI}$. Now, the change in delay between successive received signals is given by $\Delta\tau = 2\Delta z/c_o$, which can be re-expressed as

(10.1) $$\Delta\tau = \frac{2v\cos\theta}{c_o}t_{PRI}.$$ (a)

Alternatively, this can be rewritten as

(10.1) $$v = \frac{c_o\Delta\tau}{2t_{PRI}\cos\theta}.$$ (b)

Now the center frequency of the slow-time waveform can be found from $2\pi f_{pw} = d\phi/dt \approx \Delta\phi/t_{PRI}$, where $\Delta\phi$ is the phase shift of the slow-time signal. However, the fast- and slow-time signals have the same phase shift, so that $\Delta\phi = 2\pi f_c\Delta\tau$, where f_c is the center frequency of the transmitted waveform. This enables the slow-time (pulsed wave) center frequency to be written as $f_{PW} = f_c\Delta\tau/t_{PRI}$, which, after substituting for $\Delta\tau$ as given by (10.1a), becomes

(10.2) $$\boxed{f_{PW} = \frac{2v\cos\theta}{c_o}f_c.}$$

In the absence of any frequency-dependent processes, the spectrum of the reconstructed waveform from a single scatterer will be the same as that transmitted but scaled by a factor of $2v\cos\theta/c_o$. However, a number of processes combine to broaden the spectrum. For example, if the field within the sample volume is non-uniform, as is normally the case, the spectrum will be modulated by the changes in field as the scatterer traverses the sample volume. A second example arises when there are a range of scatterer velocities in the sample volume. If the transmitted waveform consists of many cycles, e.g., 8–20, the slow-time spectrum from a single scatterer in the absence of noise will be quite narrow. Thus, the presence of a distribution of velocities in the sample volume will cause the slow-time signal to have a spectral shape related to the velocity distribution.

10.2.1 Velocity Estimation Methods

The problem of estimating the mean value of a quantity under different SNR conditions is one that has been addressed in many fields. A considerable number of methods exist, and many of the most useful of these have been compared in terms of bias, variance, and speed of computation [22,23]. Perhaps the simplest are those based on measuring the frequency with which the signal crosses through zero (zero-crossing method), and those use frequency tracking [24]. However, under low SNR conditions and/or the presence of a wide spectrum of frequencies, these techniques have large biases and variances [25,26]. A straightforward technique is that based on estimating the power spectrum and using this to extract the mean, the maximum, and higher-order moments. Evans and McDicken [24, Chapter 8] have reviewed a variety of estimation methods for use in Doppler and pulsed wave ultrasound. Details of these techniques together with comparisons, based on simulated signals using various SNR conditions, have been presented by Vaitkus et al. [27,28].

Equation (10.2) shows that the mean velocity of a scatterer can be obtained by estimating the mean slow-time frequency. If the transmitted fractional bandwidth is relatively small, such a technique is often referred to as a narrowband method. A narrow bandwidth enables the SNR to be improved; however, the use of a long-duration multi-cycle transmitted pulse causes the spatial resolution in the axial direction to be diminished. Estimation methods that use much shorter-duration transmit pulses have a number of potential advantages, and these are sometimes referred to as wideband methods. Alam and Parker [29,30] have suggested that the classification of estimation methods into narrow and wideband techniques is not particularly satisfactory. They proposed the following three principal categories based on the signal models: (i) time-domain methods based on the relative change in the time at which the echo occurs (see section 10.4); (ii) frequency/phase methods based on the rate of change in phase (see sections 10.5 and 10.8); and (iii) multiple burst (tracking) methods (see section 10.9). The sections indicated will describe these methods and present examples.

As noted in Chapter 9, *spectral Doppler* is a term sometimes used to describe the method used for estimating and displaying the spectrum produced by an ensemble of moving scatterers within a sample volume. However, to be consistent with our earlier decision to use a narrow definition of the Doppler effect, we shall apply this term only for a CW system. For a pulsed wave system, the estimation and spectral display will be referred to as the *spectral flow* method. When information concerning a parameter of the signal is extracted and displayed as a 2-D color map, we shall refer to the resulting method as *pulsed wave* or *color flow imaging*. In spectral flow, the emphasis is on estimating the spectrum using the received information from many (e.g.,

40) transmissions (generally referred to as the packet size) along the same direction from one or many sample volumes. On the other hand, with color flow imaging (see section 10.7), the estimation method of choice would be one that can estimate the value of a single flow parameter along the beam direction using a relatively small number of transmissions (e.g., 4–15). In essence, each beam is divided into incremental (sample) volumes whose spacing determines the axial resolution of the measurements.

At this point, it is perhaps helpful to draw a practical distinction between spectral flow and color flow imaging. In spectral flow, the user specifies a specific sample volume, axial length, and location for interrogating the flow within the lumen of a vessel. In this case, the optimization problem is essentially how to select the best combination of the transmit waveform and receive filter (e.g., the box-car integrator illustrated in Fig. 10.3) to achieve the desired sample volume length (axial resolution) while maximizing the SNR. On the other hand, in color flow imaging, the user specifies a relatively large area of interest but not a specific range resolution, so that the problem reduces to that of finding the best combination of transmit waveform and receive filters to optimize the balance between axial resolution and SNR over the region of interest.

10.2.2 Critical Velocities

Three velocity limit values can be identified. The first relates the velocity at which aliasing first occurs to the depth of measurement. The second concerns the smallest velocity that can be successfully distinguished from clutter. The third relates to the minimum velocity needed for the slow-time waveform to be a complete copy of the fast-time waveform.

Range-Velocity Limitation

The number of samples taken from a given scatterer depends on the scatterer velocity, the size of the sample volume, and the PFR. According to the Nyquist sampling criterion, for the demodulated frequency to be unambiguously determined, two or more samples must be obtained within one period of the transmitted center frequency. This criterion enables the maximum velocity component in the beam direction to be calculated. Specifically, we first note that in one PRI, the z-distance traveled by a scatterer is given by $\Delta z = v \cos \theta / f_{PRF}$. Assuming the scatterer is moving away from the transducer, the additional time needed for the pulse to reach this new location is given by $\Delta t = 2\Delta z / c_o = 2v \cos \theta / (c_o f_{PRF})$. If aliasing is to be avoided, this time must be no greater than a half period of the fundamental transmission frequency, i.e., $\Delta t \leq 1/(2f_c)$. Consequently, the condition for no aliasing can be written as

$$(10.3) \qquad v \leq v_{max} = \pm \frac{c_o f_{PRF}}{4 f_c \cos \theta} .$$

For example, at an angle of 60 degrees for a 5 MHz pulse and a PRF of 10 kHz, this maximum velocity is given by

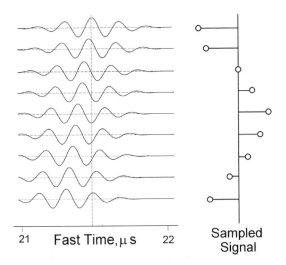

21   Fast Time, μ s   22   Sampled Signal

Figure 10.5 Similar to Fig. 10.4, except that the scatterer is moving quite slowly and toward the transducer. Note that the sampled signal consists of about one transmitted cycle for nine A-lines. This corresponds approximately to the minimum velocity that can be distinguished from stationary clutter.

$$v_{\max} = \frac{1500\,(\text{m/s}) \times 10{,}000\,(\text{Hz})}{4 \times 5.10^6\,(\text{Hz}) \times \cos 60°} = 150\,\text{cm/s}.$$

If the maximum depth over which the velocity is to be estimated is denoted by $z_{\max}$, then to allow sufficient time between pulses for the echo to reach the transducer prior to sending the next pulse,

$$1/f_{PRF} \geq 2z_{\max}/c_o.$$

By substituting this into (10.3), the *range-velocity limit* can be expressed as

(10.4) $$\boxed{z_{\max} v_{\max} = \frac{c_o^2}{8 f_c \cos\theta}.}$$

This shows that the maximum range and maximum velocity are inversely related, i.e., the velocity at which aliasing first occurs reduces as the measurement depth is increased. Using the values assumed in the previous example, the maximum depth at which the velocity can be unambiguously determined is given by

$$z_{\max} = \frac{\left[1500\,(\text{m/s})\right]^2}{8 \times 5.10^6\,(\text{Hz}) \times 1.5\,(\text{m/s}) \times \cos 60°} = 7.5\,\text{cm}.$$

Minimum Velocity

As indicated in Fig. 10.5, the minimum velocity that can be detected is determined by the requirement that at least one period of the transmitted waveform must be sampled. The scatterer would have moved a distance of $\Delta z = Nt_{PRI}v\cos\theta$ over N transmissions, and over this time interval the received pulse would be delayed by

$$\Delta t = 2\Delta z/c_o = 2Nt_{PRI}v\cos\theta/c_o$$

Thus, to observe the transmitted pulse for at least one period, ($\Delta t \geq 1/f_c$), requires that

(10.5)
$$v \geq v_{min} = \frac{c_o f_{PRF}}{2Nf_c\cos\theta}.$$

For example, consider a 5 MHz pulse with a PRF of 10 kHz and a scatterer moving at 60 degrees to the beam. If the spectrum is calculated every 50 PRIs, the minimum velocity that can be distinguished from clutter is given by

$$v_{min} = \frac{1500\,(\mathrm{m/s})\times 10{,}000\,(\mathrm{Hz})}{2\times 50\times 5.10^6\,(\mathrm{Hz})\times\cos 60^\circ} = 6\,\mathrm{cm/s}.$$

Minimum Velocity Needed to Reproduce the Transmit Waveform

Suppose that the transmitted waveform consists of M cycles of the center frequency. If there are N transmissions and the PRI is t_{PRI}, the scatterer velocity needed to ensure that the entire transmit waveform is reproduced as a slow-time waveform can be found from (10.5) as

(10.6)
$$v \geq v_M = \frac{Mc_o f_{PRF}}{2Nf_c\cos\theta}.$$

For example, if the same values are assumed as in the previous example and $M = 5$, the minimum velocity is given by

$$v \geq \frac{1500\,(\mathrm{m/s})\times 5\times 10{,}000\,(\mathrm{Hz})}{2\times 50\times 5.10^6\,(\mathrm{Hz})\times\cos 60^\circ} = 30\,\mathrm{cm/s}.$$

In addition, for the same assumed values, the maximum velocity for no aliasing can be obtained from (10.3) as 150 cm/s.

10.3 Simplified Theory

Based on the simplified block diagram of Fig. 10.3, expressions for the sampled signal will be obtained with the help of Fig. 10.6 [5,7,10]. This figure contains the space-time equations for the transmitted δ-function pulse and the received pulse. For example, if the transmit pulse path intersects a scatterer moving with a velocity of v_z at a depth of z_s, then the scattered pulse will arrive at the transducer at a time t_r.

Our objective is to derive an expression for the received signal due to a point scatterer moving with a velocity of $\mathbf{v}$ when a sequence of identical pulses

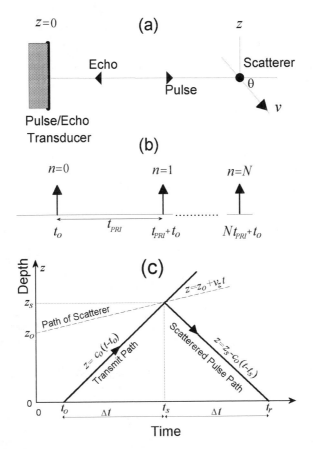

Figure 10.6 Calculation of the received signal due to a scatter moving with a velocity v through a plane wave consisting of a transmitted δ-function. (a) Assumed geometry. (b) Transmission of N pulses (δ-functions) with a pulse repetition interval of t_{PRI}. (c) Time/depth graph giving the equations for the scatterer, transmission pulse, and received pulse. The scatterer is at the location z_s when the transmitted pulse, emitted at time t_o, intercepts it. Note the symmetry about the time t_s when the transmitted pulse intercepts the scatterer.

are transmitted with a pulse repetition interval of t_{PRI}. We shall neglect the effects of attenuation and associated dispersion and assume that the transmitted pulse consists of a plane wave. Our starting point is to consider the transmission of a single impulse at a time t_o as expressed by $\delta(t - t_o)$ and suppose that at time $t = 0$, the z-coordinate of the scatterer is z_0. First, we shall determine the time t_s at which the impulse arrives at the scatterer. By this time, the scatterer will have moved to a new z-location given by $z_s = z_0 + t_s v \cos \theta = z_0 + v_z t_s$, where $v_z = v \cos \theta$. Consequently, the impulse reaches the scatterer at its new location at a time given by

$$t_s = t_o + \frac{z_s}{c_o} = t_o + \frac{z_0 + v_z t_s}{c_o} = \frac{c_o t_o + z_0}{c_o - v_z}.$$

The time interval for it to arrive at this new location is

$$\Delta t = t_s - t_o = \frac{c_o t_o + z_0}{c_o - v_z} - t_o$$

$$= t_o \left(\frac{c_o}{c_o - v_z} - 1 \right) + \frac{z_0}{c_o - v_z} = \frac{t_o v_z}{c_o - v_z} + \frac{z_0}{c_o - v_z}.$$

Because the echo pulse takes exactly the same time to arrive back at the transducer, the echo will be detected at a time of

$$t_r = t_o + 2\Delta t = t_o + \frac{2 t_o v_z}{c_o - v_z} + \frac{2 z_0}{c_o - v_z}.$$

Thus, the impulse response is given by

$$h(t) = \delta\{t - t_r\} = \delta\{(t - t_0) - (t_r - t_0)\}$$

(10.7)
$$= \delta\left\{ t - t_0 \left(\frac{c_o + v_z}{c_o - v_z} \right) - \frac{2 z_0}{c_o - v_z} \right\}.$$

In this equation, the factor of $(c_o + v_z)/(c_o - v_z)$ corresponds to time-scale expansion or contraction depending on the direction of v_z.

Now consider a sampled version of the transmitted waveform $G(t)$, sampled at regular intervals of τ and expressed by

$$G_\delta(t) = \sum_{n=-\infty}^{\infty} G(n\Delta\tau)\delta(t - n\Delta\tau).$$

Here, the nth sample is a δ-function weighted by the value of $G(t)$ at a time of $n\Delta\tau$, i.e., $G(n\Delta\tau)\delta(t - n\Delta\tau)$. It is important to recognize that each point in the discretized signal has its own start time (t_o) that can be recognized as $n\Delta\tau$. Thus, the received waveform can be expressed as

$$R_C(t) = \sum_{n=-\infty}^{\infty} G(n\Delta\tau)\delta\left\{ t - n\Delta\tau \left(\frac{c_o + v_z}{c_o - v_z} \right) - \frac{2 z_0}{c_o - v_z} \right\}.$$

In the limit as $\Delta\tau \to 0$, this becomes

$$R_C(t) = \int_{-\infty}^{\infty} G(t_o)\delta\left\{ t - t_o \left(\frac{c_o + v_z}{c_o - v_z} \right) - \frac{2 z_0}{c_o - v_z} \right\} dt_o,$$

which can be evaluated to yield[2]

2. In eqn. 4 of [7], the received signal can be rewritten as: $R_N(t) = \sum_{n=0}^{N} G\left\{ \left(\frac{c_o - v_z}{c_o + v_z} \right) t - t_{PRI} n \right.$

$\left. - \frac{2 z_o}{c_o + v_z} \right\}$. If there is just one pulse ($n = 0$), this reduces to $R_1(t) = G\left\{ \left(\frac{c_o - v_z}{c_o + v_z} \right) \left(t - \frac{2 z_0}{c_o - v_z} \right) \right\}$,

which, apart from the amplitude factor, is the same as (10.8) derived above, and is also the same as eqn. 5 in [6]. It differs from eqn. 12 in [9] but can be reconciled by assuming the definition that was given for α should have been that for $1/\alpha$.

$$(10.8) \qquad R_C(t) = \left(\frac{c_o - v_z}{c_o + v_z}\right) G\left[\left(\frac{c_o - v_z}{c_o + v_z}\right)\left(t - \frac{2z_0}{c_o - v_z}\right)\right].$$

Here again, the factor of $(c_o + v_z)/(c_o - v_z)$, which is present as an argument of G, corresponds to the expansion or dilation of the time scale, as originally observed by Newhouse and Amir [5].

Consider a transmit waveform consisting of a square wave of unit amplitude given by $G(t) = \mathcal{H}(t)\mathcal{H}(T - t)$, where $\mathcal{H}(.)$ denotes a Heaviside step function that starts at $t = 0$ and ends at $t = T$. The received waveform can be obtained from (10.8) and is given by

$$(10.9) \qquad R_C(t) = \left(\frac{c_o - v_z}{c_o + v_z}\right)\mathcal{H}\left[t - \frac{2z_0}{c_o - v_z}\right]\mathcal{H}\left[\frac{2z_0}{c_o - v_z} + T\frac{c_o + v_z}{c_o - v_z} - t\right].$$

As illustrated in Fig. 10.7b, the pulse arrives after a delay of $2z_o/(c_o - v_z)$ and has a duration of $T(c_o + v_z)/(c_o - v_z)$, corresponding to an expansion if $v_z > 0$ and a contraction if $v_z < 0$. This small change in duration arises from the classic Doppler effect.

As a second example, consider two transmitted pulses each of duration T, the second pulse occurring at a time t_{PRI}. In this case, the received waveform can be written as

$$(10.10) \qquad R_C(t) = \left(\frac{c_o - v_z}{c_o + v_z}\right)\left\{ \begin{aligned} &\mathcal{H}\left[t - \frac{2z_0}{c_o - v_z}\right]\mathcal{H}\left[\frac{2z_0}{c_o - v_z} + T\left(\frac{c_o + v_z}{c_o - v_z}\right) - t\right] + \\ &\mathcal{H}\left[t - \frac{2z_0}{c_o - v_z} - t_{PRI}\left(\frac{c_o + v_z}{c_o - v_z}\right)\right] \times \\ &\mathcal{H}\left[\left(\frac{c_o + v_z}{c_o - v_z}\right)(T + t_{PRI}) + \frac{2z_0}{c_o - v_z} - t\right] \end{aligned} \right\},$$

which is shown in Fig. 10.7d. It can be seen that the interval between the transmitted pulses and their duration have been changed by a factor of $(c_o + v_z)/(c_o - v_z)$. Thomas and Leeman [7] pointed out that this minor time-scale change is a direct result of the Doppler effect and is caused by the relative movement of the source and scatterer.

To show that the Doppler-induced time shift is indeed small compared to the difference in arrival times of the received pulse for successive transmissions, which forms the primary basis of pulsed wave velocity estimation methods, we proceed as follows. In the example illustrated in Fig. 10.7d, the time interval between the two received pulses is given by

$$\Delta t_{PRI} = \left(\frac{c_o + v_z}{c_o - v_z}\right)t_{PRI} - t_{PRI} \approx \frac{2v_z}{c_o}t_{PRI}, \text{ for } v_z \ll c_o.$$

In addition, the change in pulse duration due to the Doppler term is

$$\Delta T = \left(\frac{c_o + v_z}{c_o - v_z}\right)T - T \approx \frac{2v_z}{c_o}T, \text{ for } v_z \ll c_o.$$

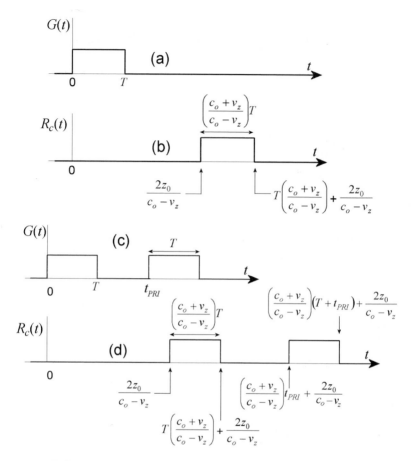

Figure 10.7 Pulse-echo waveforms for a plane wave incident on a small scatterer moving with a velocity of v whose component in the z-direction is v_z. (a) Rectangular transmit wave of duration T. (b) Received waveform from a small scatterer that is at a depth of z_0 at $t = 0$. (c), (d) Same as (a) and (b) but with two pulses having a repetition interval of t_{PRI}. The waveforms in (b) and (d) correspond to (10.9) and (10.10), respectively.

Thus, the ratio of the two effects is given by $\Delta T/\Delta t_{PRI} = T/t_{PRI}$. For instance, if $T = 1\,\mu s$ and $t_{PRI} = 100\,\mu s$, corresponding to a PRF of 10 kHz, the Doppler artifact is about 1% of the change in the time interval between successive pulses, which is sufficiently small to be neglected.

As a final example we consider the important case of a sequence of N transmit pulses with a repetition interval of t_{PRI}, as illustrated in Fig. 10.8. The received signal from a scatterer whose axial location is z_0 at $t = 0$ is given by

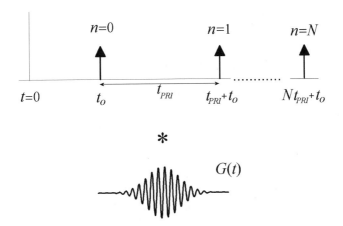

Figure 10.8 Convolution of a sequence of δ-functions separated by t_{PRI} with the transmit waveform to produce a sequence of $N + 1$ transmit pulses.

$$R_C(t) = \sum_{n=0}^{N} \int_{-\infty}^{\infty} G(t_o)\delta\left\{t - \left(nt_{PRI} + t_o\right)\left(\frac{c_o + v_z}{c_o - v_z}\right) - \frac{2z_0}{c_o - v_z}\right\}dt_o$$

(10.11)
$$= \left(\frac{c_o - v_z}{c_o + v_z}\right)\sum_{n=0}^{N} G\left\{\left(\frac{c_o - v_z}{c_o + v_z}\right)\left[\left(t - nt_{PRI}\right) - \frac{2\left(z_0 + v_z nt_{PRI}\right)}{c_o - v_z}\right]\right\}.$$

Doppler Time Time shift due to
effect change scatterer movement

Apart from the amplitude factor, which is very near unity, this expression is identical to that given by Thomas and Leeman [9, equation 12].

For the purpose of simplifying the analysis in the next two subsections, it is helpful to re-express (10.11) by writing $t \to t_F + nt_{PRI}$, i.e., by using a fast-time scale that resets to zero every transmitted pulse so that $0 \le t_F < t_{PRI}$. Substitution for t enables the received scattered signal to be expressed as

$$R_C(t_F, n) = \left(\frac{c_o - v_z}{c_o + v_z}\right)G\left\{\left(\frac{c_o - v_z}{c_o + v_z}\right)\left[t_F - \frac{2\left(z_0 + v_z nt_{PRI}\right)}{c_o - v_z}\right]\right\}.$$

Further simplification results by putting $A = \dfrac{c_o - v_z}{c_o + v_z}$ and $B = \dfrac{2z_0}{c_o - v_z}$, yielding

(10.12)
$$R_C(t_F, n) = A\,G\left[A\left(t_F - \frac{2nt_{PRI}v_z}{c_o - v_z} - B\right)\right],$$

which will be used in the next section.

10.3.1 Demodulation by Direct RF Signal Sampling

Thomas and Leeman [9] pointed out that the essence of a pulsed system can be understood by assuming that each RF A-line signal is sampled at the same instant of time following emission[3] (see Fig. 10.4). An analog output signal can then be obtained by using a circuit that maintains the same amplitude until the next transmission. In the following analysis we shall assume a non-directional system and δ-function sampling of the RF received signal for a scatterer moving with a constant velocity through the sample volume.

Consider the sampling function of $\delta(t_F - \tau)$, which can be used to extract the values of $R_C(t_F, n)$ at a time τ following the transmission of each pulse. From (10.12)

$$R_S(\tau, n) = R_C(t_F, n)\delta(t_F - \tau) = AG\left[A\left(\tau - \frac{2nt_{PRI}v_z}{c_o - v_z} - B\right)\right].$$

For a sinusoidal pulse whose envelope is $\alpha(t)$ and with a center angular frequency of ω_c, the discrete time demodulated signal is

$$(10.13) \quad R_F(\tau, n) = a\left[A\left(-\frac{2nt_{PRI}v_z}{c_o - v_z} - B + \tau\right)\right]\cos\left[\omega_c A\left(\frac{2nt_{PRI}v_z}{c_o - v_z} + B - \tau\right)\right].$$

For $v_z \ll c_o$ this equation reduces to

$$R_F(\tau, n) = a\left(\tau - \frac{2v_z nt_{PRI}}{c_o} - \frac{2z_o}{c_o}\right)\cos\left[\omega_c\left(\tau - \frac{2v_z nt_{PRI}}{c_o} - \frac{2z_o}{c_o}\right)\right],$$

which shows that if sufficient transmissions are used, the demodulated signal replicates the sampled transmitted pulse but is scaled in time by a factor of $2v_z/c_o$. If the number of transmission is insufficient, the spectral bandwidth will be greater than that of the transmitted waveform, i.e., spectral broadening will be present.

10.3.2 Phase-Quadrature Demodulation

Virtually all earlier pulsed flow systems used demodulation to baseband frequency. A coherent analog phase-quadrature demodulator, similar to that used in CW systems (see subsection 9.4.2), can be used as the first stage for extracting the spectrum for both forward and reverse flow. As illustrated in Fig. 10.9a, the in-phase and quadrature outputs can then be sampled using range-gates that are opened at a time determined by the starting location of the sample volume. An intuitive choice, originally suggested by Peronneau et al. [31], is to make the range-gate duration equal to the transmit burst duration and to integrate the signal envelope over this duration, as opposed to sampling at a specific instant of time as described in the previous subsection. By this means, significant SNR improvements can be achieved (see subsection 10.3.3).

An alternative approach is to use a quadrature scheme in which the RF signal (or an intermediate frequency) is sampled twice in each center frequency period: once at a time t and subsequently at a time of $t + 1/(4f_c)$. The

---

3. The velocity direction remains ambiguous with a single sample. As described in subsection 10.3.2, quadrature sampling of the RF signal enables the direction to be recovered.

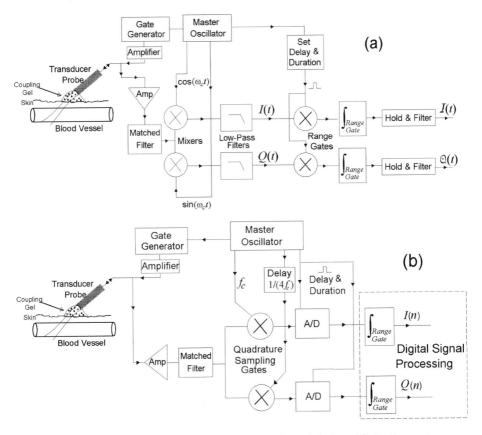

Figure 10.9 Pulsed-wave system using quadrature demodulation. (a) Analog system. (b) Digital scheme using quadrature sampling in which the RF signal is sampled twice per period. The receive filter is not restricted to an integrator for either spectral flow or color flow imaging.

second sample amplitude in relation to the first enables the flow direction to be determined. Such a scheme is illustrated in Fig. 10.9b.

We start by considering just the in-phase process and will assume a sinusoidal pulse with a center angular frequency of ω_c and an envelope of $\alpha(t)$, i.e.,

$$G(t) = a(t)\cos(\omega_c t).$$

Ignoring the amplitude factor in this and subsequent equations, (10.12) becomes

$$(10.14) \quad R_C(t_F, n) = a\left[A\left(t_F - \frac{2nt_{PRI}v_z}{c_o - v_z} - B\right)\right]\cos\left[\omega_c A\left(t_F - \frac{2nt_{PRI}v_z}{c_o - v_z} - B\right)\right].$$

Multiplying this by $\cos(\omega_c t_F)$ enables the in-phase demodulated signal to be obtained as

$$R_D(t_F, n) = a\left[A\left(t_F - \frac{2nt_{PRI}v_z}{c_o - v_z} - B\right)\right]\cos\left[\omega_c A\left(t_F - \frac{2nt_{PRI}v_z}{c_o - v_z} - B\right)\right] \times \cos(\omega_c t_F).$$

Using the relation $2\cos A \cos B = \cos(A - B) + \cos(A + B)$ to expand the product of the two cosine terms yields

$$R_D(t_F, n) = a\left[A\left(t_F - \frac{2nt_{PRI}v_z}{c_o - v_z} - B\right)\right] \times$$
$$\left\{ \cos\left[\omega_c\left(t_F(A-1) - nt_{PRI}\frac{2Av_z}{c_o - v_z} - AB\right)\right] \right.$$
$$\left. + \cos\left[\omega_c\left(t_F(A+1) - nt_{PRI}\frac{2Av_z}{c_o - v_z} - AB\right)\right] \right\}.$$

Now the argument of the second cosine term contains the term $\omega_c t_F(A + 1)$ which for $v_z \ll c_o$ is approximately equal to $2\omega_c t_F$. Consequently, the second cosine term can be eliminated by using a low-pass filter, leaving[4]

$$R_I(t_F, n) = a\left(\frac{c_o - v_z}{c_o + v_z}t_F - \frac{2nt_{PRI}v_z}{c_o + v_z} - \frac{2z_o}{c_o + v_z}\right)\cos\left[\frac{2\omega_c}{c_o + v_z}(t_Fv_z + nt_{PRI}v_z + z_o)\right]$$

For $v_z \ll c_o$ (as is usually the case), and recalling that $0 \le t_F < t_{PRI}$, this simplifies to

$$R_I(t_F, n) \approx a\left(t_F - \frac{2nt_{PRI}v_z}{c_o} - \frac{2z_o}{c_o}\right)\cos\left[\frac{2\omega_c}{c_o}(t_Fv_z + nt_{PRI}v_z + z_o)\right].$$

If the received signal for each transmission is integrated over the duration of a sample gate that extends from τ_F to $\tau_F + \Delta\tau$, the sample values are given by

$$(10.15) \quad R_I(n) \approx \cos\left[\frac{2\omega_c}{c_o}(nt_{PRI}v_z + z_o)\right]\int_{\tau_F}^{\tau_F + \Delta\tau} a\left(\left[t_F - \frac{2nt_{PRI}v_z}{c_o} - \frac{2z_o}{c_o}\right]\right)^2 dt_F.$$

This equation was obtained by making use of the fact that over the sample-gate duration the cosine term is nearly constant and can therefore be taken outside the integral sign.

For example, suppose that the transmitted envelope is the Gaussian function $\exp(-\sigma_\omega^2 t^2)$ where the −6-dB (0.5) fractional bandwidth is equal to $3.33\sigma_\omega/\omega_c$. Then, from (10.15)

$$R_I(n) \approx \cos\left[\frac{2\omega_c}{c_o}(nt_{PRI}v_z + z_o)\right] \times$$

(10.16)
$$\int_{\tau_F}^{\tau_F + \Delta\tau} \exp\left(-\sigma_\omega^2\left[t_F - \frac{2nt_{PRI}v_z}{c_o} - \frac{2z_o}{c_o}\right]^2\right)dt_F.$$
(a)

---

4. This is identical to the nth term in eqn. 12 of [7].

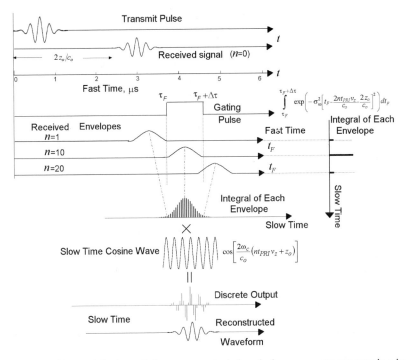

Figure 10.10 Demodulation of the range-gated signals from a scatterer moving in the z-direction. A Gaussian modulated sinusoidal transmit pulse of approximately 1-μs duration (four cycles of 4 MHz) was assumed. The reconstructed waveform assumed a range-gate duration of 1 μs and a single scatterer moving with a high velocity through the sample volume. In arriving at the discrete output as given by (10.16), each envelope of the received demodulated signal is integrated over range-gate duration and each value is then multiplied by the slow-time cosine wave for that time.

In a similar manner, multiplying (10.14) by $\sin(\omega_c t_F)$ enables the quadrature-demodulated signal to be obtained as

$$R_Q(n) \approx \sin\left[\frac{2\omega_c}{c_o}\left(nt_{PRI}v_z + z_o\right)\right] \times$$

(10.16)
$$\int_{\tau_F}^{\tau_F+\Delta\tau} \exp\left(-\sigma_\omega^2\left[t_F - \frac{2nt_{PRI}v_z}{c_o} - \frac{2z_o}{c_o}\right]^2\right)dt_F.$$
(b)

Examination of either of these results reveals that for a given n, the received envelope is integrated in fast time over the range-gate to yield a single value. When this is multiplied by the value of the trigonometric term for the corresponding n-value, the final slow-time sampled signal is obtained. For the in-phase component and a four-cycle Gaussian transmitted pulse, these steps are illustrated in Fig. 10.10. Moreover, as the gate duration is increased, so the effect of envelope truncation decreases, causing the bandwidth of the output signal to be reduced. Alternatively, if the gate duration is reduced, to improve the axial spatial resolution, the spectral broadening is increased.

It should be noted that the above result assumed that the scatterer moves in a uniform transmit/receive field throughout the entire interrogation process. In practice, as the scatterer moves through the sample volume, the field variations will modulate the received signal in a different manner to that caused by range-gating of the demodulated signal. Consider, for example, a cylindrically symmetric geometry with a transmit/receive profile denoted by $M(r,z)$ and a scatterer whose initial position is (r_o, z_o). To account for the additional modulation introduced by a scatterer with velocity components of v_r and v_z, the function $M[r_o + v_r(t_F + nt_{PRI}), z_0 + v_z(t_F + nt_{PRI})]$ must be placed under the integral sign of (10.15).

10.3.3 Axial Resolution, SNR, and Range-Gate Duration

The axial resolution is primarily governed by the characteristics of the transmitted pulse and the duration of the receive range-gate. As noted in the last subsection, a good choice is to make the duration of the range-gate and transmit pulse equal to one another. Depending on the SNR conditions and the sample volume length required, the transmit pulse might consist of between 5 and 20 cycles. Under ideal conditions, the information provided by just two transmit firings could be used to estimate the velocity, but in practice many more are needed to achieve a good estimate.

A useful starting point is a 1-D analysis in which it is assumed that the transmitted and scattered waves are confined to the same straight line and that ignores the effects of noise and statistical fluctuations in the received signal. With the help of these assumptions, a qualitative understanding can be obtained as to how the axial resolution and sensitivity are related and how the sample volume axial length depends on the transmit pulse and range-gate duration. This simplified model will be followed by a more accurate analysis that accounts for the 3-D nature of the sample volume.

For this 1-D analysis, we also assume a transmit pulse with a rectangular envelope and duration of T. Thus, the distance from the transducer to the start of the sample volume is given by

$$z_S = c_o(\tau_S - T)/2,$$

where τ_S is the interval from the start of the transmit pulse to the opening of the range-gate. Similarly, the end of the sample volume can be expressed as

$$z_E = c_o(\tau_S + \Delta\tau)/2,$$

where $\Delta\tau$ is the range-gate duration. It follows from the above equations that the sample volume length is given by

(10.17)
$$z_E - z_S = c_o(T + \Delta\tau)/2,$$

which shows that the length can be increased by increasing the transmit pulse duration, the range-gate duration, or both.

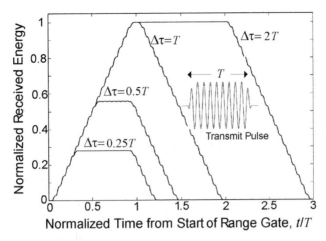

Figure 10.11 1-D simulation results showing the effect of four different range-gate to transmit durations ($\Delta\tau/T$) on the sensitivity within the sample volume axial length. The simulation assumed a nine-cycle sine-tapered transmit pulse with a 13% fractional bandwidth propagating in a medium with no attenuation.

An improved 1-D model is that first presented by Peronneau et al. [31], and that more recently described by Evans and McDicken [24, p. 48]. Such a model takes account of the partial truncation of the signal by the range-gate. Shown in Fig. 10.11 are the computed results for a nine-cycle burst, tapered at the two ends by a sine function and having a duration of T. To obtain this graph, the range-gated received signal for a scatterer placed at a given location was first determined. The energy was then obtained by multiplying the received signal FFT by its complex conjugate and integrating. This process was repeated for all scatterer locations that contributed energy. Plots are shown for the same transmit pulse amplitude for four different values of $\Delta\tau/T$. Time, normalized to the duration of the transmit signal, is shown on the horizontal axis. It can be converted to the axial position within the sample "volume" by multiplying by $c_o T/2$. The vertical axis is proportional to the gated received energy. It can be seen that when the range-gate duration $\Delta\tau \gg T$ or $\Delta\tau \ll T$, the response over the sample volume becomes more uniform compared to that when $\Delta\tau = T$. However, because the transmitted pulse amplitude was held constant, the signal energy is reduced as $\Delta\tau/T$ is reduced beyond unity.

Noise is a major factor limiting the spatial resolution. There are two primary sources: clutter caused by stationary or near-stationary scatterers, and thermal noise generated in the receiver system, particularly in the preamplifier. Vessel wall and adjacent tissue motion is often considered to be source of clutter though, as noted in Chapter 8, the information as to the wall displacement over the cardiac cycle can be an important means of assessing the vessel elasticity. For small sample volumes close to the vessel wall or long sample volumes that encompass the entire vessel, a clutter reduction filter is needed (see subsection 10.8.2). A simple high-pass filter could be used, as could a means for subtracting successive A-line signals, in the form of a delay-line canceller. As will be seen, a tradeoff exists between the SNR and axial resolution. In an important paper, Kristoffersen [32] addressed the question as to the best value for the ratio $\Delta \tau / T$ for the optimal combination of sample volume resolution and SNR.

Cathignol [33] pointed out that the SNR of any measurement system depends on the total energy received over the measurement interval. He also noted that for pulsed velocity measurement systems, improvements in the SNR could only be achieved by: (i) increasing the peak power, (ii) increasing the transmission pulse duration, and (iii) increasing the packet size. Increasing the peak power is permissible within limits that may be governed by safety considerations and the onset of nonlinear effects. Increasing the transmission pulse duration decreases the spatial resolution, as expressed in (10.17). Finally, if the packet size is increased for the same number of lines per frame and PRF, the frame rate will be decreased.

When the transmit duration is reduced to improve the axial resolution, a greater signal bandwidth will be needed, which can be achieved by increasing the preamplifier and/or the matched filter bandwidth. To compensate for the reduction in SNR associated with the increased bandwidth of the shorter transmit pulse, its amplitude should be increased. From a patient safety standpoint, it can be argued that such an increase can be in proportion to the reduction in pulse duration so that the same average power is maintained. However, as noted above, patient safety, as well as the onset of nonlinear effects, sets certain limits on the peak power.

10.3.4 Shape of the Sample Volume

The sample volume can be defined as that region over which the received gated signal power is a specified number of dB's below the peak value. Such a definition takes into consideration the fact that noise will be present and will limit the volume over which a useful backscattered signal can be obtained. A reasonable choice is a threshold of $-12\,dB$, and this will be assumed in the discussion that follows. The shape is determined primarily defined by the transmit waveform, the receive gate duration, and the characteristics of the transducer beamforming system. For a simple disk transducer, the sample volume will be cylindrically symmetric. However, for a 1-D array of the type typically used in B-mode imaging, the shape will have a lower order of symmetry, and as a result numerical methods are generally needed to determine its contours.

Work on characterizing the nature and properties of the sample volume was first described in the 1973/74 publications of Morris et al. [34], Baker et al. [35], and Jorgenson and Garbini [36]. Simplified 1-D models were generally used in which the transmit waveform incident on a scatterer was assumed to be in the form of a teardrop.[5]

---

5. In the literature the 3-D shape of the sample volume is sometimes inappropriately assumed to be similar to a teardrop.

For a 1-D model, the sample "volume" is simply the segment of a line whose boundaries correspond to the $-12\,dB$ points of the gated received signal power. These points can be determined from the sample "volume" sensitivity function, which can be found with the help of Fig. 10.12. In the time/depth graph of (a), it is assumed that scatterers are distributed throughout the medium. Also assumed is a rectangular receive gate that has a duration the same as the transmitted pulse and that starts at time t_1. Two transmitted waveforms are shown: a rectangular pulse and a teardrop pulse. Within the receive gate, the time/depth path of the transmit pulse leading edge corresponds to the lines marked with the filled black arrows, while those for the trailing edge are marked with the gray arrows. It can be seen that information first arrives at time t_1 due to the scattering of the leading edge by a scatterer at z_2. In fact, all scatterers that lie between z_1 and z_2 will simultaneously contribute receive components at t_1 due to scattering of the remaining portion of the transmitted pulse. Similarly, at time t_2, information arrives from all scatterers in the region from z_2 to z_3 by scattering of the leading through to the trailing edge of the transmitted pulse. The process whereby the received signal within the receive gate is generated corresponds to convoluting the transmit and receive waveforms, and this is illustrated in (b) for the two assumed transmit waveforms. Thus, the sample "volume" sensitivity function can be found by convoluting, giving a time-domain waveform, and then converting from time to depth.

A considerably more complex situation arises when the 3-D nature of the sample volume must be considered: generally, numerical methods must be used, especially when the source/receiver geometry is complex such as for a 1-D array. The result of such computations for a linear phased array have been described by Steinman et al. [37], and contours for regions of constant energy for various planes for a phased linear array are illustrated in Fig. 10.13. Note especially that for a fixed focus lens, the sample volume in the elevation/axial plane is much greater than that in the azimuth/axial plane, especially when the azimuth focus is well away from the elevation focus.

10.3.5 Ensemble of Scatterers

Up to now, the passage of a single point scatterer has been studied as it passes through the sample volume. A more complex situation arises when the sample volume contains an ensemble of moving scatterers, such as that illustrated in Fig. 10.14. In this case, the received signal consists of a superposition of individual backscattered signals. Moreover, movement of the ensemble causes the sample volume to contain less of the original pattern, until ultimately the entire original ensemble has been replaced. An efficient way of computing the backscattered signal is to make use of the hybrid model (see subsection 5.9.4) in which the fluid is divided into voxels with volumes of $(\lambda_o/20)^3$. The number of RBCs in a given voxel is a Gaussian variable whose variance depends on the hematocrit though (5.69). Knowledge of the point spread function of the measurement system and the backscattering cross-section for each voxel within the sample volume enables the backscattered signal to be estimated.

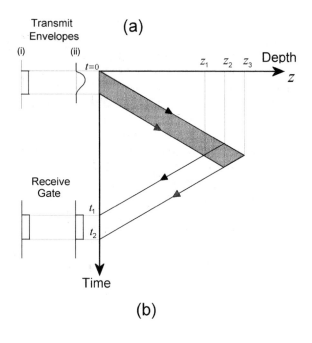

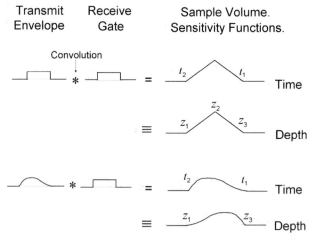

Figure 10.12 1-D model for estimating the characteristics of the sample "volume." (a) Depth/time diagram enabling the sample "volume" sensitivity function to be estimated. Examples are shown for a transmit waveform consisting of (i) a rectangular pulse and (ii) a teardrop-shape waveform. A rectangular receive gate of the same duration has been assumed. (b) Sample volume sensitivity functions. The vertical axis gives the sensitivity as a function of the z-position. Note that the shape extends from z_1 to z_3, where z_3 corresponds to the leading edge of the transmit pulse and z_1 to the trailing edge.

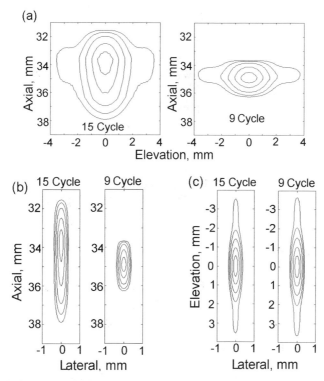

Figure 10.13 Sample volume characteristics obtained using a 3-D simulation model for a 5-MHz, 58-element array at the azimuthal focus of 35 mm. The array elements were 0.27 mm wide and 4 mm high in the elevation direction, and the kerf was 0.03 mm. Propagation was into a medium with an attenuation of 0.7 dB/(MHz.cm). A lens with a focus at 11.25 mm was assumed in the elevation plane. The transmitted excitation pulse was a tapered 5-MHz multi-cycle sine wave with 9 cycles (1.5 mm axial length) and 15 cycles (5.0 mm). The receive gate had the same duration as the transmitted pulse. Contours correspond to relative total energies of −1, −3, −6, −9, and −12 dB. Lateral F-number = 2. (a) Axial versus elevation. (b) Axial versus lateral. (c) Elevation versus lateral at a depth of 35 mm. ((a) and (b) reprinted by permission of Elsevier from Steinman et al. [37], *Ultrasound Med. Biol.*, 30, 1409–1418, ©2004 World Federation of Ultrasound in Medicine and Biology.)

10.3.6 Coded Excitation

Soon after the first publications appeared describing pulsed velocity systems, methods of improving the sensitivity by using coded excitation were discussed [38,39]. These and subsequent developments, together with the basis principles, were discussed in section 8.4. However, not discussed there was the use of frequency modulation as a means for extracting range and velocity information from a moving target. As with many ideas for improving the performance of medical ultrasound systems, this technique was first developed and

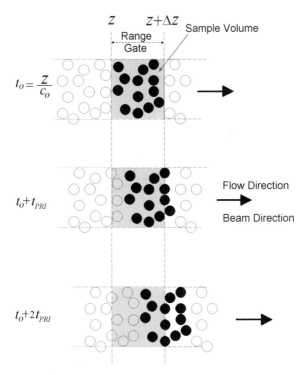

Figure 10.14 How decorrelation arises with successive A-lines. For simplicity, it has been assumed that flow is in the direction of the range-gated ultrasound beam. A certain ensemble of scatterers that is wholly within the sample volume when the first transmit pulse reaches it at time t_o is shown as filled circles. As it moves away from the transducer in the z-direction, it is gradually replaced by a new ensemble (empty circles), causing decorrelation of successive range-gated samples. The scatterer arrangements in the sample volume are also shown at times of $t_o + t_{PRI}$ and $t_o + 2t_{PRI}$.

used for improving the performance of radar systems [4, pp. 448–456; 40]. In 1974 McCarty and Woodcock [41,42] proposed that if the transmitted signal was frequency modulated, the problems arising from the lack of range discrimination in CW Doppler ultrasound could be circumvented. As illustrated in Fig. 10.15a, they examined the use of a continuous signal, frequency modulated in a linear periodic manner. For a fixed scatter at a depth z_o, it can be seen that the sawtooth, representing the instantaneous frequency of the received signal, is displaced in time. If the repetition period of the transmitted waveform is greater than $2z_o/C_o$ and if the rate of change of the transmitted frequency is constant, the instantaneous frequency difference between the transmitted and received signals is given by

$$\Delta f = \frac{2z_o}{c_o}\frac{df_t}{dt},$$

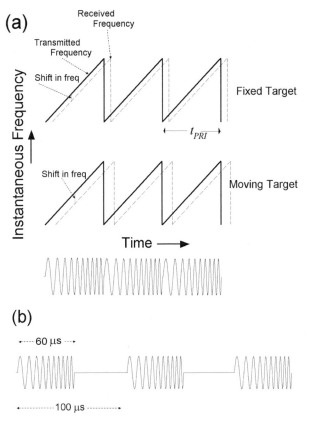

Figure 10.15 Frequency modulation schemes. (a) The CW, linear FM scheme proposed by McCarty and Woodcock [41,42]. (b) Scheme described by Wilhjelm and Pedersen [44] that uses a long FM pulse that might have a duration of 60 µs and be repeated every 100 µs.

where df_t/dt is the rate of change of the transmitted frequency. Thus, the axial location of a fixed scatterer can be determined by measuring Δf. If the scatterer is moving, the Doppler effect will cause the received instantaneous frequency to differ from Δf. In this case, if the demodulator consists of a multiplier whose inputs are the transmitted and received signals, then the low-pass filtered signal at its output will have an instantaneous frequency of

$$(10.18) \qquad \Delta f(t) = \frac{2z_o}{c_o}\frac{df_t}{dt} \pm f_D(t),$$

where $f_D(t)$ is the Doppler frequency shift. Because the instantaneous frequency of the incident wave changes with time, the Doppler frequency will also be time-dependent, making Δf a function of time. In (10.18) there are two unknowns: the depth of the scatterer and its axial velocity component (through

Δf_D). The ambiguity can be resolved by extracting additional information through frequency-domain analysis.

In radar, the range/velocity ambiguity for a single target can be resolved through frequency-domain analysis [40]. However, Bertram [43] found that in a blood vessel, where a multiplicity of scatterers can move with different velocities through the sample volume, the ambiguity could not be resolved using the transmit scheme of Fig. 10.15a. Subsequently, Wilhjelm and Pedersen [44,45] proposed the use of the relatively long linearly modulated FM pulses shown in Fig. 10.15b. As with the previous scheme, separate transmit and receive transducers were required. They showed that the center frequency difference between successive demodulated signals was directly proportional to the axial velocity component. This difference was determined by cross-correlation of successive real spectra [45]. Using a fluid seeded with small scatterers, they demonstrated that the system was capable of measuring flow velocity profiles. They also compared the performance with that of a more conventional pulsed wave system that used cross-correlation to determine the time shift (see section 10.4) and found similar levels of performance.

10.4 Velocity Estimation using Time-Shift Cross-Correlation

Estimation of the distance traveled by a scatterer in a specified interval of time forms the basis of the time-shift method for estimating its mean velocity. This distance can be estimated from the pulse-echo transit-time difference between successive transmitted pulses. Denoting this difference by $\Delta \tau$, the scatterer velocity can be obtained by rewriting (10.1) as

(10.19)
$$v = \frac{c_o \Delta \tau}{2 t_{PRI} \cos \theta}.$$

A significant advantage of this method in comparison to methods based on frequency or phase is the elimination of aliasing. Under ideal circumstances, the maximum velocity that can be estimated is limited by the need for the scatterer to remain within the sample volume for several PRIs. However, if the target is blood, signal decorrelation between successive PRIs must be sufficiently small that the time delay can be reliably estimated. In practice, delay estimate errors can arise from noise. The false peaks created by this source can be removed by nonlinear processing; however, the jitter errors arising from sampling effects remain [46]. Nonetheless, as noted by Jensen [47], under favorable SNR conditions the maximum velocity can be several times greater than the aliasing velocity as expressed by (10.3).

10.4.1 Time-Delay Estimation

By the 1960s, it was generally accepted [48] that the cross-correlation function provided an excellent method for estimating the relative delay between two partially correlated signals in the presence of uncorrelated noise. The application of this technique to estimate $\Delta\tau$ and hence to obtain the velocity using (10.19) was first described by a group working in Milan. Dotti et al. [49], in a 1976 paper, described a correlation system they used for measuring the flow velocity profile of blood flowing in an 8 mm diameter tube. A more detailed description that included improvements to the measurement system was presented by the same group [50] in 1979. In vitro results from their steady and pulsatile flow velocity profile measurements using blood, together with in vivo measurements of the velocity profile on a superficial arm vein and from a common carotid artery, were subsequently published [51]. Nearly ten years later two other research groups announced the development of similar velocity measurement systems: one focused on its use for volumetric blood flow estimation [54,55], the second for use in color flow imaging [8,56]. The first proposal for estimating tissue displacement by cross-correlating successive A-scans appears to be that reported by Dickenson and Hill [52] in 1982 (see section 8.8). Since then, estimation of soft tissue movement and its velocity in 1-D and 2-D by cross-correlation has been extensively investigated. In a 1993 review, Hein and O'Brien [53] discussed a variety of estimation methods and assessed their relative advantages.

In essence, the cross-correlation method consists of taking a range-gated portion of the received signal and searching for the time shift that gives the best match with a subsequent A-line signal. Two successive received RF A-line signals are shown in Fig. 10.16. These simulated echoes were produced with a wideband transmit pulse whose fractional bandwidth was about 50%, propagating into a simulated blood-like medium. The range-gated portion of the first echo is cross-correlated with the second echo to yield a lag waveform whose maximum has a lag equal to the delay between the two echoes in the gate region. To obtain an estimate of the flow velocity with a relatively small variance, the average time shift over several (e.g., 5–10) transmissions must be used. Because the echo signal will usually be in the form of sampled data, the cross-correlation estimate will be in a discrete form. For two successive signals $y_n(t)$ and $y_{n+1}(t)$, the cross-correlation estimate over the range-gate is given by

$$\hat{R}_{n,n+1}(s, N_{\tau_o}) = \frac{1}{N_S} \sum_{l=0}^{N_S-1} y_n(N_{\tau_o} + l)y_{n+1}(N_{\tau_o} + l + s),$$

where N_{τ_o} denotes the sample number at the beginning of the range-gate, i.e., $\tau_o = N_{\tau_o}/f_s$, f_s is the sampling frequency, s/f_s corresponds to the lag, N_s is the number of samples within each range gate, and the hat on R is used to indicate that it is an estimated value.

As discussed by Foster et al. [55] and Jensen [61], several error sources can be identified that detract from the reliability with which the velocity can be estimated. For low SNR conditions, maxima in the cross-correlation can occur for time delays that are unrelated to the true velocity. By restricting the range over which the cross-correlation is performed, e.g., to the regions between the two side lobe peaks of the cross-correlation function [47], the probability of detecting a false maximum can be reduced. However, this also limits the

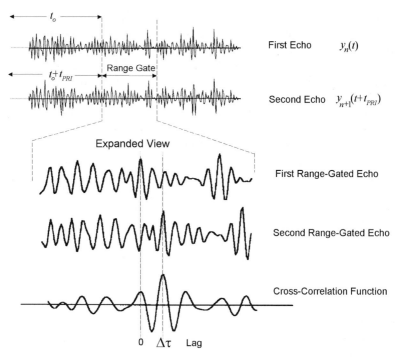

Figure 10.16 The cross-correlation method for estimating the time delay from range-gated portions of successive A-lines. The location of the maximum is equal to the delay. By using a multiplicity of A-lines, the probability of correctly estimating the delay can be improved. (Reproduced, with permission, from Vaitkus [57].)

maximum velocity that can be estimated. By limiting the range to the two side lobe peaks, this maximum may be no better than the aliasing velocity as given by (10.3).

Limitations on the sampling rate are likely to cause the maximum value of the cross-correlation lag to differ from the true delay value $\Delta\tau$. Foster et al. [55] proposed that around the maximum the sample values could be fitted to a parabola, enabling the true maximum to be estimated with improved accuracy.

10.4.2 Effects of Decorrelation

When cross-correlation is used for estimating the blood flow velocity, decorrelation of the signature produced by a particular ensemble of scatterers is of considerable importance in determining the accuracy with which the velocity can be estimated.[6] The influence of decorrelation was first mentioned by

---

6. Decorrelation has been proposed as a means for estimating blood flow using intravascular side-view imaging probes (see subsection 8.10.4).

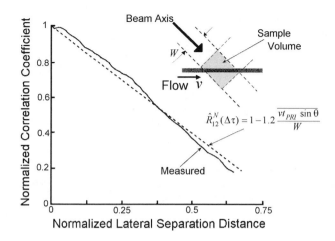

Figure 10.17 The manner in which an initial ensemble of scatterers becomes decorrelated in the sample volume because some scatterers will exit and new ones will enter between PRIs. The solid line is based on measurements. The normalized lateral separation distance is 1.2 $\overline{vt_{PRI} \sin\theta}/W$. Measured and empirical results are those obtained by Foster et al. [55].

Bassini et al. [50] and was more fully discussed by Bonnefous [58] and Foster et al. [55]. Bonnefous derived an expression for the estimated maximum value of the normalized cross-correlation coefficient $\hat{R}_{12}^N(\Delta\tau)$ as a function distance that an ensemble of scatterers moves in one PRI and velocity dispersion. If velocity dispersion can be ignored, her expression for the correlation maximum can be written as

$$(10.20) \qquad \hat{R}_{12}^N(\Delta\tau) = 1 - \frac{\overline{vt_{PRI} \sin\theta}}{W},$$

where W is the beam width at the measurement site, θ is the angle the flow velocity makes to the beam axis (same as the Doppler angle), and the quantity under the bar is the mean distance traveled by the ensemble in one PRI. This equation shows that the maximum value falls off linearly with the lateral distance traveled by the scatterers. Modulation of the RF signal by the beam profile and velocity dispersion caused by turbulence in the sample volume can be expected to further reduce $\hat{R}_{12}^N(\Delta\tau)$. The measurements shown in Fig. 10.17 indicate that up to a normalized lateral distance of 0.6, the behavior is close to linear, though a factor of 1.2 was needed in the second term of (10.20) to obtain a good fit.

To account for the effects of noise on the time delay estimate, Foster et al. [55] used a number of simplifying assumptions to develop an approximate equation for the variance of the time delay estimate. If $\Delta\tau$ denotes the true delay, then for high SNRs and long spatial windows compared to a wavelength, the standard deviation of the estimate is given by

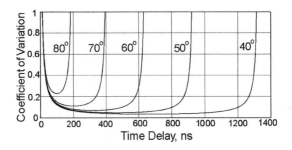

Figure 10.18 Variation in estimating the time delay when using the cross-correlation method versus the true time delay as calculated from (10.22). The sample volume was assumed to have a width of 1 mm, bandwidth 2.0 MHz, and SNR 10. The angle is θ is defined in Fig. 10.17.

$$(10.21) \qquad \sigma_{\Delta\hat{t}} \approx \frac{\sqrt{2}}{2\pi\Delta f \hat{R}_{12}^{N}(\Delta\tau)SNR},$$

where Δf is the bandwidth. A useful normalized indicator of the imprecision with which the delay can be estimated is the coefficient of variation. Also known as the normalized random error, it can be defined by [59] $\varepsilon = \sigma_{\Delta\hat{t}}/\Delta\tau$. Substituting (10.20) into (10.21) (including the factor of 1.2) and using (10.19) to eliminate v, the coefficient of variation can be expressed as

$$(10.22) \qquad \varepsilon = \sigma_{\Delta\hat{t}} / \Delta\tau \approx \frac{W\sqrt{2}}{2\pi\Delta f(W - 0.6c_o\Delta\tau\tan\theta)SNR}.$$

The manner in which this coefficient of variation changes with the delay for various angles of incidence is shown in Fig. 10.18. With shorter time delays, the effect of noise dominates, while for much longer delays and small angles of incidence, decorrelation also contributes to the coefficient increase. For intermediate delays, the coefficient of variation reaches a minimum and, in the absence of any bias, the best estimates of the true delay are achieved.

A further source of estimation error arises from non-uniformity of the pulse-echo response over the sample volume [55]. As the ensemble of scatterers within the sample volume moves between successive transmissions, each RBC will see a different incident pressure, causing the received signal to change.

The maximum measurable flow velocity can be estimated from the equation describing the effect of decorrelation. If it is assumed that a good estimate of the time shift requires that the correlation coefficient between two successive A-mode transmissions be ≥0.5, then from (10.20)

$$(10.23) \qquad v_{max} = \frac{Wf_{PRF}}{2\sin\theta}.$$

For example, if $W = 1$ mm, $f_{PRF} = 5$ kHz, and $\theta = 60$ degrees, then $v_{max} = 288$ cm/s. However, the presence of noise would require several A-mode

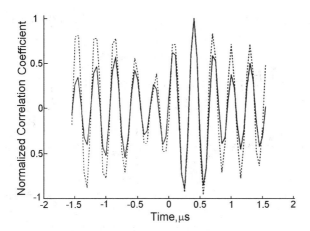

Figure 10.19 Comparison of the computed correlation coefficient using the full sampled data (solid line) from two range-gated signals with that computed using the sign of the data values (dashed line). There were 32 samples in the data that had an SNR of 10. (Reproduced, with permission of the International Federation for Medical & Biological Engineering, from Jensen [61], *Med. Biolog. Eng. Comput.*, 32, S165–S170, ©1993 IFMBE.)

transmissions to achieve acceptable accuracy. If this is taken to be five, then the maximum velocity in the above example would be 58 cm/s.

10.4.3 Approximate Method for Cross-Correlation Calculation

Determination of the cross-correlation between range-gated data involves a very significant computational burden, especially when it is desired to extract the velocity data over an entire axial region rather than over a single sample volume. An approximate method of finding the cross-correlation function for sampled data is based on first reducing the data to one-bit values, values that correspond to the sign of the sampled values. Cross-correlation is then performed using the one-bit arithmetic. Justification for this approach is based on the knowledge that for two Gaussian distributed signals with zero mean and an infinite number of samples, the sign method [10, pp. 239–240] yields the exact cross-correlation function. It appears that this method was originally used by Bassini et al. [50] in applying the cross-correlation approach for ultrasound velocity measurements, and was subsequently used by others.

The simplicity of one-bit arithmetic enables the necessary calculations to be performed in real time using custom-designed hardware [60]. For a simulated RF signal segment, Fig. 10.19 shows that the times at which the exact and approximate maxima occur are essentially the same. More sophisticated schemes with improved performance have also been described. For example, a two-bit scheme has been described by Wang et al. [62], who used an adaptively selected threshold. They reported that for reduced SNR conditions, the performance was significantly better than the one-bit scheme.

10.5 Velocity Estimation Based on Phase Shift and Frequency

One of the first techniques to be used for velocity estimation in a real-time flow imaging system was that described in 1982 by Namekawa et al. [63]. It was based on estimating the phase shift between the signals received from successive transmitted pulses by using an autocorrelation technique. Sometimes referred to as the Kasai [64] or the 1-D autocorrelation estimation method,[7] it was incorporated into the first commercially available color flow imaging system[8] and was used in many subsequent commercial systems. Its development and application was in fact preceded by important developments several years earlier, based primarily on radar techniques developed during the 1950s. Specifically, in 1975 Grandchamp [65] pointed out that by estimating the phase shift between successive A-mode lines at a given location, the flow velocity at that location could be calculated. He also pointed out that the technique was capable of estimating the velocity throughout the entire depth of the A-lines. Brandestini [66] demonstrated the practical use of this technique. Both authors recognized the importance of greatly reducing the large echo amplitudes that arise from stationary or slowly moving structures. Generally, these form a dominant part of the received signal and can seriously degrade the accuracy with which the phase difference can be estimated.

With reference to the simplified sketch of Fig. 10.4a, it should be noted that for a single scatterer, the phase shift between any pair of received signals can be estimated. If the shift lies in the range from −180 to +180 degrees (to avoid any wrap-around ambiguities) the time delay can be related to the phase shift, enabling the velocity to be estimated. Alternatively, as demonstrated in Fig. 10.4b and expressed by (10.2), the velocity can also be estimated from the center frequency of the slow-time waveform.

In the presence of a multiplicity of scatterers moving with different velocities in the sample volume, the scattered waveform will have a more complex form due to the effects of interference, as previously described in Chapter 5. Because the scatterer distribution changes between successive transmissions, it therefore becomes more difficult to extract velocity information. However, before considering phase-shift and frequency estimation methods in more detail, it may be helpful to examine some of the results from Mayo and Embree's [67] experiments, as reproduced in Fig. 10.20.

We first focus attention on the RF signal and stack gray-scale images of successive A-lines side by side to form a 2-D image. Such images were obtained

---

7. Different authors refer to this method with different names, such as the covariance estimator, the autocorrelation estimator, and the correlation phase estimator.

8. The first commercial system, the SSD-880CW, was introduced in 1983/4 by Aloka of Japan.

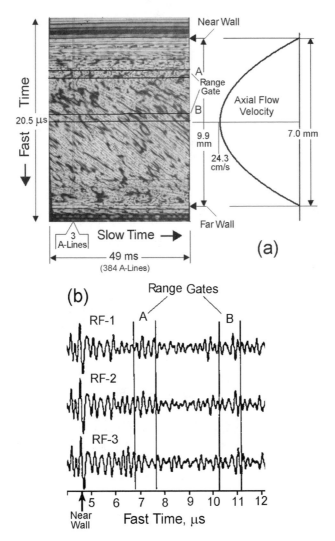

Figure 10.20 Frequency and phase methods for estimating the flow velocity. The measurements used a 5-MHz wideband transmit pulse and an ultrasound beam that intersected the flow at 45 degrees in a 7.0-mm-diameter tube. Because the beam/flow angle was 45 degrees, the path within the vessel is 9.9 mm. The fluid contained a high density of small scatterers and had a flow velocity profile that was approximately parabolic with a peak velocity of 24.3 cm/s. (a) Successive 384 RF received signals (A-lines) are displayed in gray scale side by side. (b) Portions of the three successive A-lines indicated in (a).

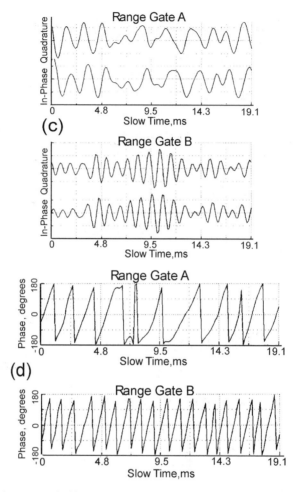

Figure 10.20 (*Continued*) (c) Complex signal obtained from two low-pass filtered range gates (A and B) of the first 150 A-lines. (d) Phase of the RF signal within the two range gates for the same 150 A-lines. (Reproduced, with permission of the International Society for Optical Engineering, from Embree and Mayo [67], pp. 70–78, in: *Int. Symp. on Pattern Recognition*, Vol. 0768, ©1987 SPIE.)

using a simple steady-flow model consisting of scatterers suspended in water flowing in a 7.0 mm diameter tube. As illustrated in Fig. 10.20a, the presence of flow causes a gray-scale pattern to emerge that is directly related to the parabolic flow velocity profile. The complex signals shown in (c), which were obtained from the first 150 lines of the two range-gates (A and B), clearly indicate their stochastic nature. It should also be noted that the mean frequency from range-gate A is much lower than that obtained from B, whose position is close to the center of the flow axis. By estimating the mean frequency of these waveforms, the mean velocities at the sample volume locations can be determined from (10.2). Note that the in-phase and quadrature signals enable the direction of flow to be determined. Specifically, because the in-phase signals lags the quadrature component, flow is directed away from the transducer whose beam/flow angle is 45 degrees. As is illustrated in (d), the presence of both components also enables the center frequency phase shift to be determined. From the slope of the phase shift, the velocity can be estimated. Techniques that can be used to achieve this are discussed in section 10.8.

10.6 Multigate Pulsed Wave Methods

In an artery, the flow changes rapidly with time, especially in the neighborhood of systole; as a result, the flow velocity profile changes over the cardiac cycle. For a considerable time, it had been realized that measurement of the profile could provide a useful means for assessing the status of a vessel. A single-channel instrument can be used to achieve this by stepping the range-gate across the vessel [68]. However, for pulsatile flow, this requires a means for synchronizing the time at which the information is obtained to the phase of the cardiac cycle. A much better scheme, and one that allows real-time profiling (Fig. 10.21a), is through the use of a multiplicity of range-gated channels.

McLeod and Anliker [69], working at Stanford University, appear to have been the first to report the development of a multigate system. Their system used transmitted pulses of 1 μs duration with a center frequency of 8 MHz and employed sixteen gates whose sample positions were automatically adjusted to provide uniform spacing along a path intersecting a flow profile. Measurements of the flow velocity profiles obtained with steady-flow models showed excellent agreement with theory. Complications arise in arterial vessels due to the elastic nature of blood vessels. The pressure changes responsible for the pulsatile flow not only cause the velocity profile to change over the cardiac cycle but also result in significant changes in the vessel diameter (Fig. 10.21b).

A detailed account of the design and application of a sixteen gate system was presented by Peronneau et al. [31,70]. Measurements of profiles for steady and pulsatile flow in tubes and for pulsatile flow in the artery of a dog were reported. About the same time (1974), Anliker's group in Zurich developed a fourteen channel pulsed system that was used extensively for profile measurements in a variety of human vessels [71,74]. Subsequent developments were reported by Fish [72], Brandestini [73], and Hoeks et al. [75]. To simplify the signal processing needed for each channel, a zero-crossing processor was often used. These time-domain processors determine the zero-crossing frequency of the demodulated signal. Under ideal SNR conditions, it can be shown [76] that the zero-crossing frequency is proportional to the RMS frequency of the input signal. However, the presence of noise can significantly degrade the performance, causing serious errors [77,78].

10.6.1 System Design

One example of a multigate system is that developed by Reneman's group in Holland [79]. It had a center frequency of 6.1 MHz, a PRF of 18 kHz, emission and gate durations of 2/3 μs, a sample volume of 1.2 to 1.7 mm^3, and 64 gates.

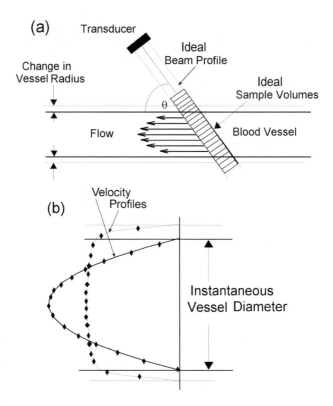

Figure 10.21 Method for using a multigate system for estimating the instantaneous flow profile. A pulsatile profile accompanied by changes in the vessel diameter is illustrated for two instants of time in the flow cycle. (a) A multiplicity of sample volumes within a blood vessel at two times in the flow cycle. (b) Velocity profiles for the same two times.

In vivo measurements from the right common carotid artery of a young volunteer are shown in Fig. 10.22 [80]. A sequence of time waveforms taken from 14 range-gates that cross the vessel is shown in (a). The waveform at the bottom shows the relative diameter changes that occur over the cardiac cycle, details of which were subsequently reported by Hoeks et al. [81]. From (b) it is clear that in the neighborhood of peak systole, the profile is relatively flat and the vessel is maximally distended.

10.6.2 Deconvolution Correction

Ideally, the sample volume should be sufficiently small that the signal obtained from a given channel represents the flow velocity component at its location. However, for most blood vessels, a typical pulsed ultrasound sample volume includes scatterers with a range of velocities; furthermore, in a multigate

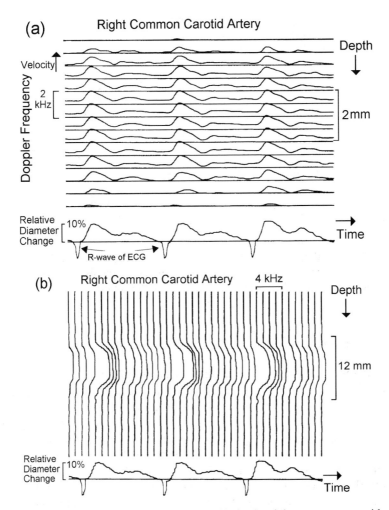

Figure 10.22 Measurement of the velocity profile in the right common carotid artery and its changes over the cardiac cycle for a young volunteer. (a) Time variations of the signal from 14 range gates; also shown are the relative changes in vessel diameter. (b) Profile variations reconstructed from the measurements shown in (a). (Reproduced, with permission of Research Studies Press, from Reneman and Hoeks [80], Chapter 4 in *Doppler Ultrasound in the Diagnosis of Cerebrovascular Disease,* ©1982 John Wiley & Sons.)

system there can be significant overlap between adjacent sample volumes, as illustrated in Fig. 10.23. A simple detector that estimates the RMS pulsed wave frequency (e.g., a zero-crossing detector) or the mean frequency takes no account of the location and relative weights of the velocities encompassed, causing the estimated velocity profile to be in error. Deconvolution procedures for obtaining a more accurate estimate were first noted by McLeod and Anliker [69] and subsequently were used by others [35,36,82].

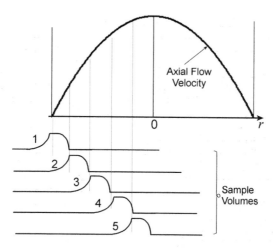

Figure 10.23 A multigate system makes possible the measurement of the flow velocity profile. The spatial locations and the sensitivity functions are shown for five sample volumes. Each encompasses a range of velocities and each overlaps the information from adjacent volumes.

10.7 Principles of CW and Pulsed Wave Flow Imaging

Of considerable importance in the diagnosis of vascular disease is the ability to image the flow and to superimpose such a flow image on the structural B-mode image. One of the initial major impediments to achieving this in real time was the problem of developing a technique for estimating the flow velocity sufficiently quickly with the computational speed then available. A number of significant developments, discussed in the first subsection, led to a method for overcoming this problem. Two examples of color flow images, superimposed on their respective gray-scale B-mode images, are shown in Fig. 10.24. The first shows the common carotid artery (shades of red) and the jugular vein (shades of blue). It was obtained with a 5 MHz linear array using beam steering. The second shows the fetal umbilical cord imaged using a curvilinear phased array. A further example is shown in Fig. 10.25. The upper portion shows a color flow display of the common carotid artery. A white marker indicates the location where a spectral flow sample volume is formed, separate from the color display, by using an aperture of adjacent array elements. The slow-wave "gray-scale" spectrum from this sample volume is shown at the bottom. It is similar to the Doppler gray-scale spectral display shown in Fig. 9.16 except that it is derived from a sample volume near the vessel center instead of from the entire vessel.

10.7.1 Historical Background

During a period when CW Doppler ultrasound was still being clinically assessed, initial steps in the development of Doppler and pulsed wave flow

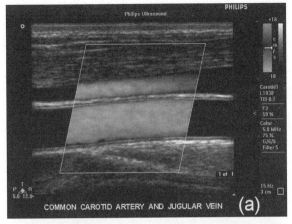

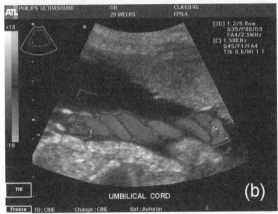

Figure 10.24 Two examples of color flow imaging. For both, the color flow image is added to the gray-scale B-mode image and the color bar scale gives the flow velocity component in the beam direction in cm/s. Vertical tick marks are 1 cm apart. (a) Common carotid artery (red scale) and the jugular vein (blue scale): 15 frames/s, 5.0-MHz center frequency; the focal point is marked by a < close to the RHS. (b) Sector scan showing the umbilical cord (two arteries and one vein) at 29 weeks: 4 frames/s, 2.5-MHz center frequency. (Courtesy Philips Ultrasound.) See color insert.

imaging were reported. In 1971/2 three brief reports appeared. Using CW Doppler ultrasound, Reid and Spencer [83] described a scheme that used a sharply focused 5 MHz transducer. As illustrated in Fig. 10.26a, the transducer was scanned over the surface, and if Doppler frequencies above 300 Hz were present at a given location, the recorded intensity was modulated by the Doppler shift frequency. A transducer position resolver was used to determine the position on the scan plane, enabling the lateral (C-mode) tracings of Fig. 10.26b to be obtained, much like those of a conventional transmission x-ray image.

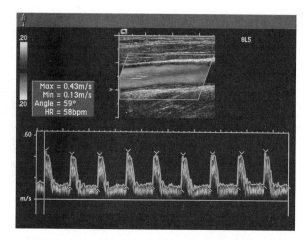

Figure 10.25 Example of a spectral flow display from a sample volume located near the center of the common carotid artery. Two small white lines mark the range-gate boundaries and the white dots show the spectral beam direction. The beam/flow angle was estimated to be 59 degrees, resulting in a peak flow velocity of 43 cm/s. The envelope of the spectral display, indicated by the gray line, gives the variation from within the sample volume of the peak flow velocity over each cycle. (Courtesy Siemens Ultrasound.) See color insert.

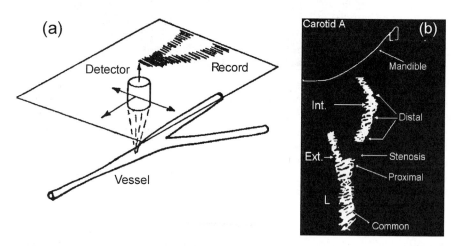

Figure 10.26 Method developed by Reid and Spencer [83] for flow mapping using CW Doppler ultrasound. (a) Schematic of scanning transducer, a vessel, and the scanned C-mode image. (Reprinted by permission of Elsevier, from Reneman and Spencer [83], *Ultrasound Med. Biol.*, 5, 1–11, ©1979 World Federation of Ultrasound in Medicine and Biology.) (b) Subsequent carotid artery recording showing a scanned right carotid artery indicating the presence of very little flow to the internal carotid artery due to the presence of a stenosis. Reproduced, with permission of *Science*, from Reid and Spencer [84], *Science*, 176, 1235–1226, ©1972 AAAS.)

About the same time, two groups described the use of pulsed wave systems for flow visualization. In the pulsed system described in 1971/2 by Hokanson et al. [87,88], a 2-D map was generated that indicated flow in the plane of the vessel, similar to that of Fig. 10.26a. On the other hand, the pulsed wave system described by Fish [85,86] generated a map to indicate the flow velocity over a vessel's cross-sectional area, i.e., normal to the plane shown in Fig. 10.26a. This system, like the other early systems, required many minutes of examination time to obtain satisfactory clinical images. Subsequently, Fish [72] described a 30-channel multigate system that was capable of imaging in several planes[9] enabling the vascular examination time to be greatly reduced.

Apart from the problem of examination time, these preliminary systems provided only a rough measure of the flow velocity, due in part to the method of display. White and Curry [89,90] made a significant improvement by color-encoding the maximum Doppler shift frequency and recording this on color film from a color CRT. Their CW Doppler system, which was manufactured[10] under the brand name of Echoflow, used a multiplicity of filters to determine the maximum Doppler frequency. Venous flow signals that might be picked up along with arterial signals were rejected by the phase-quadrature detection scheme.

Over the period 1975 to 1982 a number of schemes were proposed for more rapidly estimating the flow velocity component in the beam direction over the entire length of an A-line echo, and extending this to a 2-D map. The work of Grandchamp [65] and Brandestini [66], previously mentioned in section 10.5, was an important step toward achieving real-time flow imaging. Specifically, they demonstrated how the velocity component at a succession of locations along an A-line could be estimated by measuring the phase shift between successive A-lines. In 1978, Brandestini and Forster [91] described how this technique could be used to produce flow images in which the velocity field was color-encoded and superimposed on a gray-scale B-mode image. A subsequent publication from the same group [92] showed the color images that are reproduced in Fig. 10.27. To obtain these images they used a modified Duplex system with a scan head consisting of three rapidly rotating transducers for generating B-mode images, and these were coupled to the tissue via a water-filled boot. In addition, a single-element pulsed wave transducer was used for flow velocity estimation, and this was mounted on a pivot, enabling its direction to be manually adjusted.

A composite color-encoded flow image of a common carotid artery is shown in Fig. 10.27a. Originally published in 1981 [92], many of the features of this image are similar to those obtained with subsequent commercial systems.[8] It

---

9. MAVIS (Movable Arterial and Venous Imaging System), a range-gated scanner, was one of the first commercially available multigate systems. It was based on the design by Fish [72] and produced by GEC Medical Equipment Ltd. in the latter part of the 1970s. As described by Woodcock and Atkinson [21, Chapter 4, pp. 129–133], the MAVIS C contained imaging capability along with the ability to compute the velocity profile and the volumetric flow rate.

10. Diagnostics Electronics, Lexington, MA.

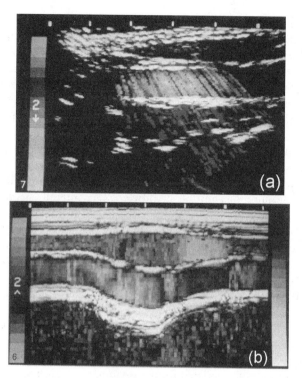

Figure 10.27 Early color-encoded flow images. (a) Common carotid artery flow image superimposed on a gray-scale B-mode image. (b) Three-second M-mode recording showing the movement of tissue and vessel walls in gray scale and blood flow in color. The beam passes through the jugular vein (blue) and then through the common carotid artery. (Reprinted by permission of Elsevier, from Eyer et al. [92], *Ultrasound Med. Biol.*, 7, 21–31, ©1981 World Federation of Ultrasound in Medicine and Biology.) See color insert.

shows the color-encoded flow velocity along approximately 25 lines superimposed on a gray-scale B-mode image. The instantaneous phase along a given A-line was estimated from the real and complex parts of the received signal. By subtraction, phase differences were determined, enabling the velocity to be estimated. For each probe direction, the velocity was color-encoded using the velocity/color scale shown on the left, and then superimposed on the stored B-mode image whose scale is shown on the right. The image shown in (b) contains a color-encoded M-mode recording over a three second period during a Valsalva maneuver. Because the beam passes through both the jugular vein (on top) and common carotid artery (below), it displays the blood velocity component in the beam direction. This image is superimposed on a conventional gray-scale pulse-echo M-mode recording showing movement of the tissue. Because a fixed beam direction was used, the composite display shows the tissue movement and the component velocity along the beam as a function of time.

A closely related pulsed wave technique for generating a velocity estimate as a function of depth is that described by Nowicki and Reid [93] in 1981. Like Brandistini [66], they recognized the importance of achieving a high degree of stationary echo cancellation. Using two analog (delay-line) moving target filters in series, reductions of around 50 dB were reported. Moreover, their technique was sensitive to flow direction. Another technique for flow imaging is that described by Arenson et al. [94,95] in 1980/82. It used a linear array of 32 elements in which each transducer element was mounted at 30 degrees to the surface. Groups of six elements were used for reception and phased transmission. A mirror driven by a stepper motor provided scanning normal to the linear elements. Using a long-pulse Doppler CW system, flow imaging was achieved at five frames per second, with each frame consisting of 10×27 pixels.

As noted in section 10.5, one of the first real-time flow imaging systems to be described was that reported in 1982 by Namekawa et al. [63]. This group, working at the Aloka Institute in Japan, initially used a mechanical scanning transducer but changed to a phased array in the middle of 1983. In 1982, Bommer and Miller [96] from the University of California also reported the development of a 2-D color flow imaging system. The flow image had 64×156 sample-sites per plane and a frame frequency of 60 Hz, and the final image contained a superimposed B-mode frame. They reported cardiac measurements on dogs and normal subjects as well as patients with tricuspid valve regurgitation and demonstrated significant enhancement of the signal level by using contrast agents. These and other developments have been summarized in Omoto's valuable historical review [97] that recounts the early development of color flow mapping, its commercialization, and clinical application.

10.7.2 Pulsed Wave Color Flow Imaging

Of central importance in the initial development of real-time flow imaging in the presence of pulsatile flow was a means for rapidly estimating the mean flow velocity along each A-line direction. Such estimators should have relatively small bias and variance, especially under the relatively poor SNR conditions that are often encountered in practice. Some of the methods discussed earlier, e.g., time-delay correlation and phase shift detection, have been successfully used in commercial systems, and details of these, along with some alternative approaches, will be presented. However, before considering the details, the basic principles underlying color flow imaging will first be described.

10.7.3 Principles

A sequence of five A-mode RF signals obtained from transmissions in the same beam direction is shown in Fig. 10.28. As noted earlier, in the absence of noise just two lines are sufficient, but from 5 to 20 may be needed to obtain a sufficiently good velocity estimate within each segment into which the received signals have been divided. To extract the required information, each

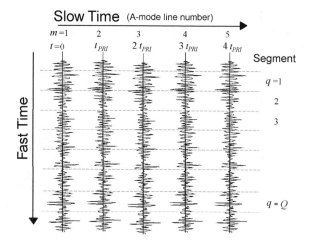

Figure 10.28 A sequence of five RF received signals are shown, each of which is divided into Q range-gated segments. The signal in each segment is sampled and integrated over the segment duration.

received signal can be quadrature demodulated (see subsection 10.3.2) to obtain its in-phase and quadrature components. These are then sampled and integrated over the range-gated segment duration. For eight such lines and a selected segment, the in-phase and quadrature analog signals, together with the sampled and integrated signals, are illustrated in Fig. 10.29 (a) to (d). The magnitude of the complex signal obtained from eight lines is shown in (e). As illustrated in (f), the superposition of these signals on a common time axis clearly shows that movement of an ensemble of scatterers within the sample volume produces a phase shift. From this, the mean scatterer velocity in the beam direction can be estimated for this particular segment. By repeating this process for all segments and then encoding this information in color, a single line of color-encoded flow can be displayed. By repeating this entire process so as to cover an entire region, a single frame of color-encoded velocity information can be displayed. As will be described, to successfully extract and display this information, the effects of stationary or slowly moving tissue must be either eliminated or greatly reduced.

10.8 One-Dimensional Autocorrelation Methods

As noted earlier, the first successful real-time color flow imaging system was based on an algorithm first described by Namekawa et al. [63,64].[11] Funda-

---

11. In the context of this and related sections, the names "1-D" and "2-D" refer to the nature of the input data, not to the spatial dimensions.

mentally, the method is a phase-domain technique that provides an estimate of the mean pulsed wave frequency and variance from the autocorrelation function and its derivative at zero lag. Namekawa and Kasai may not have been aware of a highly relevant paper by Miller and Rochwarger [98] published some 10 years earlier. It described how the moments of the spectral density of a complex Gaussian signal process could be estimated from the complex signal of successive A-mode transmissions. As will be seen, the computational complexity of this approach for estimating the mean and variance is considerably less than that based on estimating the power density spectrum and, from this, estimating the moments.

Now the range-gated sampled signal from a single scatterer moving with velocity v is that illustrated in Fig. 10.4b, and its velocity is related to the slow-time frequency by (10.2). Consequently, for a distribution of scatterers the signal will have a mean pulsed wave angular frequency of $\bar{\omega}_{PW}$ that is related to the spatial mean velocity and the incident center frequency (ω_c) by

$$(10.24) \qquad \bar{v} = \frac{c_0 \bar{\omega}_{PW}}{2\omega_c \cos\theta}.$$

By definition, the mean angular frequency $\bar{\omega}$ (temporally dropping the subscript on ω) and its variance are given by

$$(10.25) \qquad \bar{\omega} = \frac{\int_{-\infty}^{\infty} \omega \Phi(\omega) d\omega}{\int_{-\infty}^{\infty} \Phi(\omega) d\omega}, \qquad \xi^2 = \frac{\int_{-\infty}^{\infty} (\omega - \bar{\omega})^2 \Phi(\omega) d\omega}{\int_{-\infty}^{\infty} \Phi(\omega) d\omega},$$

where $\Phi(\omega)$ the power density spectrum of the noise-free sampled complex signal. Now the Wiener-Khinchin relation [99, pp. 206–207] provides a fundamental link between the time- and frequency-domain properties of complex processes. Specifically, it states that the autocorrelation function $R(\tau)$ and the power density function $\Phi(\omega)$ form a Fourier transform pair. One member of this pair is

$$(10.26) \qquad R(\tau) = \frac{1}{2\pi} \int_{-\infty}^{\infty} \Phi(\omega) e^{j\omega\tau} d\omega.$$

From this it can be seen that $R(0)$ is the average signal power. Differentiating this once and twice with respect to τ gives

$$\dot{R}(\tau) = \frac{\partial R(\tau)}{\partial \tau} = \frac{1}{2\pi} \int_{-\infty}^{\infty} j\omega \Phi(\omega) e^{j\omega\tau} d\omega,$$

$$(10.27)$$

$$\ddot{R}(\tau) = \frac{\partial^2 R(\tau)}{\partial \tau^2} = \frac{-1}{2\pi} \int_{-\infty}^{\infty} \omega^2 \Phi(\omega) e^{j\omega\tau} d\omega.$$

Consequently, setting $\tau = 0$ in (10.26) and (10.27) and substituting these into (10.25) results in

$$(10.28) \qquad \bar{\omega}_{PW} = -j \frac{\dot{R}(0)}{R(0)}, \quad \xi^2 = \left[\frac{\dot{R}(0)}{R(0)}\right]^2 - \frac{\ddot{R}(0)}{R(0)}.$$

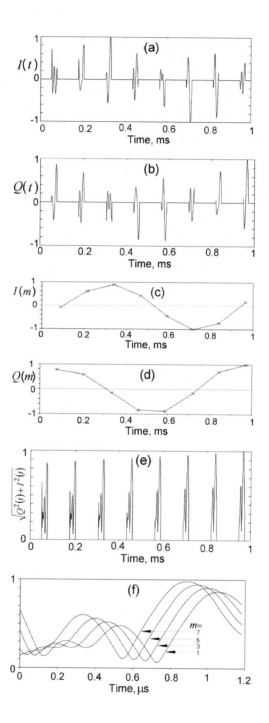

Both equations were derived by Miller and Rochwarger [98]. Because they require reasonably accurate estimates of the zero-lag autocorrelation function and its first and second derivatives, there are considerable difficulties in implementing this technique with discrete data. An alternative approach described by Miller and Rochwarger is to first express the covariance function in polar form, i.e.,

$$(10.29) \qquad R(\tau) = A(\tau)\exp[j\phi(\tau)],$$

where $A(\tau) = |R(\tau)|$ is a real even function and $\phi(\tau)$ is a real odd function of τ. Using this, (10.28) yields

$$\overline{\omega}_{PW} = -j\dot{R}(0)/R(0) = \dot{\phi}(0)$$

Since the velocity of the target can be assumed constant during the interval between two pulses t_{PRI}, the phase derivative is approximately given by

$$(10.30) \qquad \begin{aligned} \overline{\omega}_{PW} &\cong \left\{ \frac{\phi(t_{PRI}) - \phi(0)}{t_{PRI}} \right\} = \frac{\phi(t_{PRI})}{t_{PRI}} \\ &= \frac{1}{t_{PRI}}\arctan\left\{ \frac{\text{Im}[R(t_{PRI})]}{\text{Re}[R(t_{PRI})]} \right\} \equiv \frac{1}{t_{PRI}}\arg R(t_{PRI}). \end{aligned}$$

To determine the variance, according to (10.28) the first and second derivatives of the covariance function must be evaluated for zero lag. The derivatives can then be obtained from (10.29) as

$$\dot{R}(0) = jA(0)\dot{\phi}(0) \qquad \text{and} \qquad \ddot{R}(0) = \ddot{A}(0) - A(0)[\dot{\phi}(0)]^2,$$

where use has been made of the fact that $\dot{A}(0) = 0$ and $\ddot{\phi}(0) = 0$. Consequently, (10.28) for the variance can be written as

$$(10.31) \qquad \zeta^2 = -\frac{\ddot{A}(0)}{A(0)} \approx \frac{2}{t_{PRI}^2}\left[1 - \frac{A(t_{PRI})}{A(0)} \right] = \frac{2}{t_{PRI}^2}\left[1 - \frac{|R(t_{PRI})|}{R(0)} \right],$$

Figure 10.29 Scatterer simulation results to illustrate the properties of the received complex envelope over eight transmission cycles. Following phase-quadrature demodulation, eight successive range-gated portions (1.2-µs duration) of the in-phase $I(t)$ and a quadrature $Q(t)$ signal are shown in (a) and (b), respectively. If these are then integrated over the receive gate duration and sampled, the resulting sample values $[I(m), Q(m)]$ are shown as the crosses in (c) and (d). The magnitude $\sqrt{Q^2(t) + I^2(t)}$ of the range-gated complex envelope is shown in (e). Shown in (f) are the waveforms from $m = 1$ to 7 of the range-gated pulse trains in (e) using a common time axis. With increasing m, the time-shift arises from the movement of the scattering ensemble through the sample volume toward the transducer. In (a), (b), and (e), the time scales of each waveform have been expanded from the true duration to enable the form of each waveform to be seen. For this simulation $t_{PRI} = 0.128\,\text{ms}$ and $f_c = 5.0\,\text{MHz}$ ($\text{BW}_{-3\,\text{dB}} = 2.5\,\text{MHz}$). (Reproduced, with permission, from Vaitkus [57].)

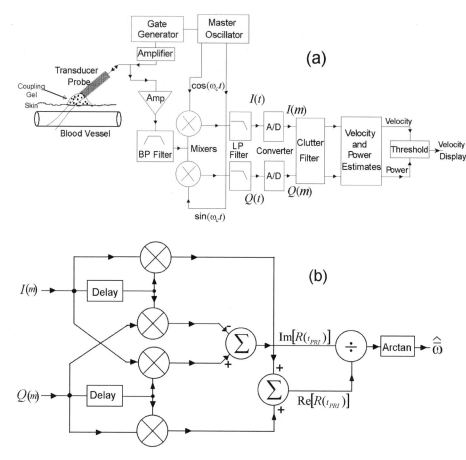

Figure 10.30 Method for estimating and displaying a color flow velocity images. (a) Overall scheme that can be used to estimate and display the velocity corresponding to a given image display pixel. (b) Estimating the mean pulsed-wave angular frequency using the Kasai algorithm. (Based on a similar diagram in Evans and McDicken [24, p. 252].)

in which the approximation made consists of expanding $A(\tau)$ as a series, neglecting third- and higher-order terms, and inserting $\tau = t_{PRI}$.

Equations (10.30) and (10.31) show that the mean angular frequency and the variance of the slow-time signal can be estimated from the magnitudes and phases of the autocorrelation function at lags of 0 and t_{PRI}. Miller and Rochwarger [98] showed that maximum-likelihood estimates can be obtained from successive pairs of samples of the complex received signal, and this is the basis of the practical scheme described below.

Consider the signal processing scheme of Fig. 10.30a in which the RF signal is phase-quadrature demodulated to baseband. After filtering, the analog in-phase and quadrature signals are converted to digital form. Each signal pair gives the flow velocity information for a given segment (see Fig. 10.28), and consequently the signals obtained from the sequence of M firings that make up a packet can be expressed as a complex vector of M elements. To improve the SNR, filtering (e.g., integration over the segment duration) can be used prior to A/D conversion. As discussed in subsection 10.8.2, the high-amplitude, low-frequency clutter caused by vessel wall movement should be removed before estimating the mean flow velocity. Moreover, because the color flow image is usually displayed as a superposition on the corresponding B-mode image, a threshold must be used to determine whether or not the flow information should be written on the corresponding image pixel. One method of achieving this is to use a threshold based on the signal power for each pixel.

The complex signal at a particular range for successive A-lines can be written as $g(m) = I(m) + jQ(m)$, where $I(m)$ and $Q(m)$ are the in-phase and quadrature signal amplitudes for the mth A-line. If M transmissions (the packet size) are used for making the velocity estimate ($M > 1$), then the correlation function estimates (denoted by hats) at lags of 0 and t_{PRI} can be written as

$$\hat{R}(0) = \frac{1}{2(M-1)} \sum_{m=1}^{M-1} |g(m-1)|^2 + |g(m)|^2 \text{ and } \hat{R}(t_{PRI}) = \frac{1}{M-1} \sum_{m=1}^{N-1} g(m)g^*(m-1).$$

When these equations, along with the definitions given above for $g(m)$, are substituted into (10.30) and (10.31), the estimated mean velocity, as given by (10.24), can be expressed as

(10.32)
$$\hat{\bar{v}} = \frac{c_o}{2t_{PRI}\omega_c \cos\theta} \tan^{-1}\left(\sum_{m=1}^{M} Q(m)I(m-1) - Q(m-1)I(m) \middle/ \sum_{m=1}^{M-1} I(m)I(m-1) + Q(m)Q(m-1) \right),$$

and its variance by

(10.33)
$$\hat{\xi}_v^2 = \frac{c_o}{t_{PRI}^2\omega_c \cos\theta}\left[1 - \frac{1}{\hat{\overline{W}}_{1D}}\left\{ \left[\frac{1}{M-1}\sum_{m=1}^{M-1} Q(m)I(m-1) - Q(m-1)I(m) \right]^2 \right.\right.$$
$$\left.\left. + \left[\frac{1}{M-1}\sum_{m=1}^{M-1} I(m)I(m-1) + Q(m-1)Q(m) \right]^2 \right\}^{1/2} \right],$$

where

(10.34)
$$\hat{\overline{W}}_{1D} = \frac{1}{M-1} \sum_{m=0}^{M-1} Q^2(m) + I^2(m)$$

is the estimated average power. Thus, the velocity can be estimated from successive sample pairs obtained at the same depth. It should be noted that the Kasai estimation scheme illustrated in Fig. 10.30b corresponds to (10.32) and that the power estimate used in the thresholding scheme of Fig. 10.30a makes use of (10.34). Although the variance can be reduced by increasing the packet size, as noted earlier, movement of the scatterers through the sample volume causes the signal from within this volume to become decorrelated. Moreover, for a given measurement depth, increasing M causes the number of lines per frame and/or the frame rate to be decreased.

The range over which the velocity can be unambiguously determined depends on the algorithm used for the arctan operation in (10.32). By preserving the signs of both the numerator and denominator in the argument, a four-quadrant arctan algorithm achieves a range from $-\pi$ to $+\pi$. Consequently, by replacing the arctan function by these limit values, the unambiguous velocity range is given by

$$(10.35) \qquad\qquad v_{\max} = \pm \frac{c_o f_{PRF}}{4 f_c \cos\theta},$$

which is identical to (10.3). The latter was derived by using the Nyquist sampling criterion for unambiguously determining the slow-time demodulated center frequency.

An important advantage of the autocorrelation approach is the absence of any bias, even under poor SNR conditions. Sirmans and Bumgarner [22] compared the autocorrelation method to an FFT technique in which the noise spectrum is subtracted from the signal spectrum. They showed that at very low SNR conditions the variance of the autocorrelation method is superior, while for other SNR conditions it is equal. Moreover, they found the influence of noise on the variance to be negligible for SNRs of greater than 15 dB.

An alternative method for obtaining an expression for the instantaneous frequency estimate can be obtained by first noting that the instantaneous frequency is the derivative of the phase. Between the mth and $m - 1$ transmissions, it is given by

$$\omega_{m,PW} = \frac{\partial \phi_m}{\partial t} \approx \frac{\phi_m - \phi_{m-1}}{t_{PRI}}$$

$$= \frac{1}{t_{PRI}} \{ \tan^{-1}[Q(m)/I(m)] - \tan^{-1}[Q(m-1)/I(m-1)] \},$$

as proposed by Grandchamp [65] and used by Brandestini [66] in a multigate pulsed system. By combining the two arctan functions, Barber et al. [100] pointed out that the above expression can be written as

$$\omega_{m,PW} = \frac{1}{t_{PRI}} \tan^{-1}\left[\frac{Q(m)I(m-1) - Q(m-1)I(m)}{I(m)I(m-1) + Q(m)Q(m-1)} \right],$$

which has the same form as a single component of (10.32). This derivation clearly shows that the autocorrelation method is based on measuring the phase-shift information from a multiplicity of sampled data pairs.

10.8.1 Effects of Frequency-Dependent Attenuation and Scattering

As shown in Chapter 1, frequency-dependent attenuation causes a reduction in the center frequency of a wideband signal, whereas the opposite is true for frequency-dependent scattering. For Doppler (CW) ultrasound under linear propagation conditions, neither the narrowband transmitted signal nor the scattered signal will be affected. However, for pulsed wave ultrasound flow measurement systems, the influence of frequency-dependent processes on the bias and variance of estimation methods needs to be considered. Newhouse et al. [1] considered their influence on a pulsed random and pseudo-random blood flowmeter system. Subsequent work by others [101,102] has confirmed that depth-dependent errors in the mean velocity estimate can occur with certain methods. Assuming a circular transducer operating in the far field, Ferrara et al. [102] conducted a theoretical investigation of four estimation techniques. They concluded that of the three estimation categories (see subsection 10.2.1), frequency/phase methods can give rise to significant depth-dependent errors, whereas time-domain and multiple burst (tracking) methods do not. In addition to the influence of frequency-dependent scattering and attenuation, the effect of dispersion, which accompanies attenuation as a consequence of the Kramers-Knonig relations (see subsection 3.10.1), should be considered. In their examination of the influence of all three phenomena, Fish and Cope [103] pointed out that dispersion should not cause a change in the pulse energy spectrum. However, because it changes the phase relations between various frequency components, it can affect the pulse shape, and this could be significant for very small sample volumes.

In time-domain correlation methods, cross-correlations are made between successive received signal segments to estimate the time delay, which is then used in (10.19) to calculate the velocity. Because the transmit/receive paths lengths are almost the same for the two transmissions, shifts in the spectrum will affect the two received signals in a virtually identical manner, causing essentially no error. However, for phase/frequency estimation methods, an error can arise from frequency-dependent attenuation in combination with frequency-dependent scattering. In the analysis given below, we shall consider just the effects of attenuation when α is proportional to frequency ($n = 1$) and the transmitted pulse is a Gaussian modulated sinusoid.

In Chapter 1 it was shown {see (1.126)} that when transmitted signal has a Gaussian envelope and that propagation is in a medium whose attenuation increases in proportional to the frequency, the two-way change in frequency due to a frequency-independent scatterer at a depth z can be expressed as $\Delta f_c = -\alpha_o z (2.66 BW f_c)^2/(4\pi^2)$. In this, $BW = \sigma_\omega/(2.66 f_c)$ is the –6-dB fractional bandwidth. Now in section 10.2 it was shown that the slow-time center frequency for a single scatterer is scaled by a factor of $2v\cos\theta/c_o$. Consequently, center-frequency error is given by (10.2), i.e., $\Delta f_{PW} = 2\Delta f_c v \cos\theta/c_o$. It follows that the fractional error in the estimated velocity is given by

$$(10.36) \qquad \frac{\Delta \bar{v}}{\bar{v}} = \frac{\Delta f_c}{f_c} = -\alpha_o \frac{z}{4\pi^2} f_c (2.66 BW)^2 .$$

In other words it is proportional to the depth and the square of the bandwidth. For the case $\alpha_o = 0.5\,\text{dB/(cm·MHz)}$, $f_c = 5.0\,\text{MHz}$, and a variety of fractional bandwidths, it can be seen from Fig. 10.31 that the fractional error can be relatively large for wideband signals.

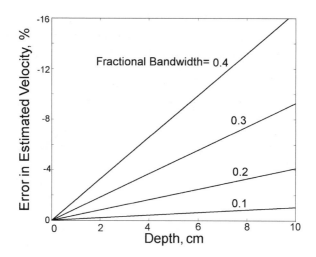

Figure 10.31 Fractional velocity estimation error caused by frequency-dependent attenuation when $n = 1$. The two-way error was calculated from (10.36) assuming a Gaussian-shaped transmit pulse. Note that z is the depth of the scatterer, so that the two-way distance is $2z$.

The assumption of a Gaussian shape, as used in the above calculation, is unlikely to be valid for the pulses generally used in narrowband frequency/phase estimation methods. Typically, they may contain from 8 to 20 cycles with tapered edges. For the nine-cycle sine-tapered pulse illustrated in Fig. 10.32, it can be seen that the velocity estimation error $(100\Delta\bar{v}/\bar{v})$ increases linearly with depth and is less than 0.7% for depths of up to 10 cm. If the effects of frequency-dependent scattering had been included, it would have been even less. Such small estimation errors are generally considered negligible in relation to other uncertainties.

For a Gaussian transmit envelope, Evans and McDicken [24, pp. 174–178] have examined the combined frequency-dependent effects as the effective number of cycles in the transmitted pulse is varied. They point out that for narrowband frequency/phase methods, the estimated velocity error is small, though if needed a depth-dependent correction can be applied.

10.8.2 Clutter Rejection Techniques

The presence of very-high-amplitude signals from the vessel wall and surrounding quasi-stationary tissue presents major difficulties in trying to estimate the flow close to the vessel wall. These clutter signals are typically 40 to 60 dB higher than that from blood. Though, because they are produced by stationary or relatively slowly moving structures, their spectrum is typically well below 1 kHz. The problem of removing their influence without introducing bias in the blood velocity estimates is a major challenge, especially since the blood flow velocity approaches zero at the vessel wall. Even when the sample

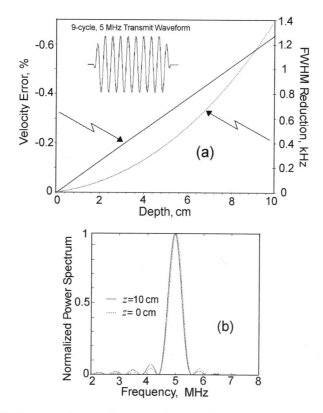

Figure 10.32 Two-way changes that occur due to a frequency-dependent attenuation of 0.5 dB/(cm.MHz). It was assumed that the transmit signal was a narrowband (13% bandwidth), nine-cycle, sine-tapered pulse with a center frequency of 5 MHz. (a) Velocity estimation error and FWHM reduction. (b) Power spectral density, showing the changes that occur when the transmitted signal is backscattered at a distance of 10 cm from the source.

volume is well away from tissue, the beam side lobes may produce significant clutter.

Many of the high-pass filter schemes initially examined were those developed for Doppler radar, where a similar problem of extracting the signal from a background of low-frequency clutter exists. A major difficulty with the choice and design of an effective filtering scheme arises from the transient nature of the digital signals to be filtered. A reasonable frame rate with adequate spatial resolution over a given area can be achieved only by limiting the number of packets sent in each direction (typically from 5 to 16). Because of the transient nature of this signal, a filter with a poor transient response can introduce serious bias and variance in the velocity estimate. On the other hand, a filter with a fast response is likely to have unsatisfactory roll-off characteristics. Many of these issues have been reviewed in Evans and McDicken [24, pp. 246–250] and in Bjaerum et al. [104].

Papers that initially addressed the problem of optimizing the design primarily considered FIR (finite impulse response) and IIR (infinite impulse response) filters [105–107]. Filters of the FIR class are non-recursive, in that the current output is derived from the current and past inputs and their non-zero response to an impulse is finite [108]. On the other hand, an IIR filter is recursive in that the output is derived from the present and past inputs and outputs. Because of its feedback nature, its response to an impulse can be infinite. However, associated with this is a relatively poor transient response that can cause serious bias to the estimated mean frequency. To minimize transient effects, various schemes have been investigated for providing appropriate initial conditions for the filter; these include step, zero, projection, exponential, and zero initialization schemes. Their purpose is to compensate for the fact that there is no prior input and no output when the first input arrives.

A different class of clutter filter, first investigated by Hoeks et al. [106] and subsequently by Kadi and Loupas [109], are regression filters. In these, the clutter signal component is fitted to a polynomial by performing a least-squares analysis. Once this has been achieved, the clutter signal is then subtracted from the total signal, leaving the blood flow signal and higher-frequency noise. A further class of this filter is based on methods that can adapt to the characteristics of the received signal [110,111]. In one such form, the clutter mean frequency over a packet is first estimated, and then, using this frequency as the reference, the entire signal is downshifted so that the clutter spectrum is centered around zero. A high-pass filter with a narrow stop-band can then be used, enabling significantly lower blood flow velocities to be estimated. Alternatively, the average clutter signal can be subtracted from each firing and the flow velocity estimated from the residual.

10.9 Two-Dimensional Methods

In the previous discussion of the color flow system shown in Fig. 10.30a, it was noted that one method for obtaining a pair of digital I and Q values from a given segment is to integrate the analog in-phase and quadrature signals over the segment duration. For a given packet size the information for this segment can be stored as a complex vector whose elements form a 1-D set. In the Kasai method, an autocorrelation approach is used to process this vector, enabling the velocity estimate to be obtained. The integration process reduces the noise and at the same time averages out the received signal. For a narrowband transmitted pulse there should be no loss of information. However, for wideband transmission it can be argued that information is lost. In 1988, Mayo and Embree [112] proposed a method for velocity estimation based on using all the information available over a segment duration rather than basing it on a single value.[12] Independent work by Wilson [114], published in 1991, described a similar approach.

---

12. It is perhaps of interest to note that in a patent applied for in 1987, Kim [113] described a method for velocity estimation based on making better use of the available information. Arguably, it can be regarded as a 2-D approach.

RF Signal

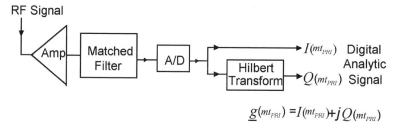

$$\underline{g}(mt_{PRI}) = I(mt_{PRI}) + j\,Q(mt_{PRI})$$

Figure 10.33 Digital signal processing scheme for color flow imaging. The quadrature-sampling scheme illustrated in Fig. 10.9b could also have been used.

To describe the above technique it is helpful to consider the front-end structure shown in Fig. 10.33 and the received RF signal segments between the depths of z_0 and z_{N-1} for the packet shown in Fig. 10.34. If each signal in the segment is sampled N times and there are M signals in a packet, there will be a total of $M \times N$ sample values. Moreover, for an analytic signal whose real and imaginary components are denoted by I and Q, each matrix element can be denoted by $g(m,n) = I(m,n) + jQ(m,n)$, where the first index (m) indicates the row number and the second (n) the column number. This complex matrix can be written as

$$(10.37) \qquad \underline{\mathbf{G}} = \begin{bmatrix} \underline{g}(0,0) & \underline{g}(0,2) & \cdots & \underline{g}(0,N-1) \\ \underline{g}(1,1) & \underline{g}(1,2) & \cdots & \underline{g}(1,N-1) \\ \vdots & \vdots & \ddots & \vdots \\ \underline{g}(M-1,1) & \underline{g}(M-1,2) & \cdots & \underline{g}(M-1,N-1) \end{bmatrix}.$$

A single column of this matrix is a *snapshot* of the analytic signal at a specific time with respect to the start of each gate segment and can be written as

$$\mathbf{g}(n) = \left[\underline{g}(0,n), \underline{g}(1,n), \ldots \underline{g}(M-1,n) \right]^{T}.$$

Thus, $\underline{\mathbf{G}}$ is a complex snapshot matrix that contains all the sample values within the segment for the entire packet. On the other hand, a row vector gives the sample values on a particular received waveform segment. By integrating along all the rows, a single column vector is produced, one element of which is given by

$$\mathbf{g}(m) = \sum_{n=0}^{N-1} \underline{g}(m,n) = \sum_{n=0}^{N-1} I(m,n) + jQ(m,n).$$

As described in section 10.8, the elements of this vector were used for the 1-D autocorrelation velocity estimator.

As pointed out in [116], the number of statistically independent snapshot vectors in the matrix $\underline{\mathbf{G}}$ is determined by the spatial time-bandwidth product of the portion of the backscattered echo from the segment. This product can be thought of as an indication of the "richness" of information contained in

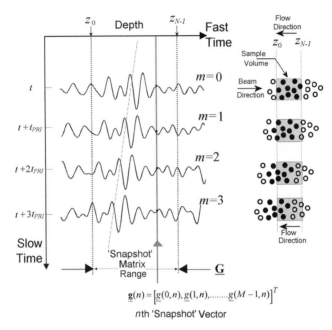

$$\underline{\mathbf{g}}(n) = \left[\underline{g}(0,n), \underline{g}(1,n), \ldots \underline{g}(M-1,n)\right]^{T}$$

nth 'Snapshot' Vector

Figure 10.34 Relationship between backscattered echoes and the 2-D Doppler signal snapshot matrix. By stacking portions of successive RF backscattered echoes, a matrix **G** of column vectors is obtained. Each column corresponds to samples of the RF signal taken at the same time (with respect to the sample gate) from each received signal of the packet. A packet containing four realizations is illustrated. Note that it is actually the complex (analytic) form of the echo signal that corresponds to each matrix element, yielding a complex matrix **G**. (Reproduced, with permission from Vaitkus and Cobbold [116], *IEEE Trans. Ultrason. Ferroelec. Freq. Contr.*, 45, 939–954, ©1998 IEEE 1998.)

the signal. It can be compared with the number of realizations or independent samples needed to estimate the probability density function of a stochastic process. The spatial time-bandwidth product or "effective" number of independent snapshot vectors over the segment is given by $N_{eff} = N\Delta f/f_s$, where f_s is the sampling frequency and Δf is the RF echo bandwidth. The estimation variance is inversely related to N_{eff}. For example, if $B = 2.5\,\mathrm{MHz}$, $f_S = 50\,\mathrm{MHz}$, and the receive gate window is $1.2\,\mu s$, there will be 60 vectors in total, but the number of statistically independent vectors will be only three.

10.9.1 Discrete Fourier Transform Methods

By taking the 2-D Fourier transform of the discrete data contained in the matrix **G**, Mayo and Embree [112] showed how a velocity estimate could be extracted in a very straightforward manner. The discrete Fourier transform of such an array yields an array of values that, depending on the sampling rate and scatterer velocity, can exhibit aliasing. To provide a simplified explanation, the approach given by Wilson [114] allows these complications to be avoided. He assumed that the returned signal $g(z,\tau)$ was real, continuous, and infinite with respect to fast and slow time. Consequently, this 2-D function can be expressed as a 1-D function $g_o(z)$ that moves along the z-axis with a velocity of $v_\varepsilon = 2v\cos\theta/c_o$, i.e., $g(z,\tau) = g_o(z + v_\varepsilon\tau)$. From Appendix B, the 2-D Fourier transform can be written as

$$\Im\{g(z,\tau)\} = G(k_z, k_\tau) = \iint\limits_{-\infty}^{\infty} g_o(z + v_\varepsilon\tau)e^{-j(k_z z + k_\tau \tau)}dz\,d\tau.$$

Denoting the Fourier transform of $g_o(z)$ by $G_o(k_z)$ and using the shifting property of the Fourier transform, this simplifies to

(10.38) $\Im\{g(z,\tau)\} = G_o(k_z)\displaystyle\int\limits_{-\infty}^{\infty} e^{jk_z v_\varepsilon \tau}e^{-jk_\tau \tau}d\tau = 2\pi G_o(k_z)\delta(k_z v_\varepsilon - k_\tau).$

A sketch of this function is shown in Fig. 10.35a, where the horizontal and vertical axes correspond to frequencies of slow time and fast time, respectively. It can be seen that the 2-D Fourier transform of the continuous data in the packet is zero everywhere except on the straight line through the origin. The slope, which can be expressed as $\hat{v}_\varepsilon = \hat{f}_{PW}/f_c = \tan\hat{\varphi}$, enables the scatterer velocity to be estimated from

(10.39) $$\hat{v} = \frac{c_o\hat{f}_{PW}}{2f_c\cos\theta} = \frac{c_o\tan\hat{\varphi}}{2\cos\theta}$$

Mayo and Embree [112] proposed that φ could be estimated by performing line integrals (projections) along radial lines from the origin and searching for the angle that yields a maximum. For an analytic signal, the elements in **G** are complex and its discrete 2-D Fourier transform consist of a 2-D array of points on a rectangular grid. Because the radial lines do not generally intersect these points, interpolation is needed to perform the line integrals.

A spectrum of frequencies in the transmitted pulse, along with the finite number of transmissions and decorrelation, results in a spread on the frequency plane. This can be seen in Fig. 10.36, which illustrates the 2-D transform for 16 A-lines obtained for wideband transmitted pulse [117]. The spread is also represented by the contours in the aliased 2-D transform of Fig. 10.35.

Frequency-dependent effects such as attenuation, scattering, the transducer bandwidth, and nonlinear propagation, cause the received signal center frequency to change from that transmitted. Moreover, the stochastic nature of the signal produces fluctuations in the estimated center frequency. From Fig. 10.35a, it is clear that the location where the power is a maximum enables the center frequency of the received pulse to be estimated. If f_c in (10.39) is replaced by this estimated center frequency, the accuracy with which the scatterer velocity can be estimated should be improved. Loupas and Gill [118] have proposed that the information available from the full range of frequencies present in the transmitted bandwidth can be used by taking slices through

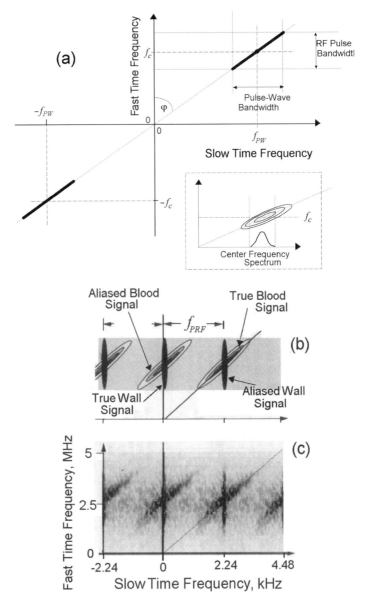

Figure 10.35 Sketches illustrating the 2-D Fourier transform of the matrix **G**. The slope of the line corresponding to the maximum value of the line integral gives the velocity estimate. (a) Simplified sketch showing the transform to the frequency plane for a continuous signal of infinite duration (see text). The insert shows the contours and the spectrum corresponding to a 1-D slice. Panel (b) provides an interpretation of the aliased signal in (c). Panel (c) is the 2-D spectrum of the signal from a normal human artery when the mean slow-time frequency is equal to f_{PRF}. Because a high-pass filter was not used, the wall movement spectrum and its aliased components were retained. The effects of aliasing on both spectra are evident. (Reprinted by permission of Elsevier from Torp and Kristoffersen [115], *Ultrasound Med. Biol.*, 21, 937–944, ©1995 World Federation of Ultrasound in Medicine and Biology.)

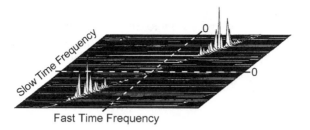

Figure 10.36 2-D Fourier transform of simulation data consisting of 16 A-lines created by a wideband transmitted pulse. (Reproduced, with permission, from Jones [117], *Critical Reviews in Biomed. Eng.*, 21, 399–483, ©1993 CRC Press.)

the 2-D transform parallel to the slow-frequency axis. Each slice would then give the spectrum corresponding to a particular RF frequency, as illustrated by the insert of Fig. 10.35a. The information obtained in this way should provide a reduction in the velocity variance. Either direct sampling of the analytic RF signal or quadrature demodulation and processing of the I and Q signals (Fig. 10.30a) can be used. In the latter case, the RF frequency spectrum is translated about zero.

Several authors have addressed the relation between the 1-D and 2-D approach. As noted earlier, for the 1-D method, integration is performed along the rows of the complex matrix $\mathbf{G}$. According to the projection-slice theorem (see subsection 8.7.1), the vector that results from a projection (integral) along each row of $\mathbf{G}$ corresponds to a slice through the Fourier transform plane. For the demodulated signal, this corresponds to a slice along the slow-frequency axis.

10.9.2 Two-Dimensional Autocorrelation Methods

One problem that arises from using the 2-D discrete Fourier transform on data derived from stochastic signals concerns the issue of stability. In 1995, Loupas et al. [119] proposed a new approach based on 2-D autocorrelation. Although prior proposals exist for 2-D autocorrelation methods [120,121], the method developed by Loupas et al. enabled the mean received RF frequency for each row of data within the segment to be estimated. Because of the stochastic nature of the signal, variations of this estimate should be matched by the corresponding variations of the mean slow-wave frequency estimate. Since the velocity estimate is proportional to the ratio of these two mean frequency estimates, the variance of the velocity estimate should be reduced.

A useful starting point for obtaining an expression for the estimated velocity is to proceed in an analogous manner to that used for the 1-D autocorrelation and to follow the analysis given by Loupas et al. [119]. We shall assume that the $M \times N$ matrix $\mathbf{G}$ is a snapshot of a zero-mean multivariate stationary Gaussian process. First, it is necessary to write down expressions for the mean RF and the mean slow-wave angular frequencies in terms of the 2-D power density spectrum {see (10.25)}. These will be denoted by $\bar{\omega}_{RF}$ and $\bar{\omega}_{pw}$, respectively. Now the 2-D autocorrelation and the 2-D spectrum form a 2-D Fourier transform pair. This enables the two mean frequencies to be written in terms of the autocorrelation function and a derivative. The sampling period along the rows is denoted by t_S and that for the columns corresponds to the PRI (i.e., t_{PRI}). In a similar manner to the method used in obtaining (10.28), Loupas et al. have shown that the estimated mean pulsed wave and RF angular frequencies are given by

$$(10.40) \quad \widehat{\bar{\omega}}_{pw} = -j\frac{\left[\partial\hat{\underline{R}}(m',n')/\partial m'\right]_{m'=n'=0}}{t_{PRI}\,\hat{\underline{R}}(0,0)} \,, \quad \widehat{\bar{\omega}}_{RF} = -j\frac{\left[\partial\hat{\underline{R}}(m',n')/\partial n'\right]_{m'=n'=0}}{t_S\,\hat{\underline{R}}(0,0)} \,,$$

where $\hat{\underline{R}}(m',n')$ denotes the 2-D discrete autocorrelation function of the elements in $\mathbf{G}$ at lags of m' and n'.

Following the same procedure used for the 1-D derivation and making use of the properties of $\mathbf{G}$, expressions for the mean scatterer velocity can be obtained. By expressing the autocorrelation function in polar form, it can be shown that both expressions in (10.40) can be written in terms of a partial derivative of the phase angle. For the smallest available lag the ratio of the two angular frequencies can be obtained, enabling the estimated mean scatterer velocity to be expressed as

$$
\hat{\bar{v}} = \frac{c_o}{2\cos\theta}\frac{\widehat{\bar{\omega}}_{PW}}{\widehat{\bar{\omega}}_{RF}} \approx \frac{c_o}{2\cos\theta}\frac{t_S}{t_{PRI}}\arctan\left\{\frac{\mathrm{Im}\left[\hat{\underline{R}}_a(t_{PRI},0)\right]}{\mathrm{Re}\left[\hat{\underline{R}}_a(t_{PRI},0)\right]}\right\}\Bigg/
$$

$$(10.41) \qquad \arctan\left\{\frac{\mathrm{Im}\left[\hat{\underline{R}}_a(0,t_S)\right]}{\mathrm{Re}\left[\hat{\underline{R}}_a(0,t_S)\right]}\right\},$$

where $\hat{\underline{R}}_a(\tau,\mathcal{R})$ is the autocorrelation function of the analytic signal for time and radial lags of τ and $\mathcal{R}$, respectively.

Loupas et al. [119] also applied the 2-D autocorrelation method for a phase-quadrature demodulated signal. If the reference angular frequency is denoted by ω_{Ref}, then the mean velocity estimate is given by

$$
\hat{\bar{v}} = \frac{c_o}{2\cos\theta}\frac{\widehat{\bar{\omega}}_{PW}}{\widehat{\bar{\omega}}_{RF}} \approx \frac{c_o}{2\cos\theta}\frac{t_S}{t_{PRI}}\arctan\left\{\frac{\mathrm{Im}\left[\hat{R}_d(t_{PRI},0)\right]}{\mathrm{Re}\left[\hat{R}_d(t_{PRI},0)\right]}\right\}\Bigg/
$$

$$(10.42) \qquad \left\{t_S\omega_{Ref}+\arctan\left\{\frac{\mathrm{Im}\left[\hat{R}_d(0,t_S)\right]}{\mathrm{Re}\left[\hat{R}_d(0,t_S)\right]}\right\}\right\},$$

where $\hat{R}_a(\tau,\mathcal{R})$ is the autocorrelation function of the demodulated complex signal.

In both of the above expressions, the real and imaginary components of the autocorrelation function can be written in terms of the real and imaginary components of the elements of $\mathbf{G}$, similar to that for (10.32). Evans and McDicken (10.24, Chapters 8 and 11), in their comprehensive review of color flow imaging methods, point out that when the change in center frequency is not accounted for, (10.41) is equivalent to that used by Hoeks et al. [120] and Torp et al. [121].

In an experimental evaluation reported by Loupas et al. [122], the results of the 2-D method were compared to those obtained with the 1-D autocorrelation technique. They also examined the effect of including the frequency correction and showed that, depending on the incident angle, the two velocity estimates were quite closely correlated. In comparison with the 1-D method, they found that the 2-D estimation method gave consistently better velocity and power estimates. Power estimates, which can be calculated from the zero-lag autocorrelation coefficients, were also compared. For the 1-D case it is given by (10.34) and for 2-D case by

$$\hat{\overline{W}}_{2D} = \frac{1}{N-1} \sum_{m=0}^{M-1} \sum_{n=0}^{N-1} Q^2(m,n) + I^2(m,n).$$

As with the velocity estimate, the 2-D power estimate showed significant improvements over the 1-D estimate.

10.9.3 Target Tracking Techniques

Movement of the scatterers between successive transmissions causes changes in the received signal. Methods based on finding the best match between a model of these changes and the actual received signals have been called tracking methods. If the scatterers can be assumed to move with a constant flow velocity over the packet duration, a relatively straightforward model can be used. The velocity can then be estimated by finding the velocity that provides a best match between the received signals and the model. In fact, as pointed out by Alam and Parker [29], the 2-D Fourier transform method described in subsection 10.9.1 can be considered as a tracking method since it involves a search for the 2-D transform of the signal that best matches the true trajectory. A more direct tracking approach is the scheme originally proposed by Ferrara and Algazi [123] in 1989 and subsequently detailed in their journal publications [124,125]. It uses a model of the range-gated complex envelope of the backscattered signal to produce a mean velocity estimate. By searching over all possible trajectories, the maximum likelihood velocity is found from the trajectory that produces a best match. It is a matched filter approach, and consequently its performance depends on accurate prior knowledge of the signal model.

Tracking approaches that make direct use of the 2-D slow/fast time waveforms have been described by Torp and Kristoffersen [115] as well as by Alam and Parker [126]. Torp and Kristoffersen showed that if the power is summed along a line that matches the scatterer velocity, a peak in the spectrum should occur at a value corresponding to the scatterer velocity. This is illustrated in Fig. 10.37, in which 13 successive RF signals are shown for a scatterer moving away from the transducer. They showed that this spectral estimation method is equivalent to integrating the 2-D spectrum along lines of differing slope that pass though the origin. Evans and McDicken [24] have pointed out that the

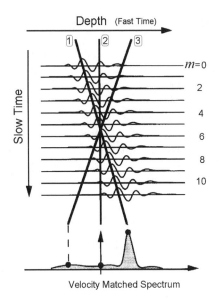

Figure 10.37 The method described by Torp and Kristoffersen [115] in which a matrix of values was obtained for a scatterer moving with a uniform velocity. The power is estimated along line ① by summing the values. Because the slope matches the scatterer velocity, the power will be a maximum. The power estimated along other lines, such as ② and ③, yields much smaller values. (Reprinted by permission of Elsevier from Torp and Kristoffersen [115], *Ultrasound Med. Biol.*, 21, 937–944, ©1995 World Federation of Ultrasound in Medicine and Biology.)

method is also equivalent to the method proposed by Loupas and Gill [118]. The "butterfly search" technique developed by Alam and Parker is similar to the above in that the power associated with each possible slow/fast time trajectory is estimated. Other estimation techniques, based on the radar method for determining the direction of arrival of an incoming signal to a passive array, have also been proposed and evaluated [57,116,127,128]. It can be seen that the dashed line in Fig. 10.34 has the appearance of a 2-D wavefront whose direction can be characterized by the wavenumber vector **k**. It is evident that the wavefront direction is directly related to the velocity. Vaitkus et al. [128] have investigated the performance of a root-MUSIC (MUltiple SIgnal Classification) algorithm to estimate the direction of **k** for both simulated and in vivo ultrasound signals under different SNR conditions.

The 2-D approach to velocity estimation provides a number of opportunities for resolving the ambiguity problem when the maximum velocity is beyond the Nyquist limit. Wilson [114], in his 1991 paper, proposed a scheme to enable the spectrum to be displayed without contamination by aliasing artifacts. For pulsatile arterial blood flow containing velocities well beyond the Nyquist limit, Torp and Kristoffersen [115] demonstrated that their technique, as illustrated in Fig. 10.37, enables major improvements to be made in the quality of the gray-scale spectral display.

Table 10.1. Color Flow Display and Estimation Techniques

Technique	Typical Display Method	Method
Color Flow Imaging	Red and blue hues used to indicate the forward and reverse velocities. Display is superimposed on a gray-scale B-mode image.	The mean velocity component is estimated from successive A-mode transmissions over an area.
Color Power Flow Imaging	Color Power Image in which the hue indicates power without regard to direction. Shades of orange are often used. It may be superimposed on a gray-scale B-mode image.	Total backscattered power above a certain threshold is estimated from both forward and reverse flow and the sum is displayed in color.
Directional Color Power Flow Imaging	Same as for *color power flow imaging* except that two colors are used whose hue indicate the power in the forward and reverse directions.	Same as above, but with power of both flow components estimated and displayed using separate colors.
Harmonic Flow Imaging	Velocity is encoded in color and displayed on a gray-scale B-mode background.	Nonlinear oscillations of contrast agent microbubbles generate second harmonic signal. Velocity distribution is displayed.
Harmonic Power Flow Imaging	The second harmonic power produced by a contrast agent or by tissue is estimated and displayed in color.	Same as above, but the harmonic power is estimated and displayed using a single color hue.
Color M-Mode Flow Imaging	The *velocity* or *power* is encoded in color and displayed as a depth versus time 2-D color-encoded image.	Multiple transmissions along a single path are used and the velocity or power is estimated. Their variation with depth and time is displayed.
Color Tissue Imaging and Color M-Mode Tissue Imaging	Same as for *color flow imaging* or *color M-mode flow imaging*, but the blood flow velocity signals are suppressed. The tissue *velocity* or *power* is encoded in color and displayed.	To suppress blood flow signals, either a low-pass filter can be used or the gain threshold can be increased. The clutter filter cutoff is lowered to enable tissue velocity or power to be displayed.

10.10 Enhanced Flow Imaging Methods

A variety of techniques has been developed to improve the flow image quality, to enhance the sensitivity to small flow rates and for real-time imaging of soft tissue velocity distributions. Some of these make use of contrast agents that were previously discussed in relation to linear and nonlinear B-mode imaging (see subsection 8.6.1). Table 10.1 provides a summary of the primary techniques, details of which are provided in the following subsections.

10.10.1 Color Flow Imaging: Frame Rate Considerations

Up to this point in the current section our discusion has focused on conventional color flow imaging. However, some aspects relating to the frame rate were not considered, and these are especially important when the imaged volume undergoes rapid changes, as in cardiac flow imaging. The area to be imaged, the spatial and velocity resolution needed, and the maximum acceleration of the blood or tissue all relate directly to the minimum frame rate needed. Furthermore, an appropriate strategy must be used for acquiring both color flow and structural B-mode images. As noted earlier, color flow images require a significant number (packet size) of transmissions (5–15) for each line of information, and the choice is directly related to the SNR. Consequently, it may not be possible to obtain a sufficiently high-quality color flow map in real time over the region seen with B-mode. Moreover, the mapped area may also be limited by transducer geometric considerations. While it is possible to achieve B-mode frame frequencies of over 100 Hz and flow imaging frequencies exceeding 40 Hz, if a superimposed display of both images is needed, considerably lower rates may have to be used, though there will likely be some loss in spatial and temporal resolution.

10.10.2 Power Flow Imaging

Estimating the average flow velocity for each sample volume is particularly challenging when the flow is small and the vessels are at a considerable distance from the transducer. Even if a vessel is relatively straight, the presence of noise can result in a color-encoded velocity image with a somewhat mottled appearance. Moreover, obtaining color flow images of structures that contain networks of smaller vessels can be quite confusing due to the variety of angles they make to the beam direction. The priority encoding software used to determine whether the velocity or the B-mode signal for a pixel should be displayed can also contribute to border jaggedness. As described below, many of these problems can be overcome by using *color power flow imaging* (also called *color power angiography*). However, quantitative information on the flow velocity and its variations is forfeited and flow changes that occur over a cardiac cycle may be lost. Thus, color power flow imaging gives primary emphasis to detecting the presence or absence of flow with the best sensitivity and resolution.

Shortly after the introduction of color flow imaging,[13] it was recognized that certain qualitative advantages over conventional color velocity imaging could be achieved when the total backscattered power in each volume segment was encoded and displayed. This information can be readily obtained from the zero-lag autocorrelation function as shown by (10.26). In a key paper

---

13. It seems that several early commercial color flow imaging systems incorporated a power mode. For example, the Toshiba and Diasonics systems both incorporated this feature. An earlier description is the 1989 book chapter by Moore [129].

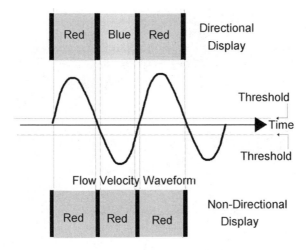

Figure 10.38 Color power flow imaging scheme. Simplified binary display method in which the backscattered power in the forward and reverse flow directions is each encoded in fixed colors—e.g., red and blue for directional, red for nondirectional. The use of a clutter filter has been assumed such that when the power falls below a certain level, the corresponding flow cycle regions are encoded in black. Many cycles can be averaged to enhance the sensitivity.

published in 1994, using machines that incorporated modified signal processing, Rubin et al. [130] provided convincing evidence of the potential advantages of power mode display, and this revitalized interest in its use. They demonstrated that highly tortuous vessels and complex vascular networks, such as those in the kidney, could be more readily identified and that the presence of much smaller vessels could be detected.

The advantages of power flow imaging are a combination of several factors. First, as noted in Chapter 5, provided that turbulence and the effects of aggregation can be ignored, the backscattered power from blood is essentially independent of the flow conditions. Second, the backscattered power is independent of the beam-to-flow angle. Third, with conventional color flow imaging the stochastic nature of the backscattered signal causes fluctuations in the color pattern, while in the power mode, using a display with a single color, such fluctuations are far less evident. Finally, because the background noise spectrum for each segment volume is also integrated along with the flow spectrum, the SNR is improved, thereby improving the sensitivity.

Because directional information is not displayed, aliasing effects are no longer seen, enabling the PRF to be reduced. This allows much smaller flow velocities to be measured. Moreover, because no attempt is made to display pulsatile flow variation, the signal can be averaged over many cardiac cycles, thereby greatly improving the sensitivity.

As illustrated in Fig. 10.38, if the flow velocity is greater than the threshold set by the clutter filter, the power mode image will consist of a constant inten-

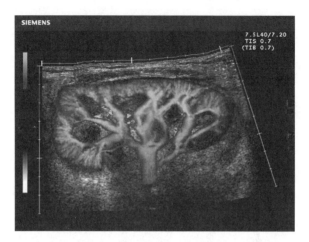

Figure 10.39 Nondirectional power flow image of a kidney. The hue and brightness of the colors indicate the relative power. Note that close to the vessel walls, where the segment volume is only partially in the vessel, the power falls and, in this region, the power scale merges from orange to purple through to black. (Courtesy Siemens Ultrasound.) See color insert.

sity region. At the edge of the vessel, where the segment volume partially intersects the flow region, the power is diminished and, when a continuous range of colors are used, the vessel edge has a smoother appearance compared to the conventional color velocity flow image. An example is shown in Fig. 10.39.

A significant problem that is particularly troublesome for power flow imaging of deep rapidly moving structures is the "flash" artifact that appears as a transient flash in certain regions of the display. It arises from the tissue motion that occurs between successive transmissions, resulting in a failure to achieve proper cancellation of the large tissue signal. As subsequently noted, the use of harmonic contrast flow imaging largely avoids this.

10.10.3 Tissue Imaging

The development of methods for imaging tissue movement in real time based on the flow estimation methods described in this chapter is of particular potential significance in the assessment of impaired myocardial function. Other techniques for imaging tissue movement based on speckle tracking (see section 8.8) and contrast agent perfusion studies (see subsection 8.6.1) have already been discussed. However, one method that makes use of many standard flow imaging techniques is of considerable potential importance. It is based on the realization that the tissue signal, normally regarded as clutter in blood flow imaging, has a much higher amplitude (20–40 dB) than that due to blood flow, and the associated velocities are relatively small. For healthy volunteers, myocardium contractile velocities from 6 to 10 cm/s have been reported,

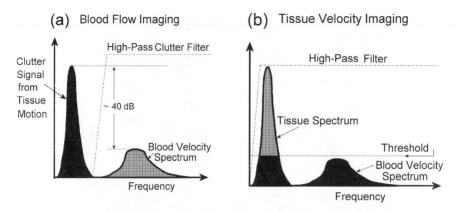

Figure 10.40 Sketches used to illustrate the different approaches used for blood flow and tissue velocity imaging. (a) In blood flow imaging, the clutter arising from tissue motion is removed. (b) For tissue velocity imaging, the blood flow signal can be removed either by a threshold adjustment or by a low-pass filter. (Based on a similar figure in Yamazaki [146].)

whereas blood velocities in the ventricular cavities might range from 10 to 100 cm/s.

The above differences between blood and tissue regions, which are qualitatively illustrated in Fig. 10.40, have enabled real-time tissue velocity imaging of the myocardium to be made. McDicken et al. [141–143] first (1992) reported the developments needed to achieve this along with a myocardial color image. An example of such an image is shown in Fig. 10.41. Independent work in Japan, initially reported in 1993 by Miyatake et al. [144], and subsequently in more detail by Yamazaki et al. [145,146], was also followed by trials to determine its clinical value. Because infarcted areas of the myocardium should show much reduced or zero velocities, the method offers the potential for identifying damaged areas without requiring the use of contrast agents. By using a power display method (see subsection 10.10.2), improvements to the sensitivity and less color fluctuations should enable infarcted areas to be more readily identified.

In their initial account, McDicken et al. [141] reported using a modified commercial flow imaging system. The modifications included are those suggested in Fig. 10.40b, together with a reduced PRF. The latter was needed to accommodate the smaller velocities while maintaining a sufficiently high frame rate and resolution. The PRF reduction was made possible by the fact that tissue SNR is much greater than that for blood.

10.10.4 Contrast Flow Imaging

As discussed in Chapter 8 (section 8.6), B-mode harmonic imaging can be based either on the nonlinearity of the tissue response to high-amplitude pres-

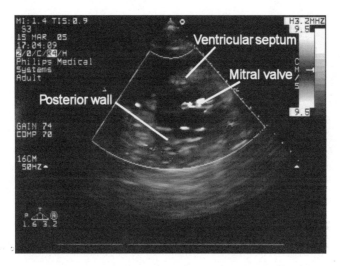

Figure 10.41 Color-encoded tissue velocity image of the heart. The time in the cardiac cycle at which the image was obtained is indicated by the bottom line. A low-pass filter has been used to suppress the blood flow information. (Courtesy Professor McDicken.) See color insert.

sures, or on the nonlinear response of contrast agents in the form of encapsulated microbubbles [131]. Suitable contrast agents for clinical use consist of encapsulated gas bubbles whose diameters are sufficiently small to enable them to pass through the lung capillaries. Conventional flow imaging of small vessels is limited by the effects of clutter, which place a lower bound on the velocities that can be satisfactorily estimated. By using the nonlinear response of injected microbubbles to generate harmonics of the incident frequency, the flow in small vessels can be detected. In collaboration with others, Burns [132–134] has made important contributions to the development of these ideas and their clinical application. The basic ideas follow directly from the initial work of Schrope and Newhouse [135] published in 1992/3 on second harmonic flow measurements. As shown in the following subsections, a variety of techniques have been developed specifically for use with ultrasound contrast agents. Much of this has been reviewed by Burns [136].

Harmonic and Power Harmonic Flow Imaging

The basic principles of harmonic flow imaging are illustrated in Fig. 10.42. If a high-amplitude transmit pressure pulse with a center frequency of f is incident on the microbubbles, a second harmonic signal at $2f$ will be generated. In addition, scattered signals at the fundamental frequency will be produced by the vessel wall, RBCs, and the microbubbles. The second harmonic component can be separated from the fundamental by means of an RF filter, though some clutter remains due to tissue nonlinearity and filter

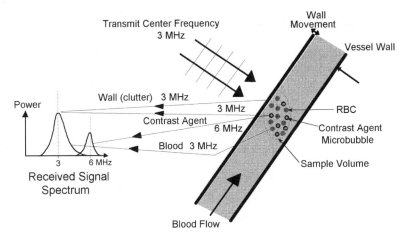

Figure 10.42 Principles of contrast agent harmonic flow imaging. By separating the second harmonic signal from the fundamental, the clutter can be rejected, leading to improved imaging close to the wall and the ability to measure smaller flow velocities. The large sample volume shown is for the purpose of illustration.

imperfections. Nonetheless, the sensitivity improvement is sufficient to enable flow in much smaller vessels to be detected.

The imaging sensitivity can be further enhanced by using the power mode technique to display the second harmonic power rather than attempting to display the velocity variations. Burns et al. [134,137] first described this method in 1994, and reported that it enabled flow to be detected in vessels that were about 10 times smaller than the system imaging resolution. They also noted that the flash artifact, caused by tissue movement (see subsection 10.10.2), was greatly reduced. Subsequently, Hope Simpson et al. [138] pointed out that because of the correlation between the RF and slow-time signals for both the bubbles and tissue, by properly coordinating the RF and clutter filter designs, the contrast could be significantly improved.

Pulse Inversion Methods

A limitation of harmonic flow imaging using contrast agents arises from some overlap between the fundamental and second harmonic spectra. Linear scattering by tissue will cause a portion of the received fundamental spectrum to overlap the second harmonic spectrum produced by microbubble contrast agents. This reduces the contrast produced by the microbubbles. To improve the contrast, a higher transmit intensity could be used to increase the second harmonic signal relative to the fundamental. However, due to contrast agent destruction (see subsection 8.6.1), this reduces the microbubble lifetime. On the other hand, if a narrower bandwidth transmit pulse is used to reduce the extent of spectral overlap, the spatial resolution will be degraded. A method for overcoming these limitations was proposed in 1997 by Hope Simpson and Burns [139], which they called *pulse inversion Doppler* (also known as power pulse inversion imaging). It is a generalization of the pulse inversion imaging method described in subsection 8.6.1 and consists of a frequency-domain method for distinguishing between the echoes from bubbles and moving tissue.

In the above scheme, multiple pulses are transmitted with alternate pulses being inverted. We shall first consider the echoes from a scatterer that responds in a linear manner. If the pulse repetition frequency is denoted by $f_{PRF} = 1/T$, successive received pressure echoes from a scatterer moving with a velocity v in the ultrasound beam direction can be written as [140]

$$p_{n+1}^L[t - T(n-1)] = -p_n^L[t - Tn - \Delta\tau],$$

where $\Delta\tau = 2\Delta z/c_o$, Δz is the change in z-location of the scatterer in the interval T, the superscript L indicates a linear scattering process, and n is the pulse index number. The phase shift between successive echoes is given by $\Delta\phi = 2\pi f_c \Delta\tau + \pi$, where the additional π corresponds to the inversion of successive pulses and f_c is the center frequency of the transmitted pulse. Because the fast- and slow-time phase shifts are identical, the estimated pulsed wave frequency is given by

(10.43) $$f_{PW}^L = (2v_\theta / c_o)f_c + f_{PRI} / 2,$$

where $v_\theta = v\cos\theta$. This shows that the pulsed wave spectrum is now centered about the Nyquist frequency rather than about zero, as is normally the case.

Consider now the case of a nonlinear scatterer. The echoes for normal and inverted pulses can be decomposed into even and odd components. Thus, for the two transmitted pulses, the echoes can be written as

$$p_N^{NL}(t) = p_N^{NL,Even}(t) + p_N^{NL,Odd}(t)$$
$$p_I^{NL}(t) = p_I^{NL,Even}(t) - p_I^{NL,Odd}(t),$$

where NL indicates the nonlinear scattered echo, N the normal transmitted pulse, and I the inverted version. As noted in subsection 8.6.1, this equation shows that the even and odd components can be extracted by addition and subtraction. The pulsed wave center frequencies can be extracted from these two components, yielding

(10.44) $$f_{PW}^{NL,Odd} = (2v_\theta / c_o)f_c + f_{PRI} / 2$$
$$f_{PW}^{NL,Even} = (2v_\theta / c_o)f_c.$$

This shows that the odd component pulsed wave frequency is identical in form to that of linear scattering, as given by (10.43). On the other hand, the even term yields a frequency identical that of a conventional pulsed wave system, i.e., it is centered about zero and is the same as (10.2). Thus, provided all the pulsed wave spectra are less than half the Nyquist frequency ($f_{PRI}/2$), echoes from stationary or moving linear and nonlinear scatterers will appear at different regions of the pulsed wave spectrum, as illustrated in Fig. 10.43. This

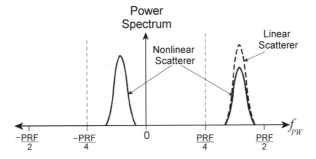

Figure 10.43 Idealized pulse inversion pulsed-wave spectra for linear and nonlinear scatterers. (Reproduced, with permission, from Simpson et al. [140], ©1999 IEEE 1999.)

enables various combinations of the scattered components to be extracted with the help of appropriate filters [138].

An important advantage of this pulsed wave inversion method is the ability to reduce the mechanical index (*MI*) to a level where contrast bubble destruction is no longer an issue, e.g. *MI* ≤ 0.1 [136]). This enables dynamic imaging of contrast agent perfusion to be performed without causing the images to be affected by ultrasound-enhanced microbubble destruction. For example, some initial work demonstrated the dynamics of myocardial perfusion at *MI* = 0.15 and a frame rate of 15 Hz [136]. The lower frame rate is a direct consequence of the longer pulse sequence needed for each A-line measurement.

10.11 Volume Flow Estimation Techniques

Accurate noninvasive measurement of the volume flow rate in blood vessels and its variation over a cardiac cycle is an important goal that can provide useful diagnostic information and lead to a better understanding of the underlying physiology. Of particular importance for monitoring patients, especially those in intensive care, is the development of a noninvasive method of measuring cardiac output (approximately equal to the integral of the volume flow in the ascending aorta over a cardiac cycle). Although many techniques have been proposed and tested [147,148], few offer the possibility of noninvasive measurement with sufficient accuracy. Of these, methods based on MRI and ultrasound offer the prospect for measurements on different-size vessels but are unlikely to be useful for long-term cardiac output monitoring. On the other hand, electrical impedance methods, based primarily on the work initially described in 1966 by Kubicek et al. [151], offers an attractive alternative. It uses a small high-frequency current (e.g., 2 ma, at 100 kHz) applied between electrodes placed on the thorax for measuring the first derivative of electrical impedance. Several commercial systems based on this technique have been evaluated [152] and found to give good agreement with the Fick method [148, pp. 306–308]. The latter is a catheter-based method, generally regarded as a gold standard.

Of considerable diagnostic importance is the measurement of tissue perfusion. This is generally defined as the volume flow of blood through a given mass or volume of tissue, e.g., units of ml/(min.100 g). For a limb, which of course involves both small and large blood vessels, a variety of methods have been used, such as strain-gauge plethysmography and radioactive tracer clearance techniques [148, pp. 301–306]. However, quantitative measurement of localized perfusion in the strict sense has proven to be a challenging problem.

It seems that in a 1981 conference presentation Hertz was the first to suggest that Doppler ultrasound might be used for measuring tissue perfusion [149]. Subsequently it was shown that high-frequency CW Doppler and pulsed wave ultrasound methods enable flow to be detected in microvessels, e.g., 40 μm, but adapting these techniques for perfusion measurements is difficult. In part, problems arise from the pseudo-random nature of the microvascular structure and the 3-D flow directions involved. In their extensive review of ultrasound perfusion techniques developed prior to 2000, Jansson et al. [150] point out that qualitative assessment is possible and can yield helpful results, especially when contrast agents are used (see subsection 10.10.4).

A large number of noninvasive ultrasound methods have been proposed and tested for volume flow measurements, but inaccuracies and implementation problems have hampered widespread clinical acceptance. Several attempts have been made to develop a satisfactory method for measuring cardiac output, but the success in clinical practice has been rather limited. One of the more promising noninvasive techniques is the attenuation compensation method described in subsection 10.11.3. Intravascular ultrasound methods for flow estimation are also of importance. As noted in Chapter 8 (see subsection 8.10.4), methods used for intravascular imaging can also be adapted to extract the flow rate. Specifically, it was shown that by using the effects of blood flow decorrelation, the flow velocity distribution could be estimated. This, together with the geometry as determined by B-mode imaging, enables the flow rate to be estimated.

Many volume flow estimation methods depend on knowing the beam/vessel angle and the vessel cross-sectional area and make a number of assumptions concerning the direction of the flow velocity vectors and vessel geometry. One of the first reviews, including an analysis of the sources of error, is contained in [16, pp. 237–254]. Subsequently, several authors [16,153–155] have addressed and reviewed this problem. Of particular importance is that presented by Evans and McDicken [24, Chapter 12].

The volume flow rate through a vessel is the volume of fluid per unit time passing through any surface that intersects the vessel, and whose periphery surrounds it. For simplicity, a plane surface that intersects a cylindrical vessel is shown in Fig. 10.44. If the area is divided into N incremental regions, then the volume flow rate is given by

$$(10.45) \qquad Q(t) = \sum_{i=1}^{N} \mathbf{v}_i \cdot \Delta \mathbf{A}_i,$$

where the summation is performed over the entire surface area. In general, due to the vessel elasticity and the pulsatile nature of the flow, v_i is a function

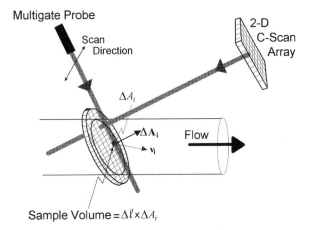

Sample Volume $= \Delta\ell \times \Delta A_i$

Figure 10.44 Two methods for estimating the volume flow rate in a vessel. With the multigate system, the beam/vessel angle must be determined. On the other hand, the C-scan system using a 2-D array is angle-independent.

of time, making the flow rate time-dependent. Thus, the mean volume that flows over one cardiac cycle of duration T can be written as

$$\overline{Q_T} = \frac{1}{T} \int_t^{T+t} \sum_i (\mathbf{v}_i \cdot \Delta\mathbf{A}_i)dt.$$

10.11.1 Local Mean Velocity Methods

Shortly following their pioneering work on the development of pulsed wave flow velocity methods, Peronneau et al. [156] described how the flow rate in a vessel could be estimated from the velocity profile. Subsequently, Histland et al. [68] reported the results for arterial measurements in anesthetized dogs and found good agreement with the results obtained using electromagnetic flow probes.

The 1-D flow profile method is based on a number of assumptions concerning the vessel and flow. Specifically, it is assumed that the vessel is cylindrical, that the flow velocity vector points in the axial direction and that the vessel axis in relation to the ultrasound beam can be determined. Using pulsed ultrasound, the mean velocity can be estimated within incremental volume regions that lie on a line of symmetry that passes through the vessel. With reference to Fig. 10.45 it should be noted that $\Delta r = \Delta\ell \sin\theta$, $\ell_i = r_i \sin\theta$ and from (10.2), $\bar{v}_i(t) = \bar{f}_i(t)c_o/(2f_c \cos\theta)$. Moreover, the volume flow rate through the incremental area is given by $\Delta Q(t) = \pi r_i \Delta r_i v_i(t)$. These relations, together with (10.45), enable the volume flow rate to be written as

(10.46)
$$Q(t) = \frac{\pi c_o \Delta\ell \sin^2\theta}{2f_c \cos\theta} \sum_i \ell_i \bar{f}_i(t).$$

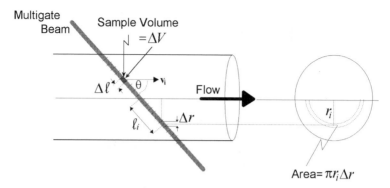

Figure 10.45 Volume flow estimation using a multigate pulsed system to determine the 1-D velocity profile of a cylindrical vessel.

From (10.46) it can be seen that the accuracy with which the flow rate can be estimated depends critically on the accuracy with which θ can be estimated. Errors also arise because the size of the sample volume may not be small compared to the vessel, and as a result the local mean velocity can be distorted. As noted in subsection 10.6.2, a deconvolution process can be used to make corrections. In addition, close to the vessel wall, where the sample volume encloses blood together with the moving vessel wall, a distorted flow signal results. Baker et al. [16] pointed out that the velocity profile method is best suited to larger vessels. For smaller vessels, errors arising from the size of the sample volume and the partial volume effects at the vessel/blood boundary become much more significant.

An extension to the 1-D flow profile method is illustrated in Fig. 10.44. It makes use of a multigate pulsed flow system to scan the flow over a surface area that intersects the vessel. Because the component of the velocity along the beam direction is estimated at each location, the assumption of axisymmetric flow is not required. However, axial flow must still be assumed and the beam/vessel angle needs to be estimated.

Fish and Walters [153] addressed the problem of estimating the beam/vessel angle and reviewed various approaches in terms of their accuracy and feasibility. In addition, as illustrated in Fig. 10.46, they proposed a method to account for the 3-D vessel/beam geometry. This scheme was incorporated into the MAVIS-C,[9] the first commercially available multigate flow imaging system [21, pp. 129–133]. A single-element, position-resolved probe was used to perform multigate scans on two planes axially separated by about 10 mm. By determining the average flow velocity at each sample location, the center of gravity on each plane can be estimated. The line joining these positions was taken as an estimate of the vessel axis direction, enabling the beam/flow angle to be found.

A potentially useful method based on C-mode flow scanning (often referred to as C-mode Doppler) is also illustrated in Fig. 10.44. The mean velocity

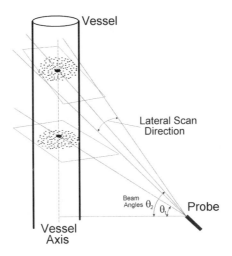

Figure 10.46 The method developed by Fish [154] for estimating the beam/vessel angle. The dots represent the presence of flow as detected by the multigate system. The center of gravity on the two scan planes gives the vessel axis direction.

component in the beam direction is determined for all sample volume elements that lie on a surface that intersects the entire vessel cross-section. Thus, $(\bar{\mathbf{v}}_i \cdot \Delta\mathbf{A}_i/\Delta A_i)$ is determined for each elementary sample volume, as required by (10.45), and consequently the method is angle-independent. Moreover, the method is independent of the vessel cross-sectional geometry and direction of the velocity vectors. The 2-D scan can be performed by using a 2-D transducer array as originally proposed in 1978 by Hottinger [157], or by a fixed range-gate transducer that is mechanically scanned. Poulsen [158] has described four C-mode methods that make use of mechanical scanning; however, limitations of the scanning speed make it unlikely that such methods could be used for pulsatile blood flow estimation. The development of a 2-D transducer array system for volume flow measurement was described by Moser et al. [159] in 1992. Using a 6×6 array and employing a synthetic aperture scheme on reception, they reported [160] that the 2-D velocity distribution could be computed within 10 to 30 ms. However, partial volume effects at the vessel wall caused the volume flow rate to be overestimated. Subsequently, Liu and Burns [161] described a method for correcting such errors by using the power information from each voxel to scale each mean velocity value.

10.11.2 Power Spectrum Methods

It was noted in Chapter 9 that the volume flow rate in a uniformly insonated cylindrical vessel can be determined from an estimate of the mean CW Doppler frequency, the Doppler angle, and the vessel radius. For a cylindrical vessel and a uniform scattering, the estimated flow rate can be expressed as

(10.47) $$\hat{Q}(t) = \pi R(t)^2 \hat{\bar{v}}(t).$$

In this equation, because of the time-dependent pressure combined with the vessel elasticity, the vessel radius $R(t)$, is a function of time. Brody [162] and Art and Roevros [163] independently showed that the mean velocity can be expressed in terms of the normalized first moment of the Doppler power spectral density.[14] Their derivations, which assumed that the flow velocity vectors all point in the same direction, yielded

(10.48) $$\hat{\bar{v}} = \frac{c_o}{2 f_o \cos \theta} \int_{f_D^{min}}^{f_D^{max}} f_D \Phi(f_D) df_D \left/ \int_{f_D^{min}}^{f_D^{max}} \Phi(f_D) df_D \right. ,$$ (a)

where f_D^{max} is the frequency above which noise dominates, f_D^{min} is determined by the wall-thump filter characteristics, and the power density spectrum $\Phi(f_D)$, is taken to be real. They also noted that this equation is independent of the shape of the flow velocity profile.

Based on the above relations, a number of CW flow estimation methods have been developed that should be independent of the beam/flow angle. Generally, these involve the use of an additional Doppler probe that subtends a different angle to the insonated region but whose orientation with respect to the other Doppler probe is well defined, enabling the angle variable to be eliminated. This, together with an A-mode probe to determine the vessel diameter, enables the flow rate to be estimated. Fahrbach [164,165] was probably the first to describe such a scheme. He used two CW probes (each with separate transmit and receive crystals) mounted at 90 degrees to one another, and determined the two mean Doppler frequencies. Using analog processing, both results were combined to yield an output proportional to the velocity but independent of the Doppler angle. It can be readily shown that if one probe has a Doppler angle of θ_1 and the second probe makes an angle of φ to the first, then the mean flow velocity can be expressed as

(10.49) $$|\bar{v}| = \frac{c_o}{2 f_o \sin \varphi} \sqrt{\bar{f}_1^2 + \bar{f}_2^2 - 2 \bar{f}_1 \bar{f}_2 \cos \varphi} ,$$ (a)

where $\bar{f}_1$ and $\bar{f}_2$ are the two mean Doppler frequencies and the Doppler angle is given by

(10.49) $$\theta_1 = \tan^{-1}[(\cos \varphi - \bar{f}_2 / \bar{f}_1)/ \sin \varphi].$$ (b)

For the case in which the two probes are at right angles to one another, these equations reduce to those given by Fahrbach. Details of this and other multi-probe methods can be found in Evans and McDicken [24, Chapter 12] and Dunmire et al. [166].

A modified form of (10.48a) can also be used as the basis for estimating the pulsed wave mean velocity at the location of the sample volume. Moreover,

---

14. It should be remarked that Peronneau et al. [13] in 1970 presented the same form of equation, though without proof.

multiprobe techniques can also be used to eliminate the angle dependence. Gill [167] has shown that when used in combination with B-mode imaging, quantitative flow measurements can be performed on relatively small, deep-lying vessels. By defocusing the incident beam and extending the sample volume axial length, a reasonably uniform intensity can be achieved. If the power density spectrum is complex, the mean velocity can be expressed as

(10.48)
$$\hat{\bar{v}} = \frac{c_o}{2f_c \cos\theta} \int_{-f_{PRF}/2}^{f_{PRF}/2} f\Phi(f)df \bigg/ \int_{-f_{PRF}/2}^{f_{PRF}/2} \Phi(f)df.$$
(b)

If the average vessel diameter and the beam/vessel angle can be determined from the B-mode image, this equation, when substituted into (10.47), enables the mean flow rate to be estimated.

10.11.3 Compensation Methods

In 1979, Hottinger and Meindl [168] described a noninvasive method for measuring volumetric flow that was based on the use of two pulsed flow sample volumes. One sample volume intersected the entire vessel cross-section, while the second was a much smaller volume entirely within the vessel lumen. By combining the results from these two measurements, they showed how the effects of attenuation and scattering could be compensated for, enabling the absolute flow rate to be determined independent of the beam angle. They called this scheme an attenuation-compensated flowmeter. To generate the two sample volumes they proposed the use of an annular array, an idea that was subsequently implemented by Fu and Gerzberg [169].

A practical realization of this technique, designed for noninvasively measuring cardiac output, was subsequently described by Evans et al. [170]. They used a two-element annular transducer appropriately apodized to generate the two sample volumes. Using an experimental version, they reported [171] excellent correlation ($r = 0.96$) in 54 patients using either a dye or thermodilution technique as the basis of comparison. A commercial version of this system, first marketed in 1986 under the trade name of Quantascope (Vital Science Ltd.), was clinically evaluated by a number of groups. However, some of the results reported were less encouraging [172], and in comparison to the thermodilution method, at least one group reported results that were significantly inferior to the simpler electrical impedance method [173]. A version of this scheme intended for intravascular flow measurement has been proposed and evaluated by Gibson et al. [174]. It used a semispherical transducer that could produce a semispherical sample volume that entirely intersected the vessel. Compensation for the effects of scattering and attenuation was achieved by estimating the power and moment of the spectra from two sample volumes that entirely intersected the vessel and were at differing radial distances from the transducer.

The basic theory of the compensation method can be discussed with the help of Fig. 10.47a. Consider a small element of area ΔA_i on an arbitrary

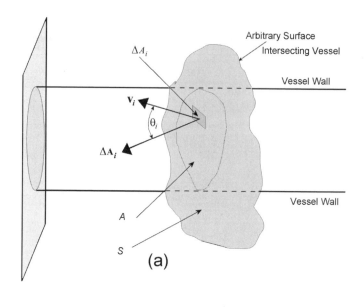

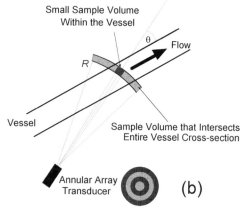

Figure 10.47 The attenuation-compensated method for volume flow rate estimation. (a) A surface S intersecting the vessel such that the cross-sectional area of the vessel projected onto the surface is A. The sample volume surface is assumed to coincide with S. (b) Using a phased annular array, two sample volumes are produced: one intersecting the entire vessel, the other within the vessel.

surface S whose periphery is a continuous line that surrounds the vessel and coincides with the sample volume surface. The volume flow-rate though ΔA_i can be expressed as

$$(10.50) \qquad \Delta Q_i(t) = \Delta \mathbf{A}_i \cdot \mathbf{v}_i = \Delta A_i v_i \cos \varphi_i,$$

where $\mathbf{v}_i$ is the flow velocity vector. The total volume flow rate through the vessel can be obtained by summing over all such elementary areas over the area S, yielding

(10.51)
$$Q(t) = \sum_i \Delta A_i v_i \cos \varphi_i.$$

Now the baseband pulsed wave signal power contributed by the flow through the elemental area ΔA_i can be written as $\Delta W_i = \Gamma_1(R)\Delta A_i$, where $\Gamma_1(R)$ is a depth-dependent proportionality constant that depends on the round-trip attenuation, the backscattering coefficient, and the pulse-echo response in the absence of attenuation. But, because the signal power can also be written as $\Delta W_i = \int \Phi_i(f)df$, we obtain the relation

(10.52)
$$\int \Phi_i(f)df = \Gamma_1(R)\Delta A_i,$$

which enables the first moment of the power density spectrum to be written as

(10.53)
$$\int f\Phi_i(f)df = f\Gamma_1(R)\Delta A_i.$$

Assuming that the beam sample volume coincides with the surface S, then, from (10.2), for each incremental area the pulse-wave frequency/velocity relation can be expressed as

$$f_{PW} = \frac{2v_i \cos \varphi_i}{c_o} f_c,$$

where f_c is the center frequency of the transmitted waveform. Consequently (10.53) can be written as

$$\int f\Phi_i(f)df = \frac{2f_c v_i}{c_o} \cos \varphi_i \Delta A_i \Gamma_1(R).$$

If, as shown in Fig. 10.47b, all elementary areas are at the same distance from the transducer, summation yields

$$\sum_i \int f\Phi_i(f)df = \frac{2f_c \Gamma_1(R)}{c_o} \sum_i \Delta A_i v_i \cos \varphi_i.$$

By substituting this into (10.51), the volume flow rate can be expressed in terms of the first moment of the spectrum and is given by

(10.54)
$$Q(t) = \frac{c_o}{2f_c \Gamma_1(R)} \int f\Phi_1(f)df.$$

It follows that the flow rate is independent of the direction of the velocity vectors over the sample volume surface and is proportional to the first moment of the spectrum.

To determine the volumetric flow using (10.54), $\Gamma_1(R)$ which relates the power to the sample volume, must be found. This can be achieved by employing a second sample volume measurement in which the sample volume is at the same distance R from the transducer and has the same axial length. This sample volume has a much smaller area to ensure that it lies entirely within the vessel (see Fig. 10.47b). The baseband signal power from this volume can be written as (see 10.52)

(10.55)
$$W_2(R) = \int \Phi_2(f)df = \Gamma_2(R)A_2(R),$$

where A_2 is the cross-sectional area.

As noted earlier, $\Gamma_2(R)$ is the product of three terms: one that accounts for the round-trip attenuation, one that depends on the backscattering coefficient, and one that characterizes the pulse-echo sensitivity in the absence of attenuation. If the first two terms can be assumed to be identical for both sample volumes and the third terms are denoted by $\Theta_1(R)$ and $\Theta_2(R)$, then, from (10.54) and (10.55), the flow rate is given by

(10.56)
$$Q(t) = \frac{c_o}{2f_c}\left(\frac{A_2(R)\Theta_2(R)}{\Theta_1(R)}\right)\int f\Phi_1(f)df \Big/ \int \Phi_2(f)df.$$

Because the term in braces is a range-dependent constant that can be determined by calibration, the flow rate can be estimated by measurement of the power density spectrum for the two sample volumes.

10.12 Velocity Vector Estimation Methods

In curved or tortuous arteries or at vessel discontinuities, the flow profile is no longer axisymmetric and the vectors generally point in non-axial directions. The three-dimensional nature of the flow field in many blood vessels has long been recognized to be of possible physiological importance in the formation and progression of arterial diseases. Furthermore, it is a source of error in some ultrasound techniques for estimating the volume flow rate. The development of in vivo methods for estimating the vector flow field could be of value in eliminating these errors and providing information that would improve our understanding of vascular physiology.

At least three different classes of ultrasound techniques have been developed for estimating two or all components of the velocity field. Peronneau et al. [156] in 1971/72 were probably the first to report the use of pulsed wave techniques for determining two of the velocity components. Since then, various pulsed and CW vector reconstruction techniques, in which the vector components are estimated directly, have been reviewed by Dunmire et al. [166] and Evans and McDicken [24, pp. 325–336]. A second class is based on tracking the speckle movements between successive B-mode images. As described in section 8.8, by cross-correlating two images taken at a known time interval apart, the 2-D vector components can be recovered. The third class, which does not require the presence of scatterers, makes use of the changes in the ultrasound propagation path. This was first described by Johnson et al. [175] in the mid 1970s. In subsection 9.3.1 it was noted that the path taken by an ultrasonic ray depends on the velocity field encountered. Consequently, the transit time from a source to a receiver, which can be expressed as the line integral over the path, will depend on the velocity field encountered. By making transit time measurements over a multiplicity of such paths, in a similar manner to ultrasound transmission tomography (see section 8.7), and inverting the line integrals, reconstruction of the velocity field is possible.

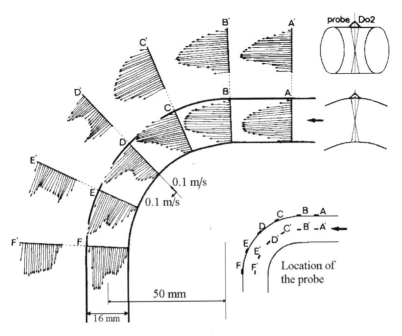

Figure 10.48 Velocity vector distribution in a 0.8-cm-radius curved pipe with a radius of curvature of 5 cm using a pulsed-wave ($f_c = 4$ MHz) ultrasound system. These appear to be the first reported 2-D pulsed measurements. They were made using a pair of transducers mounted on the exterior surface of the pipe at 90 degrees to one another. Steady flow (3.5 l/min) conditions were used with a fluid having a kinematic viscosity of 5×10^{-6} m²/s. Each arrow indicates the magnitude and direction of velocity at the position indicated. (Reproduced from Peronneau et al. [156], Chapter 2, in *Blood Flow Measurement*, ©1972, Sector Publishing Limited.)

10.12.1 Velocity Reconstruction Techniques

A number of different pulsed wave techniques have been proposed for estimating two or all velocity vector components at a point, on a line, on a plane, or over a 3-D volume. Using pulsed wave ultrasound, Peronneau et al. [156] reported in vitro 2-D velocity measurements of flow in tubes of various shapes. Using a pair of pulse-echo transducers connected to a two-channel pulsed wave system, they performed measurements of steady flow in curved tube. As illustrated in Fig. 10.48, the transducer elements were mounted at an angle to one another and placed symmetrically at the indicated locations on the tube surface. Shortly following this report, they [70,176] developed a multigate 16-channel system that they used for in vivo (pulsatile flow) measurements of the velocity field in the aortic arch flow of a dog during acute open-chest experiments.

Some of the vector methods evaluated make use of several individual transducer elements;[15] others are based on the use of a phased array. In fact, the first

15. The use of two single-element transducers for angle-independent estimation of the volume flow rate was considered in subsection 10.11.2, where it was shown that the magnitude and direction of the velocity is given by (10.49).

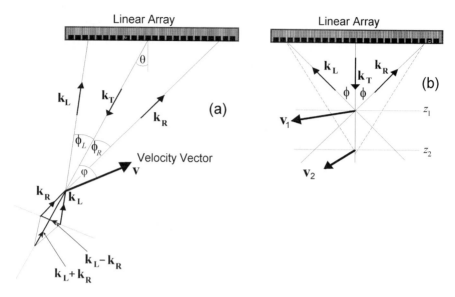

Figure 10.49 Geometry used for 2-D velocity reconstruction using a linear array. (a) Steered at an angle θ. (b) When the transmit beam is normal to the transducer face, reconstruction of the velocity along this path by dynamic steering and focusing using the two reception array apertures.

report of the use of a phased array is contained in the 1981 patent granted to Papadofrangakis et al. [177]. The flexibility realized by using a phased array provides the opportunity to implement a variety of transmit/receive schemes without altering the transducer design and without the need to reposition the transducer.

Following closely the analysis presented by Papadofrangakis et al. [177], we start by considering the linear array illustrated in Fig. 10.49 in which three subarrays of elements are identified. Suppose that the two outer ones are used as phased-array receivers and the central ones as a phased-array transmitter. Consider a scatterer moving with a velocity $\mathbf{v}$ whose instantaneous location is shown in the figure. At the scatterer the transmitted beam direction is given by the wave vector $\mathbf{k_T}$; moreover, the two receive directions are denoted by $\mathbf{k_L}$ and $\mathbf{k_R}$ (left and right). Following the same vector procedure as given in section 9.3 for calculating the Doppler shift, it can be seen that at the left and right receivers the slow-time angular frequencies are given by $\omega_L = \mathbf{v} \cdot \mathbf{k_L} + \mathbf{v} \cdot \mathbf{k_T}$ and $\omega_R = \mathbf{v} \cdot \mathbf{k_R} + \mathbf{v} \cdot \mathbf{k_T}$, respectively. These enable the sum and difference frequencies to be expressed as

$$\omega_L + \omega_R = \mathbf{v} \cdot (\mathbf{k_L} + \mathbf{k_R} + 2\mathbf{k_T}), \quad \omega_L - \omega_R = \mathbf{v} \cdot (\mathbf{k_L} + \mathbf{k_R}).$$

To simplify the analysis we shall assume that both receivers are positioned such that $\phi_L = \phi_R = \phi$. As a result (see Fig. 10.49), the vector $(\mathbf{k_L} + \mathbf{k_R} + 2\mathbf{k_T})$ will be in the transmit beam direction, and consequently its dot product with $\mathbf{v}$ gives the slow-time angular frequency of the velocity component in the transmit beam direction, i.e.,

(10.57) $$\omega_{//} = \mathbf{v} \cdot (\mathbf{k}_L + \mathbf{k}_R) + 2\mathbf{v} \cdot \mathbf{k}_T.$$

Similarly, the slow-time angular frequency perpendicular to the transmit beam direction is given by

(10.58) $$\omega_\perp = \mathbf{v} \cdot (\mathbf{k}_L - \mathbf{k}_R).$$

Noting that the magnitudes of all the wave vectors are equal to $\omega_0/c_o = k$, from Fig. 10.49 it follows that

$$\mathbf{v} \cdot \mathbf{k}_L = kv\cos(\varphi + \phi), \quad \mathbf{v} \cdot \mathbf{k}_R = kv\cos(\varphi - \phi), \quad \text{and} \quad \mathbf{v} \cdot \mathbf{k}_T = -vk\cos\varphi.$$

When these relations are substituted into (10.58) and (10.60), the two slow-time frequencies can be expressed as

$$\omega_{//} = v\frac{\omega_0}{c_o}\left[\cos(\varphi + \phi) + \cos(\varphi - \phi) + 2\cos\varphi\right]$$

$$= v\frac{\omega_0}{c_o}2\cos\varphi(1 + \cos\phi) = v_{//}\frac{\omega_0}{c_o}2(1 + \cos\phi)$$

$$\omega_\perp = v\frac{\omega_0}{c_o}\left[\cos(\phi + \varphi) - \cos(\phi - \varphi)\right]$$

$$= v\frac{\omega_0}{c_o}2\sin\varphi\sin\phi = v_\perp\frac{\omega_0}{c_o}2\sin\phi$$

Consequently, the velocity components parallel and perpendicular to the transmit beam direction can be written as

(10.59) $$v_{//} = \frac{\omega_{//}}{2(1 + \cos\phi)}\frac{c_o}{\omega_0}, \qquad v_\perp = \frac{\omega_\perp}{2\sin\phi}\frac{c_o}{\omega_0}.$$

From the estimates of $\omega_{//} = \omega_L + \omega_R$ and $\omega_\perp = \omega_L - \omega_R$, these equations enable the magnitude and direction of $\mathbf{v}$ to be calculated.

It should be noted that (10.59) are essentially the same as those originally derived for linear arrays by Papadofrangakis et al. [177] and subsequently by Hall and Bernardi [178]. The latter also considered a number of other possible transmit/receive subarray arrangements. Overbeck et al. [179], in considering three single-element focused transducers, also derived the same equation.

10.12.2 Reconstruction Algebra

The method used in color flow imaging systems for estimating [177] a single component of the velocity distribution over a plane can be extended to two or all three vector components. The ability to electronically change the direction in which the color flow scan is performed enables the two flow velocity components on a plane to be mapped without the need for any mechanical movement. This was first demonstrated by Tamura et al. [180,181] in 1990 using a commercial color flow imaging system with beam steering and extended by Maniatis et al. [182]. With a modified commercial system in which the linear array was mounted in a motor-driven harness, Rickey et al. [183] demonstrated the possibility of 3-D velocity reconstruction over a volume.

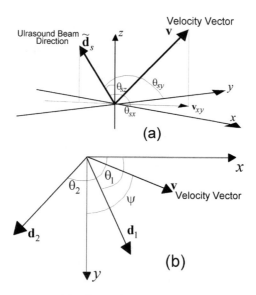

Figure 10.50 Geometry used for flow velocity reconstruction in (a) 3-D and (b) 2-D.

Following the analysis presented by Maniatis et al. [184], we consider three transducer arrays that are used to perform flow measurements of the velocity components in three different scan planes. Provided the three planes intersect along a line, the 3-D vectors can be reconstructed along that line. For the particular case in which two of the scan planes coincide but their scan directions differ, then the reconstruction line will correspond to the intersection of the third scanning plane with the coincident planes. For this case, 3-D velocity vector reconstruction over an entire plane can be achieved by a multiplicity of parallel scans in the third plane such that the intersections with the coincident planes form a set of "scan" lines. In the coordinate system shown in Fig. 10.50a, the velocity vector is denoted by $\mathbf{v}$ and the direction of the beam for the s'th measurement is the unit vector $\tilde{\mathbf{d}}_s$. The component of $\mathbf{v}$ in the direction of $\tilde{\mathbf{d}}_s$ is

$$v_{d_s} = \mathbf{v} \cdot \mathbf{d}_s = v_x \cos\theta_{sx} + v_y \cos\theta_{sy} + v_z \cos\theta_{sz},$$

where θ_{sx}, θ_{sy}, and θ_{sz} are the angles subtended by the beam to the coordinate axes x, y, and z, respectively. These are related by

$$\cos^2\theta_{sx} + \cos^2\theta_{sy} + \cos^2\theta_{sz} = 1.$$

If three measurements are made from linearly independent directions, then the three velocity components (v_x, v_y, v_z) can be found from

$$(10.60) \qquad \begin{bmatrix} v_{d_1} \\ v_{d_2} \\ v_{d_3} \end{bmatrix} = \begin{bmatrix} \cos\theta_{1x} & \cos\theta_{1y} & \cos\theta_{1z} \\ \cos\theta_{2x} & \cos\theta_{2y} & \cos\theta_{2z} \\ \cos\theta_{3x} & \cos\theta_{3y} & \cos\theta_{3z} \end{bmatrix} \begin{bmatrix} v_x \\ v_y \\ v_z \end{bmatrix},$$

a result that was also given by Rickey et al. [183].

If measurements are made from just two linearly independent observation directions $\mathbf{d}_1$ and $\mathbf{d}_2$, as shown in Fig. 10.50b, only two components of the velocity can be found. Specifically, if the two directions lie on the x-y plane, then from (10.60)

$$v_{d_1} = v_x \cos\theta_{1x} + v_y \sin\theta_{1x}$$

$$v_{d_2} = v_x \cos\theta_{2x} + v_y \sin\theta_{2x}.$$

Solving the above system and dropping the subscript x from θ yields

(10.61)
$$v_x = \frac{v_{d_1}\sin\theta_2 - v_{d_2}\sin\theta_1}{\sin(\theta_2 - \theta_1)}$$

$$v_y = \frac{v_{d_2}\cos\theta_1 - v_{d_1}\cos\theta_2}{\sin(\theta_2 - \theta_1)},$$

enabling the magnitude and angle with respect to the x-axis to be found from $|v| = \sqrt{v_x^2 + v_y^2}$ and $\Psi = \tan^{-1}(v_y/v_x)$, respectively.

An illustration of the above technique is given in Fig. 10.51 for a bypass graft model under steady flow conditions. The fluid consisted of an aqueous glycerol solution with the addition of cornstarch as a scattering medium. Color flow images were obtained using beam steering at −20, 0, and +20 degrees. By

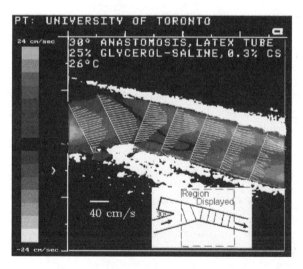

Figure 10.51 Image of a bypass graft model with superimposed vectors showing the 2-D velocity distribution for steady flow (1.4 l/min, Reynolds number = 1600). The B-mode image (7 MHz) and the flow image (5 MHz) are those obtained with a linear-array transducer with the beam in the vertical direction. The flow image scale gives the flow velocity component in the horizontal direction. The 2-D vectors were calculated from information obtained from color flow images obtained at −20, 0, and +20 degrees. (Reprinted by permission of Elsevier from Maniatis et al. [182], *Ultrasound Med. Biol.*, 20, 559–569, ©1994 World Federation of Ultrasound in Medicine and Biology.) See color insert.

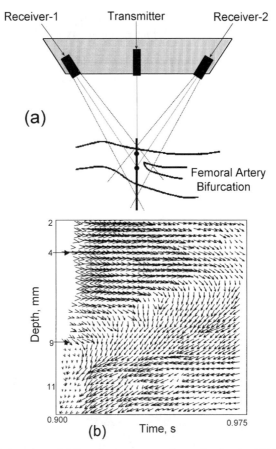

Figure 10.52 Estimation of 2-D velocity vectors from the femoral bifurcation. (a) Probe containing two wide-angle receiver transducers and a narrow beam transmitter. Superimposed is the outline of a femoral bifurcation on which are marked two dots that approximately correspond to depths of 4 and 9 mm from the near wall. In (b) are shown the 2-D vectors for a 75-ms interval in late systole. (Reproduced, with permission of The International Society for Optical Engineering, from Dunmire et al. [187], pp. 70–78 in *Medical Imaging 2001: Ultrasonic Imaging and Signal Processing*, Vol. 4325, ©2001 SPIE.)

digitizing these images and using the color to velocity scale, the information needed to calculate the magnitude and direction of the vectors was obtained. These are shown as lines whose lengths are proportional to the vector magnitudes and whose directions indicate the angles.

In vivo application of the use of color flow imaging system to 2-D vector reconstruction over a scan plane was reported by Hoskins et al. [185] in 1994 and by the same group [186] in 1996. These publications clearly demonstrated the presence of spiral flow patterns in the common femoral arteries of normal healthy subjects. An alternative approach for acquiring the information needed for 2-D vector reconstruction is that described by Dunmire et al. [187].

As illustrated in Fig. 10.52a, the probe contains three transducer elements: two receivers and a focused transmitter that ideally produces a pencil-like beam. The former have fairly wide fields of view, enabling the scattered signal produced throughout the intersection of the transmitted pulse with the vessel to be sensed. It should be noted that the probe geometry is essentially the same in Fig. 10.49b, and consequently the equations needed for reconstructing the two velocity components are given by (10.59). The in-phase and quadrature components of the velocity components $v_{//}$ and $v_\perp$ were obtained from the demodulated signals using essentially the same method as that described by Papadofrangakis et al. [177]. Using data collected over a 3-s period from the femoral bifurcation, 2-D vectors were calculated and displayed over a segment of time. For example, the vectors at depths from 2 to 12 mm over a 75-ms interval in late systole are displayed in Fig. 10.52b.

References

1. Newhouse, V.L., Ehrenwald, A.R., and Johnson, G.F., The effect of Rayleigh scattering and frequency dependent absorption on the output spectrum of Doppler flowmeters, pp. 1181–1191 in: *Ultrasound in Medicine*, Vol. 3B, D. White, and R.E. Brown (Eds.), Plenum Press, New York, 1977.

2. Round, W.H., and Bates, R.H.T., Modification of spectra of pulses from ultrasonic transducers by scatterers in non-attenuating and attenuating media, *Ultrasonic Imaging*, 9, 18–28, 1987.

3. Gill, T.P., *The Doppler Effect*, Academic Press, New York, 1965.

4. Schleher, D.C., *MTI and Pulsed Doppler Radar*, Artech House, Boston, 1991.

5. Newhouse, V.L., and Amir, I., Time dilation and inversion properties and the output spectrum of pulsed Doppler flowmeters, *IEEE Trans. Sonics Ultrason.*, 30, 174–179, 1983.

6. Thomas, N., and Leeman, S., The double Doppler effect, pp. 164–168 in: *Acoustic Sensing and Imaging*, IEE Publn. 369, London, 1993.

7. Thomas, N., and Leeman, S., The attenuation effect in pulsed Doppler flowmeters, pp. 543–552, *Acoustical Imaging*, Vol. 21., J.P. Jones (Ed.), Plenum Press, New York, 1995.

8. Bonnefous, O., and Pesque, P., Time domain formulation of pulse-Doppler ultrasound and blood velocity estimation by cross correlation, *Ultrasonic Imaging*, 8, 73–85, 1986.

9. Thomas, N., and Leeman, S., Mean frequency via zero crossings, pp. 1297–1300 in: *IEEE Ultrasonics Symp. Proc.*, 1991.

10. Jensen, J.A., *Estimation of Blood Velocities Using Ultrasound*, Cambridge Univ. Press, Cambridge, UK, 1996.

11. Peronneau, P.A., Recording ultrasonic flowmeter for blood vessels, US Patent 3,554,040, Jan. 12, 1971 (filed in US April 8, 1968, and in France April 7, 1967).

12. Peronneau, P.A., and Leger, F., Doppler ultrasonic pulsed blood flowmeter, Paper 10–11 (1-page Digest of papers) in: *Proc. 8th Int. Conf. Medical and Biol. Eng.*, Chicago, 1969.

13. Peronneau, P.A., Hinglais, J.R., Pellet, H.M., and Leger, F., Velocimetre sanguin par effet Doppler a emission ultra-sonore pulsee. A: Description de l'appareil, resultats, *L'Onde Electrique*, 50, 369–384, 1970.

14. Baker, D.W., and Watkins, D., A phase coherent pulse Doppler system for cardiovascular measurements, Paper 27-2 (1-page Digest of papers) in: *Proc. 20th Ann. Conf. on Eng. Med. Biology*, Boston, Nov. 1967.

15. Baker, D.W., Pulsed ultrasonic Doppler blood-flow sensing, *IEEE Trans. Sonics Ultrasonics*, 17, 170–185, 1970.

16. Baker, D.W., Forster, F.K., and Diagle, R.E., Doppler principles and techniques, Chapter 3, pp. 161–287 in: *Ultrasound: its Applications in Medicine and Biology*, Part 1, F.F. Fry (Ed.), Elsevier, Amsterdam, 1978.

17. Flaherty, J.J., and Strauts, E.J., Ultrasonic pulsed Doppler instrumention, Paper 10-10 (1-page digest) in: *Proc. 8th Int. Conf. Medical and Biol. Eng.*, Chicago, 1969.

18. Wells, P.N.T., A range-gated ultrasonic Doppler system, *Med. Biolog. Eng.*, 7, 641–652, 1969.

19. Barber, F.E., Baker, D.W., Nation, A.W.C., et al., Ultrasonic duplex echo-Doppler scanner, *IEEE Trans. Biomed. Eng.*, 21, 109–113, 1974.

20. Phillips, D.J., Powers, J.E., Eyer, M.K., et al., Detection of peripheral vascular disease using the Duplex Scanner III, *Ultrasound Med. Biol.*, 6, 205–218, 1980.

21. Atkinson, P. and Woodcock, J.P., *Doppler Ultrasound and its Use in Clinical Measurement*, Academic Press, London, 1982.

22. Sirmans, D., and Bumgarner, B.W.C., Numerical comparison of five mean frequency estimators, *J. Appl. Meteorology*, 14, 991–1003, 1975.

23. van Leeuwen, G.H., Hoeks, A.G.P., and Reneman, R.S., Simulation of real-time estimators for pulsed Doppler systems, *Ultrasonic Imaging*, 8, 252–271, 1986.

24. Evans, D.H., and McDicken, W.N., *Doppler Ultrasound: Physics, Instrumentation and Signal Processing*, 2nd Ed., Wiley, New York, 2000.

25. Lunt, M.J., Accuracy and limitations of the ultrasonic Doppler blood velocimeter and zero crossing detector, *Ultrasound Med. Biol.*, 2, 1–10, 1975.

26. Burckhardt, C.B., Comparison between spectrum and time interval histogram of ultrasound Doppler signals, *Ultrasound Med. Biol.*, 7, 79–82, 1981.

27. Vaitkus, P.J., and Cobbold, R.S.C., A comparative study and assessment of Doppler ultrasound spectral estimation techniques: Part I, Estimation methods, *Ultrasound Med. Biol.*, 14, 661–672, 1988.

28. Vaitkus, P.J., Cobbold, R.S.C., and Johnston, K.W., A comparative study and assessment of Doppler ultrasound spectral estimation techniques: Part II, Methods and results, *Ultrasound Med. Biol.*, 14, 673–688, 1988.

29. Alam, S.K., and Parker, K.J., Color flow mapping, *Ultrasound Med. Biol.*, 24, 607–611, 1998.

30. Alam, S.K., and Parker, K.J., Implementation issues in ultrasonic flow imaging, *Ultrasound Med. Biol.*, 29, 517–528, 2003.

31. Peronneau, P.A., Bournat, J.-P., Bugnon, A., et al., Theoretical and practical aspects of pulsed Doppler flowmetry: real-time application to the measure of instantaneous velocity profiles in vitro and in vivo, Ch. 6, pp. 66–84 in: *Cardiovascular Applications of Ultrasound*, R.S. Reneman (Ed.), North-Holland Pub., Amsterdam, 1974.

32. Kristoffersen, K., Optimal receiver filtering in pulsed Doppler ultrasound blood velocity measurements, *IEEE Trans. Ultrason. Ferroelect. Freq. Contr.*, 33, 51–58, 1986.

33. Cathignol, D., Pseudo-random correlation flow measurement, Chapter 7, pp. 247–279 in: *Progress in Medical Imaging*, V.L. Newhouse (Ed.), Springer-Verlag, New York, 1988.

34. Morris, R.L., Histand, M.B., and Miller, C.W., The resolution of the ultrasound pulsed Doppler for blood velocity measurements, *J. Biomechanics*, 6, 701–710, 1973.

35. Baker, D.W., Jorgensen, J.E., and Campau, D.N., The characteristics of the pulsed ultrasonic Doppler flowmeter, pp. 1389–1400 in: *Flow: its Measurement and Control in Science and Industry*, Vol. 1., Part 3, R.B. Dowdell (Ed.), Instr. Soc. of Am., Pittsburgh, 1974.

36. Jorgensen, J.E., and Garbini, J.L., An analytical procedure of calibration for the pulsed ultrasonic Doppler flowmeter, *Trans. ASME: J. Fluids Enginering*, 96, 158–167, 1974.

37. Steinman, A.H., Lui, E.Y.L., Johnston, K.W., and Cobbold, R.S.C., Sample volume shape for pulsed flow velocity estimation using a linear array, *Ultrasound Med. Biol.*, 30, 1409–1418, 2004.

38. Ohtsuki, S., and Okujima, M., Ultrasonic Doppler velocity meter by M-sequence modultaion method [in Japanese], *J. Acoust. Soc. Japan.*, 29, 347–355, 1973. See also two Japanese Conference presentations in 1970, as referenced in: Takeuchi, Y., *Ultrasonics*, 17, 175–182, 1979.

39. Waag, R.C., Myklebust, J.B., Rhoads, W.L., and Gramiak, R., Instrumentation for noninvasive cardiac chamber flow rate measurement, pp. 74–77 in: *IEEE Ultrasonics Symp. Proc.*, 1972.

40. Fiocco, G.D., Frequency modulated Doppler radar system, US Patent 3,19,330, Sept. 1964 (filed Nov. 1959).

41. McCarty, K., and Woodcock, J.P., The ultrasonic Doppler shift flowmeter—a new development, *Biomed. Eng.*, 9, 336–341, 1974.

42. McCarty, K., and Woodcock, J.P. Frequency modulated ultrasonic Doppler flowmeter, *Med. Biolog. Eng.*, 13, 59–64, 1975.

43. Bertram, C.D., Distance resolution with the FM-CW ultrasonic echo-ranging system, *Ultrasound Med. Biol.*, 5, 61–67, 1979.

44. Wilhjelm, J.E., and Pedersen, P.C., Target velocity estimation with FM and PW echo ranging Doppler systems, *IEEE Trans. Ultrason. Ferroelect. Freq. Contr.*, 40, 366–372, 1993.

45. Wilhjelm, J.E., and Pedersen, P.C., Analytical and experimental comparisons between the frequency-modulated-frequency-shift measurement and the pulsed-wave-time-shift measurement Doppler systems, *J. Acoust. Soc. Am.*, 100, 3957–3970, 1996.

46. Walker, W.F., and Trahey, G.E., A fundamental limit on the performance of correlation based phase correction and flow estimation techniques, *IEEE Trans. Ultrason. Ferroelect. Freq. Contr.*, 41, 644–654, 1994.

47. Jensen J.A., Range/velocity limitations for time-domain blood velocity estimation, *Ultrasound Med. Biol.*, 19, 741–749, 1993.

48. Woodward, P.M., *Probability and Information Theory, with Applications to Radar*, Pergamon Press, London, 1953.

49. Dotti, D., Gatti, E., Svelto, V., et al., Blood flow measurements by ultrasound correlation techniques, *Energia Nucleare*, 23, 571–575, 1976.

50. Bassini, M., Dotti, D., Gatti, E., et al., An ultrasonic non-invasive blood flowmeter based on cross-correlation techniques, pp. 273–278 in: *Ultrasonics International Proc.*, 1979.

51. Bassini, M., Gatti, E., Longo, T., et al., *In vivo* recording of blood velocity profiles and studies *in vitro* of profile alterations induced by known stenoses, *Texas Heart Inst. J.*, 9, 185–194, 1982.

52. Dickinson, R.J., and Hill, C.R., Measurement of soft tissue motion using correlation between A-scans, *Ultrasound Med. Biol.*, 8, 263–271, 1982.
53. Hein, I.A., and O'Brien, W.D., Current time-domain methods for assessing tissue motion by analysis from reflected ultrasound echoes-a review, *IEEE Trans. Ultrason. Ferroelect. Freq. Contr.*, 40, 84–102, 1993.
54. Embree, P.M., The accurate ultrasonic measurement of the volume flow of blood by time domain correlation, pp. 963–966 in: *IEEE Ultrasonics Symp. Proc.*, 1985.
55. Foster, S.G., Embree, P.M., and O'Brien, W.D., Flow velocity profile via time-domain correlation: error analysis and computer simulation, *IEEE Trans. Ultrason. Ferroelect. Freq. Contr.*, 37, 164–175, 1990.
56. Bonnefous, O., Pesque, P., and Bernard, M., A new velocity estimator for color flow mapping, pp. 855–860 in: *IEEE Ultrasonics Symp. Proc.*, 1986.
57. Vaitkus, P.J., A new time-domain narrowband velocity estimation technique for Doppler ultrasound flow imaging, Ph.D. thesis,University of Toronto, 1995.
58. Bonnefous, O., Statistical analysis and time correlation processes applied to velocity measurement, pp. 887–892 in: *IEEE Ultrasonics Symp. Proc.*, 1989.
59. Bendat, J.S., and Piersol, A.G., *Random Data Analysis and Measurement Procedures*, 2nd ed., Wiley, New York, 1986.
60. Jensen J.A., Implementation of ultrasound time-domain cross-correlation blood velocity estimators, *IEEE Trans. Biomed. Eng.*, 40, 468–474, 1993.
61. Jensen J.A., Artifacts in blood velocity estimation using ultrasound and cross-correlation, *Med. Biolog. Eng. Comput.*, 32, S165–S170, 1993.
62. Wang, L-M., Shung, K.K., Camps, O.I., Two bit correlation—an adaptive time delay estimation, *IEEE Trans. Ultrason. Ferroelect. Freq. Contr.*, 43, 473–481, 1996.
63. Namekawa, K., Kasai, C., Tsukamoto, and M., Koyano, A., Real-time blood flow imaging system utilizing auto-correlation techniques, pp. 203–208 in: *Proc. Ultrasound '82*, R.A. Lerski, and P. Morley, (Eds.), Pergamon Press, New York, 1982.
64. Kasai, C., Namekawa, K., Koyano, A., and Omoto, R., Real-time two dimensional blood flow imaging using an autocorrelation technique, *IEEE Trans. Sonics Ultras.*, 32, 458–464, 1985.
65. Grandchamp, P.A., A novel pulsed directional Doppler velocimeter: the phase detection profilometer, pp. 137–143 in: *Ultrasonics in Medicine* (Proc. 2nd European Congress) E. Kazner, M. de Vieger, H.R. Muller, and V.R. McCready (Eds.), Exerpta Medica, Amsterdam, 1975.
66. Brandestini, M., Application of the phase detection principle in a transcutaneous velocity profile meter, pp. 144–152 in: *Ultrasonics in Medicine* (Proc. 2nd European Congress) E. Kazner, M. de Vieger, H.R. Muller, and V.R. McCready (Eds.), Exerpta Medica, Amsterdam, 1975.
67. Embree, P.M., and Mayo, W.T., Ultrasonic M-mode display technique with application to flow visualization, pp. 70–78 in: *Int. Symp. Pattern Recognition*, SPIE Vol. 0768, 1987.
68. Histland, M.B., Miller, C.W., and McLeod, F.D., Transcutaneous measurement of blood velocity profiles and flow, *Cardiovasc. Res.*, 7, 703–712, 1973.
69. McLeod, F.D., and Anliker, M., Multiple gate pulsed Doppler flowmeter, p. 51 in: *IEEE Ultrasonics Symposium* (Abstract of Papers), 1971.
70. Peronneau, P.A., Pellet, M.M., Xhaard, M.C., and Hinglais, J.R., Pulsed Doppler ultrasonic blood flowmeter. Real-time instantaneous velocity profiles, pp. 1367–1376 in: *Flow: its Measurement and Control in Science and Industry*, Vol. 1., Part 3, R.B. Dowdell (Ed.), Instr. Soc. of Am., Pittsburgh, 1974.

71. Brunner, H.H., Bollinger, A., Anlinker, M., et al., Bestimmung instantaner Stromungsgeschwindigkeitsprofile in der A. femoralis communis mit gepulstem Doppler-ultraschall bei stenosen und verschlussen der beckenarterien, [Measurement by pulsed Doppler ultrasound of instantaneous flow velocity profiles in the common femoral artery of patients with stenoses or occlusion of the pelvic arteries]. *Deutsche Medizinische Wochenschrift*, 99, 3–12, 1974.
72. Fish P.J., Multichannel, direction-resolving Doppler angiography, pp. 153–159 in: *Ultrasonics in Medicine* (Proc. 2nd European Congress) E. Kazner, M. de Vieger, H.R. Muller, and V.R. McCready (Eds.), Exerpta Medica, Amsterdam, 1975.
73. Brandestini, M., Topoflow—a digital full range velocity meter, *IEEE Trans. Sonics Ultrasonics*, 25, 287–293, 1978.
74. Anliker, M., Diagnostic analysis of arterial flow pulses in man, pp. 113–123 in: *Cardiovascular System Dynamics*, J. Baan, A. Noordergraaf, and J. Raines (Eds.), MIT Press, Cambridge, MA, 1978.
75. Hoeks, A.G.P., Reneman, R.S., and Peronneau, P.A., A multigate system with serial data processing, *IEEE Trans. Sonics Ultrasonics*, 28, 242–247, 1981.
76. Rice, S.O., Mathematical analysis of random noise, *Bell System Tech. J.*, 23, 282–332, 1944.
77. Lunt, M.J., Accuracy and limitations of the ultrasonic Doppler blood velocimeter and zero crossing detector, *Ultrasound Med. Biol.*, 2, 1–10, 1975.
78. Johnston, K.W., Maruzzo, B.C., and Cobbold, R.S.C., Errors and artifacts of Doppler flowmeters and their solution, *Arch. Surg.*, 112, 1335–1342, 1977.
79. Reneman, R.S., van Merode, T., Hick, P., and Hoeks, A.P.G., Cardiovascular applications of multi-gate pulsed Doppler systems, *Ultrasound Med. Biol.*, 12, 357–370, 1986.
80. Reneman, R.S., and Hoeks, A.P.G., Doppler ultrasound—Principle, advantages and limitations, Chapter 4, pp. 77–101 in: *Doppler Ultrasound in the Diagnosis of Cerebrovascular Disease*, R.S. Reneman, and A.P.G. Hoeks (Eds.), Research Studies Press (Wiley), Chichester, UK, 1982.
81. Hoeks, A.G.P., Ruissen, C.J., Hick, P., and Reneman, R.S., Transcutaneous detection of relative changes in artery diameter, *Ultrasound Med. Biol.*, 11, 51–59, 1985.
82. Flaud, P., Bensalah, A., and Peronneau, P., Deconvolution process in measurement of arterial velocity profiles via ultrasonic pulsed Doppler velocimeter for evaluation of the wall shear rate, *Ultrasound Med. Biol.*, 23, 425–436, 1997.
83. Reid, J.M., and Spencer, M.P., Ultrasonic Doppler technique for imaging blood vessels, *Science*, 176, 1235–1226, 1972.
84. Reneman, R.S., and Spencer, M.P., Local Doppler audio spectra in normal and stenosed carotid arteries in man, *Ultrasound Med. Biol.*, 5, 1–11, 1979.
85. Fish, P.J., Visualizing blood vessels by ultrasound, Chapter 3, pp. 29–32 in: *Blood Flow Measurement*, C. Roberts (Ed.), Williams & Wilkins, Baltimore, 1972.
86. Fish, P.J., Kakkar, V.V., Corrigan, T., and Nicolaides, A.N., Arteriography using ultrasound, *Lancet*, 1, (June 10th) 1269–1270, 1972.
87. Hokanson, D.E., Mozersky, D.J., Sumner, D.S., and Strandness, D.E., Ultrasonic arteriography: a new approach to arterial visualization, *Biomed. Eng.*, 6, 420, 1971.
88. Hokanson, D.E., Mozersky, D.J., Sumner, D.S., et al., Ultrasonic arteriography: a noninvasive method of arterial visualization, *Radiology*, 102, 435–436, 1972.
89. White, D.N., and Curry, G.R., Colour coded ultrasonic differential velocity carotid bifurcation scanner, pp. 85–87 in: *IEEE Ultrasonics Symp. Proc.*, 1976.
90. Curry, G.R., and White, D.N., Colour coded ultrasonic differential velocity arterial scanner (echoflow), *Ultrasound Med. Biol.*, 4, 27–35, 1978.

91. Brandestini, M.A., and Forster, F.K., Blood flow imaging using a discrete-time frequency meter, pp. 348–352 in: *IEEE Ultrasonics Symp. Proc.*, 1978.

92. Eyer, M.K., Brandestini, M.A., Phillips, D.J., and Baker, D.W., Color digital echo/Doppler image presentation, *Ultrasound Med. Biol.*, 7, 21–31, 1981.

93. Nowicki, A., and Reid, J.M., An infinite gate pulse Doppler, *Ultrasound Med. Biol.*, 7, 41–50, 1981.

94. Arenson, J.W., Cobbold, R.S.C., and Johnston, K.W., A linear stepped Doppler ultrasound array for real-time two-dimensional blood flow imaging, pp. 775–779 in: *IEEE Ultrasonics Symp. Proc.*, 1980.

95. Arenson, J.W., Cobbold, R.S.C., and Johnston, K.W., Real-time two-dimensional blood flow imaging using a Doppler ultrasound array, pp. 529–538 in: *Acoustical Imaging*, Vol. 12., E.A. Ash, and C.R. Hill (Eds.), Plenum Press, New York, 1982.

96. Bommer, W.J., and Miller, L., Real-time two-dimensional color-flow Doppler: enhanced Doppler flow imaging in the diagnosis of cardiovascular disease [abstract]., *Am. J. Cardiol.*, 49, 944, 1982.

97. Omoto, R., History of color flow mapping technologies, Ch. 1, pp. 1–6, in: *Texbook of Color Doppler Echocardiology*, N.C. Nanda (Ed.), Lea & Febiger, Philadelphia, 1989.

98. Miller, S.K., and Rochwarger, M.M., A covariance approach to spectral moment estimation, *IEEE Trans. Inform. Theory*, 18, 588–596, 1972.

99. Peebles, P.Z., *Probability, Random Variables, and Random Signal Processing*, 3rd Ed., McGraw-Hill, New York, 1993.

100. Barber, W.D., Eberhard, J.W., and Karr, S.G., A new time domain technique for velocity measurements using Doppler ultrasound, *IEEE Trans. Biomed. Eng.*, 32, 213–229, 1985.

101. Embree, P.M., and O'Brien, W.D., Pulsed Doppler accuracy assessment due to frequency-dependent attenuation and Rayleigh scattering sources, *IEEE Trans. Biomed. Eng.*, 37, 322–326, 1990.

102. Ferrara, K.W., Algazi, V.R., and Liu, J., The effect of frequency dependent scattering and attenuation on the estimation of blood velocity using ultrasound, *IEEE Trans. Ultrason. Ferroelect. Freq. Contr.*, 39, 754–767, 1992.

103. Fish, P.J., and Cope, J.A., Effect of frequency dependent processes on pulsed Doppler sample volume, *Ultrasonics*, 29, 275–282, 1991.

104. Bjaerum, S., Torp, H., and Kristoffersen, K., Clutter filter design for ultrasound color flow imaging, *IEEE Trans. Ultrason. Ferroelect. Freq. Contr.*, 49, 204–216, 2002.

105. Willemetz, J.C., Nowicki, A., Meister, J.J., et al., Bias and variance in the estimate of the Doppler frequency induced by wall motion filter, *Ultrasonic Imaging*, 11, 215–225, 1989.

106. Hoeks, A.P.G., van der Vorst, J.J.W., Dabenkaussen, A., et al., An efficient algorithn to remove low frequency Doppler signals in digital Doppler systems, *Ultrasonic Imaging*, 13, 135–144, 1991.

107. Tysoe, C., and Evans, D.H., Bias in mean frequency estimation of Doppler signals due to wall clutter filters, *Ultrasound Med. Biol.*, 21, 671–677, 1995.

108. Parks, T.W., and Burrus, C.S., *Digital Filter Design*, Wiley, New York, 1987.

109. Kadi A.P., and Loupas, T., On the performance of regression and step-initialized IIR clutter filters for color Doppler systems in diagnostic medical ultrasound, *IEEE Trans. Ultrason. Ferroelect. Freq. Contr.*, 42, 927–937, 1995.

110. Thomas, L., and Hall, A., An improved wall filter for flow imaging of low velocity flow, pp. 1701–1704 in: *IEEE Ultrasonics Symp. Proc.*, 1994.

111. Bjaerum, S., Torp, H., and Kristoffersen, K., Clutter filters adapted to tissue motion in ultrasound color flow imaging, *IEEE Trans. Ultrason. Ferroelect. Freq. Contr.*, 49, 693–704, 2002.

112. Mayo, W.T., and Embree, M., Two dimensional processing of pulsed Doppler signals, US Patent 4,930,513, June 1990 (filed July 1988).

113. Kim, J.H., Doppler processing method and apparatus, US Patent 4,800,891, Jan. 1989 (filed Nov. 1987).

114. Wilson, L.S., Description of broad-band pulsed Doppler ultrasound processing using the two-dimensional Fourier transform, *Ultrasonic Imaging*, 13, 301–315, 1991.

115. Torp, H., and Kristoffersen, K., Velocity matched spectrum analysis: a new method for suppressing velocity ambiguity in pulsed-wave Doppler, *Ultrasound Med. Biol.*, 21, 937–944, 1995.

116. Vaitkus, P.J., and Cobbold, R.S.C., A new time domain narrowband velocity estimation technique for Doppler ultrasound flow imaging, part I: Theory, *IEEE Trans. Ultrason. Ferroelec. Freq. Contr.*, 45, 939–954, 1998.

117. Jones, S.A., Fundamental sources of error and spectral broadening in Doppler ultrasound signals, *Critical Reviews in Biomed. Eng.*, 21, 399–483, 1993.

118. Loupas, T., and Gill, R.W., Multifrequency Doppler: improving the quality of spectral estimation by making full use of the information present in the backscattered RF echoes, *IEEE Trans. Ultrason. Ferroelect. Freq. Contr.*, 41, 522–531, 1994.

119. Loupas, T., Powers, J.T., and Gill, R.W., An axial velocity estimator for ultrasound blood flow imaging, based on a full evaluation of the Doppler equation by means of a two-dimensional autocorrelation technique, *IEEE Trans. Ultrason. Ferroelect. Freq. Contr.*, 42, 672–688, 1995.

120. Hoeks, A.P.G., Brands, P.J., and Reneman, R.S., Comparison of the performance of the RF cross correlation and Doppler autocorrelation technique to estimate the mean velocity of simulated ultrasound signals, *Ultrasound Med. Biol.*, 19, 727–740, 1993.

121. Torp, H., Kristoffersen, K., and Angelsen, B.-A.-J., Autocorrelation techniques in color flow imaging: Signal model and statistical properties of the autocorrelation estimates, *IEEE Trans. Ultrason. Ferroelec. Freq. Contr.*, 41, 604–612, 1994.

122. Loupas, T., Peterson, R.B., and Gill, R.W., Experimental evaluation of velocity and power estimation for ultrasound blood flow imaging, by means of a two-dimensional autocorrelation approach, *IEEE Trans. Ultrason. Ferroelect. Freq. Contr.*, 42, 689–699, 1995.

123. Ferrara, K.W., and Algazi, V.R., Estimation of blood velocity using the wideband maximum likelihood estimator, pp. 897–900 in: *IEEE Ultrasonics Symp. Proc.*, 1989.

124. Ferrara, K.W., and Algazi, V.R., A new wideband spread target maximum likelihood estimator for blood velocity estimation—Part I: Theory, *IEEE Trans. Ultrason. Ferroelec. Freq. Contr.*, 38, 1–16, 1991.

125. Ferrara, K.W., and Algazi, V.R., A new wideband spread target maximum likelihood estimator for blood velocity estimation—Part II: Evaluation of estimators with experimental data, *IEEE Trans. Ultrason. Ferroelec. Freq. Contr.*, 38, 17–26, 1991.

126. Alam, S.K., and Parker, K.J., The butterfly search technique for estimation of blood velocity, *Ultrasound Med. Biol.*, 21, 657–670, 1995.

127. Allam, M.E., and Greenleaf, J.F., Isomorphism between pulsed-wave Doppler ultrasound and direction-of-arrival estimation—Part I: Basic principles, *IEEE Trans. Ultrason. Ferroelec. Freq. Contr.*, 43, 911–922, 1996.

128. Vaitkus, P.J., Cobbold, R.S.C., and Johnston, K.W., A new time domain narrow-band velocity estimation technique for Doppler ultrasound flow imaging, Part II: Comparative performance assessment, *IEEE Trans. Ultrasonics, Ferroelectrics & Freq. Control*, 45, 955–971, 1998.

129. Moore, G.W., Limitations of color doppler flow imaging, Chapter 8, pp. 67–73 in: *Texbook of Color Doppler Echocardiology*, N.C. Nanda (Ed.), Lea & Febiger, Philadelphia, 1989.

130. Rubin, J.M., Bude, R.O., Carson, P.L., et al., Power Doppler US: a potentially useful alternative to mean frequency-based color Doppler US, *Radiology*, 190, 853–856, 1994.

131. Hoff, L., *Acoustic Characterization of Contrast Agents for Medical Ultrasound Imaging*, Kluwer Academic Publishers, Boston, 2001.

132. Burns, P.N., Powers, J.E., Simpson, D.H., et al., Harmonic power mode Doppler using microbubble contrast agents: an improved method for small vessel flow imaging, pp. 1547–1550 in: *IEEE Ultrasonics Symp. Proc.*, 1994.

133. Burns, P.N., Harmonic imaging with ultrasound contrast agents, *Clin. Radiol.*, 51 (suppl. 1), 50–55, 1996.

134. Powers, J.E., Burns, P.N., and Souquet, J., Imaging instrumentation for ultrasound contrast agents, Chapter 8, pp. 139–170 in: *Advances in Echo Imaging Using Contrast Enhancement*, N.C. Nanda, R. Schlief, and B.B. Goldberg (Eds.), 2nd. Ed., Kluwer Academic Pub., Boston, 1997

135. Schrope, B., and Newhouse, V.L., Second harmonic ultrasonic blood perfusion measurement, *Ultrasound Med. Biol.*, 19, 567–579, 1993.

136. Burns, P.N., Instrumentation for contrast echocardiography, *Echocardiography*, 19, 241–258, 2002.

137. Burns, P.N., Powers, J.E., Simpson, D.H., et al., Harmonic power mode Doppler using microbubble contrast agents: an improved method for small vessel flow imaging, pp. 1547–1550 in: *IEEE Ultrasonics Symp. Proc.*, 1994.

138. Simpson, D.H., Burns, P.N., and Averkiou, A., Techniques for perfusion imaging with microbubble contrast agents, *IEEE Trans. Ultrason. Ferroelect. Freq. Contr.*, 48, 1483–1494, 2001.

139. Simpson, D.H., and Burns, P.N., Pulse inversion Doppler: a new method for detecting nonlinear echoes from microbubble contrast agents, pp. 1597–1600 in: *IEEE Ultrasonics Symp. Proc.*, 1997.

140. Simpson, D.H., Chin, C.T., and Burns, P.N., Pulse inversion Doppler: a new method for detecting nonlinear echoes from microbubble contrast agents, *IEEE Trans. Ultrason. Ferroelect. Freq. Contr.*, 46, 372–382, 1999.

141. McDicken, W.N., Sutherland, G.R., Moran, C.M., and Gordon, L.N., Color Doppler imaging of the myocardium, *Ultrasound Med. Biol.*, 18, 651–654, 1992.

142. Groundstroem, K.W.E., Sutherland, G.R., Moran, C.M., and McDicken, N., Myocardial imaging by color-Doppler coded velocity mapping—from regional contraction to tissue characterization, Chapter 24, pp. 375–399 in: *Advances in Echo Imaging Using Contrast Enhancement*, N.C. Nanda, and R. Schlief (Eds.), Kluwer Academic Pub., Dordrecht, Netherlands, 1993.

143. Sutherland, G.R., Doppler myocardial imaging, Chapter 9, pp. 171–186 in: *Advances in Echo Imaging Using Contrast Echo Enhancement*, N.C. Nanda, R. Schlief, and B.B. Goldberg (Eds.), 2nd Ed., Kluwer Academic Pub., Dordrecht, Netherlands, 1997.

144. Miyatake, K., Yamagishi, M., Tanaka, N., et al., A new method for evaluation of left ventricular motion by color-coded tissue Doppler echcardiography: in vitro and in vivo studies [abstract], *Circulation*, 88, Part 2, I-48, 1993.

145. Yamazaki, N., Mine, Y., Sano, A., et al., Analysis of ventricular wall motion using color-coded tissue Doppler imaging system, *Jpn. J. Appl. Physics*, 33, 3141–3146, 1994.

146. Yamazaki, N., Principles of Doppler tissue velocity measurement, Chapter 3, pp. 9–15 in: *Atlas of Tissue Doppler Echocardiography-TDE*, R. Erbel, H. Nesser, and J. Drozdz (Eds.), Steinkopff Verlag, Darmstadt, 1995.

147. Roberts, C. (Ed.), *Blood Flow Measurement*, Williams & Wilkins, Baltimore, 1972.

148. Cobbold, R.S.C., *Transducers for Biomedical Measurements:Principles and Applications*, Wiley, New York, 1974.

149. Hertz, C.H., The estimate of blood volume and blood perfusion in tissue, Abstract 295, *4th European Congress on Ultrasonics in Medicine* (Dubrovnik, May 1981), V. Latin (Ed.), Congress Series No 547, Excerpta Medica, Amsterdam, 1981.

150. Jansson, T., Persson, H.W., and Lindstrom, K., Esimation of blood perfusion using ultrasound, *Proc. Inst. Mech. Engrs.*, Part H, 213, 91–106, 1999.

151. Kubicek, W.G., Karnegis, J.N., Patterson, R.P., et al., Development and evaluation of impedance cardiac output system, *Aerospace Medicine*, 37, 1208–1212, 1966.

152. Linton, D.M., and Gilon, D., Advances in noninvasive cardiac output monitoring, *Annals Cardiac Anaesthesia*, 5, 141–148, 2002

153. Fish, P.J., and Walters, D., Beam/vessel angle problem in Doppler flow measurement, Chapter 8 in *Non-Invasive Clinical Measurement*, D.E.M. Taylor, and J. Whammond (Eds.), Pitman Medical Pub., Tunbridge Wells, UK, 1977.

154. Fish, P.J., A method of transcutaneous blood flow measurement—accuracy considerations, pp. 110–115 in: *Recent Advances in Ultrasound Diagnosis 3*, A. Kurjakn, and A. Kratochwil (Eds.), *Proc. 4th European Congress on Ultrasonics in Medicine*, Dubrovnik, May 1981.

155. Gill, R.W., Measurement of blood flow by ultrasound: accuracy and sources of error, *Ultrasound Med. Biol.*, 11, 625–641, 1985.

156. Peronneau, P.A., Xhaard, M., Nowicki, A., et al., Pulsed Doppler ultrasonic flowmeter and flow pattern analysis, Chapter 2, pp. 24–28 in: *Blood Flow Measurement*, C. Roberts (Ed.), Williams & Wilkins, Baltimore, 1972.

157. Hottinger, C.F., Volume-flow measurement using Doppler ultrasound: a unified approach, Technical Report #4959-2, Stanford University, 1978.

158. Poulsen, J.K., Four ultrasonic methods for measurement of volumetric flow with no angle correction, pp. 197–202 in: *Acoustical Imaging*, Vol. 23, S. Lees, and L.A. Ferrari (Eds.), Plenum Press, New York, 1997.

159. Moser, U., Vieli, A., Schumacher, P., et al., Ein Doppler-Ultraschall-Gerat zur Bestimmung des Blut-Volumenflusses [A Doppler ultrasound device for determining blood volume flow], *Ultraschall in der Medizin.*, 13, 77–9, 1992.

160. Moser, U., Schumacher, P.M., and Anliker, M., Benefits and limitations of the C-mode Doppler procedure, p. 509–514 in: *Acoustical Imaging*, Vol. 21, J.P. Jones (Ed.), Plenum Press, New York, 1995.

161. Liu, G.Y., and Burns, P.N., The attenuation compensated C-mode flowmeter: a new Doppler method for blood volume flow measurement, pp. 1285–1289 in: *IEEE Ultrasonics Symp. Proc.*, 1997.

162. Brody, W.R., Theoretical analysis of the ultrasonic flowmeter,Technical Report #4958-1, Stanford University, 1971.

163. Arts, M.G.J., and Roevros, J.M.J.G., On the instantaneous measurement of blood flow by ultrasonic means, *Med. Biolog. Eng.*, 10, 23–34, 1972.

164. Fahrbach, K., Ein beitrag zur blutgeschwindigkeitsmessung unter anwendungdes Dopplereffektes [A major contribution to blood speed measurement using the Doppler effect], *Elektromedizin*, 15, 26–36, 1970.

165. Fahrbach, K.E., Apparatus for measuring the speed of flowing media, US Patent 3,766,517, Oct. 1973 (filed Jan 1972).

166. Dunmire, B., Beach, K.W., Labs, K-H., et al., Cross-beam vector Doppler ultrasound for angle-independent velocity measurements, *Ultrasound Med. Biol.*, 26, 1213–1235, 2000.

167. Gill, R.W., Pulsed Doppler with B-mode imaging for quantitative blood flow measurement, *Ultrasound Med. Biol.*, 5, 223–235, 1979.

168. Hottinger, C.F., and Meindl, J.D., Blood flow measurement using the attenuation-compensated volume flowmeter, *Ultrasonic Imaging*, 1, 1–15, 1979.

169. Fu, C.-C., and Gerzberg, L., Annular arrays for quantitative Doppler ultrasonic flowmeters, *Ultrasonic Imaging*, 6, 1–16, 1983.

170. Evans, J.M., Skidmore, R., Baker, J.D., and Wells, P.N.T., A new approach to the noninvasive measurement of cardiac output using an annular array Doppler technique—I, theoretical considerations and ultrasonic fields, *Ultrasound Med. Biol.*, 15, 169–178, 1989.

171. Evans, J.M., Skidmore, R., and Wells, P.N.T., A new approach to the noninvasive measurement of cardiac output using an annular array Doppler technique—II, practical implementation and results, *Ultrasound Med. Biol.*, 15, 179–187, 1989.

172. Niclou, R., Teague, S.M., and Lee, R., Clinical evaluation of a diameter sensing Doppler cardiac output meter, *Critical Care Med.*, 18, 428–432, 1990.

173. Castor, G., Klocke, R.K., Stoll, M., et al., Simultaneous measurement of cardiac output by thermodilution, thoracic electrical bioimpedance and Doppler ultrasound, *Br. J. Anaesthesia*, 72, 133–138, 1994.

174. Gibson, W.G.R., Cobbold, R.S.C., and Johnston, K.W., Principles and design feasibility of a Doppler ultrasound intravascular volumetric flowmeter, *IEEE Trans. Biomed. Eng.*, 41, 898–908, 1994.

175. Johnson, S.A., Greenleaf, J.F., Tanaka, M., and Flandro, G., Reconstructing three-dimensional temperature and fluid velocity vector fields from acoustic transmission measurements, *Instr. Soc. Am. Trans.*, 16, 3–15, 1977.

176. Peronneau, P.A., Hinglais, J.R., Xhaard, M., et al., The effects of curvature on pulsatile flow in vivo and in vitro, pp. 203–215 in: *Cardiovascular Applications of Ultrasound*, R.S. Reneman (Ed.), North-Holland Pub., Amsterdam, 1974.

177. Papadofrangakis, E., Engeler, W.E., and Fakiris, J.A., Measurement of true blood velocity by an ultrasound system, US Patent 4,265,126, May 1981 (filed June 1979).

178. Hall, A.L., and Bernardi, R.B., Method for detecting two-dimensional flow for ultrasound color flow imaging, US Patent 5,398,216, Mar. 1995 (filed Aug. 1992).

179. Overbeck, J.R., Beach, K.W., and Strandness, D.E., Vector Doppler: accurate measurement of blood velocity in two dimensions, *Ultrasound Med. Biol.*, 18, 19–31, 1992.

180. Tamura, T., Cobbold, R.S.C., and Johnston, K.W., Determination of 2-D velocity vectors using color Doppler ultrasound, pp. 1537–1540 in: *IEEE Ultrasonics Symp. Proc.*, 1990.

181. Tamura, T., Cobbold, R.S.C., and Johnston, K.W., Determination of two-dimensional flow velocity vector fields using color Doppler ultrasound, pp. 17–20 in: *Proc. ASME Biomechanics Symposium*, Vol. 120, Columbus, OH, 1991.

182. Maniatis, T.A., Cobbold, R.S.C., and Johnston, K.W., Flow imaging in an end-to-side anastomosis model using two-dimensional velocity vectors, *Ultrasound Med. Biol.*, 20, 559–569, 1994.

183. Rickey, D.W., Picot, P.A., Holdsworth, D.W., et al., Quantitative three-dimensional true color Doppler imaging, pp. 1277–1280 in: *IEEE Ultrasonics Symp. Proc.*, 1991.

184. Maniatis, T.A., Cobbold, R.S.C., and Johnston, K.W., Two-dimensional velocity reconstruction strategies for color flow Doppler ultrasound images, *Ultrasound Med. Biol.*, 20, 137–145, 1994.

185. Hoskins, P.R., Fleming, A., Stonebridge, P., et al., Scan-plane vector maps and secondary flow motions in arteries, *Eur. J. Ultrasound*, 1, 159–169, 1994.

186. Stonebridge, P., Hoskins, P.R., Allan, P.L., and Belch, J.F.F., Spiral laminar flow in vivo, *Clin. Sci.*, 91, 17–21, 1996.

187. Dunmire, B., Beach, K.W., Labs, K-H., et al. Two-dimensional velocity map of a normal femoral bifurcation, and its implications for conventional pulsed Doppler ultrasound, pp. 272–283 in: *Medical Imaging 2001: Ultrasonic Imaging and Signal Processing*, M.F. Insana, and K.K. Shung (Eds.), Proc. SPIE, Vol. 4325, 2001.

APPENDIX A

Properties of Time- and Space-Invariant Linear Systems

Consider the system shown in Fig. A-1, in which $\mathbf{r_i}$ denotes the vector position of the input and $\mathbf{r}$ that of the output. For example, the input $s_i(.)$ could be the velocity potential at the position $\mathbf{r_i}$ and $s_o(.)$ could be the value at some output location $\mathbf{r}$. We shall assume that the system is linear, time- and space-invariant, and causal. Time-invariance implies that the system properties remain constant in time. If it is space-invariant, then its properties depend only on $(\mathbf{r_i} - \mathbf{r})$. Causality demands that there be no output for negative times, i.e., that $h(.) = 0$ for $t < 0$.

The mapping of the input into the output can be expressed by

$$s_o(\mathbf{r}{:}t) = \wp\{s_i(\mathbf{r_i}{:}t)\}, \tag{A.1}$$

where $\wp\{.\}$ denotes the (mathematical) operation of mapping. For the system to be linear it must obey the following superposition statement:

$$\wp\{a s_i(\mathbf{r_i}{:}t) + b s_o(\mathbf{r_i}{:}t)\} = a\,\wp\{s_i(\mathbf{r_i}{:}t)\} + b\,\wp\{s_o(\mathbf{r_i}{:}t)\}, \tag{A.2}$$

in which a and b are any real or complex numbers.

The sifting property of the δ-function enables the input to be written as the following multidimensional convolution integral:

$$s_i(\mathbf{r_i}{:}t) = \int\!\!\int_{-\infty}^{\infty} s_i(\mathbf{r}{:}\tau)\delta(\mathbf{r_i} - \mathbf{r}{:}t - \tau)d\mathbf{r}d\tau. \tag{A.3}$$

By substituting this into (A.1) we find that

$$s_o(\mathbf{r_i}:t) = \wp\left\{\iint\limits_{-\infty}^{\infty} s_i(\mathbf{r}:\tau)\delta(\mathbf{r_i} - \mathbf{r}:t - \tau)d\mathbf{r}d\tau\right\}$$
$$= \iint\limits_{-\infty}^{\infty} s_i(\mathbf{r}:\tau)\wp\{\delta(\mathbf{r_i} - \mathbf{r}:t - \tau)d\mathbf{r}d\tau\}, \quad (A.4)$$

where the second step follows from the first by using the linearity property, as given by (A.2). If we define the impulse response function by

$$h(\mathbf{r} - \mathbf{r_i}:t - \tau) = \wp\{\delta(\mathbf{r_i} - \mathbf{r}:t - \tau)\}, \quad (A.5)$$

so that (A.4) can be expressed as the multidimensional convolution integral

$$\boxed{s_o(\mathbf{r}:t) = \iint\limits_{-\infty}^{\infty} s_i(\mathbf{r_i}:\tau)h(\mathbf{r} - \mathbf{r_i}:t - \tau)d\mathbf{r_i}d\tau,} \quad (A.6)$$

which is the *superposition integral* for a time-invariant and spatial-invariant linear system. For brevity, this can be written in the shorthand form

$$\boxed{s_o(\mathbf{r}:t) = s_i(\mathbf{r_i}:\tau) * h(\mathbf{r} - \mathbf{r_i}:t - \tau).} \quad (A.7)$$

In this equation a single asterisk has been used to denote a multidimensional convolution: multiple asterisks are sometimes used, one for each dimension. For example, if the source plane of a 2-D imaging system is $\hat{x} - \hat{z}$ the image plane is $x - z$, and the impulse response (point spread function) is denoted by $h(x - \hat{x}, z - \hat{z})$, then for a source plane distribution of $s_i(\hat{x}, \hat{z})$ the output (image) plane distribution can be written as

$$s_o(x, z) = s_i(\hat{x}, \hat{z}) \underset{xz}{**} h(x - \hat{x}, z - \hat{z}). \quad (A.8)$$

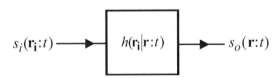

Figure A.1 A linear system with an input $s_i(.)$, an output $s_o(.)$, and whose impulse response is denoted by $h(.)$.

APPENDIX B

Function Definitions and Transform Pairs

Function Definitions and Some Properties

Dirac Delta Function:

$$\int_{x_2}^{x_1} f(x)\delta(x)dx = \begin{cases} f(0) & \text{if integration range includes } x = 0 \\ 0 & \text{if integration range excludes } x = 0 \end{cases}$$

$$\delta(ax + b) = \frac{1}{|a|}\delta\left(x + \frac{b}{a}\right), \quad \text{for } a \neq 0$$

$$\delta[f(x)] = \sum_{i=1}^{N} \delta(x - x_i) \bigg/ \left|\frac{df}{dx}\right|_{x=x_i}, \quad \text{where } x_i \text{ are the } N \text{ zeros of } f(x)$$

Other Functions:

$$\text{sinc}(\varsigma) = \frac{\text{sinc}(\pi\varsigma)}{\pi\varsigma}.$$

$$\text{rect}(\varsigma) = 1 \text{ for } |\varsigma| \leq 0.5, \text{rect}(\varsigma) = 0 \text{ elsewhere}.$$

$$\text{circ}(\varsigma) = 1 \text{ for } \varsigma \leq 1, \quad \text{circ}(\varsigma) = 0 \text{ elsewhere}.$$

$$\text{comb}(\varsigma) = \sum_{n=-\infty}^{\infty} \delta(\varsigma - n)$$

Transform Definitions and Some Properties

1-D Fourier:
$$\Im\{q(t)\} \equiv Q(\omega) = \int_{-\infty}^{\infty} q(t)e^{-j\omega t}\,dt,$$

inverse:
$$\Im^{-1}\{Q(\omega)\} \equiv q(t) = \frac{1}{2\pi}\int_{-\infty}^{\infty} Q(\omega)e^{j\omega t}\,d\omega.$$

2-D Fourier:
$$\Im\{q(x,y)\} \equiv Q(k_x,k_y) = \iint_{-\infty}^{\infty} q(x,y)e^{-j(k_x x + k_y y)}\,dx\,dy.$$

inverse:
$$\Im^{-1}\{Q(k_x,k_y)\} \equiv q(x,y) = \frac{1}{(2\pi)^2}\iint_{-\infty}^{\infty} Q(k_x,k_y)e^{j(k_x x + k_y y)}\,dk_x\,dk_y,$$

Hankel (zero-order):
$$\mathcal{H}\{q(r)\} \equiv Q(k_r) = \int_{0}^{\infty} rq(r)J_0(rk_r)\,dr$$

inverse:
$$\mathcal{H}^{-1}\{Q(k_r)\} \equiv q(r) = \int_{0}^{\infty} k_r q(k_r)J_0(rk_r)\,dk_r.$$

Hilbert:
$$\mathcal{H}\{f(t)\} \equiv g(t) = \frac{1}{\pi}\int_{-\infty}^{\infty} \frac{f(\tau)}{\tau-t}\,d\tau = -\frac{1}{\pi t} * f(t),$$

inverse:
$$\mathcal{H}^{-1}\{g(t)\} \equiv f(t) = -\frac{1}{\pi}\int_{-\infty}^{\infty} \frac{g(\tau)}{\tau-t}\,d\tau = \frac{1}{\pi t} * g(t),$$

where the Cauchy principal value is taken in each integral. The convolution form enables the spectrum to be readily found and related to the Hilbert transform of $f(t)$. For example, if $f(t) = \delta(t)$, then $g(t) = -1/(\pi t)$.

$$\text{Noting that } \Im\left\{(-\pi t)^{-1}\right\} = -j\,\mathrm{sgn}(\omega), \text{ where } \mathrm{sgn}(\omega) = \begin{cases} +1 & \text{for} \quad \omega > 0 \\ 0 & \text{for} \quad \omega = 0, \\ -1 & \text{for} \quad \omega < 0 \end{cases}$$

the convolution theorem enables the Fourier transform of the Hilbert transform to be written as $G(\omega) = -j\,\mathrm{sgn}(\omega) \times F(\omega)$. This specifies a filter whose transfer function is given by $H(\omega) = G(\omega)/F(\omega) = -j\,\mathrm{sgn}(\omega)$. Thus, the Hilbert transform is equivalent to a filter that leaves the amplitudes unchanged but changes the phase by $-\pi/2$ for $\omega > 0$ and by $+\pi/2$ for $\omega < 0$.

Correlation and Autocorrelation Function Definitions

If the functions $f(t)$ and $g(t)$ are complex, then the cross- and autocorrelation functions can be defined by:

$$R_{fg}(t) = \int_{-\infty}^{\infty} f^*(\tau-t)g(\tau)\,d\tau = \int_{-\infty}^{\infty} f^*(\tau)g(\tau+t)\,d\tau,$$

$$R_{ff}(t) = \int_{-\infty}^{\infty} f^*(\tau-t)f(\tau)\,d\tau = \int_{-\infty}^{\infty} f^*(\tau)f(\tau+t)\,d\tau$$

Convolution and Product Theorems

<u>1-D Definition:</u> $f(t) * g(t) = \int_{-\infty}^{\infty} f(t-\tau)g(\tau)d\tau = \int_{-\infty}^{\infty} f(\tau)g(t-\tau)d\tau$

If $\Im\{f(t)\} = f(\omega)$ and $\Im\{g(t)\} = G(\omega)$ then

$$\Im\{f(t) * g(t)\} = F(\omega)G(\omega),\ \Im^{-1}\{F(\omega)G(\omega)\} = f(t) * g(t)$$

and $\Im^{-1}\{F(\omega) * G(\omega)\} = 2\pi f(t)g(t),\ F(\omega) * G(\omega) = 2\pi\Im\{f(t)g(t)\}$

<u>2-D Definition:</u> $f(x,y) * g(x,y) = \iint_{-\infty}^{\infty} f(x-x_0, y-y_0)g(x_0, y_0)dx_0dy_0$

If $\Im\{f(x,y)\} = F(p,q)$ and $\Im\{g(x,y)\} = G(p,q)$ then

$$\Im\{f(x,y) * g(x,y)\} = F(p,q)G(p,q),\ f(x,y) * g(x,y) = \Im^{-1}\{F(p,q)G(p,q)\}$$

Table B.1. One-Dimensional Fourier Transform Pairs

$q(t) \equiv \Im^{-1}\{Q(\omega)\}$	$Q(\omega) \equiv \Im\{q(t)\}$
$\alpha\delta(t)$	α
$\delta(t-\tau)$	$e^{-j\omega\tau}$
$\sum_{n=-\infty}^{\infty} \delta(t-n\tau)$	$\dfrac{2\pi}{\tau} \sum_{n=-\infty}^{\infty} \delta\left(\omega - \dfrac{2\pi n}{\tau}\right)$
α	$2\pi\alpha\delta(\omega)$
$\cos(\alpha t)$	$\pi[\delta(\omega-\alpha) + \delta(\omega+\alpha)]$
$\sin(\alpha t)$	$\pi j[\delta(\omega+\alpha) - \delta(\omega-\alpha)]$
$\text{rect}(t/\tau)$	$\tau\text{sinc}(\omega\tau/2\pi)$
$\Omega\text{sinc}(\Omega t)$	$\text{rect}(\omega/2\pi\Omega)$
$e^{j\omega_o t}$	$2\pi\delta(\omega - \omega_o)$
$e^{-t^2/4\tau^2}$	$2\tau\sqrt{\pi}e^{-\tau^2\omega^2}$
$e^{\pm jt^2/4\tau^2}$	$\tau(1 \pm j)\sqrt{2\pi}e^{\mp j\tau^2\omega^2}$

Table B.2. Two-Dimensional Fourier Transform Pairs

$q(x,y) \equiv \Im^{-1}\{Q(k_x, k_y)\}$	$Q(k_x, k_y) \equiv \Im\{q(x,y)\}$
$\delta(x/\alpha, y/\beta)$	$|\alpha\beta|$
$\text{rect}(x/\alpha)\,\text{rect}(y/\beta)$	$|\alpha\beta|\text{sinc}(\alpha k_x/2\pi)\,\text{sinc}(\beta k_y/2\pi)$
$\text{comb}(x/\alpha)\,\text{comb}(y/\beta)$	$|\alpha\beta|\text{comb}(\alpha k_x/2\pi)\,\text{comb}(\beta k_y/2\pi)$
$e^{j(\alpha x+\beta y)}$	$4\pi^2\delta(k_x - \alpha, k_y - \beta)$
$e^{-(x^2/\alpha^2+y^2/\beta^2)/4}$	$4\pi|\alpha\beta|e^{-(\alpha^2 k_x^2+\beta^2 k_y^2)}$
$e^{j(x^2/\alpha^2+y^2/\beta^2)/4}$	$j4\pi|\alpha\beta|e^{-j(\alpha^2 k_x^2+\beta^2 k_y^2)}$
$\dfrac{e^{-jk\left(x^2+y^2+z^2\right)^{1/2}}}{\left(x^2+y^2+z^2\right)^{1/2}}$	$-2\pi j\,\dfrac{e^{-jz\left[k^2-\left(k_x^2+k_y^2\right)\right]^{1/2}}}{\left[k^2-\left(k_x^2+k_y^2\right)\right]^{1/2}}$

Table B.3. Zero-Order Hankel Transforms

$q(r) \equiv \mathcal{H}^{-1}\{Q(k_r)\}$	$Q(k_r) \equiv \mathcal{H}\{q(r)\}$
circ(r/a)	$aJ_1(ak_r)/k_r$
$1/r$	$1/k_r$
$\delta(r-a)$	$aJ_0(ak_r)$

Table B.4. Hilbert Transforms

$f(t) \equiv \mathcal{H}^{-1}\{g(t)\}$	$g(t) \equiv \mathcal{H}\{f(t)\}$
$\cos t$	$-\sin t$
$\sin t$	$\cos t$
$\delta(t)$	$-1/(\pi t)$

References

1. Champeney, D.C., *Fourier Transforms and their Physical Applications*, Academic Press, New York, 1973. (Contains useful pictorial representations of the transform pairs.)
2. Bracewell, R.N., *The Fourier Transform and its Applications*, 3rd Ed., McGraw-Hill, New York, 2000.

APPENDIX C

Some Integral and Function Relations

Various Forms of the Fresnel Integral

The Fresnel integral can be defined by: $F(\rho) = \int_0^\rho e^{-j\pi x^2/2} dx$

Now $\int_{-\infty}^\infty e^{-\alpha x^2} dx = \sqrt{\pi/\alpha}$, and consequently if $\alpha = j\pi/2$ then

$\int_{-\infty}^\infty e^{-\alpha x^2} dx = \sqrt{2/j} = \sqrt{2} e^{-\pi/2} = e^{-\pi/4}\sqrt{2} = 1 - j = 1/(1+j)$; it therefore follows that

$(1+j)\int_0^\infty e^{-j\pi x^2/2} dx = (1+j)\int_{-\infty}^0 e^{-j\pi x^2/2} dx = 1$

Bessel Functions: Values and Relations

$$J_0(0) = 1, J_0(\infty) = 0,$$
$$J_1(0) = 0, J_1(\infty) = 0, \underset{\lim x \to 0}{J_1(x)/x = 1/2}$$

For real x: $J_n(-x) = J(x)$

$$J_n(x) = j^{-n} J_n(jx),$$
$$J_n(x) = j^n J_n(-jx)$$

$$\frac{dJ_n(x)}{dx} = \frac{1}{2}[J_{n-1}(x) - J_{n+1}(x)] = -\frac{n}{x} J_n(x) + J_{n-1}(x)$$

$$\int_0^\infty J_0(x)dx = 1$$

$$\int_0^\infty J_0(bx)\frac{e^{\left[-a\sqrt{x^2-c^2}\right]}}{\sqrt{x^2-c^2}}xdx = \frac{e^{\left[\mp jc\sqrt{a^2+b^2}\right]}}{\sqrt{a^2+b^2}}, \quad \text{(eq. 25, p. 9 in [2])}$$

$$J_0\left(a\sqrt{x^2+y^2}\right) = \frac{1}{2\pi}\int_0^{2\pi} e^{-a(x\cos\theta + y\sin\theta)}d\theta \text{ for } a \geq 0 \quad \text{(eq. 3.937.2 in [3])}$$

$$J_0(a) = \frac{1}{2\pi}\int_0^{2\pi} e^{\pm ja\cos(\theta-\varphi)}d\theta \text{ for } a \geq 0$$

$$\int_0^\infty J_0(ax)e^{-bx}xdx = b(b^2+a^2)^{-3/2} \quad \text{(eq. 6.623.20 in [3])}$$

$$aJ_1(a) = \int_0^a xJ_0(x)dx$$

$$J_n(a) = \frac{1}{j^n\pi}\int_0^\pi e^{ja\cos\theta}\cos(n\theta)d\theta$$

$$J_n(a) = \frac{e^{jn\left(\frac{\pi}{2}-\beta\right)}}{2\pi}\int_0^{2\pi} e^{-ja\cos(\theta-\beta)+jn\theta}d\theta \quad \text{(p. 372 in [4])}$$

Bessel Function Expansions

$$e^{-jax\cos\varphi} = J_0(ax) + 2\sum_{n=1}^\infty (-j)^n J_n(ax)\cos(n\varphi) \quad \text{(eq. 8.511.4 in [3])}$$

$$e^{-jax\cos\varphi} = \sqrt{\frac{\pi}{2ax}}\sum_{n=0}^\infty (-j)^n(2n+1)J_{n+\frac{1}{2}}(ax)P_n(\cos\varphi)$$

$$\qquad\qquad\qquad\qquad\qquad\qquad\qquad \text{(eq. 8.511.4 in [3])}$$

$$= \sum_{n=0}^\infty (-J)^n(2n+1)\mathcal{J}_n(ax)P_n(\cos\varphi)$$

where $\mathcal{J}_n(ax) = \sqrt{\dfrac{\pi}{2ax}}J_{n+1/2}(ax)$ is a spherical Bessel function of order n, and $P_n(.)$ is a Legendre polynomial of order n.

Integrals in Chapter 1 for the Sommerfeld Diffraction Equations

These integrals can be written as:

$$\frac{(1+j)}{2}\int_\rho^\infty e^{-j\pi x^2/2}dx = \frac{(1+j)}{2}\left[\int_0^\infty e^{-j\pi x^2/2}dx - \int_0^\rho e^{-j\pi x^2/2}dx\right] = \left[\frac{1}{2} - \frac{(1+j)}{2}\int_0^\rho e^{-j\pi x^2/2}dx\right]$$

$$\frac{(1+j)}{2}\int_{\infty}^{|\rho|}e^{-j\pi x^2/2}dx = \frac{(1+j)}{2}\left[\int_{-\infty}^{\infty}e^{-j\pi x^2/2}dx - \int_{|\rho|}^{\infty}e^{-j\pi x^2/2}dx\right]$$

$$= \left[1 - \frac{(1+j)}{2}\int_{|\rho|}^{\infty}e^{-j\pi x^2/2}dx\right]$$

$$= 1 - \frac{1}{2} + \frac{(1+j)}{2}\int_{0}^{|\rho|}e^{-j\pi x^2/2}dx = \frac{1}{2} + \frac{(1+j)}{2}\int_{0}^{|\rho|}e^{-j\pi x^2/2}dx$$

References

1. Abramowitz, M, and Stegun, I.A. (Eds.) *Handbook of Mathematical Functions*, Dover, New York, 1965.
2. Erdelyi, A. (Ed.), *Table of Integral Transforms*, Vol. 2, McGraw-Hill, New York, 1954.
3. Gradshteyn, I.S., and Ryzhik, I.M., *Table of Integrals, Series, and Products*, 5th Ed., Academic Press, New York, 1994.
4. Stratton, J.A., *Electromagnetic Theory*, McGraw-Hill, New York, 1941.

APPENDIX D

Some Vector Relations

In the relations that follow, w is a scalar field, the boldface quantities $\mathbf{u}$ and $\mathbf{v}$ are vector fields, and $\mathbf{r}$ is a position vector. All unit vectors are indicated with a tilde ~.

Cartesian Coordinate Definitions

$$\text{del} \equiv \nabla = \left(\tilde{\mathbf{x}} \frac{\partial}{\partial x} + \tilde{\mathbf{y}} \frac{\partial}{\partial y} + \tilde{\mathbf{z}} \frac{\partial}{\partial z} \right)$$

$$\nabla^2 \equiv \nabla \cdot \nabla = \frac{\partial^2}{\partial x^2} + \frac{\partial^2}{\partial y^2} + \frac{\partial^2}{\partial z^2} \text{ (Laplace's operator)}$$

$$\text{div } \mathbf{u} \equiv \nabla \cdot \mathbf{u} = \frac{\partial u_x}{\partial x} + \frac{\partial u_y}{\partial y} + \frac{\partial u_z}{\partial z}$$

$$\text{grad } w \equiv \nabla w = \tilde{\mathbf{x}} \frac{\partial w}{\partial x} + \tilde{\mathbf{y}} \frac{\partial w}{\partial y} + \tilde{\mathbf{z}} \frac{\partial z}{\partial z}$$

$$\text{curl} \equiv \nabla \times \mathbf{u} = \left(\tilde{\mathbf{x}} \frac{\partial}{\partial x} + \tilde{\mathbf{y}} \frac{\partial}{\partial y} + \tilde{\mathbf{z}} \frac{\partial}{\partial z} \right) \times \mathbf{u}$$

$$\nabla^2 w = \frac{\partial^2 w}{\partial x^2} + \frac{\partial^2 w}{\partial y^2} + \frac{\partial^2 w}{\partial z^2}$$

$$\nabla^2 \mathbf{u} = \frac{\partial^2 \mathbf{u}}{\partial x^2} + \frac{\partial^2 \mathbf{u}}{\partial y^2} + \frac{\partial^2 \mathbf{u}}{\partial z^2}$$

$$= \tilde{\mathbf{x}}\nabla^2 u_x + \tilde{\mathbf{y}}\nabla^2 u_y + \tilde{\mathbf{z}}\nabla^2 u_z$$

Expansion Formulae

$$\nabla \cdot (w\mathbf{u}) = \nabla w \cdot \mathbf{u} + w\nabla \cdot \mathbf{u}$$

$$\nabla \times (w\mathbf{u}) = \nabla w \times \mathbf{u} + w\nabla \times \mathbf{u}$$

$$\nabla \cdot (\mathbf{u} \times \mathbf{v}) = \mathbf{v} \cdot \nabla \times \mathbf{u} - \mathbf{u} \cdot \nabla \times \mathbf{v}$$

$$\nabla \times (\mathbf{u} \times \mathbf{v}) = \mathbf{v} \cdot \nabla \mathbf{u} - \mathbf{u} \cdot \nabla \mathbf{v} + \mathbf{u}\nabla \cdot \mathbf{v} - \mathbf{v}\nabla \cdot \mathbf{u}$$

$$\nabla(\mathbf{u} \cdot \mathbf{v}) = \mathbf{v} \cdot \nabla \mathbf{u} + \mathbf{u} \cdot \nabla \mathbf{v} + \mathbf{v} \times \operatorname{curl}\mathbf{u} + \mathbf{u} \times \operatorname{curl}\mathbf{v}$$

Second-Order Differential Functions

$$\nabla \cdot \nabla \times \mathbf{u} = \operatorname{div}(\operatorname{curl}\mathbf{u}) = 0$$

$$\nabla \cdot \nabla w = \operatorname{curl}(\operatorname{grad}w) = 0$$

$$\nabla \cdot \nabla w = \operatorname{divgrad}w = \nabla^2 w$$

$$\nabla \times (\nabla \times \mathbf{u}) = \nabla(\nabla \cdot \mathbf{u}) - \nabla^2 \mathbf{u}$$

Properties of r^m

Noting that $\nabla r^m = mr^{m-1}\,\tilde{\mathbf{r}}$,

it follows that $\nabla(r) = \tilde{\mathbf{r}}$ and $\nabla(1/r) = -\tilde{\mathbf{r}}/r^2$.

In addition, since $\nabla^2 r^m = m(m+1)r^{m-2}$,

it also follows that $\nabla^2 r = 2$, and $\nabla^2(1/r) = 0$.

Gauss' Divergence Theorem and Deductions

If $\tilde{\mathbf{n}}$ is a unit vector normal to a surface S and pointing in the outward direction and V denotes the volume enclosed by S, then Gauss' divergence theorem for a vector field $\mathbf{u}$ is:

$$\iiint_V \nabla \cdot \mathbf{u}\,dV = \iint_S \mathbf{u} \cdot \tilde{\mathbf{n}}\,dS.$$

From this, the following two equations can be obtained:

$$\iiint_V \nabla w\,dV = \iint_S \tilde{\mathbf{n}}w\,dS,$$

$$\iiint_V \nabla \times \mathbf{u}\,dV = \iint_S \tilde{\mathbf{n}} \times \mathbf{u}\,dS.$$

Green's Theorems

If Φ and ψ are scalar point-function functions that within and on a closed surface S have continuous first- and second-order partial derivatives, $\partial/\partial n$ denotes the partial derivative in an *outward* normal direction on S and V denotes the volume enclosed by S, then

$$\iiint\limits_V (\nabla\Psi \cdot \nabla\Phi)dV = \iint\limits_S \Phi\frac{\partial\Psi}{\partial n}dS - \iiint\limits_V \Phi\nabla^2\Psi dV,$$

which is known as Green's theorem. Also known as Green's theorem is the relation

$$\iint\limits_S \left[\Psi\frac{\partial\Phi}{\partial n} - \Phi\frac{\partial\Psi}{\partial n}\right]dS = \iiint\limits_V (\Psi\nabla^2\Phi - \Phi\nabla^2\Psi)dV.$$

List of Principal Symbols and Abbreviations

Dimensions are shown in [ ] and the MKS Units in { }.

Roman-Based Symbols

A	Cross-sectional area [L^2]
a	Radius [L]
$a(t)$	Envelope function
a	Lagrangian spatial coordinate in the x-direction (Chapter 4)
a	Parameter for limited diffraction beams
B/A	Parameter of nonlinearity
C_T	Electrical capacitance {Farads}
CW	Continuous wave
C_o	Clamped capacitance {Farads}
c	Speed of sound [LT^{-1}]
c_L	Speed of sound in Lagrangian coordinates [LT^{-1}]
c_o	Small-signal speed of sound [LT^{-1}]
c_ϕ	Phase propagation speed [LT^{-1}]
c_g	Group propagation speed [LT^{-1}]
c_E	Small-signal extensional wave speed [LT^{-1}]
c_T	Small-signal transverse wave speed [LT^{-1}]
c_L	Small-signal longitudinal wave speed [LT^{-1}]
c_R	Small-signal Rayleigh wave speed [LT^{-1}]

766

C_p	Specific heat at a constant pressure
C_v	Specific heat at a constant volume
d	General distance variable
$\mathcal{D}$	Aperture diameter [L]
D	Directivity function
D	Electric displacement {C/m^2}
D_i	Electric displacement component {C/m^2}: $i = 1, 2, 3$
D	As a superscript, it implies that D is held constant
$e(t)$	Voltage waveform {Volts}
E	Young's modulus [ML^{-1}T^{-2}]
$E[.]$	Expectation value of argument
E	Acoustic energy [ML^{2}T^{-2}] {Joules}
$\mathcal{E}_i$	Electric field component {V/m}: $i = 1, 2, 3$
$\mathcal{E}$	As a superscript, it implies that $\mathcal{E}$ is held constant.
f	Frequency [T^{-1}]
f_{PRF}	Pulse repetition frequency [T^{-1}]
f_c	Center frequency [T^{-1}]
f_D	Doppler frequency [T^{-1}]
f_{PW}	Slow-time (pulse-wave) frequency [T^{-1}]
$f(\mathbf{r}:t)$	Source strength in time domain [T^{-1}]
$F(\mathbf{r}:\omega)$	Source strength in frequency domain
F	Focal length [L]
F	Force [MLT^{-2}] {Newton}
$F(x,v:t)$	Particle velocity function: nonlinear dependence [LT^{-1}]
$FWHM$	Full width at half maximum
$\mathfrak{I}\{\cdot\}, \mathfrak{I}^{-1}\{\cdot\}$	Fourier and inverse Fourier transforms
$\mathbf{G}$	Complex snapshot matrix with elements of $g(.)$
$G(x,v:t)$	Particle velocity function: nonlinear dependence [LT^{-1}]
G	Pressure gain for a concave transducer
$G(t)$	Transmitted waveform
$G_p(\mathbf{r}|\mathbf{r_o})$	Point source (unbounded) Green's function in frequency domain
$G_D(\mathbf{r})$	Green's function for Dirichlet boundary conditions
$G_N(\mathbf{r})$	Green's function for Neumann boundary conditions
$G(\mathbf{r}|\mathbf{r_o})$	Frequency domain Green's function
$g(\mathbf{r}|\mathbf{r_o})$	Time-domain Green's function
$g_p(\mathbf{r}|\mathbf{r_o})$	Point source (unbounded) time-domain Green's function
H	Hematocrit: i.e., fractional volume occupied by scatterers ($= NV_s/V$)
H	Height of transducer [L]
$\mathcal{H}(t)$	Heaviside unit step function
$H(.)$	Spatial frequency transfer function
$\mathcal{H}_0(.)$	Hankel transform of zero order (Fourier-Bessel integral)
$h_n(.)$	Spherical Hankel function of the 2nd kind and n'th order
$h(.)$	Velocity impulse response function
$h_p(.)$	Point spread function

$h_f(\ )$	Free-space impulse response
h	Height of rim for a concave transducer [L]
Im{ }	Imaginary part of a complex quantity
$\mathbf{I}(\mathbf{r}{:}t)$	Instantaneous intensity vector [MT^{-3}] {W/m^2}
$\bar{\mathbf{I}}(\mathbf{r})$	Time-average intensity vector [MT^{-3}] {W/m^2}
$I(t)$	In-phase signal
$J(\ )$	Jacobian
$J_n(\ )$	Cylindrical Bessel function of the first kind and the nth order
$\mathcal{J}_n(\ )$	Spherical Bessel function of the n'th order
j	$= \sqrt{-1}$
k	Wave number (= $2\pi/\lambda = \omega/c$) [L^{-1}]
k	Piezoelectric coupling factor
$\mathbf{k}$	Wave vector (= $\tilde{\mathbf{k}}k$) [L^{-1}]
k_x,k_y,k_z	Spatial frequencies [L^{-1}]
K	Adiabatic bulk modulus (= $1/\kappa$) [ML^{-1}T^{-2}] {Pa}
$\mathcal{K}$	Thermal conductivity
ℓ	Distance or thickness of a layer [L]
$\mathcal{L}$	General operator
MI	Mechanical index
m	An integer
m	Packing dimension
m'	Particle dimension
n	An integer or a dimensionless variable
n	Power law exponent for the attenuation coefficient
n	Fluctuation in number of scatterers in a voxel
$\mathbf{n}$ or $\tilde{\mathbf{n}}$	Unit vector in the outward direction normal to a surface element
$n_n(\ )$	Spherical Neumann function of the nth order
N	Number of acoustic particles
N	Number of scatterers in the sample volume
N_v or N^v	Number of scatterers in a voxel
N_x	Number of voxels in the sample volume
$\mathcal{N}_n(\ )$	Cylindrical Neumann function of the nth order
P	Power [MT^{-3}L^2] {Watts}
$PDF(\ )$	Probability distribution function
$P(\mathbf{r}_i,\mathbf{r}_j)$	Pair correlation function
$\mathcal{P}_n(\ )$	Legendre polynomial of the nth order
$p(\mathbf{r}{:}t)$	Pressure [MT^{-2}L^{-1}] {Pa}
p_o	Equilibrium pressure [MT^{-2}L^{-1}] {Pa}
$p_1 = p - p_o$	Excess pressure [MT^{-2}L^{-1}] {Pa}
q	General variable
$Q(t)$	Quadrature signal
$Q(t)$	Volumetric flow rate [L^{3}T^{-1}]
Re{ }	Real part of a complex quantity
$\mathbf{r}, \mathbf{r_o}$, etc	Position vectors [L]

R	Magnitude of distance between two points [L]
$R(.)$	Autocorrelation function
R_A	Axial resolution [L]
$R_C(t)$	Received waveform
R_I	Intensity reflection coefficient
R_L	Lateral resolution [L]
$\tilde{\mathbf{R}}$	Unit vector in the direction of R
$\mathcal{R}(.)$	Radon transform operator
s	Entropy
S	Strain
$S(.)$	Aperture function
$S(.)$	Spatial frequency spectral density function
$\hat{S}(.)$	Angular spectral density function
T	Temperature
TI	Thermal Index
T_I	Intensity transmission coefficient
T	Stress $[ML^{-1}T^{-2}]$ {Pa or N/m^2}
$\mathcal{T}$	Time period [T]
t	Time [T]
t_{PRI}, T	Pulse repetition interval [T]
$\bar{t}$	Time to form a shock wave [T]
u, U	Aperture transmission function and its Fourier transform
$\text{var}(.)$	Variance of the argument
$\mathbf{v}$	Velocity vector $[LT^{-1}]$
V	Volume $[L^{-3}]$
V_v	Volume of a voxel
V_s or V^s	Scatterer volume
V	Pulse-echo sample volume
v_n	Velocity normal to a surface in an inward direction $[LT^{-1}]$
$v_z(x,y,z{:}t)$	Velocity component along the z-axis at (x,y,z) at time t (similarly for v_x, v_y) $[LT^{-1}]$
$v_{no}(.)$	Time variation component of v_n
v_o	Velocity normal to a surface $[LT^{-1}]$
W	Width of transducer [L]
W	Power $[MT^{-3}L^2]$ {Watts}
$W(m)$	Packing factor (function of the packing dimension m)
x, y, z	Cartesian coordinate system components
$\tilde{\mathbf{x}}, \tilde{\mathbf{y}}, \tilde{\mathbf{z}}$	Unit vectors along Cartesian coordinate axes
$\bar{x}$	Shock formation distance [L]
$\mathcal{X}(t)$	Source x-location (Earnshaw's solution) [L]
$\underline{Z}$	Specific acoustic impedance $[ML^{-2}T^{-1}]$ {Rayl, Pa.s/m}
Z_o	Characteristic impedance $[ML^{-2}T^{-1}]$ {Rayl, Pa.s/m}
Z_a	Acoustic impedance $[MT^{-1}]$ {N.s/m}
Z_n	Normalized distance along the z-axis
Z_F	Depth of field [L]

Greek-Based Symbols

α	Amplitude attenuation coefficient ($= \alpha_o f^n$) [L^{-1}]
α_{dB}	Attenuation coefficient expressed in dB's
α_a	Absorption contribution to the attenuation coefficient [L^{-1}]
α_s	Scattering contribution to the attenuation coefficient [L^{-1}]
α_o	Attenuation factor ($\alpha = \alpha_o f^n$) [$L^{-1}T^n$]
α'_o	Angular frequency attenuation factor ($\alpha = \alpha'_o \omega^n$) [$L^{-1}T^n$]
α	Angle subtended
α, β, γ	Plane wave direction cosines
β	Coefficient of nonlinearity ($= 1 + B/2A$)
β	Volume expansivity
γ	Ratio of specific heats ($= C_p/C_v$)
$\delta(\ )$	Dirac delta function
ε	Permittivity {Farads/m}
ε	Parameter governing Gaussian apodization
ε	Acoustic energy density {Joules/m^3}
ε_M	Mach number ($= v/c_o$)
ε_ρ	Number density (concentration) of scatterers ($= N/V$) [M^{-3}]
ς	General variable
θ	General angle
κ	Adiabatic compressibility {Pa^{-1}}
κ_T	Isothermal compressibility {Pa^{-1}}
λ	Wavelength [L]
λ_R	Rayleigh (surface) wave wavelength [L]
λ_ℓ	First Lamé constant [$ML^{-1}T^{-2}$]
μ	Coefficient of shear viscosity [$ML^{-1}T^{-1}$]
μ_B	Coefficient of bulk viscosity [$ML^{-1}T^{-1}$]
μ_ℓ	Second Lamé constant or shear modulus [$ML^{-1}T^{-2}$]
$\xi_o(\ )$	Apodization function (e.g., spatial variation of the normal velocity component)
ξ	Acoustic particle displacement [L]
ξ	Standard deviation (subsequent to Chapter 5)
$\rho(\mathbf{r}{:}t)$	Density of propagation medium [ML^{-3}]
$\rho_1 = \rho - \rho_o$	Excess density [ML^{-3}]
ρ_o	Equilibrium density [ML^{-3}]
σ	General variable
σ_f	Standard deviation
σ	Poisson's ratio
σ_{BSC}	Backscattering coefficient (BSC) {m^{-1}.sr^{-1}}
σ_b	Backscattering cross-section {m^2.sr^{-1}}
σ_t	Total scattering cross-sections {m^2}
σ_d	Differential scattering cross-sections {m^2.sr^{-1}}
σ_S	Shock parameter
τ	Retarded time ($= t - (x/c_o)$) [T]
τ	Specific instant of time [T]

τ	Stress tensor
φ	Time parameter in Earnshaw's solution
φ	General angle
$\phi(\mathbf{r}{:}t)$	Velocity potential in spatial and time domains $[L^2T^{-1}]$
$\Phi(\mathbf{r}{:}\omega)$	Velocity potential in spatial and frequency domains $[L^2T^{-1}]$
Φ	Power density spectrum
χ	Axial elastic modulus $[ML^{-1}T^{-2}]$
Ω	Solid angle
$\Omega(\ )$	Aperture function
ω	Angular frequency ($\omega = 2\pi f$) $[T^{-1}]$
ω_c	Center angular frequency $[T^{-1}]$
ω_D	Doppler angular frequency $[T^{-1}]$
ω_{PW}	Slow-time (pulse-wave) angular frequency $[T^{-1}]$

Miscellaneous Symbols, Functions, and Abbreviations

∇	Gradient operator
$\nabla\cdot$	Divergence operator
∇^2	Laplacian operator ($= \nabla\cdot\nabla$)
$\cdot$	Dot product of two vectors
$*$	Convolution, or complex conjugate
$<.>$	Time-retarded value of a quantity
$\_$	Underscore denotes a phasor quantity.
$\sim$	Overscore denotes a unit vector.
$\bar{\ }$	Bar overscore denotes average value.
$circ(\varsigma)$	Circle function, $= 1$ for $\varsigma \leq 1$ and zero elsewhere
$erf(\varsigma)$	Error function $\left(= (2/\sqrt{\pi})\int_0^\varsigma e^{-\varsigma'^2}\,d\varsigma'\right)$
$rect(\varsigma)$	Rectangular function, $= 1$ for $\varsigma \leq 1$ and zero elsewhere
$sinc(\varsigma)$	Sinc function ($= \sin(\pi\varsigma)/(\pi\varsigma)$)

Index

Page numbers followed by f refer to figures; those followed by t refer to tables; those followed by n refer to a footnote; those followed by ff indicate many succeeding pages.